SPECIALTY IMAGING™

PET/CT

ONCOLOGIC IMAGING WITH CORRELATIVE DIAGNOSTIC CT

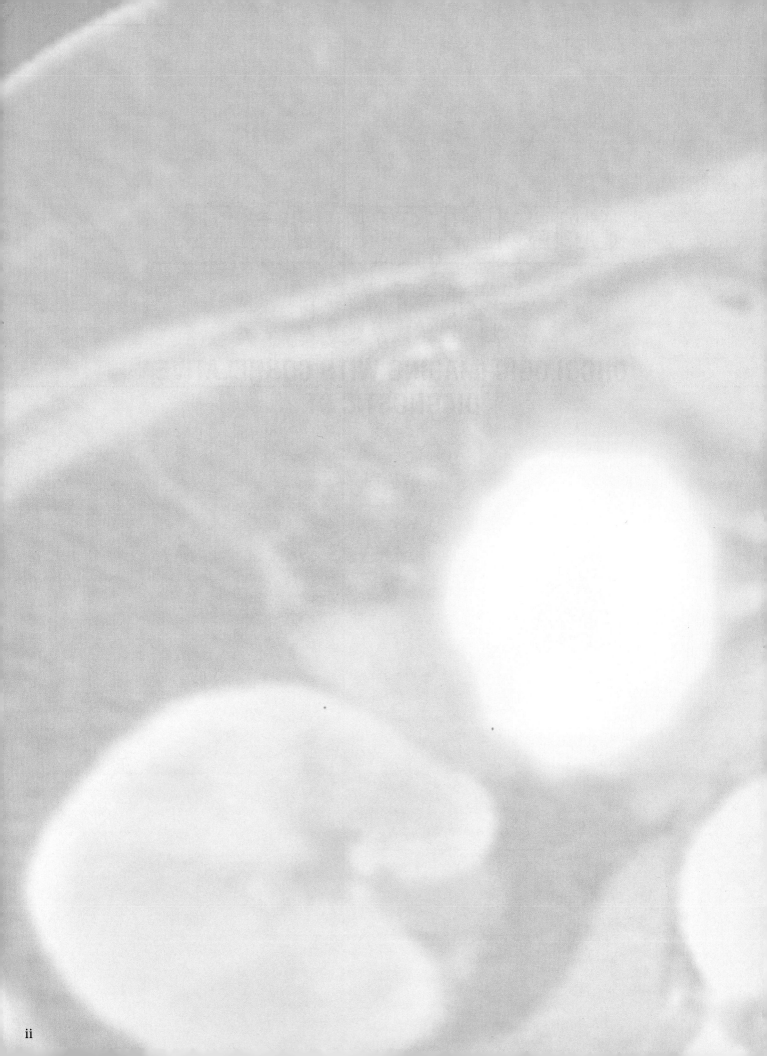

SPECIALTY IMAGING™

PET/CT

ONCOLOGIC IMAGING WITH CORRELATIVE DIAGNOSTIC CT

Todd M. Blodgett, MD
Assistant Professor of Radiology
Chief of Cancer Imaging
University of Pittsburgh Medical Center
Pittsburgh, PA

Alex Ryan, MD
Radiology Resident
University of Pittsburgh Medical Center
Pittsburgh, PA

Omar Almusa, MD
Assistant Professor of Radiology
University of Pittsburgh Medical Center
Pittsburgh, PA

Marios Papachristou, MD
Radiology Resident
University of Pittsburgh Medical Center
Pittsburgh, PA

Sanjay Paidisetty, BS
University of Pittsburgh Medical Center
Pittsburgh, PA

AMIRSYS®
Names you know. Content you trust.®

AMIRSYS®
Names you know. Content you trust.®

First Edition

Copyright © 2009 Amirsys, Inc.

Composition by Amirsys, Inc., Salt Lake City, Utah

Printed in Canada by Friesens, Altona, Manitoba, Canada

ISBN: 978-1-9318-8418-1

Notice and Disclaimer

Library of Congress Cataloging-in-Publication Data

Blodgett, Todd M.
  Specialty imaging. PET/CT oncologic imaging with correlative diagnostic CT / Todd M. Blodgett. -- 1st ed.
     p. ; cm.
  Includes bibliographical references and index.
  ISBN 978-1-931884-18-1
  1. Tumors--Tomography. I. Title. II. Title: PET/CT oncologic imaging with correlative diagnostic CT.
  [DNLM: 1. Neoplasms--radionuclide imaging--Handbooks. 2. Neoplasms--radiography--Handbooks. 3. Radiography, Dual-Energy Scanned Projection--methods--Handbooks. 4. Tomography, Emission-Computed--methods--Handbooks. 5. Tomography, X-Ray Computed--methods--Handbooks. QZ 39 B652s 2009]

  RC270.3.T65B56 209
  616.99'4075722--dc22

                          2008044383

This book is dedicated to my wife, Helene, for all of her love and support through this book.

TMB

PREFACE

Between 1998 and 2001, the University of Pittsburgh Medical Center helped evaluate the first prototype PET/CT scanner. The first scan that I remember was of a patient who had been newly diagnosed with a left-sided head and neck squamous cell carcinoma. Although the CT image alone showed only unilateral involvement, the PET/CT scan showed a single normal-sized but suspicious contralateral node. This finding altered the recommended surgical procedure and the patient's ultimately successful treatment. Indeed, the surgery confirmed what the PET/CT scan suggested: the normal-sized contralateral node was malignant. In 2001, the FDA approved PET/CT for non-experimental use, and the rest is history. More than 100,000 PET/CT scans have been performed at the University of Pittsburgh Medical Center, and I have catalogued over 4,000 teaching cases. These cases have finally found a textbook home.

The "added benefits" of the combined modality have intrigued me over the years, especially as the full power of PET/CT requires expertise in both PET and diagnostic CT. In many ways, *PET/CT: Oncologic Imaging with Correlative Diagnostic CT* is a tangible realization of that long-term interest. The book, designed for the practicing physician, includes comprehensive chapters on normal FDG uptake patterns and benign causes of FDG uptake, both of which contribute to false-positive imaging interpretations. The remainder of the chapters presents both diagnostic CT and PET findings, devoted to clinical matters rather than research topics.

I would like to thank Carolyn Meltzer and David Townsend for sparking my interest and for opening the doors of opportunity to me. I am also extremely grateful to Mike Federle for his mentorship and the introduction to Amirsys. Thanks to Ric, Mike, Kaerli, Rich, Melissa, Paula, and the rest of the Amirsys team for giving me the opportunity to do this! This book would not have happened without the help of a few individuals, in particular Alex Ryan, who worked tirelessly to make it a reality.

Finally, this book is absolutely dedicated to my beautiful wife Helene and crazy (but wonderful) kids—James, Rosie, and Elsa—for their continual support. I know that I was a virtual parent while writing this book, but that doesn't change the fundamental truth: I love you guys!

Todd M. Blodgett, MD
Assistant Professor of Radiology
Chief of Cancer Imaging
University of Pittsburgh Medical Center
Pittsburgh, PA

ACKNOWLEDGMENTS

Text Editing

Douglas Grant Jackson

Ashley R. Renlund, MA

Kellie J. Heap

Image Editing

Jeffrey J. Marmorstone

Mitch D. Curinga

Medical Text Editing

Alex Ryan, MD

Art Direction and Design

Lane R. Bennion, MS

Richard Coombs, MS

Production Lead

Melissa A. Hoopes

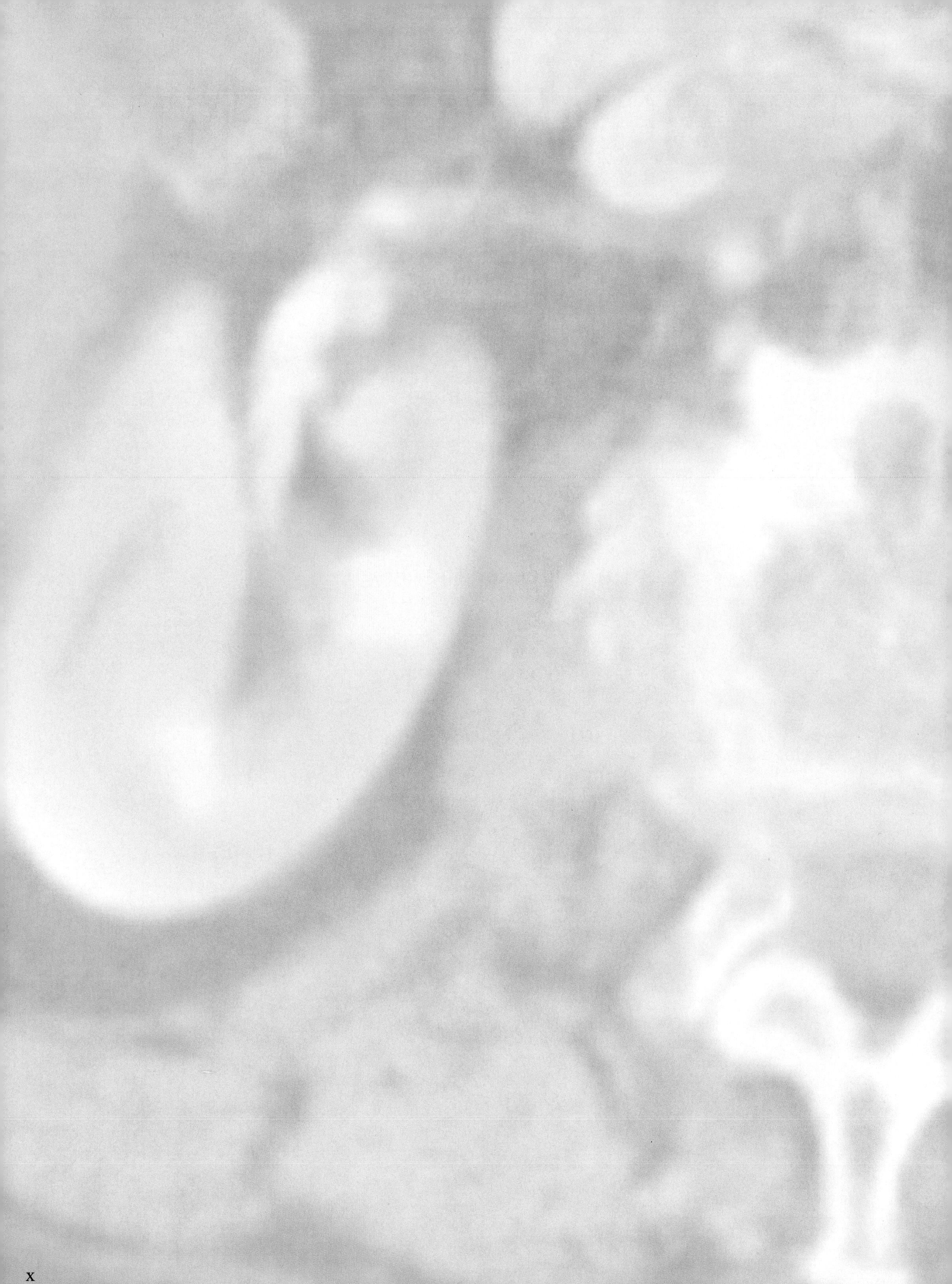

SECTIONS

Introduction to PET/CT Imaging
Clinical Applications of PET/CT
Emerging Clinical Applications of PET/CT
Pitfalls and Limitations

TABLE OF CONTENTS

SECTION 4
Pitfalls and Limitations

SPECIALTY IMAGING™

PET/CT

ONCOLOGIC IMAGING WITH CORRELATIVE DIAGNOSTIC CT

SECTION 1
Introduction to Pet/CT Imaging

Introduction and Overview

Introduction to PET/CT Imaging

INTRODUCTION TO PET/CT IMAGING

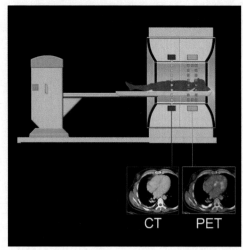

Graphic depicts a typical PET/CT scanner, which houses both CT and PET scanners in a single unit.

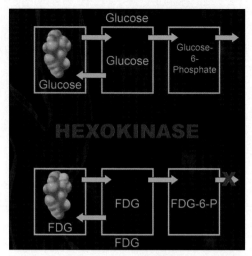

Graphic shows the metabolic pathway for FDG. It enters the cell, undergoes the first step of cellular metabolism, but is not further metabolized. FDG is trapped in the cell long enough to appear on images of the patient.

TERMINOLOGY

Abbreviations
- Fluorodeoxyglucose (FDG), standard uptake value (SUV), Hounsfield unit (HU), attenuation correction (AC), fine-needle aspiration (FNA)
- Positive predictive value (PPV), negative predictive value (NPV)

IMAGING ANATOMY

General Anatomic Considerations
- Hardware approach to image fusion allows accurate registration of anatomic and metabolic images
  - PET and CT scanners are housed in single device
  - Single gantry passes patient through both scanners without interim repositioning
  - Motion between the CT and PET portions of a PET/CT scan will cause significant misregistration

PET BIOCHEMISTRY

FDG Uptake
- Enhanced glycolysis in many malignant cells leads to increased FDG uptake
  - Glucose transmembrane transporter glut-1 is overexpressed
- Not all malignant cells overexpress glut-1 transporter
  - These malignancies may not take up significantly elevated levels of glucose or FDG
- FDG enters the cell and is a substrate for hexokinase, the first enzyme of glycolysis
- Hexokinase phosphorylates FDG to FDG-6-phosphate
- Metabolic activity of FDG ceases at that point and FDG remains trapped in the cell long enough to image the patient

PET PHYSICS

Hardware
- History
  - First PET/CT scanner became operational in 1998, and first commercial scanners appeared in 2001
  - Current state of the art incorporates multi detector row CT with high resolution PET scanners
    - Larger patient ports (70 cm or larger)
    - Aids in radiation planning and accommodates increasing dimensions of average patient in USA
- Technical considerations
  - Smaller detectors contribute to improved resolution
    - For example, 4 x 4 mm lutetium oxyorthosilicate detectors offer slightly higher PET resolution than 6 x 6 mm detectors
  - Gadolinium oxyorthosilicate and lutetium oxyorthosilicate scintillators
    - Result in lower rates of both scattered photons and random coincidences compared with bismuth germinate scintillators
    - Generally offers improved whole-body 3D imaging

Radiotracers
- Radioisotope most commonly used in PET imaging is fluorine-18
  - Can be substituted for hydrogen atoms and is incorporated into glucose as fluoro-deoxyglucose-18
  - Cyclotron-produced with half-life of 109.8 minutes
  - Long half-life is useful for transportation from remote cyclotron
- Positron emitters are neutron-deficient isotopes that achieve stability through nuclear transmutation of a proton into a neutron
  - This process involves emission of a positive electron, i.e., positron (e+) and an electron neutrino
  - F-18 is a relatively low-energy positron emitter compared to other radionuclides, with Emax of 0.633 MeV

INTRODUCTION TO PET/CT IMAGING

Introduction to PET/CT Imaging

PET Biochemistry
- FDG is taken up by many malignancies due to overexpression of glut-1
- Some malignancies may not have significant upregulation of glut-1 and may not be visualized well on FDG PET

PET Physics
- PET imaging uses positron emitting radioisotopes such as F-18
- F-18 is attached to glucose, resulting in FDG
- FDG is taken up by cells, preferentially by many malignant cells
- FDG is a marker of cellular metabolism but is not itself metabolized

AC Algorithms
- CT is used for attenuation correction with PET/CT scanners
- Obviates the need for a separate transmission scan leading to overall decease in scan times

Typical Scan Protocol
- Patients are injected with FDG and remain in a quiet room for 1-2 hours
- Patients scanned CT first then PET

PET/CT Increasingly Important in
- Diagnosis, staging, and restaging of cancer
- Image-guided radiation therapy planning
- Treatment monitoring

Imaging Considerations
- Limitations of spatial resolution in PET imaging
  - Range
    - After emission, a positron loses energy through interactions with surrounding tissues until it annihilates with an electron
  - Coincidence detection
    - Two annihilation gamma rays are emitted in nearly opposite directions and are detected in coincidence
- Physical effects contribute 2 mm or less to degradation of image resolution
  - Spatial resolution of PET scanner is limited by multiple other factors and is, at best, 6-8 mm with current technology

CT-BASED ATTENUATION CORRECTION

Protocol
- Use of CT-based attenuation correction has eliminated need for separate PET transmission scan
  - This formerly represented about 40% of the whole body study time
    - Replaced with a CT acquisition of approximately 45 seconds
  - Overall examination times of 5-10 minutes are attainable, vs. 45 minute scans typical with PET-only devices
  - Overall time will depend on body habitus and weight
    - For patients ≤ 130 pounds, a PET acquisition time of 1-2 minutes per bed position is possible
    - Larger patients will need increasing PET acquisition times, usually 3-5 minutes per bed position

AC Physics
- Scaling factors
  - Attenuation values are energy dependent
    - Scaling must be performed between mean photon energy of CT at 70-140 keV and PET energy of 511 keV
  - CT photon energy represents mean energy of a polychromatic (multi-wavelength) X-ray beam
- Attenuation
  - Bone, IV and oral contrast, metallic implants, and heavily calcified structures such as lymph nodes can heavily attenuate photons
  - Non-physiologic or unexpected physiologic areas of high attenuation can complicate image interpretation
  - Iodinated contrast agents have higher density than any physiologically encountered material
- IV contrast and oral contrast
  - Iodinated IV contrast results in 40% CT attenuation
  - At PET energy level, where the photoelectric effect is negligible, contrast has a 2% effect on attenuation
  - If contrast-enhanced pixels are identified as water-bone mix
    - Scaling factors may be incorrect and will erroneously scale, leading to artifacts
    - IV contrast artifact generally does not lead to interpretive errors
    - May be clinically relevant if a lesion is adjacent to an AC artifact
  - Newer AC algorithms allow for routine use of iodinated contrast materials with significantly fewer artifacts

AC Algorithms
- Biologic tissues other than bone can be well represented by a mixture of air and water
- Bone has calcium and phosphorus content, so a different scaling factor is required to reflect a mixture of water and cortical bone
  - Break point around 100 HU generally considered optimal

INTRODUCTION TO PET/CT IMAGING

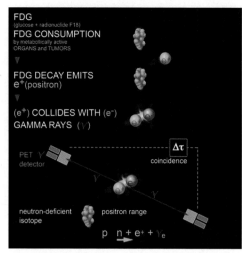

Graphic depicts the process of positron annihilation and subsequent coincidence detection.

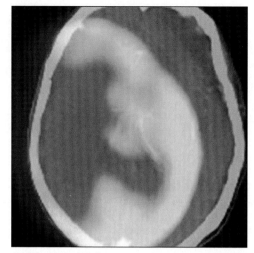

Axial fused PET/CT shows gross misregistration of the PET and CT images in this patient who moved between the CT and PET portions of a PET/CT scan. Patient motion will cause significant misregistration.

STANDARD PET/CT PROTOCOL

Major Issues Addressed by Protocols
- Respiration
- Use of IV and oral contrast
- CT operating parameters
- PET scanning time
- Optimal injected dose of FDG

General Procedure
- Questionnaire is administered to collect information regarding
  - Clinical history
    - Malignancy being evaluated
    - Date of diagnosis
    - Therapy and dates of therapy
    - Any relevant co-morbidities that may cause misinterpretation such as recent infections, inflammatory process, or trauma
  - Diabetic status; serum glucose should be less than 200 mg/dL and ideally less than 150 mg/dL
- Injection of 10-15 mCi (370-555 MBq) of FDG (3.7-5.2 MBq/kg, max dose 740 MBq)
- 1-2 hour uptake period resting quietly
  - Longer uptake times may be beneficial
- Patient is positioned in scanner
- Digital radiograph is obtained, and total ranges of PET and CT are determined according to indication
  - Consider skull base to abdomen for head and neck malignancies
  - Neck to upper thigh for most others
  - Consider head to toe for melanoma if there is extremity involvement
- Once helical CT is done, patient bed is advanced into PET field of view and PET data are acquired over same range as CT
  - CT is obtained first in craniocaudal direction
  - Once complete, PET imaging proceeds in opposite direction beginning at proximal thigh for most applications

- This method minimizes misregistration in pelvic organs that occurs due to normal peristalsis and bladder filling

Respiration Protocol
- Important to define and implement to minimize mismatch between CT and PET images
- Standard protocol calls for full breath hold during CT acquisition and shallow breathing with PET
  - Mismatch in lung bases may obscure nodules or confuse regional anatomy
- Best images are obtained when patient suspends respiration at end-tidal volume (quiet end-expiration) during CT acquisition

Positioning
- Comfort is important to minimize movement during exam
- Immobilization devices are an important part of quality control
  - Patient motion can lead to significant misregistration of CT and PET images
- Patients are held securely to scanning table with blankets and Velcro straps
- Keeping arms out of field of view is essential for CT image quality
  - For body imaging, arms are positioned above head
  - For head and neck imaging, two CT scans may be performed
    - Head and neck area with arms at sides
    - Torso with arms above head

RELATED REFERENCES

1. Beyer T et al: Optimized intravenous contrast administration for diagnostic whole-body 18F-FDG PET/CT. J Nucl Med. 46(3):429-35, 2005
2. Kinahan PE et al: X-ray-based attenuation correction for positron emission tomography/computed tomography scanners. Semin Nucl Med. 33(3):166-79, 2003

INTRODUCTION TO PET/CT IMAGING

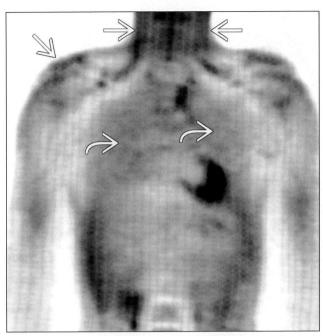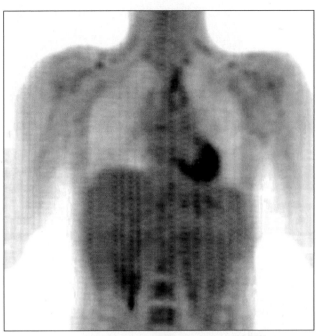

(Left) Coronal non-attenuation corrected PET image shows the typical appearance of prominent skin activity ➜ and darker lungs ➜. PET/CT scanners utilize CT for attenuation correction rather than the typical point source used on dedicated PET scanners. *(Right)* Coronal attenuation corrected PET image from the same patient shows reduction of the skin activity and apparent activity in the lungs.

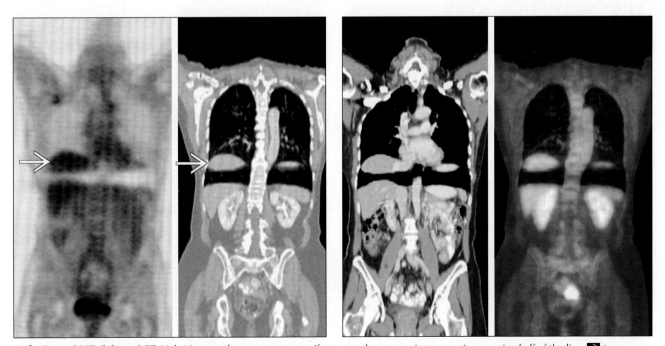

(Left) Coronal PET (left) and CT (right) images show an extreme artifact secondary to respiratory motion, causing half of the liver ➜ to appear as a mass in the lung. *(Right)* Coronal CT and PET/CT images in the same patient further illustrate the potential for artifact. Newer PET/CT scanners with faster CT will help reduce motion; however, optimized respiratory protocols can have a significant impact on image quality, particularly when there are lesions near the lung bases.

1

ADDED BENEFITS OF PET/CT

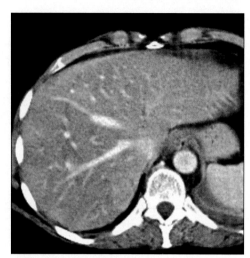

Axial CECT (with well-timed portal venous phase) of a patient with a history of breast cancer and recent rise in CA 27-29 shows no evidence of hepatic lesions.

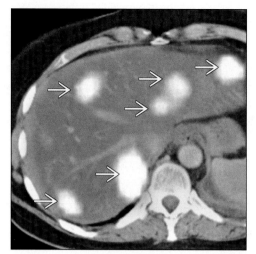

Axial fused PET/CT shows at least 6 FDG-avid bilobar hepatic metastatic lesions ➡. One of the major added benefits of PET/CT is detection of lesions not identifiable on CT, even with good contrast enhancement.

TERMINOLOGY

Abbreviations
- PET/CT benefits

Definitions
- Benefits of hardware PET/CT fusion

CLINICAL IMPLICATIONS

Clinical Importance
- Most comparative studies of PET or CT vs. combined PET/CT have shown incremental benefit of PET/CT
- Often affect clinical management
- Often reduce indeterminate lesions

GENERAL CONSIDERATIONS

DICOM Fusion Methods
- **Mental fusion**
  ○ Side-by-side inspection of PET and CT images and visual fusion
  ○ Least effective method, unless lesion is obvious on both CT and PET
- **Retrospective software coregistration**
  ○ Several proprietary software programs to register two DICOM data sets
    ▪ Even data acquired at different times on different scanners can be coregistered
  ○ Tend to work well with brain applications, including coregistration of PET and MR
    ▪ Brain is fixed in position by the skull; therefore, coregistering two independent data sets is relatively accurate
  ○ Less reliable in whole-body applications due to differences in patient positioning, internal organ movement, and technique differences
  ○ Software registration fails where it could be the most useful

- When there is a lesion on PET not visualized or present on CT
- **Hardware fusion**
  ○ Hardware fusion increases confidence level of interpreting physician for accurately localizing a lesion not visible on CT
  ○ Provides optimal coregistration of PET and CT images acquired in one imaging session
  ○ If patient moves between PET and CT portions of exam, images will have inaccurately coregistered images
    ▪ Data is acquired sequentially rather than simultaneously
    ▪ Motion restraint devices recommended

TECHNICAL ADDED BENEFITS

Decrease in Total Scan Time
- Approximately 40% less time to do PET and CT on a combined PET/CT scanner than to acquire PET and CT on a dedicated PET scanner and CT scanner
  ○ For a typical scan protocol, emission scan takes 2-5 minutes/bed position, for a total emission time of 12-30 minutes for a 6-bed-position scan
  ○ Total scan times for hardware PET/CT: Emission scan time (~ 12-30 mins) + CT scan time (1-3 minutes)
  ○ No need to perform a separate transmission scan on hardware PET/CT, as CT is used for attenuation correction
    ▪ Transmission scan performed on a dedicated PET scanner adds 12-24 minutes to the overall scan time

Consolidation of Imaging Studies
- Prior to PET/CT, patients usually scanned on separate PET and CT scanners, usually in different departments or even different hospitals
- As most patients have CT scans when first diagnosed with malignancy, performing PET and CT in single scanning session is optimal

ADDED BENEFITS OF PET/CT

Added Benefits of PET/CT Imaging

Technical Benefits
- Consolidation of patient's imaging studies
  - More convenient to patients
- Imaging times reduced by up to 40% compared to dedicated PET alone
  - Transmission scans do not need to be performed with PET/CT
  - CT used for attenuation correction
- Easy integration with radiation therapy planning

Clinical Benefits
- Detection of lesions by PET not detected on CT, even with good contrast enhancement on CT
- Detection of lesions within streak artifact or beam hardening artifact on CT
- Improved lesion localization when images are accurately coregistered, particularly when no definite abnormality on CT
- Improved biopsy localization information
- Improved radiation therapy planning
- Exclusion of suspicious lesions on other imaging modalities
- Improved differentiation of physiologic from pathologic FDG activity

Summary of PET/CT Literature
- Most comparative studies of PET or CT vs. combined PET/CT have shown incremental benefit of having accurately coregistered images
- PET/CT often has clinical impact and leads to changes in clinical management

Radiation Therapy Planning Integration
- Many patients with newly diagnosed malignancies will be candidates for radiation therapy planning
- PET and CT DICOM data sets can be imported into almost all major planning software systems
- Obviates the need for separate planning CT as long as the patient is positioned with flat "radiation therapy planning" bed

CLINICAL ADDED BENEFITS

General Added Benefits of PET/CT
- Detection of lesions by PET missed on CT, even with good contrast-enhanced CT
  - Contrast-enhanced CT more sensitive than noncontrast CT but still may miss early lesions, even with good parenchymal enhancement
  - CT very insensitive for detection of early lytic bone metastases; FDG PET more sensitive than traditional bone scanning for detection of osteolytic lesions
- For CMS covered indications, FDG PET has a higher sensitivity than CT alone for most applications

Detection of Lesions in CT Artifacts
- Fused PET/CT images allow confident detection and localization of a lesion that may be obscured by streak artifacts on CT

Improved Lesion Localization
- Reliance on accurate coregistration is essential
- Fused PET/CT images show the location of the lesion despite an anatomical abnormality on CT

Biopsy Localization Information
- Can identify the most metabolically active portion of a lesion
- Can minimize sampling error

Improved Radiation Therapy Planning
- Usually leads to decrease in gross tumor volume (GTV) and clinical tumor volume (CTV) in patients with central lung cancers and post-obstructive atelectasis by identifying tumor margins more accurately
- Usually leads to increase in GTV in planning for other tumors by identifying unsuspected additional lesions

Exclusion of Suspicious Lesions
- Patients often referred for further evaluation of a suspicious lesion on ultrasound, CT, or MR
- PET/CT can help exclude possible malignancy

Physiologic vs. Pathologic FDG Activity
- Prior to PET/CT, areas of focal muscular FDG activity and brown fat were often misinterpreted as pathology
- Many structures may have intense physiologic FDG activity
- PET/CT helps differentiate physiologic from pathologic FDG activity by allowing accurate coregistration

BRIEF REVIEW OF LITERATURE

General Oncology
- Comparative studies of PET/CT vs. PET and CT side-by-side
  - Fewer equivocal interpretations due to enhanced observer confidence
  - Most studies show PET/CT has modest but clinically relevant impact on diagnostic performance
- PET/CT provides additional information in 41-49% of patients compared to visually correlated PET and CT
- Significantly more accurate than CT alone, PET alone, and visually correlated PET and CT for T staging
  - Shown to have accuracy for TNM staging superior to other modalities
    - Accuracies of 84% for PET/CT, 76% for side-by-side, 63% for CT alone, and 64% for PET alone
- PET/CT impact on patient management
  - 6% vs. side-by-side

ADDED BENEFITS OF PET/CT

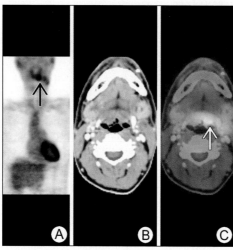

Coronal PET (A) shows focal FDG activity ➡ in this patient with metastatic squamous cell carcinoma but unknown primary. Axial CT (B) is normal. However, PET/CT (C) localizes the primary lesion ➡.

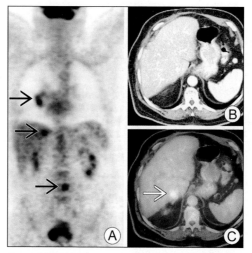

Coronal PET (A) shows 3 metastatic lesions ➡ in this patient recently discharged after a lobectomy for lung cancer. Axial CECT (B) is normal. PET/CT (C) shows hepatic metastasis ➡.

- ○ 15% vs. CT alone
- ○ 17% vs. PET alone

Head and Neck Cancer

- Receiver operating characteristic curve (ROC) analyses demonstrated that PET/CT was significantly better than FDG PET or CT alone for depiction of malignancy in the head and neck
- Sensitivity and specificity
  - ○ PET/CT: 98% and 92%
  - ○ PET alone: 87% and 91%
  - ○ CT alone: 74% and 75%
- Accuracy, PPV, NPV
  - ○ PET/CT: 94%, 88%, 99%
  - ○ PET alone: 90%, 85%, 92%
  - ○ CT alone: 74%, 63%, 83%

Colorectal Cancer

- Certainty of lesion localization and characterization: Major improvement with the combined modality
  - ○ PET/CT reduced number of lesions of uncertain location by 55% and number of equivocal and probable lesion characterizations by 50%
- Sensitivity, specificity, accuracy
  - ○ PET/CT: 86%, 67%, 83%
  - ○ PET: 88%, 56%, 83%
- Major advantage of PET/CT over PET is in overall improved staging accurately
  - ○ Number of patients incorrectly staged was reduced by half with PET/CT
  - ○ Overall accuracy of staging increased from 78% to 89%

RELATED REFERENCES

1. Benz MR et al: Treatment Monitoring by 18F-FDG PET/CT in Patients with Sarcomas: Interobserver Variability of Quantitative Parameters in Treatment-Induced Changes in Histopathologically Responding and Nonresponding Tumors. J Nucl Med. 49(7):1038-1046, 2008
2. Farma JM et al: PET/CT fusion scan enhances CT staging in patients with pancreatic neoplasms. Ann Surg Oncol. 15(9):2465-71, 2008
3. Ford EC et al: Comparison of FDG-PET/CT and CT for delineation of lumpectomy cavity for partial breast irradiation. Int J Radiat Oncol Biol Phys. 71(2):595-602, 2008
4. Gjelsteen AC et al: CT, MRI, PET, PET/CT, and ultrasound in the evaluation of obstetric and gynecologic patients. Surg Clin North Am. 88(2):361-90, vii, 2008
5. Hillner BE et al: Impact of positron emission tomography/computed tomography and positron emission tomography (PET) alone on expected management of patients with cancer: initial results from the National Oncologic PET Registry. J Clin Oncol. 26(13):2155-61, 2008
6. Kitajima K et al: Performance of integrated FDG-PET/contrast-enhanced CT in the diagnosis of recurrent ovarian cancer: comparison with integrated FDG-PET/non-contrast-enhanced CT and enhanced CT. Eur J Nucl Med Mol Imaging. 35(8):1439-48, 2008
7. Kuehl H et al: Impact of whole-body imaging on treatment decision to radio-frequency ablation in patients with malignant liver tumors: comparison of [18F]fluorodeoxyglucose-PET/computed tomography, PET and computed tomography. Nucl Med Commun. 29(7):599-606, 2008
8. Murakami R et al: Impact of FDG-PET/CT fused imaging on tumor volume assessment of head-and-neck squamous cell carcinoma: intermethod and interobserver variations. Acta Radiol. 49(6):693-9, 2008
9. Schreurs LM et al: Better assessment of nodal metastases by PET/CT fusion compared to side-by-side PET/CT in oesophageal cancer. Anticancer Res. 28(3B):1867-73, 2008
10. Tikkakoski T: Impact of FDG-PET/CT fused imaging on tumor volume assessment of head-and-neck squamous cell carcinoma. Acta Radiol. 49(6):615-6, 2008
11. Weigert M et al: Whole-body PET/CT imaging: combining software- and hardware-based co-registration. Z Med Phys. 18(1):59-66, 2008
12. Casneuf V et al: Is combined 18F-fluorodeoxyglucose-positron emission tomography/computed tomography superior to positron emission tomography or computed tomography alone for diagnosis, staging and restaging of pancreatic lesions? Acta Gastroenterol Belg. 70(4):331-8, 2007
13. Branstetter BF 4th et al: Head and neck malignancy: is PET/CT more accurate than PET or CT alone? Radiology. 235(2):580-6, 2005

ADDED BENEFITS OF PET/CT

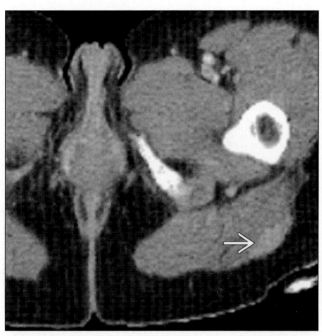 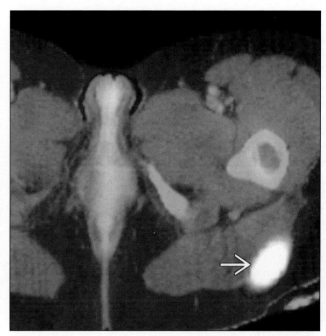

(Left) Axial CECT shows no obvious metastatic lesions, although there is questionable abnormal enhancement of the left gluteal muscle ➡ that was not called prospectively on CT. *(Right)* Axial fused PET/CT shows focal intense FDG activity correlating with the lesion in the left gluteal muscle ➡, compatible with metastatic disease.

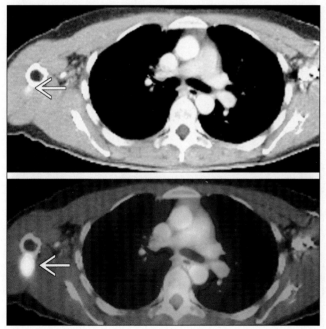 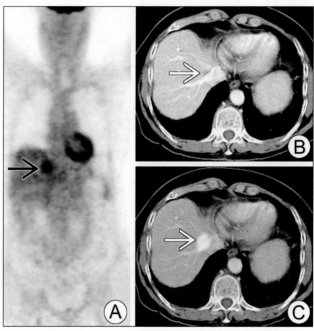

(Left) Axial CECT (top) and PET/CT (bottom) images show a focal area of intense FDG activity and mild nonspecific contrast enhancement just posterior to the right humerus ➡ in this patient with a history of melanoma, compatible with a metastatic lesion. *(Right)* Coronal PET (A) shows a focal area of intense FDG activity in the liver ➡, correlating with a subtle low attenuation lesion adjacent to the inferior vena cava ➡ on axial CT (B) and fused PET/CT images (C). The lesion was missed prospectively on CT.

ADDED BENEFITS OF PET/CT

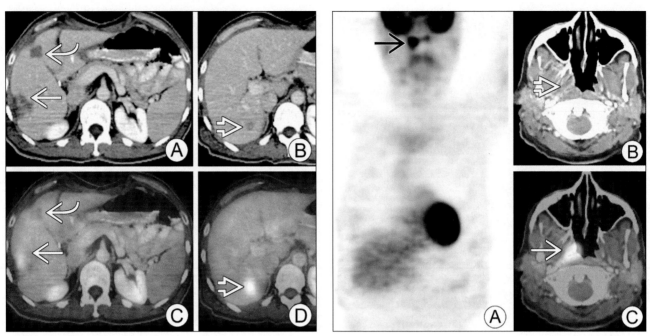

(Left) Axial CECT (A, B) and PET/CT (C, D) images show 3 lesions 10 weeks post radiofrequency ablation with one successful ablation ➔, one lesion with viable tumor anteriorly ➔, and one lesion that failed ablation ➔. *(Right)* Coronal PET (A) shows focal intense activity in the right nasopharyngeal region ➔. Axial PET/CT (C) shows intense focal activity ➔ in an area of subtle mass effect ➔ identified on the CT (B). An added benefit of combined PET/CT is identification of neoplasms, which may have subtle or equivocal findings on CT.

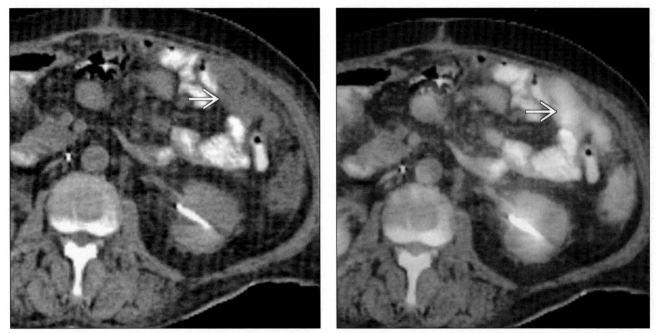

(Left) Axial CECT shows what appears to be unopacified bowel in the anterior abdomen on the left ➔. *(Right)* Axial fused PET/CT shows areas of moderately increased FDG activity corresponding to omental metastases ➔. When PET/CT is performed with oral contrast, it increases the conspicuity of lesions that sit adjacent to bowel and might otherwise be interpreted as part of bowel.

ADDED BENEFITS OF PET/CT

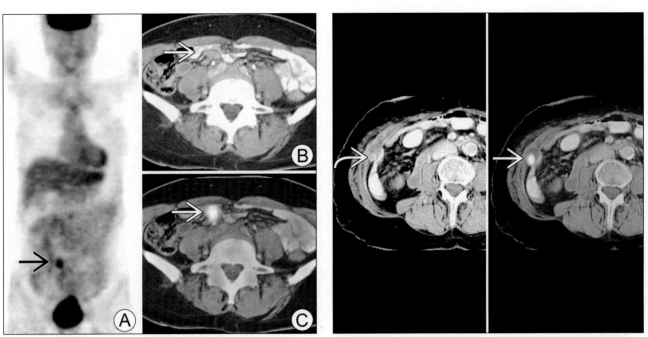

(Left) Coronal PET (A) shows a focal area of intense FDG activity in the right lower abdomen ➡, correlating with a subtle metastatic lesion just posterior to bowel ➡ on axial CT (B) and fused PET/CT (C). Identification of this lesion is facilitated by having well-opacified bowel adjacent to it. (Right) Axial CECT (left) and PET/CT (right) images show a subtly enhancing lesion in the anterior bowel wall on the right ➡ on CT, which corresponds to a lesion with focal intense FDG activity ➡ on PET/CT, compatible with metastatic disease.

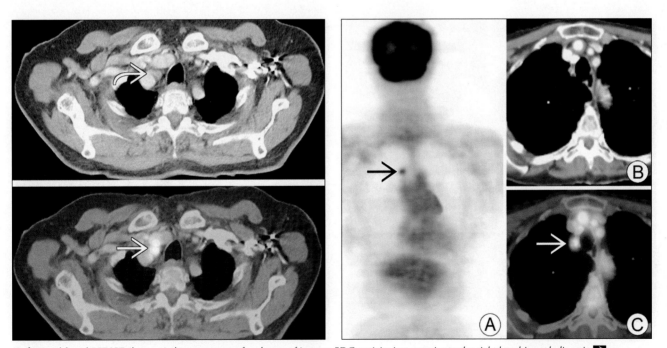

(Left) Axial fused PET/CT (bottom) demonstrates a focal area of intense FDG activity just anterior to the right brachiocephalic vein ➡, corresponding to a "normal" sized lymph node ➡ on axial CT (top). One of the added benefits of PET/CT is identification of malignant lymph nodes that are "normal" by size criteria. (Right) Coronal PET (A) shows a focal area of intense FDG activity ➡ correlating with a tiny 6 mm upper right paratracheal lymph node ➡ on axial PET/CT (C). Although PET is not currently able to detect lesions less than approximately 6 mm, it is much better than CT images, such as (B), for detecting malignancy in lesions in the 6-10 mm range.

ADDED BENEFITS OF PET/CT

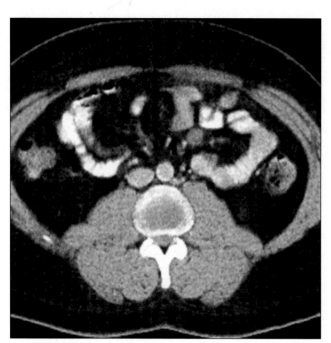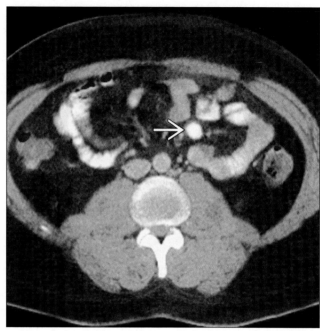

(Left) Axial CECT shows no obvious evidence for metastatic disease. (Right) Axial fused PET/CT shows focal intense FDG activity corresponding to a mesenteric lymph node ➜, compatible with metastatic disease.

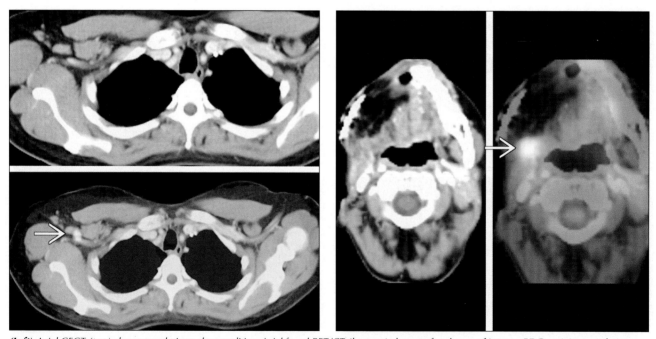

(Left) Axial CECT (top) shows no obvious abnormalities. Axial fused PET/CT (bottom) shows a focal area of intense FDG activity correlating with a normal-sized lymph node ➜, compatible with malignancy. (Right) Axial CECT (left) shows no obvious abnormality. Fused PET/CT (right) shows a subtle focal area of intense FDG activity ➜ correlating with a new lesion along the posterior flap border, compatible with residual/recurrent tumor.

ADDED BENEFITS OF PET/CT

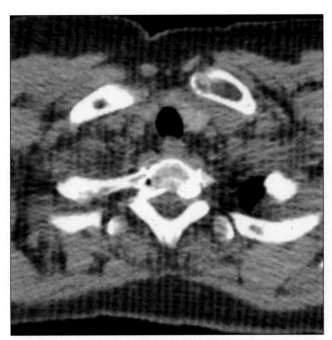 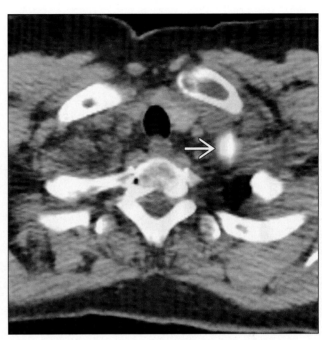

(Left) Axial NECT shows no obvious abnormalities in this patient. *(Right)* Axial fused PET/CT shows a normal-sized but malignant left supraclavicular lymph node ➔.

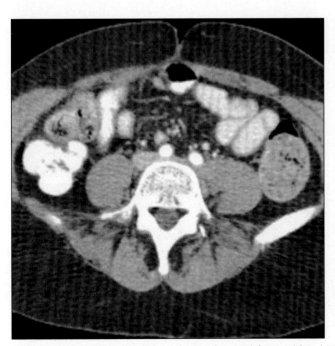 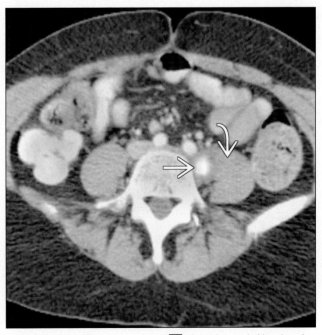

(Left) Axial CECT shows no obvious abnormalities. *(Right)* Axial fused PET/CT shows a subtle metastatic lesion ➔ along the medial border of the left psoas muscle ➔.

ADDED BENEFITS OF PET/CT

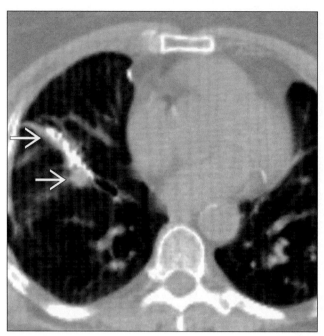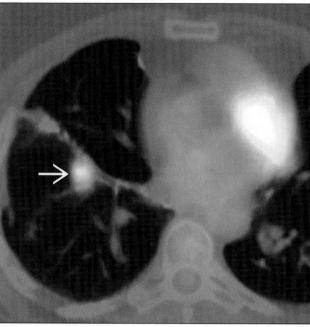

(Left) Axial CECT shows thickening along a wedge resection line ➡ in a patient with a history of lung cancer. *(Right)* Axial fused PET/CT shows focal intense FDG activity medially ➡, corresponding to recurrent tumor in this area. The fused PET/CT image helps prove the presence of tumor in an otherwise equivocal CT.

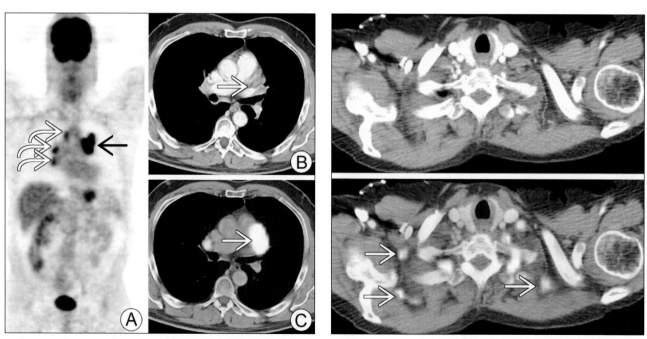

(Left) Coronal PET (A) shows intense FDG activity ➡ associated with a left-sided primary lung cancer ➡ on axial CT (B) and fused PET/CT (C). There was no evidence of contralateral or distant metastatic disease based on CT. The PET image shows at least 3 contralateral foci of intense FDG activity ➡ compatible with metastatic nodes, making this patient's disease stage IIIB and unresectable. *(Right)* Axial fused PET/CT (bottom) shows multiple areas of intense focal FDG activity ➡ in this patient with a history of lymphoma. Inspection of the axial CT image (top) confirms the lesions localize to areas of fat attenuation, compatible with physiologic brown fat.

1

ADDED BENEFITS OF PET/CT

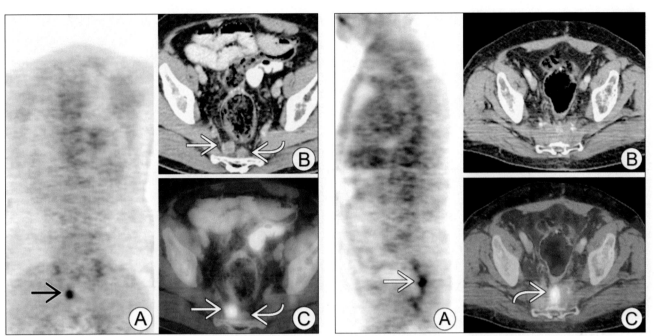

(Left) Coronal PET (A) shows a focal area of intense FDG activity ➡ posteriorly. However, axial CT (B) and PET/CT (C) show 2 presacral lesions, one with activity ➡ and one with no activity ➡. A directed CT-guided biopsy of the FDG-avid lesion showed recurrent adenocarcinoma. *(Right)* Sagittal PET (A) shows presacral FDG activity ➡ in this patient with a recent negative biopsy. Axial PET/CT (C) shows focal intense activity only in the anteromedial margin of the presacral mass ➡ seen on axial CT (B). By clearly delineating between tumor and adjacent nonneoplastic soft tissue, PET/CT can reduce sampling error that may lead to false negative biopsy results.

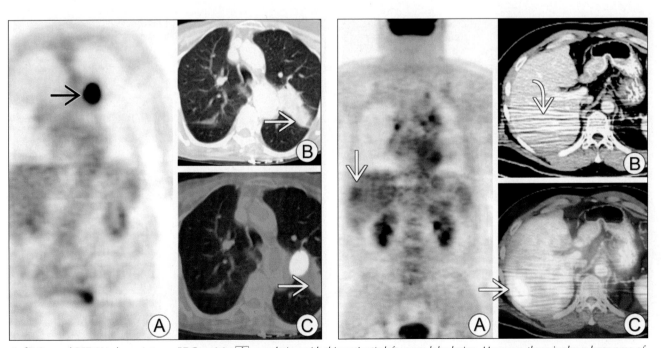

(Left) Coronal PET (A) shows intense FDG activity ➡ correlating with this patient's left upper lobe lesion. However, there is also a large area of post obstructive atelectasis ➡ without increased metabolic activity seen on axial CT (B) and fused PET/CT (C). This is particularly helpful for radiation treatment planning, as it enables the radiation oncologist to differentiate tumor from normal collapsed lung. *(Right)* Coronal PET (A) and axial PET/CT (C) demonstrate intense activity along the lateral border of the posterior hepatic segment ➡, obscured by extensive beam hardening artifact ➡ on CT (B).

ADDED BENEFITS OF PET/CT

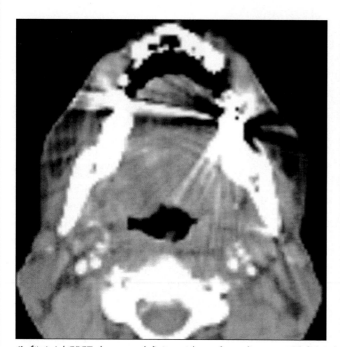 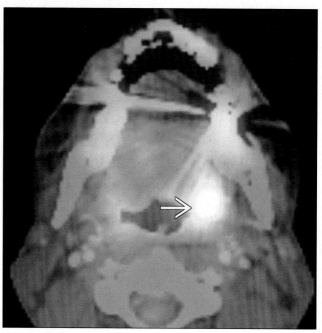

(Left) Axial CECT shows no definite evidence for malignancy. *(Right)* Axial fused PET/CT shows a focal area of intense FDG activity in the left retromolar trigone area ➡ obscured by streak artifact. One of the added benefits of PET/CT is identification of malignant lesions within areas otherwise obscured by artifact on CT.

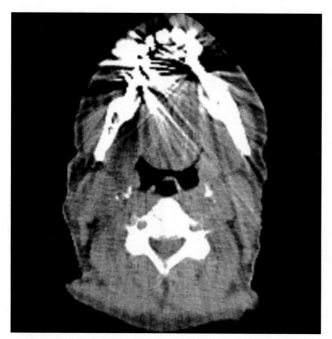 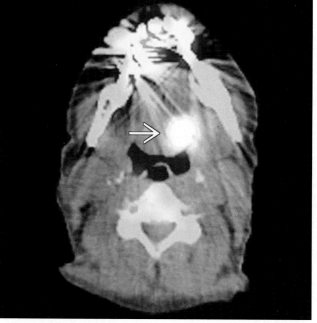

(Left) Axial NECT shows no obvious abnormalities. *(Right)* Axial fused PET/CT shows intense FDG activity involving the left base of tongue ➡, compatible with malignancy that would not be detectable by CT due to the streak artifact.

ADDED BENEFITS OF PET/CT

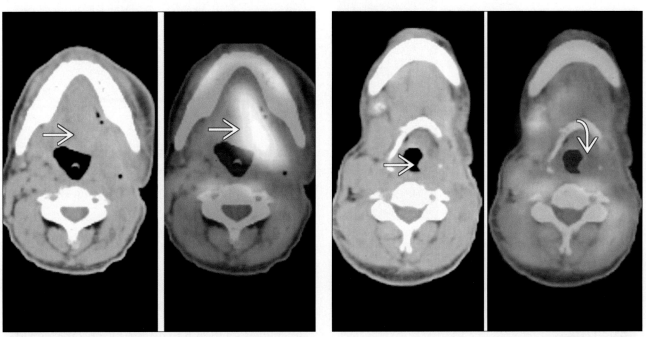

(Left) Axial NECT (left) and fused PET/CT (right) show a large area of asymmetrical intense FDG activity in the left oral tongue ➡, compatible with residual tumor. This patient with known squamous cell carcinoma was being evaluated for potential surgical resection. *(Right)* Axial NECT (left) shows a questionable lesion ➡ detected by an MR performed at an outside hospital as suspicious. However, no increased metabolic activity is seen in the lesion ➡ on axial PET/CT, making it highly unlikely that this lesion represents malignancy.

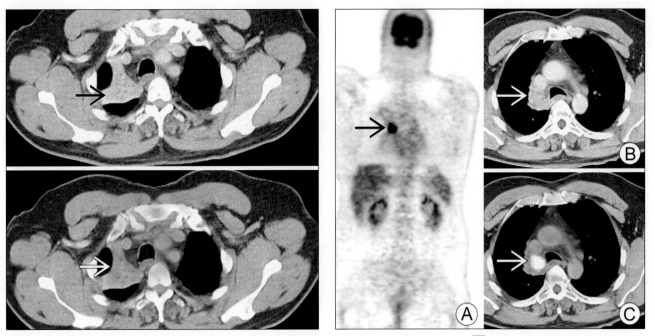

(Left) Additional axial CT (top) from the same patient shows right upper lobe post obstructive atelectasis ➡ secondary to the obstructing right hilar lesion. No abnormal FDG activity ➡ is identified on the fused PET/CT image (bottom). *(Right)* Coronal PET (A) shows intense focal FDG activity in the right hilar area ➡. Axial CT (B) and fused PET/CT (C) show a small hypermetabolic soft tissue density lesion ➡ that slightly narrows the right mainstem bronchus.

PET/CT ARTIFACTS

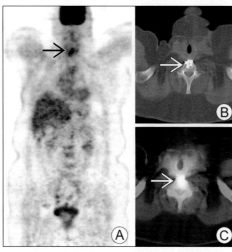

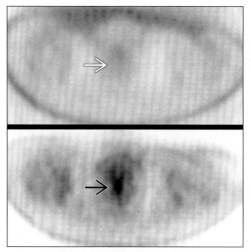

Coronal PET (A) shows a focal area of apparent increased FDG activity ⇥ correlating with an anterior fusion high attenuation orthopedic device ⇥ on axial CT (B) and fused PET/CT (C).

Axial attenuation-corrected PET image (bottom) reveals apparent uptake ⇥, which is not visualized on the uncorrected image (top) ⇥.

TERMINOLOGY

Abbreviations
- Attenuation correction (AC) artifacts, respiratory artifacts, beam hardening artifacts

Definitions
- Artifacts encountered on PET/CT images

PATHOLOGY-BASED IMAGING ISSUES

Key Concepts or Questions
- **AC artifacts**
  - Result from presence of IV and oral contrast on the CT used for AC correction
  - Advantage of PET/CT is ability to use CT for attenuation correction
    - Obviates the need for an extra transmission scan as performed on dedicated PET scanners
    - Use of CT for AC permits 40% reduction in examination time
  - AC algorithms tend to overcorrect objects with high attenuation, such as contrast agents and chemotherapy ports
  - Many artifacts are easily identified as such
    - Some presentations with atypical appearances can lead to more challenging interpretation
    - e.g., calcified lymph nodes
  - High attenuation material
    - Using older scanners may result in artifacts that mimic intense FDG uptake
    - May be clinically significant when located adjacent to true lesion
    - May occasionally appear as focal finding and mimic a malignant lymph node
    - True malignant lesion may be obscured by a contrast artifact
    - Newer scanners with better AC algorithms have lower incidence of AC artifacts

- **Methods for avoiding misinterpretation of AC artifacts**
  - Simplest solution is to inspect the uncorrected PET images
    - When a scan is positive, check the uncorrected images
    - Can be cumbersome to switch between attenuation-corrected and uncorrected images on some viewing systems
    - Some fusion systems will not allow side-by-side comparison
  - Low dose CT prior to diagnostic PET/CT
    - Noncontrast CT can be performed prior to diagnostic PET/CT imaging to be used for AC
    - Disadvantages include additional radiation exposure, costs
  - Software solution
    - Most appealing means of handling AC artifacts
    - Methods are currently being investigated
    - Most vendors have upgraded AC algorithms installed in newer scanners

Imaging Approaches
- **Oral and IV contrast issues**
  - Barium- and iodine-based oral contrast agents are highly attenuating on CT and tend to cause AC artifact
    - Water-based oral contrast agents generally do not cause artifact
  - Overlap of physiologic and artifactual bowel activity is common
    - Linear appearance of bowel activity on PET generally has limited clinical importance
    - Focal or irregular appearance should prompt inspection of uncorrected PET image
  - Clinical importance of these artifacts is unclear
    - Study results are conflicting
    - Software solutions being developed may simplify interpretation
  - Clinical importance of oral contrast
    - May be essential for differentiation of physiologic from pathologic FDG uptake

1

PET/CT ARTIFACTS

PET/CT Artifacts

AC Artifacts
- Most common AC artifacts secondary to
  - Intravenous contrast
  - Oral contrast
  - Chemotherapy ports
  - Orthopedic devices
  - Dental implants/fillings
  - Calcified structures (lymph nodes)
  - Pacemakers
  - Methylmethacrylate (vertebroplasty)
- Always check the non-AC images when there is apparent FDG activity associated with high HU
- AC artifacts may be clinically relevant if misinterpreted as true pathology
- Newer scanners have improved AC algorithms, and fewer artifacts are observed

Respiratory Artifacts
- Most common: "Mushroom" artifact at or near the diaphragm
- Consider using either a modified breath hold or performing a second CT with a breath hold

Other Issues that Negatively Affect Image Quality
- Elevated blood glucose
- Large patient body habitus
- Infiltrated FDG dose
- Beam hardening artifact when arms are down

CT Protocols
- Multiple ways to perform the CT portion of a PET/CT to optimize protocols for various malignancies

---

- Protocols based on clinical indication may be reasonable and cost effective
- **Ports and other high contrast materials**
  - Metallic objects, including orthopedic devices and chemotherapy ports
    - May demonstrate falsely elevated FDG uptake on AC PET images (with CT-based attenuation correction)
  - Small malignant lymph nodes or soft tissue lesions adjacent to such devices can be more difficult to detect
  - Patient movement between PET and CT portions of exam can produce artifactual uptake in area of orthopedic devices
    - Uptake in this pattern may be mistaken for infection or loosening
  - Dental implants and fillings can produce artifactual uptake on PET
    - May obscure or mimic true lesions
    - Particularly pertinent in patients with head and neck malignancies
- **Metallic devices**
  - Produce a photopenic area on dedicated PET
  - Produce increased apparent FDG activity on most PET/CT scanners
  - Newer scanners with improved AC algorithms may not cause artifacts
- **Calcified lymph nodes**
  - Perhaps the most clinically significant AC artifact
  - Lung cancer patients can be erroneously upstaged by the presence of a single contralateral node
    - May lead to non-surgical management if artifact is not suspected
  - High index of suspicion must be used when calcified lymph nodes are seen on CT portion of exam
    - Focal apparent FDG uptake is particularly easy to misinterpret
- **Non-AC artifacts: Diaphragmatic motion artifacts**
  - Diaphragm motion during CT scan can cause large portions of the liver to appear displaced into the thorax

- Typically due to protocol that includes deep inspiration for CT acquisition and tidal-breathing for PET acquisition
    - Modified breathing algorithms can be used, such as breath-hold at normal end-expiration for scanning through liver
  - Lesions in superior liver or lower thorax are most likely to be misinterpreted secondary to these artifacts
    - Lesions may be located to the wrong organ
    - Radiotherapy applications hinge on accurate localization
- **Other image quality considerations**
  - **Lymphangiogram effect**
    - FDG injection may accidentally be infused into subcutaneous tissue, leading to uptake into lymphatic system
    - Axillary or mediastinal lymph nodes may subsequently demonstrate intense FDG uptake
    - Study becomes non-diagnostic, and short term follow-up is recommended
  - **Patient size**
    - Photon attenuation is minimized with smaller body size
    - Results in images with good signal-to-noise ratio
    - Images quality generally degrades with increasing patient bulk
    - Consider slightly longer PET scanning times or increased FDG dose
  - **Arm positioning**
    - Arms in the imaging plane can cause significant beam-hardening and streak artifact in CT images
    - Positioning arms above thorax can lead to discomfort and motion artifact
    - However, scanning with arms up significantly improves image quality and should be performed when possible
    - Head and neck imaging can be performed separately with arms down
  - **Blood glucose and insulin**
    - Glucose competes with FDG for cellular entry, so elevated blood glucose can diminish image quality

PET/CT ARTIFACTS

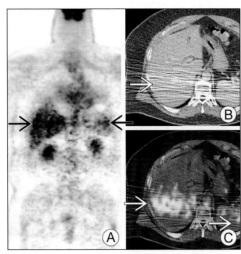

Coronal PET (A) shows areas of increased uptake in the liver and spleen ⇨ due to the arms-down position that caused beam hardening artifact ⇨ on the axial CT (B) and PET/CT (C).

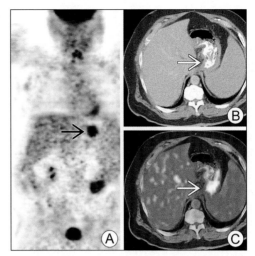

Coronal PET (A) reveals an area of apparent increased uptake in the left upper quadrant of the abdomen ⇨, correlating with the oral contrast in the stomach ⇨ on axial CT (B) and fused PET/CT (C).

- Unfortunately, insulin promotes diffuse FDG uptake that can also impair diagnostic value of PET scan
- Fat and muscle are affected, leading to diffuse linear FDG uptake in skeletal muscle
- In general, good-quality PET/CT images depend on tight glucose control prior to scanning

Imaging Protocols
- **CT-based attenuation correction**
  - Measured Hounsfield units (HU) must be transformed into corresponding quantity at higher PET photon energy of 511 keV
  - Most algorithms segment image pixels into soft tissue or bone, based on HU, and transform using scale factors
  - Other algorithms treat image pixels as mixture of two well-defined materials and transform them accordingly
- **CT portion of PET/CT examination**
  - Three approaches to this portion of the exam
    - Low current CT (~ 40 mAs): Used primarily for AC and localization
    - Normal current CT (~ 140 mAs): With or without IV/oral contrast to provide diagnostic-quality image
    - Both low and normal current CT: Noncontrast low dose scan used for AC, and normal scan used for diagnostic quality imaging

CLINICAL IMPLICATIONS

Clinical Importance
- AC artifacts may be clinically relevant when they have atypical appearances or are misinterpreted as pathology

RELATED REFERENCES

1. Hamill JJ et al: Respiratory-gated CT as a tool for the simulation of breathing artifacts in PET and PET/CT. Med Phys. 35(2):576-85, 2008
2. Nahmias C et al: Does Reducing CT Artifacts from Dental Implants Influence the PET Interpretation in PET/CT Studies of Oral Cancer and Head and Neck Cancer? J Nucl Med. 49(7):1047-1052, 2008
3. Bacharach SL: PET/CT attenuation correction: breathing lessons. J Nucl Med. 48(5):677-9, 2007
4. Chi PC et al: Design of respiration averaged CT for attenuation correction of the PET data from PET/CT. Med Phys. 34(6):2039-47, 2007
5. Cook GJ: Pitfalls in PET/CT interpretation. Q J Nucl Med Mol Imaging. 51(3):235-43, 2007
6. Kaneta T et al: High-density materials do not always induce artifacts on PET/CT: what is responsible for the difference? Nucl Med Commun. 28(6):495-9, 2007
7. Meirelles GS et al: Deep-inspiration breath-hold PET/CT: clinical findings with a new technique for detection and characterization of thoracic lesions. J Nucl Med. 48(5):712-9, 2007
8. Nehmeh SA et al: Deep-inspiration breath-hold PET/CT of the thorax. J Nucl Med. 48(1):22-6, 2007
9. Beyer T et al: Whole-body 18F-FDG PET/CT in the presence of truncation artifacts. J Nucl Med. 47(1):91-9, 2006
10. Blodgett TM et al: Positron emission tomography/computed tomography: protocol issues and options. Semin Nucl Med. 36(2):157-68, 2006
11. Carney JP et al: Method for transforming CT images for attenuation correction in PET/CT imaging. Med Phys. 33(4):976-83, 2006
12. Mawlawi O et al: PET/CT imaging techniques, considerations, and artifacts. J Thorac Imaging. 21(2):99-110, 2006
13. Mawlawi O et al: Truncation artifact on PET/CT: impact on measurements of activity concentration and assessment of a correction algorithm. AJR Am J Roentgenol. 186(5):1458-67, 2006
14. Beyer T et al: Optimized intravenous contrast administration for diagnostic whole-body 18F-FDG PET/CT. J Nucl Med. 46(3):429-35, 2005
15. Blodgett TM et al: Issues, controversies, and clinical utility of combined PET/CT imaging: what is the interpreting physician facing? AJR Am J Roentgenol. 184(5 Suppl):S138-45, 2005

PET/CT ARTIFACTS

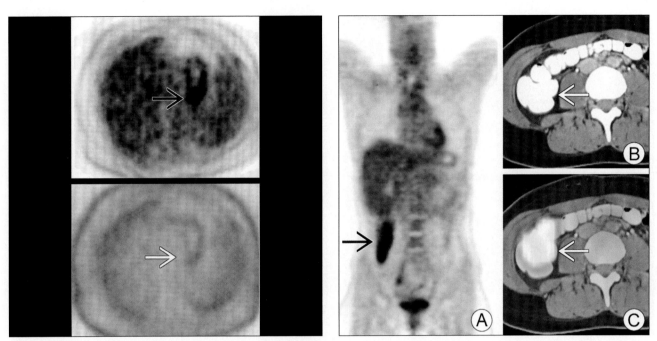

(Left) Axial attenuation-corrected PET image (top) reveals artifactual uptake in the stomach ➡, which is not apparent on the uncorrected image ➡ (bottom). **(Right)** A linear area of apparent increased FDG accumulation in the right lower quadrant ➡ is evident on the coronal PET image (A), corresponding to an area of oral contrast in the large bowel ➡ on axial CT (B) and PET/CT (C).

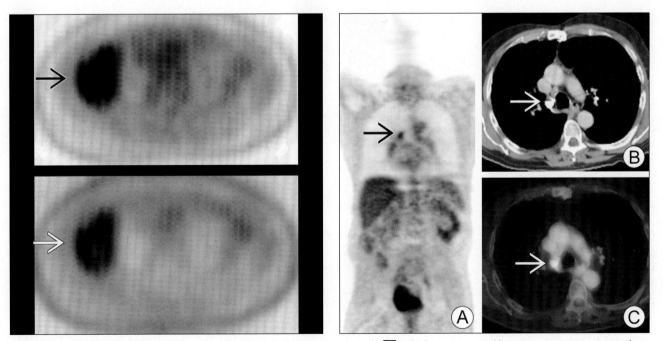

(Left) Axial uncorrected PET image (bottom) shows physiologic large-bowel uptake ➡, which is accentuated by attenuation-correction artifact ➡ on the corrected PET image (top). **(Right)** Coronal PET (A) reveals apparent focal uptake in the right lower paratracheal region ➡ that corresponds to a calcified node ➡ on axial CT (B) and fused PET/CT (C).

PET/CT ARTIFACTS

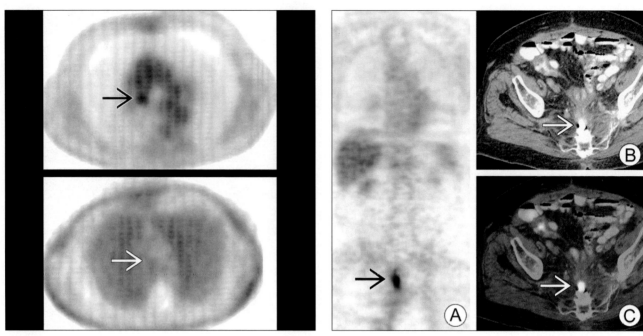

(Left) Axial attenuation-corrected PET image (top) reveals artifactual uptake in the right lower paratracheal region ➡ not visualized on the uncorrected PET ➡ (bottom). *(Right)* Coronal PET (A) shows a focal area of apparent FDG uptake in the lower mid-pelvic region ➡. On axial CT (B) and fused PET/CT (C), this correlates to extruded barium in the presacral region ➡.

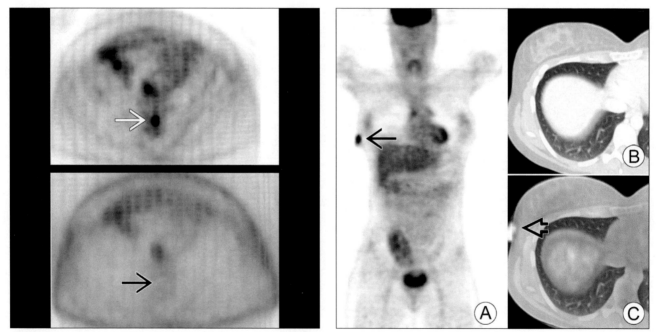

(Left) Axial attenuation-corrected PET image (top) reveals artifactual uptake in the region of the extruded barium in the pelvis ➡ that is not visualized on the uncorrected image ➡ (bottom). *(Right)* Coronal PET (A) shows a focal area of increased FDG activity in the right breast ➡. This uptake is noted overlying the skin of the right lower breast ➡ on fused PET/CT (C) without any CT correlate (B).

PET/CT ARTIFACTS

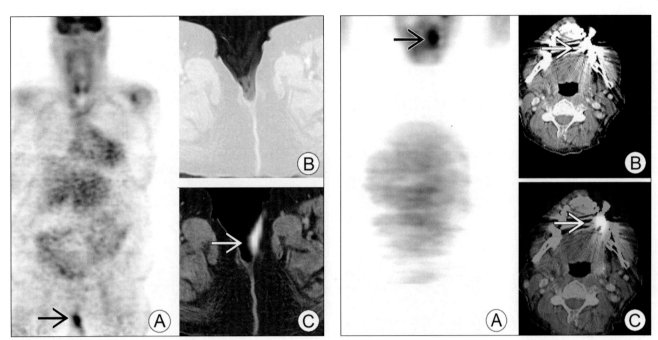

(Left) Coronal PET (A) shows a linear area of increased FDG activity in the perineum ➡, corresponding to an area overlying the skin of the medial aspect of the left proximal thigh ➡ on fused PET/CT (C) with no CT correlate (B). *(Right)* Coronal attenuation-corrected PET (A) reveals apparent focal uptake in the region of the face ➡. This corresponds to focal uptake in the region of left maxillary high-attenuation dental filling material ➡ seen on axial CT (B) and fused PET/CT (C).

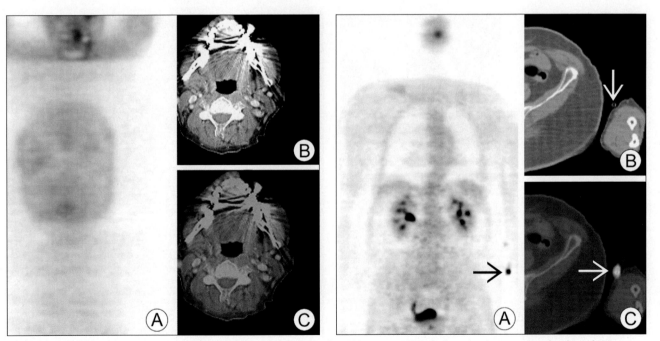

(Left) Coronal uncorrected PET (A) and corresponding CT (B) and fused PET/CT image (C) in the same patient reveal no focal uptake in the facial region. *(Right)* A focal area of uptake in the region of the left forearm ➡ seen on the coronal PET image (A) correlates with the IV injection cannula through which the tracer was injected ➡, seen on axial CT (B) and fused PET/CT (C).

PET/CT ARTIFACTS

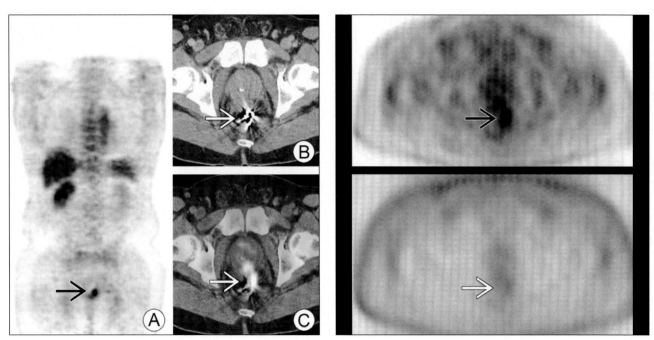

(Left) Coronal PET (A) shows a focal area of apparent FDG uptake in the lower pelvic region ➡. On axial CT (B) and fused PET/CT (C) images this area of uptake ➡ overlaps with high attenuation surgical clips. *(Right)* Axial attenuation-corrected PET (top) shows focal uptake in the deep pelvis ➡ that was not seen on the uncorrected PET image ➡ (bottom).

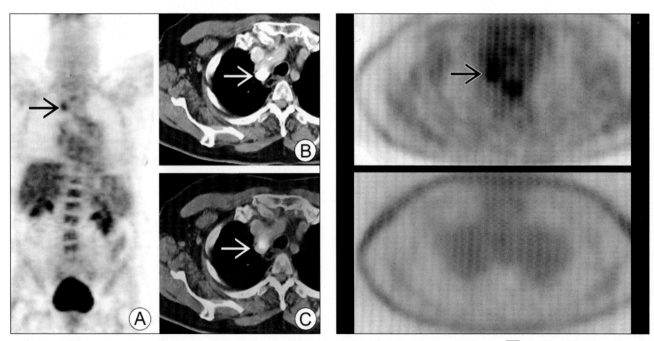

(Left) Coronal FDG PET (A) reveals an apparent area of increased uptake in the right upper paratracheal region ➡. On axial CT (B) and fused PET/CT (C) this corresponds to an area of intravenous contrast ➡. *(Right)* Axial attenuation-corrected PET image (top) demonstrates focal activity in the right upper mediastinum ➡ without any uptake on the uncorrected image (bottom).

PET/CT ARTIFACTS

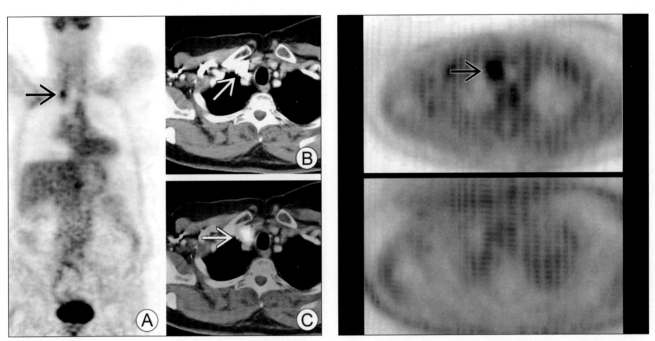

(Left) Coronal FDG PET image (A) reveals an apparent area of FDG activity ➡ in the right upper chest. On axial CT (B) and fused PET/CT (C) this correlates with an area of intravenous contrast in the right innominate vein ➡. *(Right)* Attenuation-corrected FDG PET image (top) demonstrates focal activity in the right upper paratracheal region ➡ without any uptake on the uncorrected image (bottom).

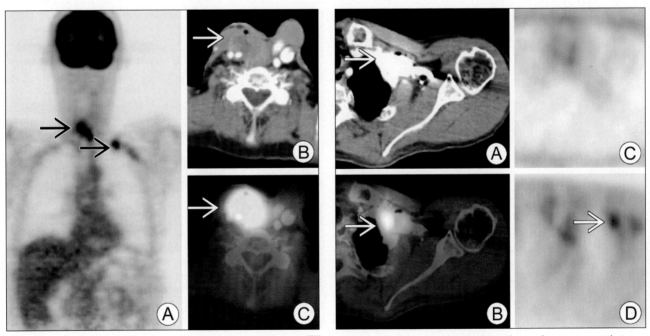

(Left) Two areas of intense focal FDG uptake are noted in the neck ➡ on the coronal PET image (A). The larger focus of tracer accumulation is noted in the lower neck mass ➡ on axial CT (B) and fused PET/CT (C). *(Right)* Axial CT (A) & fused PET/CT (B) and corrected axial PET image (D) demonstrate apparent focal intense tracer activity within IV contrast in the left subclavian vein ➡. The activity is not visualized on the uncorrected PET image (C).

PET/CT ARTIFACTS

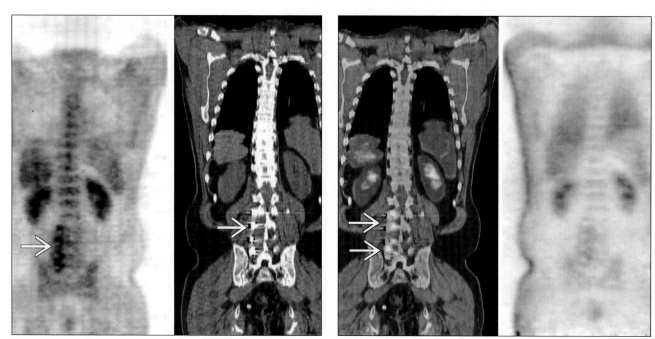

(Left) Coronal PET (left) and CT (right) depict linear uptake ➡ with central photopenic areas involving the right lateral aspect of contiguous lumbar vertebrae. *(Right)* Coronal PET/CT fused image (left) demonstrates linear uptake ➡ with central photopenic areas involving contiguous lumbar vertebrae that corresponds to orthopedic fusion metallic hardware. The uncorrected PET image (right) lacks the "uptake".

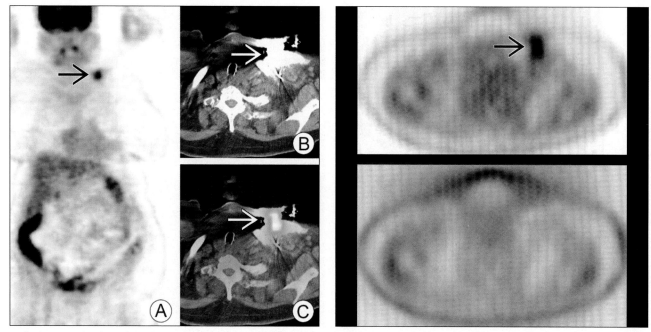

(Left) Apparent focal uptake in the left anterior chest wall ➡ is visualized on the coronal PET (A) and correlates with a pacemaker device ➡ implanted in the left anterior chest wall, as seen on axial CT (B) and fused PET/CT (C). *(Right)* Axial attenuation-corrected PET image (top) demonstrates an area of apparent focal activity in the left upper chest ➡ without any uptake on the uncorrected image (bottom).

PET/CT ARTIFACTS

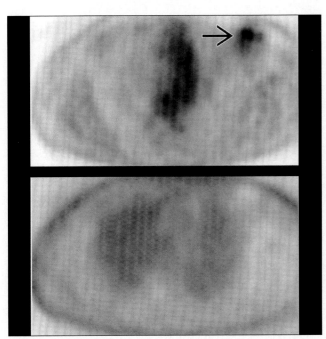

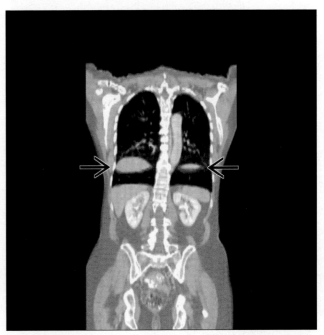

(Left) Axial attenuation-corrected PET image (top) demonstrates an area of apparent focal activity in the left upper chest ➡ without any activity on the uncorrected image (bottom). The lack of FDG activity in this area on the non-attenuation-corrected image proves this is an artifact. *(Right)* Coronal CT in lung windows reveals breathing motion artifact of the diaphragms ➡. The CT images were acquired as part of "quiet-breathing" protocol by the patient, which allows for optimal PET/CT coregistration.

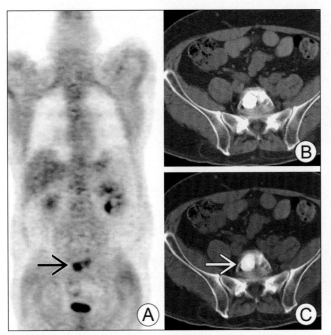

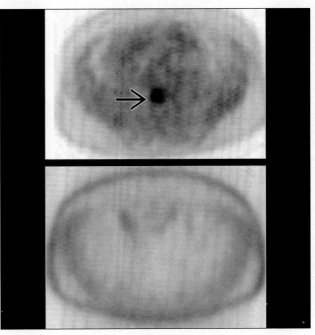

(Left) Coronal PET (A) reveals an area of apparent increase in uptake in the lower posterior pelvic region ➡, which corresponds to high density bone filling material at the site of L5 vertebroplasty ➡ on axial CT (B) and fused PET/CT (C). *(Right)* Axial attenuation-corrected PET image (top) in the same patient demonstrates an area of apparent focal activity in the posterior pelvis ➡ without any uptake on the corresponding uncorrected image (bottom) at the site of the L5 vertebroplasty.

URGENT/EMERGENT CT FINDINGS

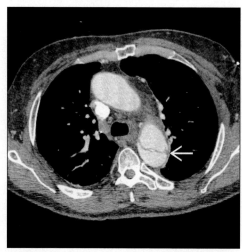

Axial CECT shows dissection within the descending aorta ➡. The proximal extent needs to be determined since it will affect management.

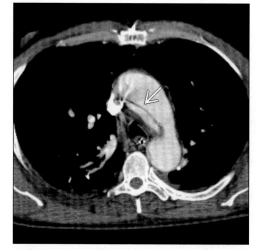

Axial CECT shows the typical appearance of a type A aortic dissection ➡, an emergent finding that is treated surgically.

BRAIN

Chronic Subdural Hematoma
- NECT
  - Density varies, depending on stage of evolution
    - Progresses from hyperdense acute subdural hematoma (SDH) to isodense (subacute) to hypodense chronic SDH over ~ 3 week period
    - Progressive increase in density &/or size of chronic SDH from 3 weeks to 3 months
    - Likely from re-bleed of fragile neocapillaries in outer membrane
    - Eventual resorption in most chronic SDH > 3 months (outer membrane "stabilizes" & thus not prone to re-bleed)
- CECT
  - Inward displacement of enhancing cortical vessels
  - Enhancement of dura & membranes

Cerebral Aneurysm
- NECT
  - Ruptured saccular aneurysms have high density blood in basal cisterns and sulci
    - Pattern of subarachnoid hemorrhage (SAH) helps localize subarachnoid (SA) location
  - Patent aneurysm
    - Well-delineated round/lobulated extra-axial mass
    - Slightly hyperdense to brain (may have mural calcifications)
  - Partially/completely thrombosed aneurysm
    - Moderately hyperdense (calcifications common)
- CECT
  - Lumen of patent SA enhances uniformly
  - Completely thrombosed SA may have reactive rim enhancement

Cerebral Edema
- NECT
  - Compressed ventricles & effaced sulci
  - Low attenuation brain parenchyma: White matter (WM) > gray matter (GM)
    - Subcortical WM less resistant to fluid accumulation than GM
    - Loss of GM-WM interfaces
  - Vasogenic more prominent in WM, cytotoxic more prominent in GM
  - ↓ Supratentorial perfusion with preservation of infratentorial perfusion → "white cerebellum" sign
  - High density hemorrhage often present in closed head injury
- CECT
  - Usually no enhancement unless blood-brain barrier disrupted

CHEST

Aortic Dissection
- Aortic dissection, CT nearly 100% accurate
  - Displacement of calcified intima
  - "Double barrel" spirals down the aorta from true and false lumen
  - True vs. false lumen
    - Connect true lumen with non-dissected portion on sequential images
  - False lumen
    - Cobwebs: Thin strands crossing lumen
    - Beak sign: Acute angle between the dissected flap and the outer wall; angle may contain thrombus
    - Largest lumen usually the false lumen
    - Delayed contrast passage through false lumen
    - Intraluminal thrombus: Entire lumen may be thrombosed
  - Intimo-intimal intussusception: Complete circumferential stripping (360°) inverts the intima like a windsock
    - Tear usually originates near coronary arteries
    - Inner lumen usually the true lumen
  - Complications
    - Obstruction pf aortic branch vessels (left renal artery most common: 25%)
    - Pericardial effusion ominous finding that suggests rupture into pericardial sac

URGENT/EMERGENT CT FINDINGS

General Review of Urgent/Emergent Findings Encountered on CT

Subdural Hematoma
- Density varies, depending on stage of evolution

Cerebral Aneurysm
- Partially/completely thrombosed aneurysm

Deep Venous Thrombosis
- Identification of clot within vessel on CECT

Pulmonary Embolism
- Directly visualizes intraluminal clot

Aortic Dissection
- "Double barrel" spirals down the aorta

Abdominal Aortic Aneurysm

- Easily detected on noncontrast CT; size of aorta crucial

Retroperitoneal Hematoma
- High attenuation fluid in the retroperitoneal area

Pneumothorax
- Direct visualization of air in the pleural space

Misplaced Tubes/Lines
- Direct visualization of tubes/lines in unexpected position/location

Acute Intramural Hematoma
- Crescent-shaped high attenuation area along the aorta

- ○ Pitfalls
  - ▪ False negatives: Poor contrast enhancement
  - ▪ False positives: Streak artifacts, large calcified atherosclerotic plaques (may mimic displaced intima), focal atelectasis adjacent to aortic wall

Acute Intramural Hematoma
- High density crescentic focal or circumferential mass in aortic wall (acute hemorrhage)
- Aortic lumen normal or compressed; intimal calcifications may be displaced
- Nonenhanced CT crucial to make diagnosis
- May be FDG avid
- May progress to dissection
  - ○ Predictive findings
    - ▪ Type A location
    - ▪ Compression of true lumen: Ratio of minimum and maximum transverse diameter of true lumen at site of maximal hematoma thickness < 0.75
    - ▪ Thickness of hematoma (> 15 mm)
    - ▪ Pericardial or pleural effusion

Penetrating Aortic Ulcer
- Contrast-filled ulcer extends into aortic wall; edges usually jagged
- Typical location: Descending aorta
- Wall usually shows extensive atherosclerotic plaque; wall is thickened and may enhance
- End result saccular aneurysm, which may rupture

Pulmonary Embolus (PE)
- NECT
  - ○ Rarely can see intravascular hyperattenuation clot in pulmonary artery
- CECT
  - ○ Directly visualizes intraluminal clot
    - ▪ High sensitivity and specificity (> 90%); high inter-observer agreement, [+LR 24, -LR 0.1]
    - ▪ Acute PE clot attenuation measures 33 ± 14 HU; chronic clot measures 90 ± 30 HU
  - ○ Acute PE: Partial intraluminal filling defects, sharp interface surrounded by contrast

- ▪ Eccentric or peripheral intraluminal filling defects; form acute angles with vessel wall
- ▪ Total cutoff of vascular enhancement; arterial occlusion may enlarge vessel caliber
- ○ Clot burden: Miller method
  - ▪ Indicates severity of PE; however, poor predictor of mortality (which depends more on the cardiopulmonary status of patient)
  - ▪ Right lung 9 segments (right upper lobe 3, right middle lobe 2, right lower lobe 4); left lung 7 segments (left upper lobe 2, lingula 2, left lower lobe 3)
  - ▪ Clot in artery = 1 point; clot proximal to segmental artery = number of segments arising distally
  - ▪ Maximum score for right lung 9, left lung 7; maximum total score 16
- ○ Right ventricular strain
  - ▪ Normal right ventricle (RV)/left ventricle (LV) short axis ratio (at level of tricuspid valve) < 0.9 (severe right ventricular strain if > 1.5)
  - ▪ Leftward septal bowing
  - ▪ Pulmonary artery diameter > 30 mm (= 20 mm Hg)
  - ▪ Increased diameter of superior vena cava or azygos vein
  - ▪ Contrast regurgitation into intrahepatic inferior vena cava
- ○ Patent foramen ovale (PFO) or atrial septal defect
  - ▪ Prevalence of PFO in normal population 25%
  - ▪ Contrast attenuation in aorta (ascending or descending) ≥ attenuation in main pulmonary artery
  - ▪ 60% will have indeterminate PE studies
  - ▪ If have emboli, at risk for paradoxical embolus
- ○ Chronic PE: Mural-based, crescent-shaped intraluminal defect
  - ▪ Defects form obtuse angles with vessel wall
  - ▪ Intimal irregularities, recanalization, webs, bands, flaps, or occlusion
  - ▪ Stenotic vessels, smaller in caliber than same order vessels that are uninvolved

1

URGENT/EMERGENT CT FINDINGS

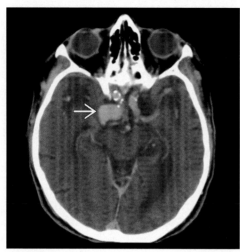

Axial CECT shows a large aneurysm of the internal carotid artery ➔ at its bifurcation into the anterior and middle cerebral arteries.

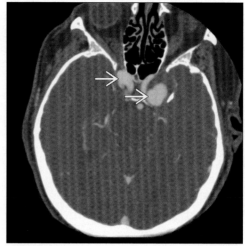

Axial CECT shows multiple large intracerebral aneurysms ➔ involving the proximal middle cerebral arteries.

- ▪ Enlarged pulmonary and bronchial arteries
- ▪ Pericardial effusion of small to moderate size
- Lung
  - ○ Mosaic perfusion pattern (50%)
    - ▪ 50% from vascular occlusion; 50% from air-trapping
  - ○ Infarcts: Pleural-based, wedge-shaped opacities with no contrast enhancement; may rarely cavitate

Pneumothorax
- NECT
  - ○ Very useful to distinguish pneumothorax from bullous emphysema or cystic lung disease
    - ▪ Important to distinguish prior to chest tube placement to avoid creating a bronchopleural fistula
  - ○ More sensitive for pneumothorax, distinguishing apical bulla, evaluating for underlying lung disease
  - ○ CT may be necessary to diagnose pneumothorax in critically ill patients in whom upright or decubitus films are not possible
  - ○ CT demonstrates focal areas of emphysema in more than 80% of patients with spontaneous pneumothorax, even in lifelong nonsmokers
    - ▪ Situated predominantly in the peripheral regions of the apex of the upper lobes

Significantly Misplaced Tubes
- Right mainstem bronchus intubation
  - ○ Atelectasis of left lung, hyperinflation right lung; sidehole may ventilate left lung; right pneumothorax
- Chest tube in the chest wall: Outer wall of chest tube is not visible
- Sidehole in chest wall may lead to massive subcutaneous emphysema or empyema necessitans
- CVL malposition: Infusion of fluid into mediastinum, heart, pericardium, liver, pleura
- CVL: Pneumothorax after placement
- Swan-Ganz catheter: Pulmonary infarction, from wedged catheter with or without clot, with or without inflated balloon tip

- Torn catheter between clavicle and first rib "osseous pinch"; embolization of catheter fragment
- Lines can change position over time; follow-up films to check for change

ABDOMEN AND PELVIS

Abdominal Aortic Aneurysm
- Best diagnostic clue
  - ○ Saccular = involvement of portion of wall
  - ○ Fusiform = circumferential involvement
  - ○ True aneurysm = all layers of weakened but intact walls
  - ○ False aneurysm = focal contained perforation
- Location
  - ○ 91% are infrarenal
  - ○ 66% extend into iliac arteries
- NECT
  - ○ Crescent sign = peripheral high mural attenuation that indicates rupture due to acute intramural hematoma
  - ○ Limited to evaluate branch vessel stenosis/occlusion
  - ○ Focal effacement of wall with retroperitoneal fluid may represent rupture
- CECT
  - ○ Depicts luminal thrombus (80%) and branch vessel stenoses
  - ○ Active leak depicted as extraluminal contrast

Retroperitoneal Hematoma
- Best diagnostic clue: High density collection in retroperitoneal space with fluid-fluid level
- Active bleeding
  - ○ Linear or flame-like appearance isodense to enhanced vessels
  - ○ Extravasation of vascular contrast (80-370 HU)
- Acute (60-80 HU): High attenuating fluid collection or hematoma
- Chronic (20-40 HU): Low density (organized clot)
- Mixed density mass (acute and chronic)

URGENT/EMERGENT CT FINDINGS

- ± Hematoma within perihepatic, perisplenic, perirenal, pararenal, &/or pelvic spaces
- ± Mass effect: Displacement of spleen anteriorly, kidney anteriorly &/or midline
- ± Extension of hematoma: Superiorly to diaphragm, inferiorly to pelvis
  - Extensive swelling of psoas & iliac muscle
- Signs of bleeding from coagulopathy or anticoagulation
  - Hematocrit effect
    - Fluid-fluid level within "mass"
  - Bleeding into several anatomic spaces (e.g., retroperitoneum, body wall muscles)
  - Bleeding out of proportion to injury

Free Intraperitoneal Air

- Presence of free gas in the peritoneum is nonspecific
  - May be the result of bowel perforation, recent surgery, or peritoneal dialysis
  - History is critical
- CT can readily depict as little as 5 cm³ of free air in the peritoneum
- In a supine position, anteriorly placed gas can generally be differentiated from gas within the bowel
- With any perforation, an outpouring of inflammatory fluid of varying quantities can be observed within the peritoneum
  - Amount depends on the site of perforation, but in general is easily detected with CT
- CT is useful in identifying even a small amount of extraluminal gas, particularly when plain radiographic findings are nonspecific
  - Less dependent than plain radiographs on the patient's position and the technique used
- Anteriorly located gas from a pneumoperitoneum is sometimes difficult to differentiate from gas in a distended bowel
- With CT, it is also difficult to localize the site of the perforation
- Often helpful to look at lung windows when examining abdomen, may help determine whether a finding is intraluminal or extraluminal
- Clinical history is paramount regarding history of surgery with CO₂ insufflation, etc.

Deep Vein Thrombosis (DVT)

- Combined CTA of pulmonary arteries and CT venography (CTV) of the lower extremity allows one session evaluation of VTE
- Direct CTV (dilute contrast injected through dorsalis pedis vein with ankle tourniquet) best modality to distinguish acute from chronic DVT
- Indirect CTV (usual peripheral intravenous injection)
  - Intravascular clot as complete, partial, or mural filling defect
  - Venous dilatation, per venous edema, soft tissue swelling
  - Enhancement of vein wall (vasa vasorum)
  - Opacification of collateral veins

Acute Cord Compression

- Location: Predominates at C3-4 through C5-6 levels
- NECT: May show disc protrusion or extrusion

- Bone CT
  - Spondylosis or congenital canal stenosis
  - Typically no fracture
  - May be normal
- CT scanning is reserved for delineating bony abnormalities or fracture
  - CT scanning with sagittal and coronal reformatting may be more sensitive than plain radiography for the detection of spinal fractures
- Perform CT scanning in the following situations
  - Plain radiography is inadequate
  - If a CT scan of the head is required, then it is usually simpler and faster to obtain a CT of the cervical spine at the same time
    - Similarly, CT images of the thoracic or lumbar spine might be easier and faster to obtain than plain radiographs
  - CT scanning provides better visualization of the extent and displacement of the fracture

Arterial Thrombosis

- Important to differentiate between arterial and venous thrombosis
- Immediate notification of referring physician required
- Patient usually symptomatic
- Superior mesenteric artery occlusion may manifest as abdominal pain and ischemic bowel
- Acute arterial thrombosis leads to multiple negative outcomes

RELATED REFERENCES

1. Chen CW et al: Massive lower gastrointestinal hemorrhage caused by a large extraluminal leiomyoma of the colon: report of a case. Dis Colon Rectum. 51(6):975-8, 2008
2. Christensen JD et al: Multimodality imaging in the diagnosis of deep vein thrombosis and popliteal pseudoaneurysm complicating a sessile osteochondroma. Pediatr Radiol. 38(8):887-91, 2008
3. Hurley KF et al: The utility of multiple imaging modalities to diagnose acute aortic dissection. CJEM. 10(1):75-80, 2008
4. Salvolini L et al: Acute aortic syndromes: Role of multi-detector row CT. Eur J Radiol. 65(3):350-8, 2008
5. von Bierbrauer A et al: Acute aortic dissection--vascular emergency with numerous pitfalls. Vasa. 37(1):53-9, 2008
6. Elabsi M et al: Colorectal intussusception secondary to sigmoid carcinoma in an adult. South Med J. 100(10):1039-41, 2007
7. Ryan A et al: Acute intramural hematoma of the aorta as a cause of positive FDG PET/CT. Clin Nucl Med. 32(9):729-31, 2007
8. Ryan A et al: Acute intramural hematoma of the aorta as a cause of positive fluorodeoxyglucose positron emission tomography/computed tomography. J Thorac Cardiovasc Surg. 134(2):520-1, 2007
9. Hamada K et al: FDG-PET imaging for chronic expanding hematoma in pelvis with massive bone destruction. Skeletal Radiol. 34(12):807-11, 2005
10. Uemura K et al: Positron emission tomography in patients with a primary intracerebral hematoma. Acta Radiol Suppl. 369:426-8, 1986

URGENT/EMERGENT CT FINDINGS

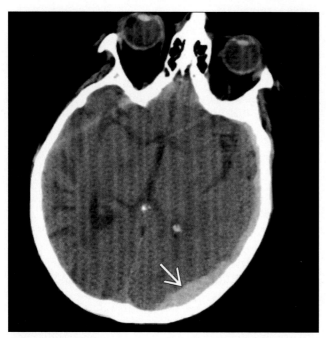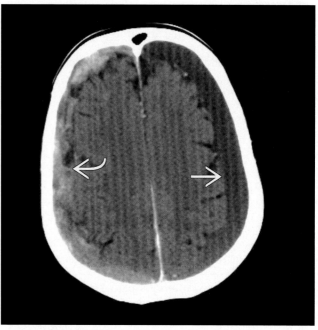

(Left) *Axial NECT shows crescentic high density material from a subdural hematoma* ➡. *(Right)* *Axial NECT shows bilateral subdural collections. The right collection* ➡ *has mixed density fluid, consistent with an acute or chronic subdural hematoma. The left subdural collection* ➡ *is water density and is consistent with a chronic subdural hematoma or a hygroma.*

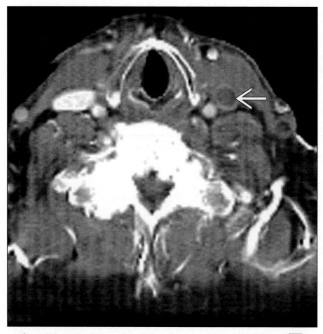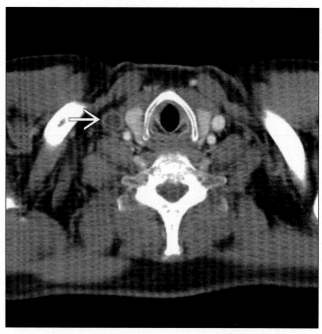

(Left) *Axial CECT shows clot within the left internal jugular vein* ➡. *Patients with neoplasm are often at risk for deep vein thromboses. Neck and upper extremity veins are also at risk because of long-term indwelling catheters.* *(Right)* *Axial CECT shows thrombosis of the right internal jugular vein* ➡.

URGENT/EMERGENT CT FINDINGS

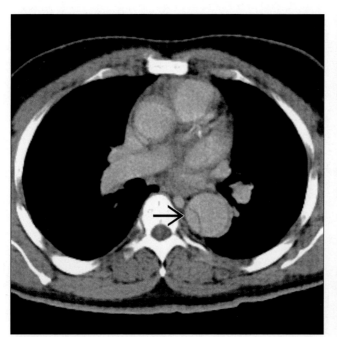 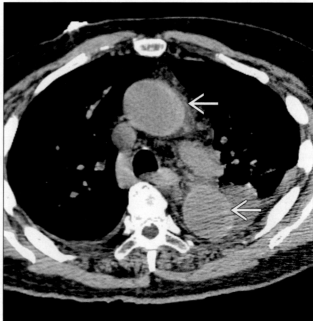

(Left) Axial CECT shows a type B aortic dissection involving the descending aorta ➡. Type B dissections are managed medically. Nonetheless, if this is a new finding, it warrants an immediate call to the referring physician. *(Right)* Axial NECT shows a high attenuation crescentic area in the aorta ➡, consistent with an acute intramural hematoma involving the ascending and descending aorta. These are typically viewed as dissections, and this patient would likely be treated surgically. Acute intramural hematomas may demonstrate increased FDG activity.

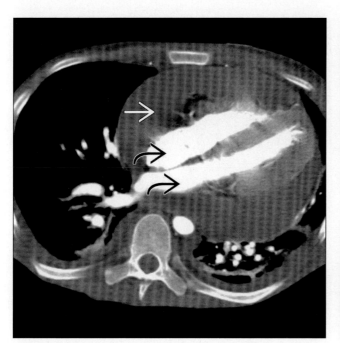 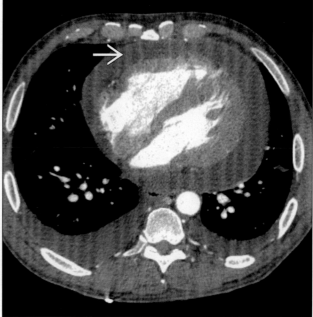

(Left) Axial CECT shows a large pericardial effusion ➡ with a tubular configuration ➡ to the ventricular chambers. This "tubulization" of the ventricles indicates tamponade physiology. *(Right)* Axial CECT shows a large pericardial effusion ➡.

URGENT/EMERGENT CT FINDINGS

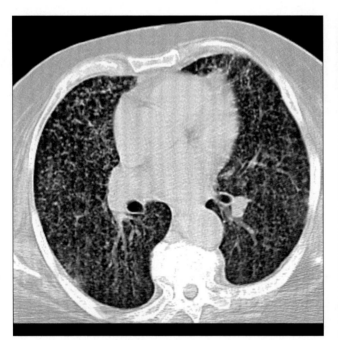
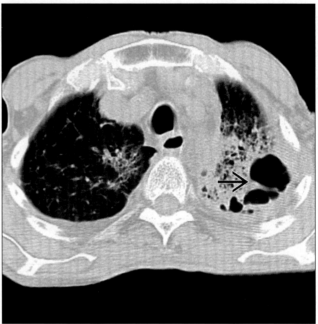

(Left) Axial NECT shows innumerable small miliary nodules bilaterally involving the lungs. The differential diagnosis includes metastatic disease, viral infection, fungal infection, and tuberculosis. This patient was diagnosed with miliary tuberculosis. *(Right)* Axial NECT shows left upper lobe cavitary lesions ➡, subsequently proven to be tuberculosis. Upper lobe or superior segment lower lobe cavitary lesions should raise at least some suspicion of tuberculosis.

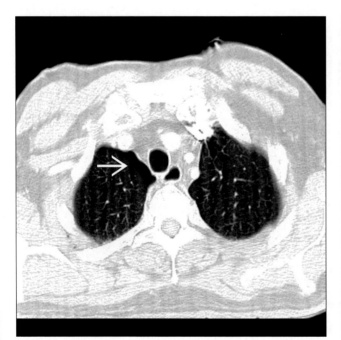
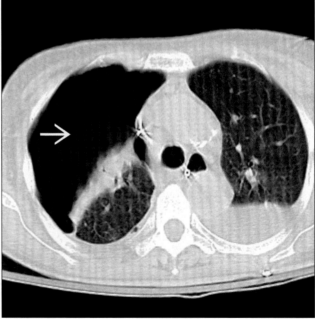

(Left) Axial CECT shows a small right apical pneumothorax ➡. Although this may be asymptomatic, it does require notification of the referring physician at the time of image interpretation. *(Right)* Axial NECT shows a much larger example of a pneumothorax ➡.

URGENT/EMERGENT CT FINDINGS

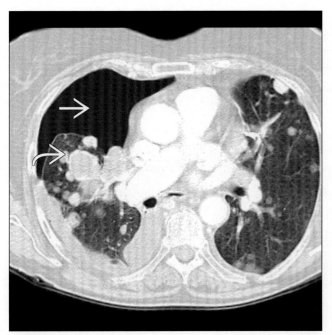 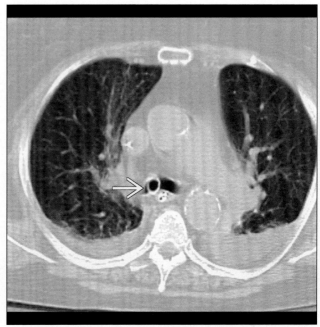

(Left) Axial CECT shows a moderate- to large-sized pneumothorax ➡ and innumerable pulmonary metastases ➡ from metastatic sarcoma. Sarcomas may cause a spontaneous pneumothorax when the metastatic lesions involve the pleura. *(Right)* Axial NECT shows a misplaced endotracheal tube in the right main stem bronchus ➡, requiring immediate notification of the referring physician.

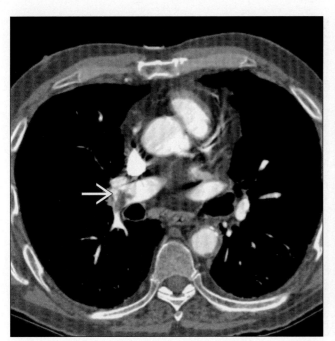 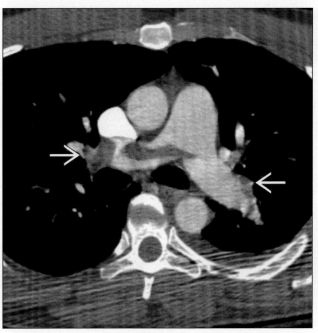

(Left) Axial CECT shows a small non-occlusive pulmonary embolism in the right main pulmonary artery ➡. *(Right)* Axial CECT shows pulmonary emboli in the main pulmonary arteries ➡. The hypercoagulable states of oncology patients place them at higher risks for deep vein thromboses and, consequently, pulmonary emboli.

URGENT/EMERGENT CT FINDINGS

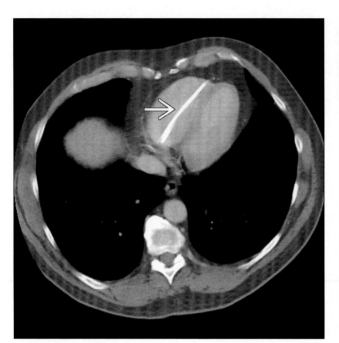 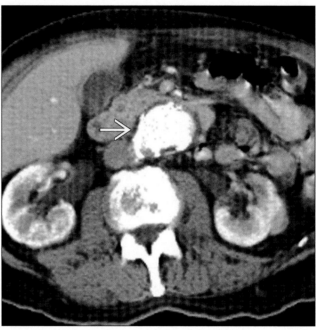

(Left) Axial CECT shows a central venous catheter that had sheared off. The distal end is now positioned in the right ventricle ➡. Immediate notification of the referring physician is required. *(Right)* Axial CECT shows an abdominal aortic aneurysm ➡. Although not an emergent finding, aneurysms should be described in detail including maximal dimensions and any findings of impending rupture.

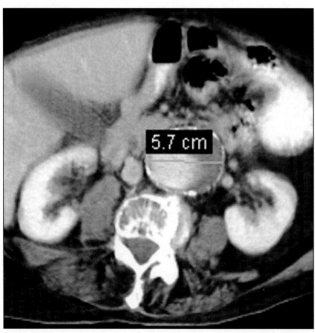 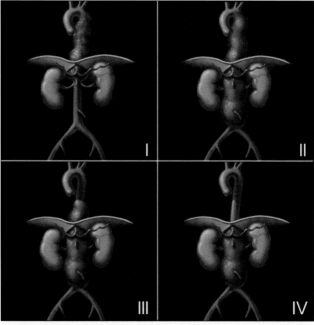

(Left) Axial CECT shows the dimensions of another abdominal aortic aneurysm. *(Right)* Graphic shows examples of various types and locations of abdominal aortic aneurysms. The most common type is an infrarenal type or type IV. Any description of an aneurysm should include type, dimensions, and extent of involvement in terms of the proximal and distal limits.

URGENT/EMERGENT CT FINDINGS

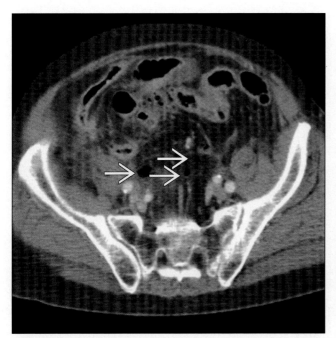 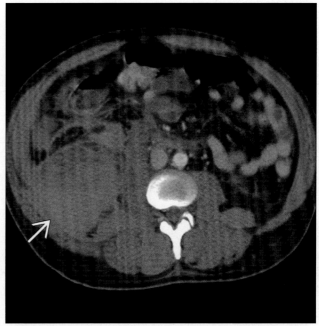

(Left) Axial CECT shows multiple locules of free air in the sigmoid mesocolon ➡. Although this may be due to a recent surgical procedure, it is important to notify the referring physician of the findings unless there is a reliable history of a very recent surgical procedure. (Right) Axial CECT shows high density material with some layering ➡, suggesting a fluid-fluid level. Retroperitoneal hematomas are common anti-coagulation bleeds that may occur in the psoas, rectus, and iliacus muscles.

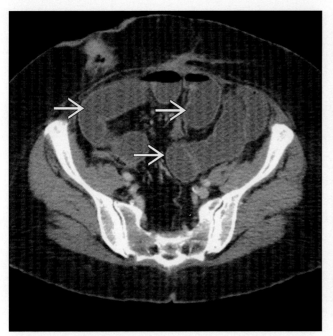 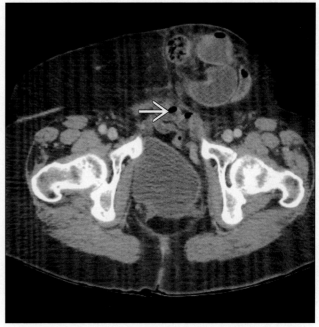

(Left) Axial CECT shows a small bowel obstruction (point of transition not shown) with multiple loops of dilated small bowel ➡. (Right) Axial CECT in the same patient shows the hernia sac and decompressed bowel loops exiting the sac ➡, indicating incarceration.

URGENT/EMERGENT CT FINDINGS

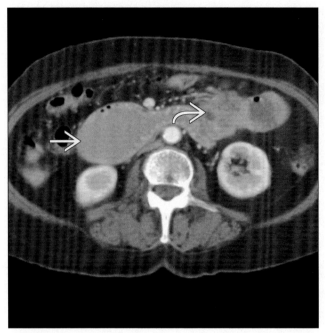 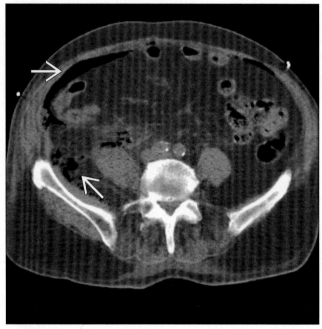

(Left) Axial CECT shows multiple loops of fluid-filled dilated small bowel loops ➡. This is secondary to a proximal small bowel obstruction secondary to a mass that involves the duodenum more distally ➡. *(Right)* Axial NECT shows free air ➡.

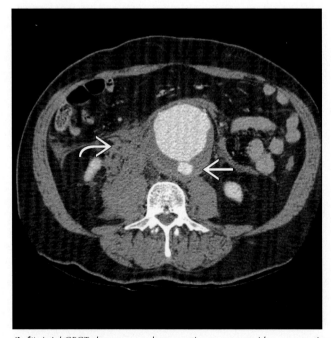 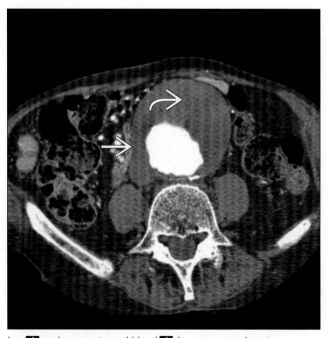

(Left) Axial CECT shows a very large aortic aneurysm with a penetrating ulcer ➡ and retroperitoneal blood ➡ from a ruptured aortic aneurysm. *(Right)* Axial CECT in a different patient shows a large abdominal aortic aneurysm ➡ with extensive intramural thrombus ➡.

URGENT/EMERGENT CT FINDINGS

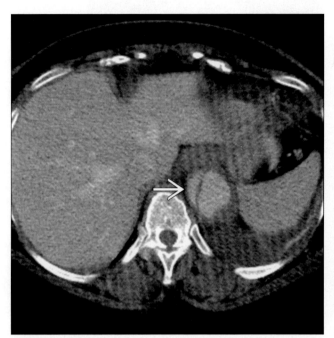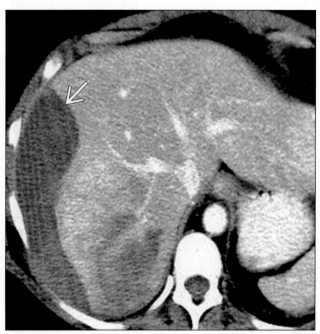

(Left) Axial CECT shows dissection involving the descending thoracic aorta ➡. (Right) Axial CECT shows a subcapsular hepatic hematoma ➡ in this patient with a recent history of a hepatic biopsy.

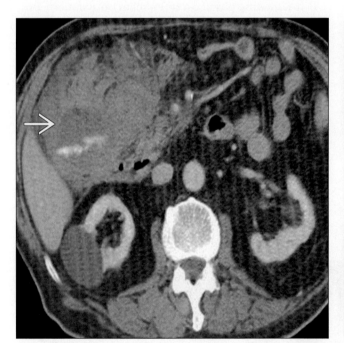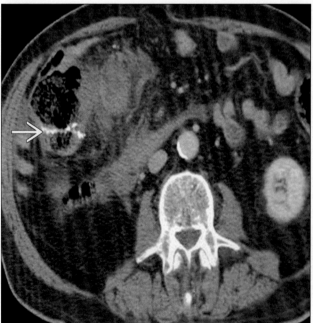

(Left) Axial CECT shows a hematoma involving the omentum ➡ in this patient who had recent colonic surgery. (Right) Axial CECT in the same patient shows the suture line ➡.

NORMAL PHYSIOLOGIC FDG UPTAKE PATTERNS

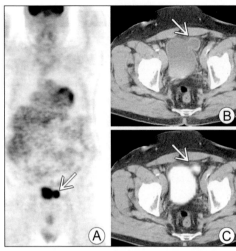

Multiple images (A, B, C) show the typical appearance of a bladder diverticulum ➡.

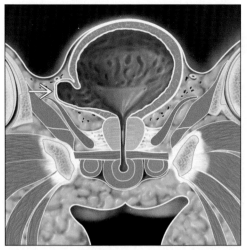

Graphic shows a representation of a right-sided bladder diverticulum ➡, similar in structure to the one depicted in the previous images.

TERMINOLOGY

Definitions
- FDG activity associated with normal anatomical structures or benign processes

IMAGING FINDINGS

General Features
- Best diagnostic clue
  - FDG uptake in primary neoplasms is usually greater than that observed in even the most metabolically active normal structures
    - However, overlap does occur & may confound interpretation
- Morphology: Any physiologic FDG activity should correlate with otherwise normal-appearing structures

Imaging Recommendations
- Best imaging tool: Correlation with CT is absolutely essential to minimize misinterpretation
- Protocol advice

- Sedation and neck immobilization may help reduce physiologic FDG activity in the skeletal muscles
  - Sedation is inconvenient for patients and may not completely eliminate physiologic uptake
- Patients generally instructed to remain quiet during FDG uptake phase to limit vocal cord uptake

Nuclear Medicine Findings
- Symmetry
  - Interpreting physician often relies on symmetry or location to differentiate between physiologic and pathologic FDG accumulations
  - Symmetry is not always a reliable indicator of physiologic processes
    - Physiologic uptake will often be asymmetrical
    - Several malignancies can present with strikingly symmetrical FDG uptake
  - Post-surgical patients often demonstrate anatomic asymmetry
    - Example: Vocal cord paralysis from prior neck surgery can cause compensatory effort and FDG uptake in unaffected cord

DDx: Focal FDG Activity

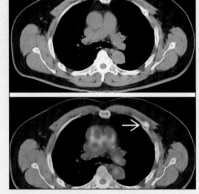

Fracture

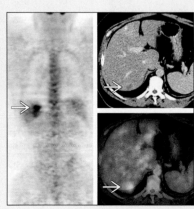

Malignancy

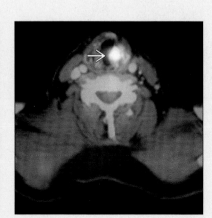

Inflammation: Teflon Granuloma

NORMAL PHYSIOLOGIC FDG UPTAKE PATTERNS

Key Facts

Terminology
- FDG activity associated with normal anatomical structures or benign processes

Imaging Findings
- FDG uptake in primary neoplasms is usually greater than that observed in even the most metabolically active normal structures
  - However, overlap does occur and may confound interpretation
- Symmetry is not always a reliable indicator of physiologic processes
- Physiologic uptake will often be asymmetrical
- Post-surgical patients often demonstrate anatomic asymmetry
- Any physiologic FDG activity should correspond to otherwise normal-appearing structures

- Correlation with CT is absolutely essential to minimize misinterpretation

Top Differential Diagnoses
- Head and Neck Structures with Variable FDG Uptake
- Pterygoid Muscles
- Lymphoid Tissue in Waldeyer Ring
- Thymus
- Fat
- Post-Operative Altered Physiologic States
- Lymphoid Tissue

Clinical Issues
- Brown fat more common in women during the winter months

  - Example: Patients who have undergone removal of gland or muscle may have asymmetrical physiologic activity in normal remaining gland

DIFFERENTIAL DIAGNOSIS

Head and Neck Structures with Variable FDG Uptake
- Nasal turbinates
- Pterygoid muscles
- Extraocular muscles
- Parotid and submandibular glands
- Lymphoid tissue in Waldeyer throat ring

Chest Structures with Variable Uptake
- Thymus
- Heart
- Thorax muscles
- Many are age- or activity-dependent

Thyroid Gland
- Normal thyroid has variable appearance using FDG PET
  - May demonstrate diffuse, focal, asymmetric, or virtually no uptake
  - Each of the above patterns may be seen in physiologic, benign, and pathologic processes
- Focal uptake
  - Relatively nonspecific
    - Malignancy, including second primary
    - Adenomatous processes
    - Toxic thyroid adenoma
  - Recommended that all patients with nodules ≥ 10 mm and all those with intense asymmetric FDG uptake be referred for biopsy
- Diffuse symmetric uptake
  - Seen in normal thyroid
  - Occasionally seen with diffuse goiter
  - Chronic autoimmune thyroiditis

Salivary Glands
- FDG is taken up by salivary glands and excreted into saliva
- Parotid and submandibular glands normally demonstrate symmetric mild-moderate uptake
  - Normal glands may also show no uptake
- Asymmetric uptake seen in
  - Patients who have undergone surgical removal of a gland
  - Patients with primary or metastatic lesions to the glands
  - FDG-avid parotid tumors include
    - Warthin tumor
    - Pleomorphic adenoma
    - Primary parotid lymphoma
- Nonmalignant uptake
  - Infectious etiologies
  - Granulomatous disorders (e.g., sarcoidosis)
- Benign and malignant parotid tumors cannot be distinguished with PET/CT alone because of high false positive rates
  - In addition, several salivary gland malignancies have little or no FDG avidity
  - Lack of FDG uptake does not exclude malignancy
- Malignancy can sometimes cause bilateral FDG uptake in the parotid or submandibular glands or in intraparotid lymph nodes
  - Mimics a physiologic pattern of uptake

Muscles of Neck and Face
- Neck muscle uptake a common diagnostic dilemma
- Muscular uptake can frequently be distinguished from malignant nodal uptake by identifying characteristic pattern of linear symmetric uptake
- However, muscles often have more focal uptake patterns
  - Fusion images often localize FDG uptake to the myotendinous junction
  - Can be difficult to distinguish from abnormal lymph nodes

NORMAL PHYSIOLOGIC FDG UPTAKE PATTERNS

- o Intense asymmetric uptake may be seen in sternocleidomastoid muscle, mimicking enlarged node
- Inspection of coronal or sagittal reconstructions may reveal linearity
- Inferior obliquus capitis muscle frequently demonstrates asymmetric tracer uptake
  - o Uptake may appear focal on coronal images
  - o Linear nature evident in axial plane
  - o Extreme posterior position of these muscles often helpful in identifying them as the source of FDG uptake
- Muscles of facial expression may also demonstrate linear FDG activity
- Close inspection of 3 orthogonal planes is essential to avoid misdiagnosis

Muscles of Oropharynx and Nasopharynx
- Symmetric physiologic uptake seen in pterygoid muscles and muscles of oral floor
  - o May mimic malignancy when asymmetric
- Lingual uptake is common and may appear as diffuse or bilateral symmetrical focal uptake
  - o Often inseparable from slightly more superior palatal mucosal uptake
  - o Can be differentiated on PET/CT images

Laryngeal Muscles
- Talking during FDG uptake period causes tracer accumulation in vocal cords and muscles of phonation
- Cricopharyngeus muscle can also appear as focal area of uptake
- Coughing during uptake period produces activity in pharyngeal constrictor muscles and vocal cords
- In patients with head and neck malignancies, thyroid cancer, or lymphoma, it can be very difficult to distinguish physiologic from pathologic uptake

Fat
- Brown fat is metabolically active and may demonstrate FDG uptake
  - o Theorized to be useful for heat generation
- Generally easily localized by PET/CT
- Brown fat can be distinguished from other tissue if Hounsfield units measure fat attenuation, -50 to -150 HU
- Warming patients may reduce uptake in this tissue
- More common in women and observed more commonly in winter months
- Commonly seen in the following areas
  - o Neck
  - o Retrocrural
  - o Perirenal
  - o Left paratracheal

Post-Operative Altered Physiologic States
- Knowledge of prior surgeries and surgical complications is essential for properly interpreting foci of FDG in the head and neck
  - o e.g., recurrent laryngeal nerve damage and intense FDG uptake by compensatory effort of contralateral vocal cord

Lymphoid Tissue
- Lymphatic structures in head and neck
  - o Waldeyer throat ring (adenoids, palatine tonsils, and lingual tonsils)
  - o Lymph nodes
  - o Lymphatic channels
- Physiologic uptake can be seen in any lymphatic structures in head and neck
  - o Related to uptake in macrophages and lymphocytes
  - o Malignancy and hyperplasia may have similar symmetric appearance
- Malignancy usually presents with asymmetric FDG uptake
  - o May appear with or without significant anatomic abnormalities
  - o Uptake in Waldeyer ring will often be asymmetric
- When accidentally infiltrated into subcutaneous tissue, FDG can be transported through lymphatic channels and produce lymphangiogram effect
  - o May accumulate in lymph nodes of axilla and supraclavicular area

Mucosa
- Mucosa of oropharynx and nasopharynx often demonstrates physiologic FDG uptake
- Rarely causes diagnostic problems because almost invariably superficial along mucosal plane in linear configuration

Esophagus
- Generally not very FDG avid
- Several benign infectious/inflammatory processes can cause spectrum of FDG uptake
  - o Distal esophagitis: Mild focal uptake
  - o Radiation injury (and other etiologies that affect entire esophagus): Diffuse linear intense FDG uptake
- Great majority of esophageal malignancies are visualized as focal to short segment areas of intense FDG uptake
  - o Exception: Some gastroesophageal junction adenocarcinomas that arise in cardia of stomach

Lung
- On attenuation-corrected (AC) images, lungs appear very light with little FDG uptake
- Benign lung lesions may mimic a malignant pulmonary nodule
  - o Tuberculosis
  - o Pneumonia (viral, bacterial, fungal)
  - o Collagen vascular diseases
  - o Vasculitides
  - o Sarcoidosis
  - o Silicosis
- Most malignant lesions > 1 cm tend to have higher SUVs (> 2.5) than benign lesions
  - o However, there are reports of benign lesions with SUVs well above 5
  - o Some malignancies are poorly FDG avid, including bronchoalveolar cell carcinoma
- PET/CT imaging allows anatomic correlation that can help secure diagnosis

NORMAL PHYSIOLOGIC FDG UPTAKE PATTERNS

Thymus
- Often visible in pediatric population as V-shaped structure just above heart on coronal image, with mild to intense FDG uptake
- In adult patients, thymus typically not visible on FDG PET or CT
- Causes of thymic uptake in adult
  - Thymic carcinoma
  - Thymic rebound after illness or chemotherapy
  - Thymic hyperplasia

Heart
- Most important factor determining heart uptake is whether patient has fasted
  - Most protocols instruct patient to fast for 4-6 hours prior to scan
  - Fasting reduces cardiac glucose dependence
- In non-fasting patient, left ventricular FDG uptake can obscure a lesion directly adjacent to left ventricle
  - Left ventricle is the only chamber with appreciable activity on PET scan

Abdominal Muscle
- Muscle generally exhibits more FDG uptake when exercised during or preceding FDG injection
- Muscles that may appear asymmetrical include crus of diaphragm and strap muscles

Stomach
- Variable physiologic FDG activity ranging from minimal to fairly intense
- Uptake typically distributed throughout gastric mucosa
- Inflammatory processes such as gastritis can increase uptake

Liver/Spleen
- Both organs have similar physiologic FDG activity, usually mild and diffuse
- Focal areas worrisome for neoplastic uptake
- Causes of diffuse splenic uptake
  - Erythropoietin
  - Chemotherapy
  - G-CSF

Bowel
- One of the most difficult structures in which to differentiate physiologic from pathologic uptake
- Typical appearance is linear in 3 orthogonal planes, ranging from mild to intense
- Focal bowel activity
  - Can be physiologic
  - Should raise suspicion of neoplastic process (particularly if the rest of the bowel has no activity)
  - Most patients should have correlation with colonoscopy or sigmoidoscopy
  - Polyps may have focal uptake irrespective of degree of malignancy
- Focal lesions adjacent to normal linear bowel uptake often cannot be separated as distinct structures

Uterus
- Patient history is crucial to interpretation

- Intense endometrial activity is seen during menstruation
  - With correct menstrual history, no follow-up is warranted
  - In postmenopausal patient, intense uptake very concerning for endometrial carcinoma
- Fibroids can have focal FDG uptake ranging from minimal to very intense in the setting of degeneration

Ovary
- Most patients do not have visible FDG uptake within ovaries
- Cases of physiologic uptake have been reported
- Benign structures such as corpus luteum cyst can have intense FDG uptake
  - Correlation with CT is important
  - Typical appearance of corpus luteum cyst: Thick rind of enhancement in otherwise normal-appearing ovary

Urinary Collecting System
- Unlike glucose, FDG is normally excreted in the urinary collecting system
- Background uptake in kidneys makes it difficult to distinguish renal masses (such as renal cell carcinoma) from background excretory FDG
- Focal ureteral stasis may appear as focal area of FDG uptake and mimic appearance of lymph node
  - Helpful to have patient void and then repeat 1-2 bed positions through area of uptake

CLINICAL ISSUES

Demographics
- Gender: Brown fat more common in women during the winter months

SELECTED REFERENCES

1. Chang JM et al: False positive and false negative FDG-PET scans in various thoracic diseases. Korean J Radiol. 7(1):57-69, 2006
2. Rosenbaum SJ et al: False-positive FDG PET uptake--the role of PET/CT. Eur Radiol. 16(5):1054-65, 2006
3. Truong MT et al: Pitfalls in integrated CT-PET of the thorax: implications in oncologic imaging. J Thorac Imaging. 21(2):111-22, 2006
4. Blodgett TM et al: Combined PET-CT in the head and neck: part 1. Physiologic, altered physiologic, and artifactual FDG uptake. Radiographics. 25(4):897-912, 2005
5. Fukui MB et al: Combined PET-CT in the head and neck: part 2. Diagnostic uses and pitfalls of oncologic imaging. Radiographics. 25(4):913-30, 2005
6. Heiba SI et al: The distinctive role of positron emission tomography/computed tomography in breast carcinoma with brown adipose tissue 2-fluoro-2-deoxy-d-glucose uptake. Breast J. 11(6):457-61, 2005
7. Nakamoto Y et al: Normal FDG distribution patterns in the head and neck: PET/CT evaluation. Radiology. 234(3):879-85, 2005
8. Subhas N et al: Imaging of pelvic malignancies with in-line FDG PET-CT: case examples and common pitfalls of FDG PET. Radiographics. 25(4):1031-43, 2005

NORMAL PHYSIOLOGIC FDG UPTAKE PATTERNS

Physiologic FDG Activity in the Neck

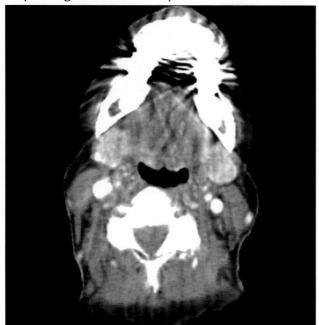 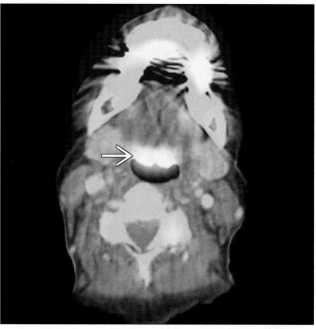

(Left) Axial CECT shows no abnormalities. *(Right)* Axial fused PET/CT shows symmetrical intense FDG activity within the lingula tonsils ➡, compatible with normal physiologic activity.

Physiologic FDG Activity in the Neck

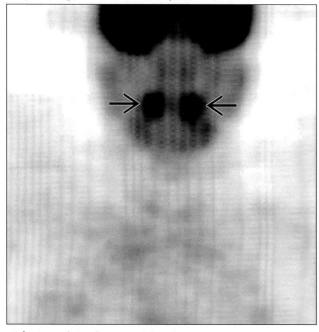 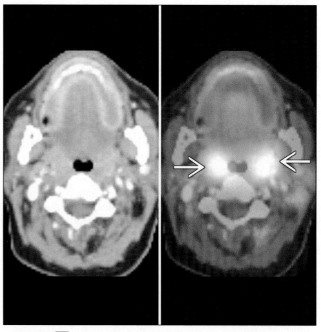

(Left) Coronal PET shows symmetrical intense FDG activity within the palatine tonsils ➡, compatible with physiologic activity. *(Right)* Axial images show normal anatomy on the axial CT (left) with corresponding focal intense FDG activity on fused PET/CT (right) in the palatine tonsils ➡, compatible with normal physiologic activity.

NORMAL PHYSIOLOGIC FDG UPTAKE PATTERNS

Physiologic FDG Activity in the Neck

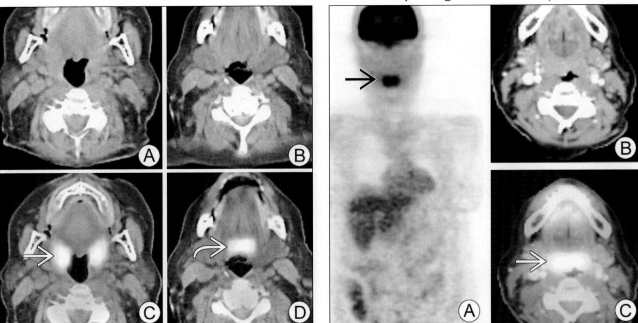

(Left) Axial CT (A, B) and fused PET/CT (C, D) show physiologic activity within the lingual tonsils bilaterally ➡ as well as the palatine tonsils ➡, compatible with normal physiologic activity. *(Right)* Coronal PET (A) shows intense FDG activity along the midline ➡, corresponding to the lingual tonsils ➡ on the fused PET/CT image (C). Note that no abnormalities are seen on the CECT (B).

Physiologic FDG Activity in the Neck

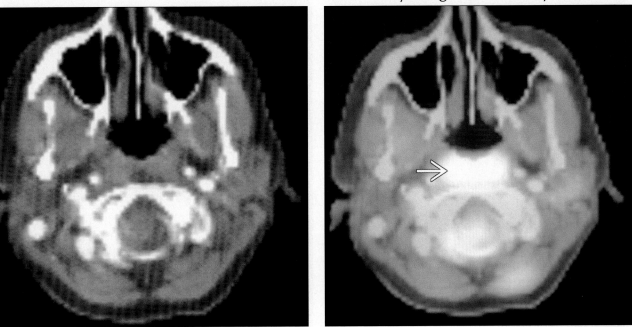

(Left) Axial CECT shows no obvious abnormalities. *(Right)* Axial fused PET/CT shows diffuse FDG activity within the adenoids bilaterally ➡, compatible with normal physiologic activity.

NORMAL PHYSIOLOGIC FDG UPTAKE PATTERNS

Physiologic FDG Activity in the Neck

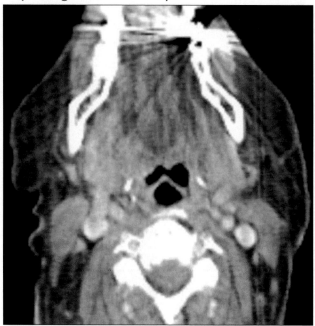 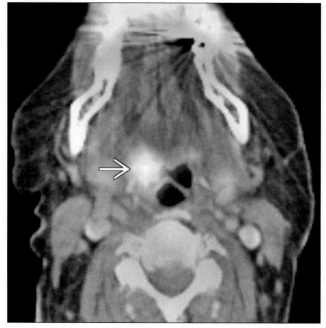

(Left) Axial CECT shows no obvious abnormalities. (Right) Axial fused PET/CT shows focal asymmetrical FDG activity in the right lingual tonsil ➡. A subsequent biopsy demonstrated hyperplasia.

Physiologic FDG Activity in the Neck

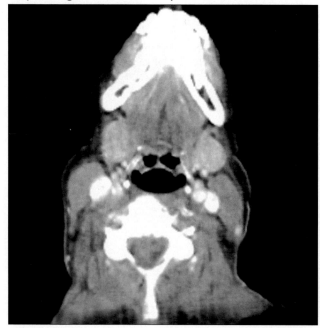 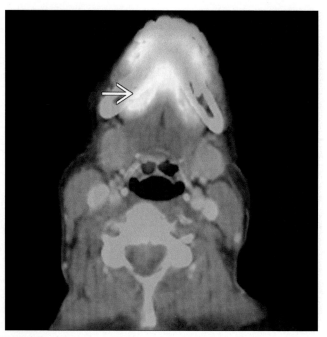

(Left) Axial CECT shows no obvious abnormalities. (Right) Axial fused PET/CT shows bilateral areas of linear intense FDG activity that correspond to the sublingual glands ➡ and are compatible with physiologic activity.

NORMAL PHYSIOLOGIC FDG UPTAKE PATTERNS

Physiologic FDG Activity in the Neck

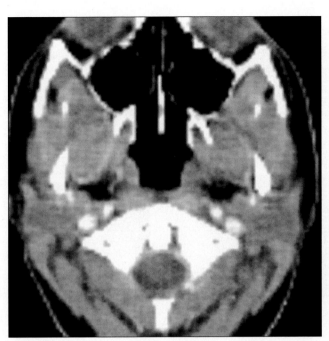 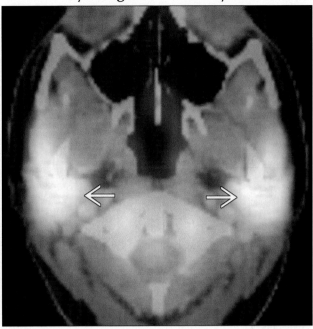

(Left) Axial CECT shows no obvious abnormalities. *(Right)* Axial fused PET/CT shows intense diffuse symmetrical activity within both parotid glands ➡, compatible with physiologic activity.

Physiologic FDG Activity in the Neck

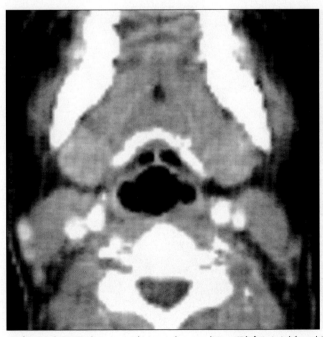 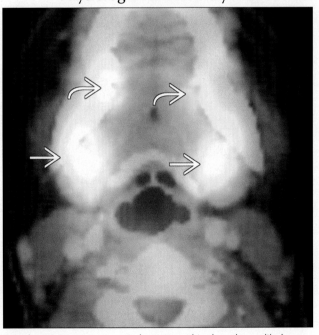

(Left) Axial CECT shows no obvious abnormalities. *(Right)* Axial fused PET/CT shows intense symmetrical activity within the submandibular glands ➡, as well as within the sublingual glands ➡, compatible with physiologic activity.

NORMAL PHYSIOLOGIC FDG UPTAKE PATTERNS

Physiologic FDG Activity in the Neck

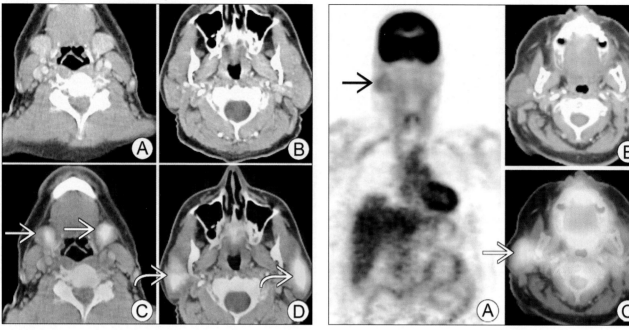

(Left) Axial CT (A, B) and fused PET/CT (C, D) demonstrate intense FDG activity within the submandibular glands ➡, as well as the parotid glands bilaterally ➡, compatible with normal physiologic activity. *(Right)* Coronal PET (A) shows asymmetrical mild to moderately increased FDG activity within the right neck ➡, corresponding to asymmetrical physiologic activity within the right parotid gland ➡ on PET/CT (C) in this patient who had a history of a left-sided parotidectomy. Axial CT (B) is normal.

Physiologic FDG Activity in the Neck

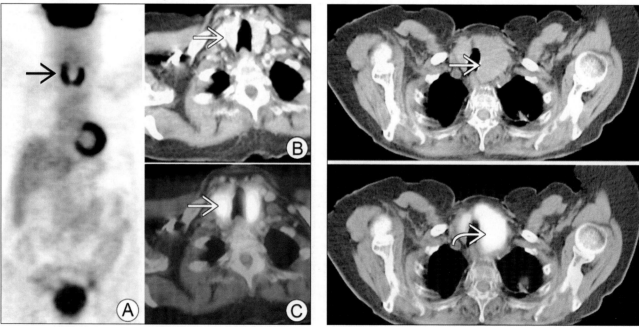

(Left) Coronal PET (A) shows diffuse intense FDG activity throughout the thyroid gland ➡, corresponding to an otherwise normal-appearing thyroid ➡ on axial CT (B) and fused PET/CT (C). Subsequent correlation with thyroid function test showed no abnormalities, suggesting physiologic activity. *(Right)* Axial fused PET/CT (bottom) shows diffusely increased FDG activity ➡ that corresponds to an enlarged left lobe of the thyroid ➡ on axial CT (top), findings compatible with a multinodular goiter.

NORMAL PHYSIOLOGIC FDG UPTAKE PATTERNS

Physiologic FDG Activity in the Neck

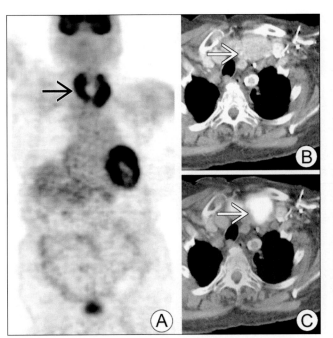
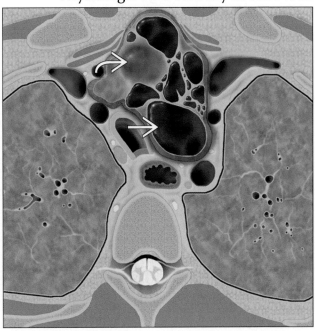

(Left) Coronal PET (A) shows diffusely increased FDG activity throughout both lobes of the thyroid gland ➡, corresponding to an unenlarged gland with multiple nodules ➡ on axial CT (B) and fused PET/CT (C), compatible with multinodular goiter. *(Right)* Graphic shows a multinodular goiter with multiple colloid cysts ➡, as well as slightly more nodular soft tissue areas ➡.

Physiologic FDG Activity in the Neck

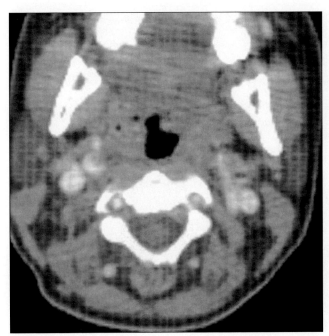
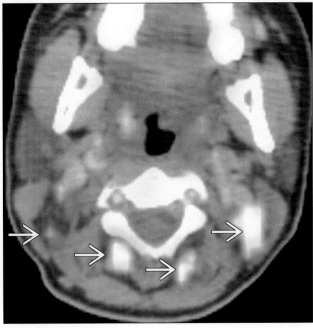

(Left) Axial CECT shows no obvious abnormalities. *(Right)* Axial fused PET/CT shows multiple foci of increased FDG activity that correspond to areas of fat attenuation ➡, compatible with physiologic brown fat.

NORMAL PHYSIOLOGIC FDG UPTAKE PATTERNS

Physiologic FDG Activity in the Neck

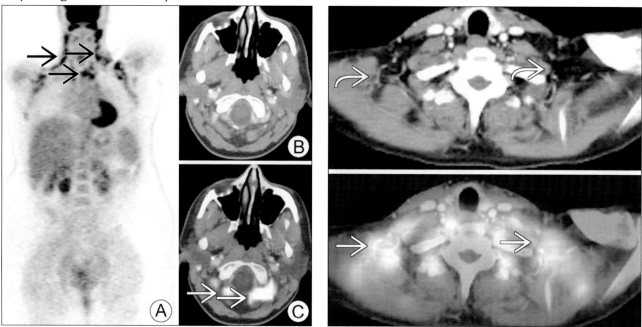

(Left) Coronal PET (A) shows extensive foci of increased FDG activity in the neck and supraclavicular/axillary areas ➡, corresponding to areas of fat attenuation ➡ on CT (B) and fused PET/CT (C), compatible with brown fat. *(Right)* Axial fused PET/CT (bottom) shows multiple foci of intense FDG activity in the supraclavicular area ➡, corresponding to areas of fat attenuation ➚ on the axial CT (top), compatible with physiologic brown fat.

Physiologic FDG Activity in the Neck

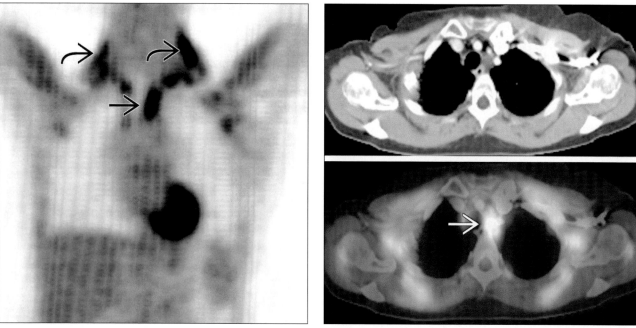

(Left) Coronal PET shows focal intense FDG activity in the left paratracheal area ➡, as well as more linear areas of activity ➚ that correspond to the sternocleidomastoid muscles. *(Right)* Axial CT (top) and fused PET/CT (bottom) show focal intense FDG activity in the left paratracheal area ➡, compatible with physiologic brown fat. The left paratracheal area is a common location for brown fat.

NORMAL PHYSIOLOGIC FDG UPTAKE PATTERNS

Physiologic FDG Activity in the Neck

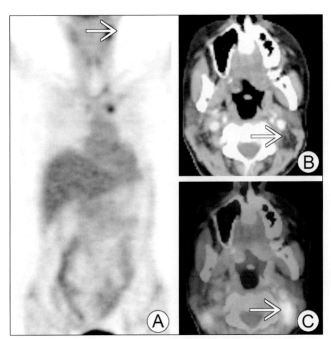

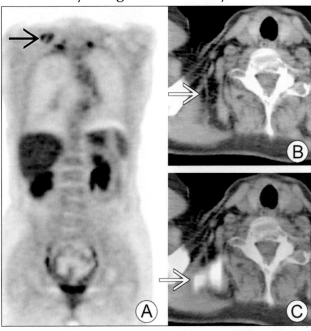

(Left) Coronal PET (A), axial CT (B) and fused PET/CT (C) show a focal area of intense FDG activity in the left posterior neck corresponding to fat attenuation ➡, compatible with brown fat. *(Right)* Coronal PET (A) shows multiple foci of intense FDG activity in the right supraclavicular area ➡, corresponding to areas of fat attenuation ➡ on axial CT (B) and fused PET/CT (C), compatible with brown fat.

Physiologic FDG Activity in the Neck

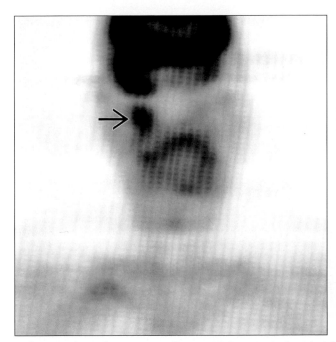

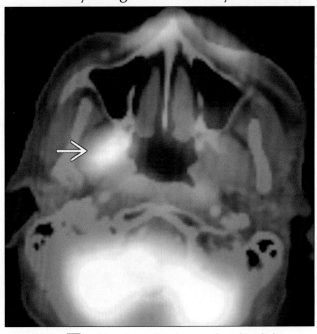

(Left) Coronal PET shows an area of intense FDG activity in the right infratemporal area ➡ in this patient with a history of a right-sided squamous cell carcinoma of the head and neck. *(Right)* Axial fused PET/CT shows linear intense FDG activity within the right pterygoid muscle ➡, compatible with physiologic activity.

NORMAL PHYSIOLOGIC FDG UPTAKE PATTERNS

Physiologic FDG Activity in the Neck

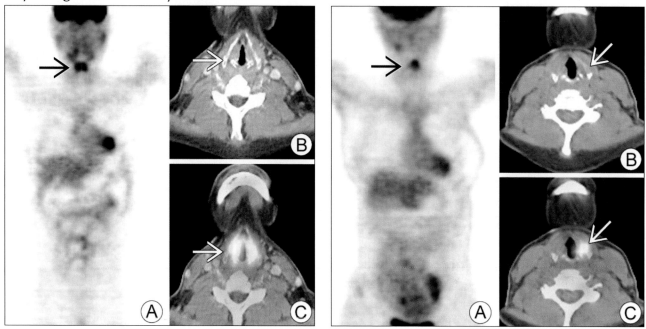

(Left) Coronal PET (A) shows two foci of intense FDG activity just lateral to midline ⮕ corresponding to the larynx ⮕ on axial CT (B) and PET/CT (C), compatible with physiologic vocal cord activity. *(Right)* Coronal PET (A) shows a single focal area of intense FDG activity just left of midline ⮕ corresponding to asymmetrical activity within the left vocal cord ⮕ on axial CT (B) and fused PET/CT (C) in this patient with a history of paralyzed right vocal cord.

Physiologic FDG Activity in the Chest

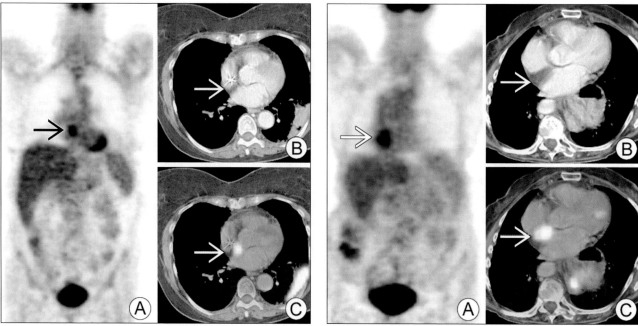

(Left) Coronal PET (A) shows focal intense FDG activity between the atria of the heart ⮕, correlating with fat attenuation in the interatrial septum ⮕ on axial CT (B) and PET/CT (C), compatible with lipomatous hypertrophy of the interatrial septum with brown fat. *(Right)* Coronal PET (A), axial CT (B) and PET/CT (C) show a large area of intense FDG activity in the right lower chest correlating with a fatty hypertrophy interatrial septum ⮕, compatible with physiologic activity.

NORMAL PHYSIOLOGIC FDG UPTAKE PATTERNS

Physiologic FDG Activity in the Chest

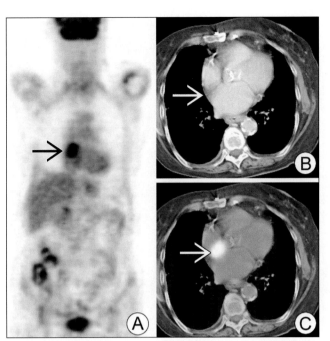

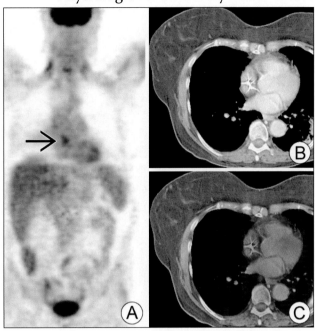

(Left) Multiple images show a focal area of intense FDG activity ➨ on coronal PET (A), corresponding to lipomatous hypertrophy of the interatrial septum ➨ on axial CT (B) and fused PET/CT (C). *(Right)* Coronal PET (A), axial CT (B) and fused PET/CT (C) show the same patient approximately 3 months after the previous images. Note the almost complete interval resolution of the brown fat activity in the intra-atrial septum ➨.

Physiologic FDG Activity in the Chest

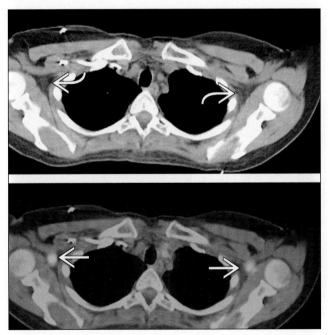

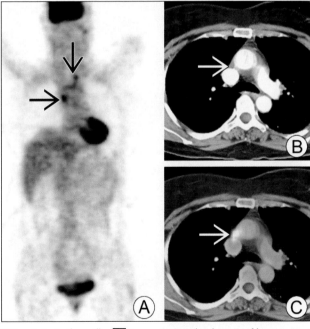

(Left) Axial fused PET/CT (bottom) shows bilateral areas of intense focal FDG activity in the axillae ➨ in a patient with a history of breast cancer. However, inspection of the axial CT (top) shows areas of fat attenuation ➨, compatible with brown fat. *(Right)* Coronal PET (A) shows focal areas of increased metabolic activity in the mediastinum ➨, correlating with small fat attenuation areas, compatible with brown fat. One such area between the superior vena cava and descending aorta ➨ is noted on axial CT (B) and PET/CT (C).

1

NORMAL PHYSIOLOGIC FDG UPTAKE PATTERNS

Physiologic FDG Activity in the Chest

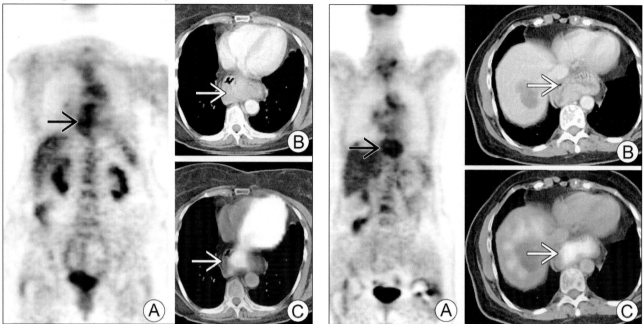

(Left) Coronal PET image (A) shows moderately increased FDG activity ➡ found posterior to the heart ➡ on axial CT (B) and fused PET/CT (C), correlating with a moderate-sized hiatal hernia. *(Right)* Coronal PET (A) shows moderately increased FDG activity just superior to the diaphragm ➡ and posterior to the heart ➡ on axial CT (B) and fused PET/CT (C), correlating with a moderate-sized hiatal hernia.

Physiologic FDG Activity in the Chest

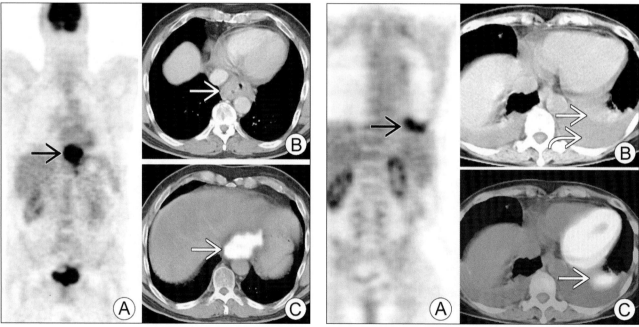

(Left) Coronal PET (A) shows moderate to intense FDG activity in the stomach ➡, representing normal physiologic activity in a hiatal hernia ➡ on axial CT (B) and PET/CT (C). *(Right)* Coronal PET (A) shows a moderate to intense FDG-avid area in the left lower chest ➡, correlating with a normal-appearing but slightly atelectatic left lower lobe ➡ with accompanying bilateral pleural effusions ➡ seen on axial CT (B) and fused PET/CT (C). Normal atelectatic lung can have variable amounts of FDG activity.

NORMAL PHYSIOLOGIC FDG UPTAKE PATTERNS

Physiologic FDG Activity in the Chest

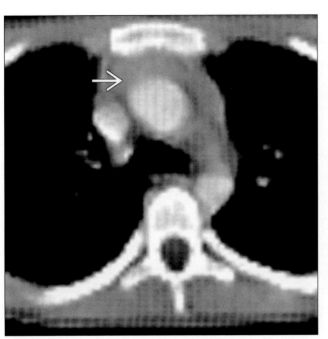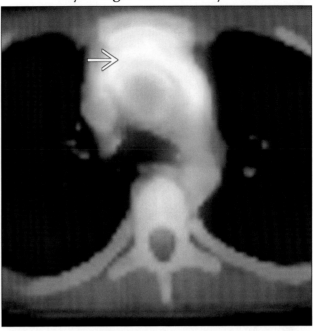

(Left) Axial CECT shows homogeneous linear soft tissue attenuation in the anterior mediastinum ➡, compatible with a normal-appearing thymus. *(Right)* Axial fused PET/CT shows linear intense FDG activity ➡ in the anterior mediastinum, correlating with the thymus in this 18 year old patient. Findings are compatible with physiologic thymic activity.

Physiologic FDG Activity in the Chest

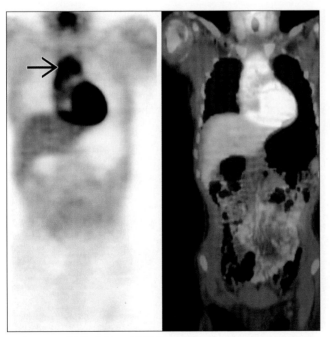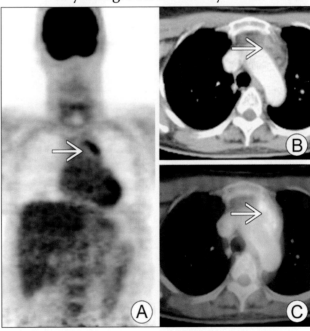

(Left) Coronal PET (left) and PET/CT (right) show the typical linear inverted "V" appearance of the normal thymus ➡ in this 18 year old patient. In general, physiologic thymic activity decreases with age. *(Right)* Coronal PET (A), axial CT (B) and PET/CT (C) show a linear-appearing area of increased metabolic activity anterior to the aortic arch ➡, which correlates with a nodular soft tissue attenuation lesion seen in this 35 year old patient approximately 6 months post-chemotherapy. Resection showed thymic hyperplasia.

NORMAL PHYSIOLOGIC FDG UPTAKE PATTERNS

Physiologic FDG Activity in the Chest

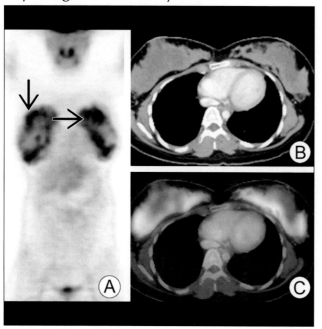
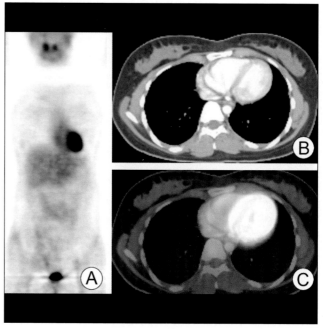

(Left) Coronal PET (A) shows patchy heterogeneous bilateral areas of intense FDG activity within both breasts ⇨ in this patient who was lactating. This is a typical appearance of lactating breasts on CECT (B) and PET/CT (C). *(Right)* Follow-up coronal PET (A), axial CT (B) and fused PET/CT (C) of the same patient shows complete resolution of the FDG activity within the breast after discontinuation of breast feeding.

Physiologic FDG Activity in the Chest

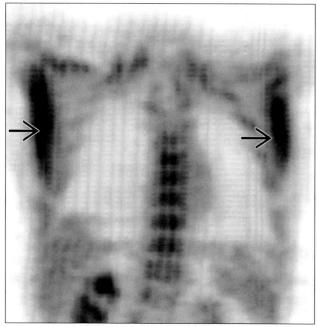
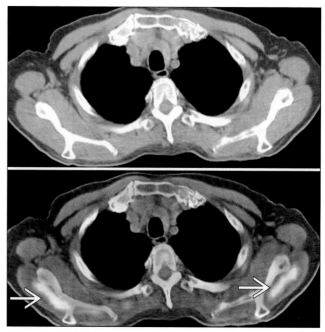

(Left) Coronal PET shows linear areas of intense FDG activity in the upper posterior back ⇨ in this patient who reported exercising 6 hours prior to the FDG injection. *(Right)* Axial CT (top) and fused PET/CT (bottom) images in the same patient show the linear areas of FDG activity that correspond to the posterior back muscles ⇨, with prominent activity within the infraspinatus muscles.

NORMAL PHYSIOLOGIC FDG UPTAKE PATTERNS

Physiologic FDG Activity in the Abdomen and Pelvis

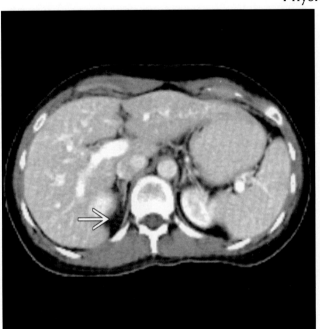 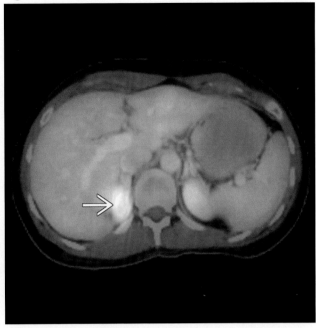

(Left) Axial CECT shows no obvious abnormalities. Note the suprarenal area of fat attenuation ➡. (Right) Axial fused PET/CT in the same patient shows focal intense FDG activity in the right suprarenal area ➡, a common location for brown fat. This patient was newly diagnosed with cervical carcinoma.

Physiologic FDG Activity in the Abdomen and Pelvis

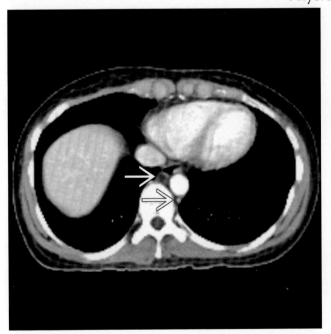 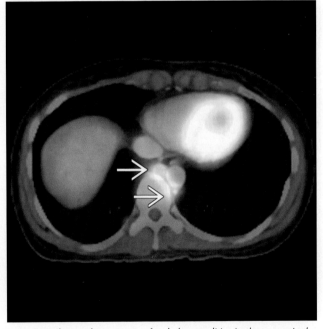

(Left) Axial CECT shows no obvious abnormalities. However, as the following image shows, there are two focal abnormalities in the paraspinal area correlating with areas of fat attenuation ➡. (Right) Axial fused PET/CT in the same patient shows two focal areas of intense FDG activity in the paraspinal areas ➡, compatible with brown fat.

1

NORMAL PHYSIOLOGIC FDG UPTAKE PATTERNS

Physiologic FDG Activity in the Abdomen and Pelvis

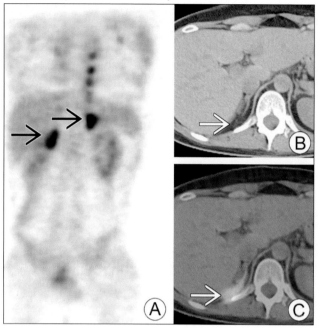

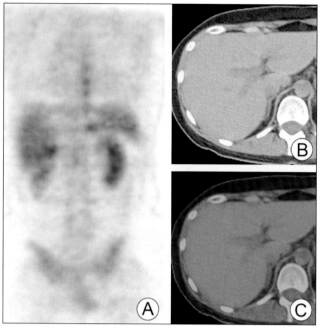

(Left) Coronal PET (A) shows bilateral intense FDG activity in the suprarenal areas ➡, mimicking bilateral adrenal metastases. However, axial CT (B) and PET/CT (C) demonstrate a correlative linear area of fat attenuation ➡ posterior to the liver and right adrenal gland and superior to the right kidney, confirming suprarenal brown fat. *(Right)* Coronal PET (A), axial CT (B) and PET/CT (C) in the same patient 6 months later show resolution. The patient received no treatment.

Physiologic FDG Activity in the Abdomen and Pelvis

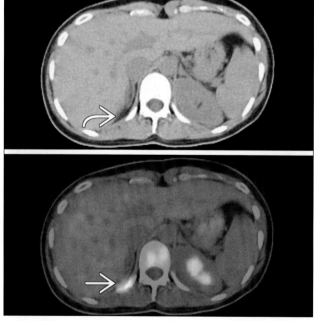

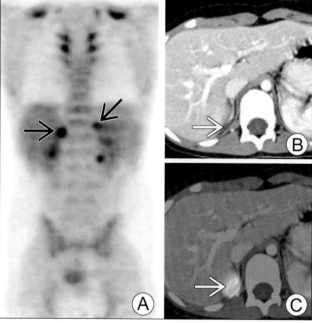

(Left) Axial fused PET/CT (bottom) shows linear and intense FDG activity posterior to the liver & right adrenal gland and superior to the right kidney ➡, correlating to an area of fat attenuation ➡ on CT (top), compatible with brown fat. *(Right)* Coronal PET (A) shows focal areas of intense FDG activity bilaterally in the suprarenal areas ➡. Axial CT (B) and fused PET/CT (C) localized the focal area to a linear area of fat attenuation in the suprarenal area ➡, compatible with brown fat.

NORMAL PHYSIOLOGIC FDG UPTAKE PATTERNS

Physiologic FDG Activity in the Abdomen and Pelvis

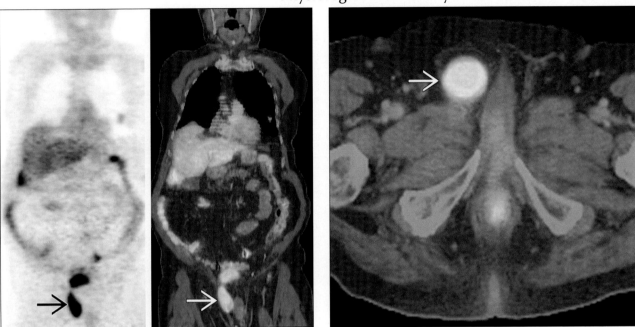

(Left) Coronal PET (left) image shows a teardrop-shaped area of intense FDG activity in the right inguinal canal ➡, corresponding to an atypical cystocele ➡ shown on the fused PET/CT image (right). *(Right)* Axial fused PET/CT shows FDG activity corresponding to a fluid attenuation area in the right groin ➡, compatible with a cystocele.

Physiologic FDG Activity in the Abdomen and Pelvis

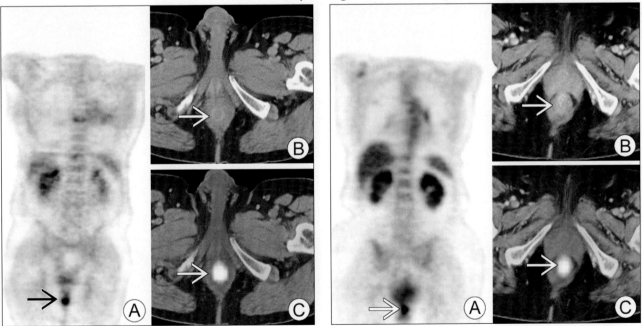

(Left) Coronal PET (A) shows focal intense FDG activity in the pelvis ➡, correlating with focal intense activity at the anorectal junction ➡ on axial CT (B) and PET/CT (C), compatible with physiologic activity. Although a small rectal carcinoma could have a similar appearance, physiologic activity at the anorectal junction is very common. *(Right)* Coronal PET (A), axial CT (B) and PET/CT (C) show focal but physiologic FDG activity at the anorectal junction ➡.

NORMAL PHYSIOLOGIC FDG UPTAKE PATTERNS

Physiologic FDG Activity in the Abdomen and Pelvis

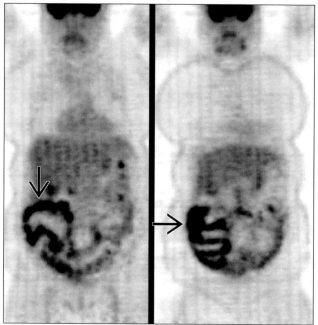
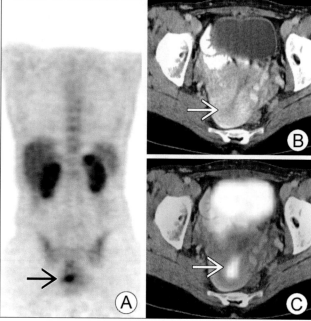

(Left) Coronal PET shows diffuse linear intense FDG bowel activity ➡, compatible with physiologic activity. Inflammatory bowel disease could have a similar appearance but was not reported by the patient. *(Right)* Coronal PET (A) shows focal intense FDG activity within the pelvis ➡, corresponding to fluid within the endometrial canal ➡ on axial CT (B) and fused PET/CT (C) of a patient who was menstruating.

Physiologic FDG Activity in the Abdomen and Pelvis

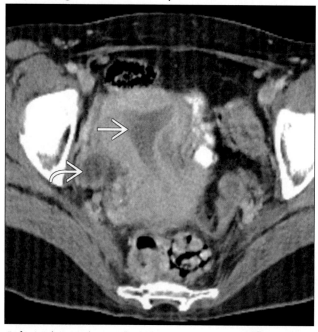
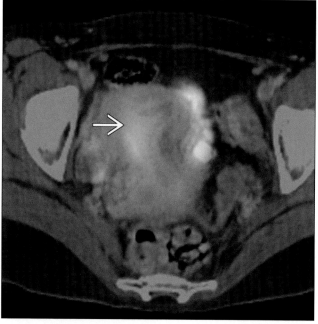

(Left) Axial CECT shows a fluid-filled endometrial canal ➡ in a patient with a reported history of active menstruation. Incidental note is also made of a right adnexal cyst ➡. *(Right)* Axial fused PET/CT shows diffuse mildly increased FDG activity ➡ correlating with the fluid or blood within the endometrial canal. During menstruation, the endometrial canal may have variable FDG activity, including intense activity.

NORMAL PHYSIOLOGIC FDG UPTAKE PATTERNS

Physiologic FDG Activity in the Abdomen and Pelvis

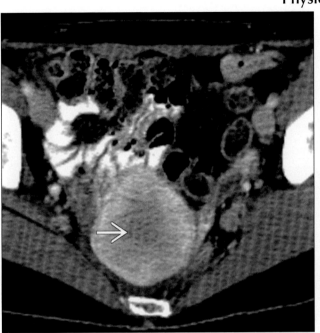 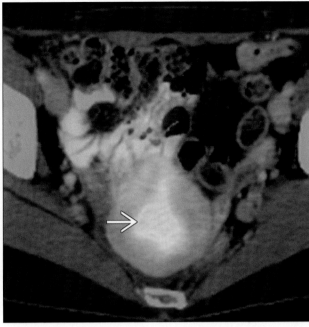

(Left) Axial CECT shows the fluid-filled endometrial canal ➡ of a patient during active menstruation. *(Right)* Axial fused PET/CT shows intense FDG activity ➡, corresponding to the fluid within the endometrial canal and compatible with active menstruation. With a good history of active menstruation in a young patient, follow-up is usually not necessary. However, the same appearance in a postmenopausal patient should raise the suspicion of endometrial carcinoma.

Physiologic FDG Activity in the Abdomen and Pelvis

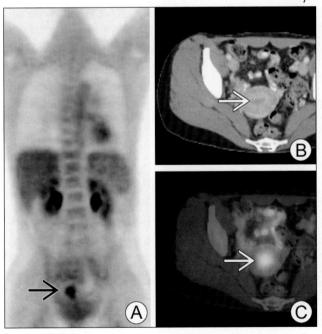 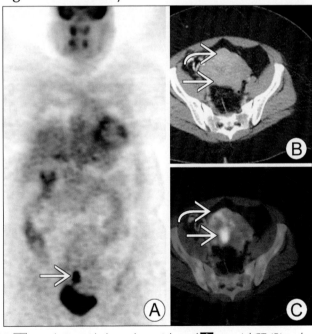

(Left) Coronal PET (A) demonstrates focal intense FDG activity in the pelvis ➡ correlating with the endometrial canal ➡ on axial CT (B) and fused PET/CT (C), compatible with active menstruation. *(Right)* Coronal PET (A) shows a focal area of intense FDG activity superior to the bladder ➡, correlating with an intramural leiomyoma on axial CT (B) and fused PET/CT (C). Multiple other leiomyomas demonstrate only mildly increased FDG activity ➡.

NORMAL PHYSIOLOGIC FDG UPTAKE PATTERNS

Physiologic FDG Activity in the Abdomen and Pelvis

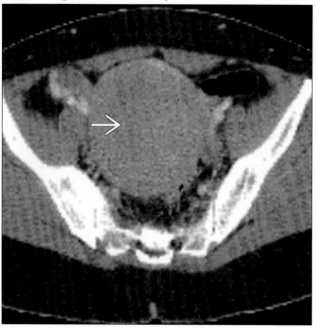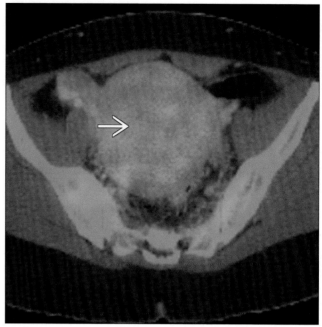

(Left) Axial CECT shows a large pelvic mass ➡ in a patient with known large uterine fibroids. *(Right)* Axial fused PET/CT shows mildly increased homogeneous activity throughout the uterine fibroid ➡. Variable FDG activity can be seen within uterine fibroids, ranging from minimal to intense. Although leiomyosarcoma should be a differential consideration, the rarity of this entity usually obviates the need for further evaluation.

Physiologic FDG Activity in the Abdomen and Pelvis

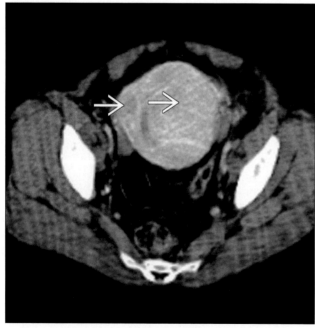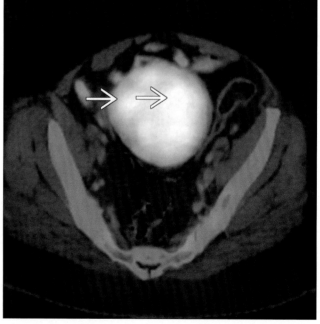

(Left) Axial CECT shows multiple masses ➡ of different attenuation within the uterus, compatible with leiomyomas. *(Right)* Axial fused PET/CT shows intense FDG activity ➡ correlating with the uterine leiomyomas. This is a typical appearance of uterine fibroids on FDG PET, although there is a wide range of FDG activity that may be encountered.

NORMAL PHYSIOLOGIC FDG UPTAKE PATTERNS

Physiologic FDG Activity in the Abdomen and Pelvis

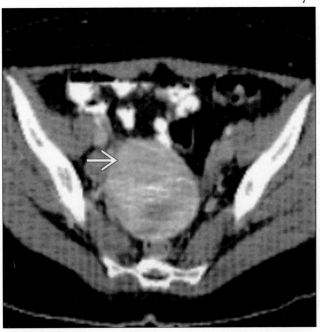 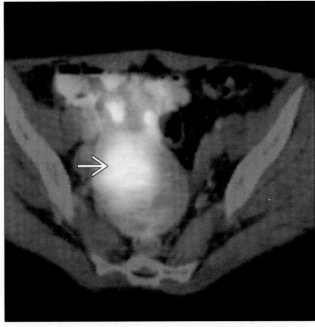

(Left) Axial CECT shows a moderate-sized homogeneous mass ➡ within the anterior aspect of the uterus, compatible with a uterine fibroid. *(Right)* Axial fused PET/CT shows intense FDG activity ➡ correlating with the uterine fibroid.

Physiologic FDG Activity in the Abdomen and Pelvis

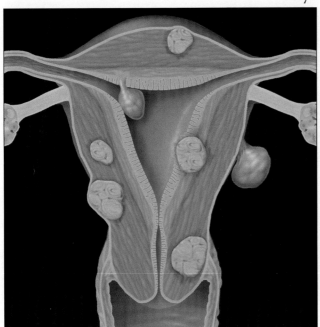 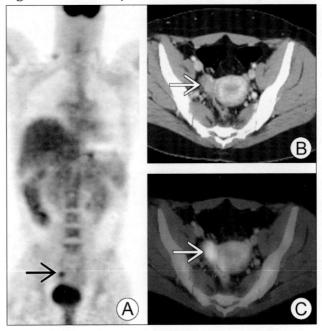

(Left) Graphic shows various locations in which uterine leiomyomas may arise. *(Right)* Coronal PET (A) shows mild to moderate focally increased FDG activity within the right pelvis just superior to the bladder ➡, corresponding to a normal-appearing ovary ➡ on axial CT (B) and fused PET/CT (C). Ovaries may demonstrate increased physiologic activity.

NORMAL PHYSIOLOGIC FDG UPTAKE PATTERNS

Physiologic FDG Activity in the Abdomen and Pelvis

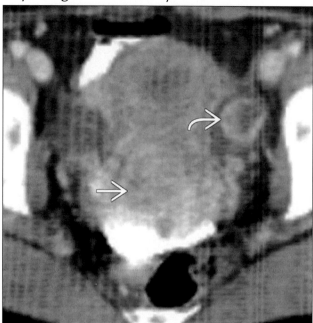 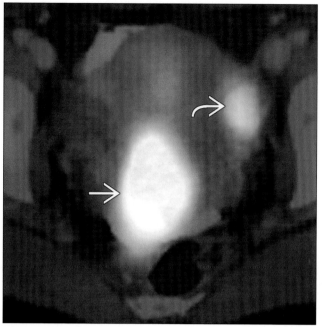

(Left) Axial CECT shows an abnormally enhancing cervical mass ➔ in a patient with newly diagnosed cervical carcinoma. In addition, there is a ring-enhancing lesion within the left ovary ➔, a characteristic finding of a corpus luteal cyst. *(Right)* Axial fused PET/CT shows intense diffuse FDG activity within the right cervical carcinoma ➔ in addition to moderately increased FDG activity within the corpus luteal cyst ➔. Subsequent pathology showed a hemorrhagic corpus luteal cyst on the left.

Physiologic FDG Activity in the Abdomen and Pelvis

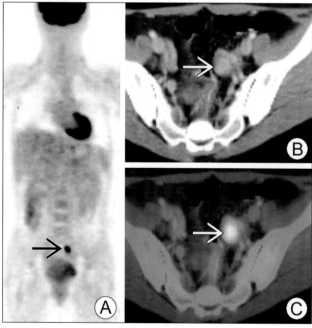 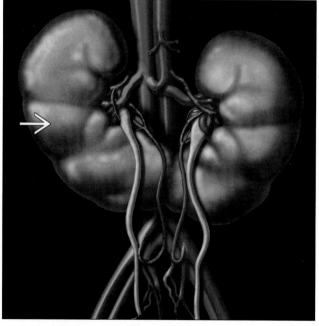

(Left) Coronal PET (A) shows a focal area of moderate to intense FDG activity in the left adnexal area ➔, correlating with a higher attenuation lesion within the left ovary ➔ on axial CT (B) and fused PET/CT (C). A follow-up PET/CT performed 6 weeks later showed complete resolution, compatible with a probable hemorrhagic corpus luteal cyst. *(Right)* Graphic shows a typical appearance of a "horseshoe" kidney ➔.

NORMAL PHYSIOLOGIC FDG UPTAKE PATTERNS

Physiologic FDG Activity in the Abdomen and Pelvis

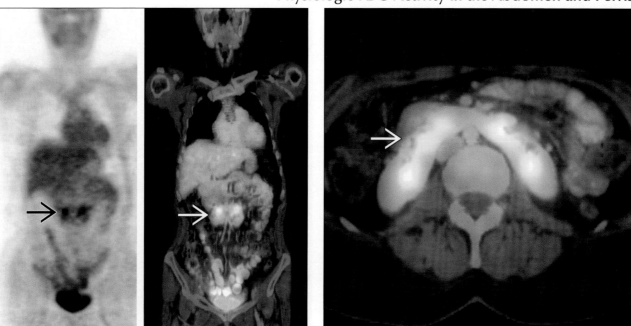

(Left) Coronal PET (left) shows an atypical appearance of FDG activity within the kidneys ➡, correlating with a horseshoe kidney ➡ on coronal fused PET/CT (right). *(Right)* Axial fused PET/CT shows the typical appearance of a horseshoe kidney ➡ with intense excretory FDG within the collecting system.

Physiologic FDG Activity in the Abdomen and Pelvis

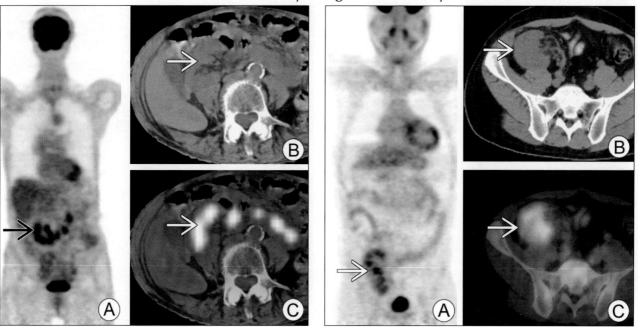

(Left) Coronal PET (A) shows a peculiar appearance of multiple focal areas of intense FDG activity within the mid-abdomen ➡, corresponding to aortic kidney ➡ on axial CT (B) and fused PET/CT (C). *(Right)* Coronal PET (A), axial CT (B) and fused PET/CT (C) show the typical appearance of a transplanted right pelvic kidney ➡.

NORMAL PHYSIOLOGIC FDG UPTAKE PATTERNS

Physiologic FDG Activity in the Abdomen and Pelvis

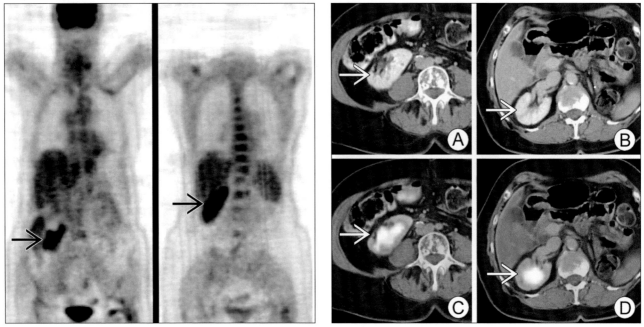

(Left) Coronal PET images show two large areas of FDG activity in the abdomen ⇨, corresponding to kidneys with fused ectopia. (Right) Axial CECT (A, B) and fused PET/CT (C, D) show a typical appearance of crossed fused ectopic kidneys ⇨.

Physiologic FDG Activity in the Abdomen and Pelvis

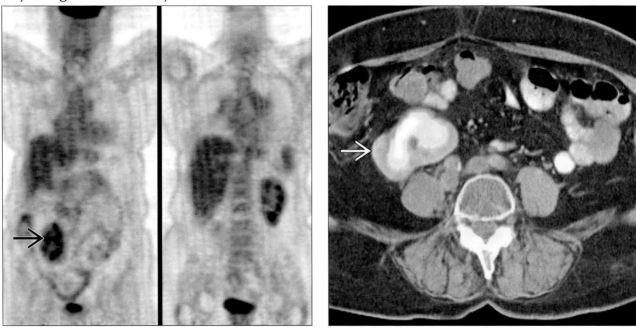

(Left) Coronal PET images show an abnormally positioned but otherwise normal-appearing right kidney ⇨. (Right) Axial fused PET/CT in the same patient shows an ectopic and rotated right kidney ⇨, more inferiorly positioned than an atypical normal kidney.

NORMAL PHYSIOLOGIC FDG UPTAKE PATTERNS

Physiologic FDG Activity in the Abdomen and Pelvis

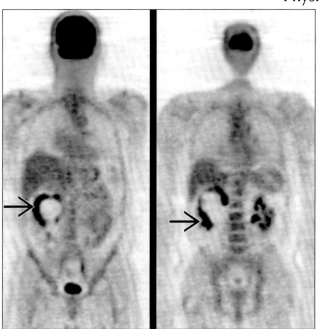
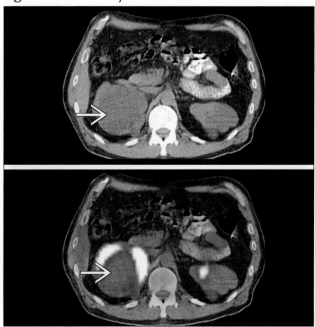

(Left) Coronal PET shows a peculiar distribution of FDG in the abdomen on the right ➡ that does not show the typical pattern of excretory FDG within the right kidney. *(Right)* Axial CT (top) and fused PET/CT (bottom) images show bilateral large renal cysts ➡, which cause the unusual linear appearance of FDG on the previous coronal PET images.

Physiologic FDG Activity in the Abdomen and Pelvis

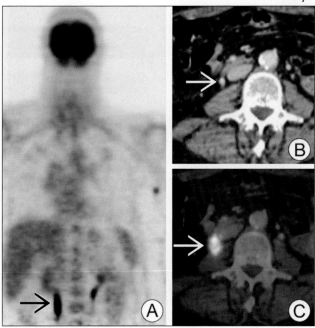
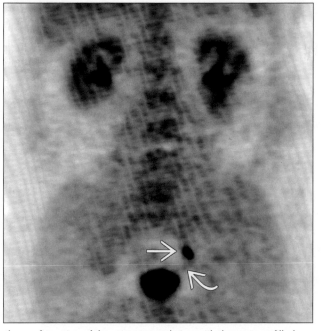

(Left) Coronal PET (A) shows linear areas of increased FDG activity ➡ in the configuration of the ureters, correlating with the contrast-filled ureters ➡ on the axial CT (B) and fused PET/CT (C), compatible with excretory FDG. *(Right)* Coronal PET shows a focal area of intense FDG activity in the left lower pelvis ➡ representing normal excretory FDG in the ureter. Note faint activity in the distal ureter leading to the bladder ➡.

NORMAL PHYSIOLOGIC FDG UPTAKE PATTERNS

Physiologic FDG Activity in the Abdomen and Pelvis

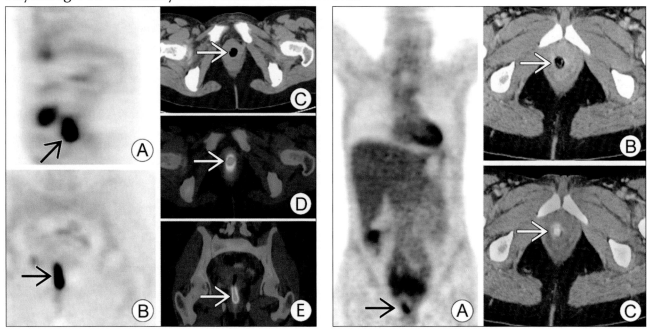

(Left) Sagittal (A) and coronal PET (B) show FDG activity in the pelvis ➔, correlating to the vaginal canal ➔ on axial CT (C) and PET/CT (D, E) in this patient reporting active menstruation. Axial CT image shows subtle mass effect, compatible with a tampon. *(Right)* Coronal PET (A) shows increased FDG ➔ inferior to the bladder, corresponding to area of mass effect ➔ on the axial CT (B) and PET/CT (C), compatible with menstrual blood around a tampon.

Physiologic FDG Activity in the Abdomen and Pelvis

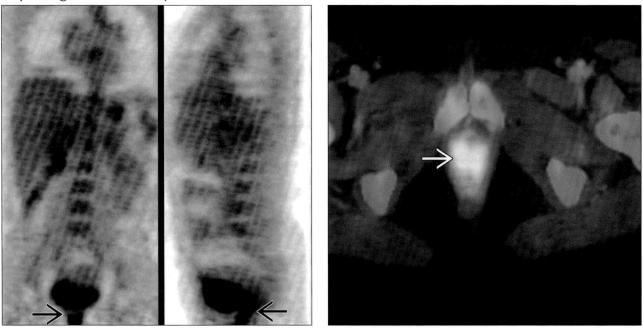

(Left) Coronal (left) and sagittal (right) PET images show focal, intense, somewhat linear activity inferior and posterior to the bladder ➔ in this multiparous women. *(Right)* Axial fused PET/CT shows intense activity in the vaginal canal ➔. Further discussion with the patient elicited a long history of stress incontinence.

NORMAL PHYSIOLOGIC FDG UPTAKE PATTERNS

Physiologic FDG Activity in the Abdomen and Pelvis

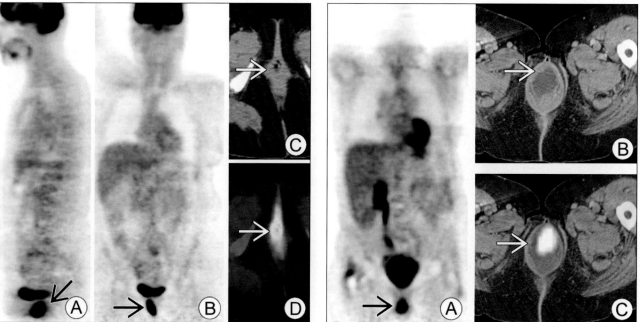

(Left) Sagittal (A) and coronal (B) PET images show intense FDG activity inferior to the bladder ➡, correlating with the vaginal canal ➡ on axial CT (C) and fused PET/CT (D) in this patient with known incontinence. *(Right)* Multiple images show FDG activity ➡ inferior to the bladder on coronal PET (A), corresponding to a large cystocele ➡ on axial CT (B) and fused PET/CT (C).

Physiologic FDG Activity in the Abdomen and Pelvis

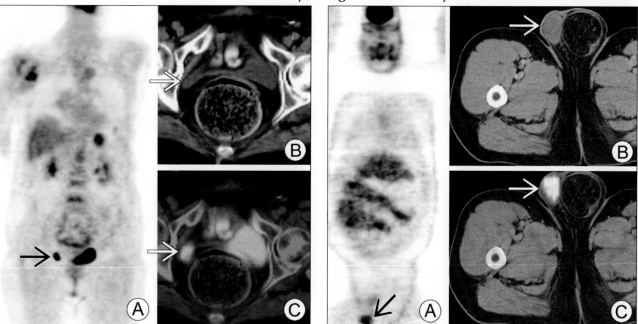

(Left) Coronal PET (A) shows a focal area of intense FDG activity appearing to be separate from the urinary bladder ➡, possibly representing a metastatic lesion. Axial CT (B) and PET/CT (C) show a slightly atypical configuration of the bladder ➡. *(Right)* Coronal PET (A) shows asymmetrical physiologic FDG activity ➡, correlating with the right testis ➡ on axial CT (B) and fused PET/CT (C) in this patient who has a fat-containing left-sided scrotal hernia.

NORMAL PHYSIOLOGIC FDG UPTAKE PATTERNS

Physiologic FDG Activity in the Abdomen and Pelvis

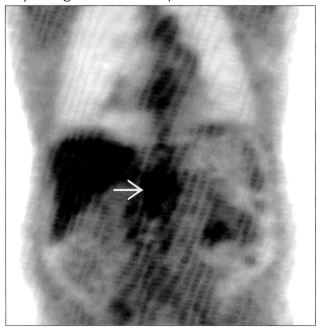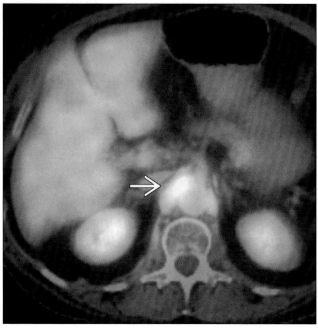

(Left) Coronal PET shows a linear area of FDG activity ➡ in this patient with a history of lymphoma. *(Right)* Axial fused PET/CT in the same patient shows intense FDG activity ➡ that correlates with asymmetrical physiologic FDG activity in the right crus of the diaphragm.

Physiologic FDG Activity in the Abdomen and Pelvis

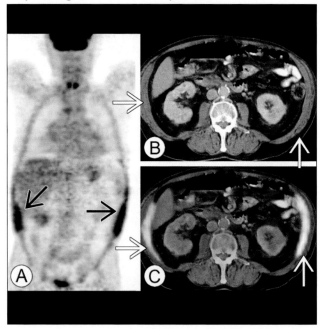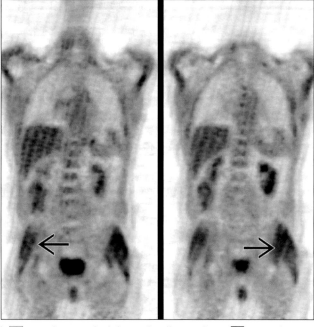

(Left) Coronal PET (A) shows linear areas of intense FDG activity bilaterally ➡, correlating with abdominal wall musculature ➡ on axial CT (B) and fused PET/CT (C) in this patient who reports doing abdominal exercises the night before. *(Right)* Coronal PET shows relatively symmetrical moderate to intense FDG activity ➡ bilaterally in the lower pelvis.

NORMAL PHYSIOLOGIC FDG UPTAKE PATTERNS

Physiologic FDG Activity in the Abdomen and Pelvis

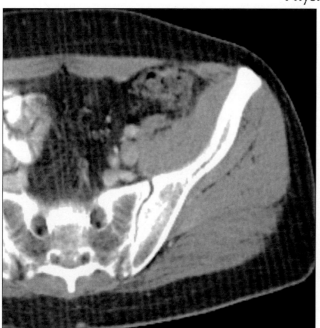
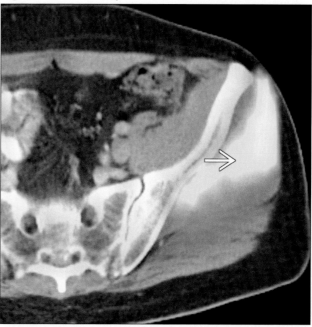

(Left) Axial CECT shows no definite abnormality. *(Right)* Axial fused PET/CT shows diffusely increased metabolic activity within the gluteal muscles on the left ➡ in this patient who reported doing squats the night before the examination.

Physiologic FDG Activity in the Abdomen and Pelvis

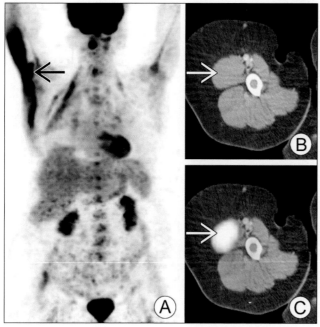
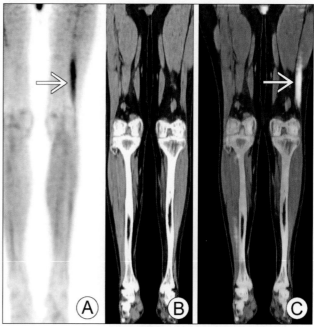

(Left) Coronal PET (A) shows intense linear activity within the right arm ➡, corresponding to musculature ➡ on CECT (B) and fused PET/CT (C) in this patient with a recent throwing injury. *(Right)* Coronal PET (A), CT (B), and fused PET/CT (C) show linear FDG activity along the iliotibial band ➡ in this patient with a clinical history of iliotibial band syndrome.

1

71

SECTION 2
Clinical Applications of PET/CT

PRIMARY BRAIN NEOPLASMS

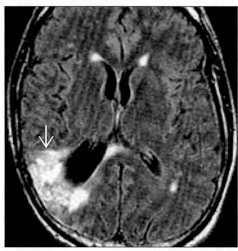

Axial FLAIR MR shows abnormal signal ➡ in a patient with a glioblastoma multiforme treated with gamma knife. Differential is radiation necrosis vs. recurrent tumor.

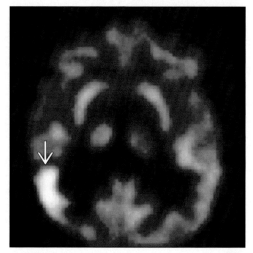

Axial PET shows correlative intense FDG activity ➡, compatible with residual/recurrent tumor rather than radiation necrosis.

TERMINOLOGY

Abbreviations and Synonyms
- Low grade gliomas (LGG)
- Astrocytomas
- Glioblastoma multiforme (GBM)
- Other primary brain neoplasms

Definitions
- Imaging of neoplasms of glial or astrocyte origin
- **World Health Organization (WHO) grade I**
  - Most are benign
  - Example: Pilocytic astrocytoma
- **WHO grade II**
  - Benign to semi-benign
  - Example: Astrocytoma and oligoastrocytoma
- **WHO grade III**
  - Semi-benign to malignant
  - Example: Astrocytoma
- **WHO grade IV**
  - Malignant
  - Example: GBM
  - Two types
    - Primary (de novo)
    - Secondary (degeneration from lower grade tumors)

IMAGING FINDINGS

General Features
- Best diagnostic clue
  - MR shows variable amounts of enhancement
    - Most low grade gliomas show little if any enhancement
    - High grade tumors show extensive enhancement
  - MRS shows abnormal choline-to-creatine (Cho:Cr) ratio and decreased N-acetylaspartate (NAA)
  - FDG PET shows little activity in low grade gliomas and increasing amounts of FDG uptake in higher grade tumors
- Location
  - Intra-axial
  - 2/3 supratentorial and 1/3 infratentorial for low grade gliomas
  - Most anaplastic astrocytomas and GBMs are hemispheric
- Size

DDx: Enhancing Lesions on MR Evaluated with PET

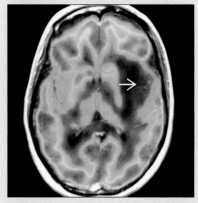

Low Grade Glioma

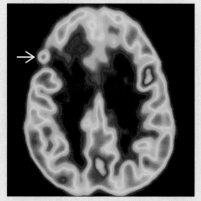

Glioblastoma Multiforme

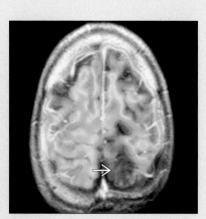

Post-Radiation Necrosis

PRIMARY BRAIN NEOPLASMS

Key Facts

Terminology
- Low grade gliomas (LGG), astrocytomas, glioblastoma multiforme (GBM)

Imaging Findings
- MR shows variable amounts of enhancement, with most low grade gliomas showing little if any enhancement
- High grade tumors with extensive enhancement
- FDG PET shows little activity in low grade gliomas and increasing amounts of FDG uptake in higher grade tumors
- MR is first choice to show position and extent of tumor
- MR: FLAIR images show extent of vasogenic edema
- FDG PET: Increased uptake in higher grade gliomas & astrocytomas, pilocytic astrocytomas

- GBM will typically enhance and may have necrosis centrally
- Low grade gliomas should have no enhancement
- CNS lymphoma, high grade glioma, and metastatic tumor show enhancement on MR
- Low grade gliomas show mild FDG uptake, generally more than normal white matter, much less than normal cortex

Top Differential Diagnoses
- Metastases
- Abscess
- Infarct
- Radiation Necrosis

Diagnostic Checklist
- Initial imaging evaluation should include MR with contrast ± FDG PET

- o Variable, from a few millimeters to several centimeters
- o Smaller tumors < 6 mm often not visualized by FDG PET
- Morphology
  - o Variably sized intra-axial tumor ± enhancement with surrounding vasogenic edema
  - o Gliomas tend to be diffuse without sharp border, especially WHO grade II tumors

Imaging Recommendations
- Best imaging tool
  - o MR is first choice to show location and extent of tumor
  - o MR
    - Primary tumor usually demonstrates extent of enhancement
    - Low grade tumors may not show abnormal enhancement
    - FLAIR images show extent of vasogenic edema
    - May show mass effect, hemorrhage, necrosis, and signs of increased intracranial pressure
  - o FDG PET
    - Increased uptake in pilocytic astrocytomas and higher grade gliomas & astrocytomas
    - Can estimate grade and malignancy of tumor before operation, as well as show tumor extent and heterogeneity
- Protocol advice
  - o FDG PET
    - Minimize auditory and visual stimulation during FDG uptake phase
    - Dynamic acquisition
- Additional nuclear medicine imaging options
  - o SPECT
- Other PET tracers for neurooncology (investigational)
  - o C-11 Methionine: Amino acid transport
  - o C-11 Tyrosine: Amino acid transport
  - o C-11 Choline: Membrane synthesis, proliferation
  - o F-18 Fluorothymidine: Proliferation
- Correlative imaging features

- o CT: Variable appearance, difficult to see without contrast unless large
- o MR: Most primary CNS tumors will show some enhancement, except low grade gliomas (grade I-II); usually accompanied by vasogenic edema

CT Findings
- **General**
  - o NECT
    - Ill-defined mass occasionally with calcifications (up to 20% in LGG, rare in anaplastic and GBM)
    - Often mass may not be visible on a noncontrast study
  - o CECT
    - Low grade gliomas should have no enhancement
    - GBM will typically enhance and may have necrosis centrally
- **GBM**
  - o NECT
    - Irregular isodense or hypodense mass with central hypodensity representing necrosis
    - Marked mass effect and surrounding edema/tumor infiltration
    - Hemorrhage not uncommon
    - Calcification rare (related to low grade tumor degeneration)
  - o CECT
    - 95% have strong heterogeneous irregular rim enhancement
- **Low grade astrocytoma**
  - o NECT
    - Ill-defined homogeneous hypo-/isodense mass
    - 20% calcified; cysts are rare
    - Calvarial erosion in cortical masses (rare)
- CECT
  - o No enhancement or very minimal
    - Enhancement should raise suspicion of focal malignant degeneration

MR Findings
- FLAIR

PRIMARY BRAIN NEOPLASMS

○ Typically will show a larger area of involvement representing edema
- T1 C+
  ○ No enhancement with low grade tumor
  ○ Variable amounts of enhancement, mass effect, and central necrosis with GBM
- MRS
  ○ Elevated Cho:Cr ratio and decreased NAA
- CNS lymphoma, high grade glioma, and metastatic tumor show enhancement on MR

Nuclear Medicine Findings
- Metabolic activity in primary glial and astrocytic tumors correlates with tumor grade and prognosis
- Low grade gliomas show mild FDG uptake
  ○ Generally more than normal white matter, much less than normal cortex
- Higher grade tumors have increasing FDG activity, with GBM being very FDG avid, as much or more than normal cortex
- PET/CT neuronavigation-guided surgery can achieve total tumor resection in 31% of cases vs. 19% in conventional operation
- High grade gliomas show significantly higher SUV average and SUV maximum than metastatic tumors
  ○ However, considerable overlap between these two tumors exists
  ○ FDG accumulation alone is unlikely to be adequate in clinical setting
- SUV max of 15 used for cutoff of high grade glioma and lymphoma
- Using cutoff SUV of 15, lymphoma can be excluded, and differential can be narrowed to high grade glioma vs. metastatic brain tumor
- SUV max most accurate parameter for distinguishing CNS lymphoma from other brain tumors
  ○ CNS lymphoma typically has highest uptake of primary brain tumors
- SUV in primary brain tumor dependent on variety of factors
  ○ Plasma glucose level, steroid treatment, tumor size and heterogeneity, time after injection, and previous irradiation
  ○ Steroid treatment may decrease FDG uptake in CNS lymphoma

DIFFERENTIAL DIAGNOSIS

Metastases
- Primary cannot be differentiated from a metastatic lesion by imaging
  ○ Whole-body FDG PET can help identify primary lesion if outside the brain
- Multiple ring-enhancing lesions
- History of malignancy makes this diagnosis the most likely

Abscess
- Usually cannot be differentiated by imaging
- Patients usually have other infectious symptoms such as fever and elevated white blood cell count

Infarct
- Little or no FDG uptake
- May conform to a vascular distribution

Multiple Sclerosis (MS)
- Tumefactive MS can look similar to an intracranial neoplasm

Radiation Necrosis
- PET negative in most cases
- In contrast, high grade tumors tend to have increased levels of FDG uptake

Vasculitis
- Usually multiple smaller areas of involvement
- Usually no enhancement

PATHOLOGY

General Features
- Genetics: Loss, mutation, or hypermethylation of tumor suppressor gene TP53
- Etiology: Variable
- Epidemiology
  ○ **Gliomas**
    - Incidence is 6-8/100,000, with 50% being malignant subtypes
  ○ **GBM**
    - 3-4/100,000; ≈ 50% of all gliomas are GBM
  ○ Younger patients tend to have lower grade gliomas with grade increasing in older age groups

Gross Pathologic & Surgical Features
- Tumor is difficult to distinguish from normal or edematous brain tissue at operation
  ○ Percentage of complete removal by routine surgery is disappointing, leading to poor prognosis
  ○ Genuine total removal of glioma probably impossible because of diffuse growth and location

Microscopic Features
- Grade depends on
  ○ Degree of cellularity
  ○ Cellular pleomorphism
  ○ Mitotic figures
  ○ Necrosis
  ○ Vascular proliferation

CLINICAL ISSUES

Presentation
- Most common signs/symptoms
  ○ Various neurologic symptoms
    - Headaches
    - Seizures
    - Visual disturbances
- Other signs/symptoms: Other symptoms related to mass effect or hemorrhage

Demographics
- Age

PRIMARY BRAIN NEOPLASMS

- o Low grade gliomas typically occur in younger patients
- o Higher grade tumors typically occur in older patients
- Gender: Males and females equally affected

Natural History & Prognosis

- Overall prognosis poor
  - o 5 year survival 30% for all astrocytomas
  - o Worse with increasing age
  - o Worse for GBM; 5 year survival 2%
- Spread along tracts, along surfaces, and across the meninges
- Some GBMs may arise from lower grade tumors
  - o PET often helpful if baseline shows low/absent FDG activity in tumor and follow-up shows intense uptake

Treatment

- Combination of primary surgical resection with chemoradiation
- FDG PET has 75-88% sensitivity and 81% specificity for detecting recurrent tumor as opposed to radiation necrosis

DIAGNOSTIC CHECKLIST

Consider

- Initial imaging evaluation should include MR with contrast ± FDG PET
- Primary roles for FDG PET are tumor grading, prognosis, and differentiating recurrent tumor from radiation necrosis

Image Interpretation Pearls

- Low grade gliomas may have only mildly increased FDG uptake compared to normal white matter
- Small lesions < 1 cm may not be seen due to the large amount of FDG activity in normal brain and partial volume averaging
- Areas of intense FDG uptake in a patient with a low grade glioma likely represent tumor transformation to higher grade (i.e., GBM)
- FDG PET generally very good for differentiating radiation necrosis from recurrent tumor
- Areas of decreased FDG activity can be seen following radiotherapy

SELECTED REFERENCES

1. Kato T et al: Metabolic assessment of gliomas using 11C-methionine, [18F] fluorodeoxyglucose, and 11C-choline positron-emission tomography. AJNR Am J Neuroradiol. 29(6):1176-82, 2008
2. Terakawa Y et al: Diagnostic accuracy of 11C-methionine PET for differentiation of recurrent brain tumors from radiation necrosis after radiotherapy. J Nucl Med. 49(5):694-9, 2008
3. Gumprecht H et al: 11C-Methionine positron emission tomography for preoperative evaluation of suggestive low-grade gliomas. Zentralbl Neurochir. 68(1):19-23, 2007
4. Levivier M et al: Integration of functional imaging in radiosurgery: the example of PET scan. Prog Neurol Surg. 20:68-81, 2007
5. Moulin-Romsée G et al: Non-invasive grading of brain tumours using dynamic amino acid PET imaging: does it work for 11C-methionine? Eur J Nucl Med Mol Imaging. 34(12):2082-7, 2007
6. Pötzi C et al: [11C] methionine and [18F] fluorodeoxyglucose PET in the follow-up of glioblastoma multiforme. J Neurooncol. 84(3):305-14, 2007
7. Roelcke U et al: Metabolic deactivation of low-grade glioma during chemotherapy. J Neurol. 254(5):668-9, 2007
8. Wyss MT et al: Uptake of 18F-Fluorocholine, 18F-FET, and 18F-FDG in C6 gliomas and correlation with 131I-SIP(L19), a marker of angiogenesis. J Nucl Med. 48(4):608-14, 2007
9. Xiangsong Z et al: Differentiation of recurrent astrocytoma from radiation necrosis: a pilot study with 13N-NH3 PET. J Neurooncol. 82(3):305-11, 2007
10. Andersen PB et al: A prospective PET study of patients with glioblastoma multiforme. Acta Neurol Scand. 113(6):412-8, 2006
11. Douglas JG et al: [F-18]-fluorodeoxyglucose positron emission tomography for targeting radiation dose escalation for patients with glioblastoma multiforme: clinical outcomes and patterns of failure. Int J Radiat Oncol Biol Phys. 64(3):886-91, 2006
12. Kwon JW et al: Paediatric brain-stem gliomas: MRI, FDG-PET and histological grading correlation. Pediatr Radiol. 36(9):959-64, 2006
13. Meyer MA: Positron-emission tomography in cancer therapy. N Engl J Med. 354(18):1958-60; author reply 1958-60, 2006
14. Miyamoto J et al: Surgical decision for adult optic glioma based on [18F]fluorodeoxyglucose positron emission tomography study. Neurol Med Chir (Tokyo). 46(10):500-3, 2006
15. Saga T et al: Evaluation of primary brain tumors with FLT-PET: usefulness and limitations. Clin Nucl Med. 31(12):774-80, 2006
16. Wang SX et al: FDG-PET on irradiated brain tumor: ten years' summary. Acta Radiol. 47(1):85-90, 2006
17. Floeth FW et al: The value of metabolic imaging in diagnosis and resection of cerebral gliomas. Nat Clin Pract Neurol. 1(2):62-3, 2005
18. Minn H: PET and SPECT in low-grade glioma. Eur J Radiol. 56(2):171-8, 2005
19. Torii K et al: Correlation of amino-acid uptake using methionine PET and histological classifications in various gliomas. Ann Nucl Med. 19(8):677-83, 2005
20. Van Laere K et al: Direct comparison of 18F-FDG and 11C-methionine PET in suspected recurrence of glioma: sensitivity, inter-observer variability and prognostic value. Eur J Nucl Med Mol Imaging. 32(1):39-51, 2005
21. Giammarile F et al: High and low grade oligodendrogliomas (ODG): correlation of amino-acid and glucose uptakes using PET and histological classifications. J Neurooncol. 68(3):263-74, 2004
22. Engelhard HH et al: Oligodendroglioma and anaplastic oligodendroglioma: clinical features, treatment, and prognosis. Surg Neurol. 60(5):443-56, 2003
23. Hara T et al: Use of 18F-choline and 11C-choline as contrast agents in positron emission tomography imaging-guided stereotactic biopsy sampling of gliomas. J Neurosurg. 99(3):474-9, 2003
24. Etzl MM Jr et al: Positron emission tomography in three children with pleomorphic xanthoastrocytoma. J Child Neurol. 17(7):522-7, 2002
25. Levivier M et al: The integration of metabolic imaging in stereotactic procedures including radiosurgery: a review. J Neurosurg. 97(5 Suppl):542-50, 2002
26. Ross DA et al: Imaging changes after stereotactic radiosurgery of primary and secondary malignant brain tumors. J Neurooncol. 56(2):175-81, 2002

PRIMARY BRAIN NEOPLASMS

Typical

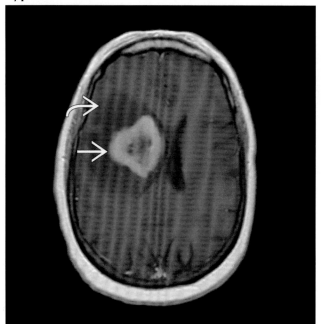 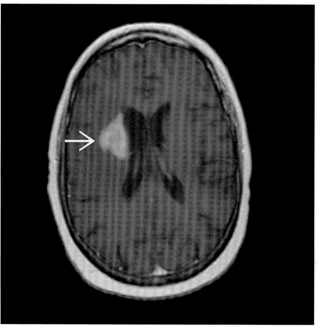

(Left) Axial T1 C+ MR shows a large enhancing right frontal lobe mass ➡ with surrounding vasogenic edema ➡ in this patient with primary CNS lymphoma. *(Right)* Axial T1 C+ MR following 3 cycles of chemotherapy shows interval decrease in size of the enhancing right frontal lobe mass ➡ as well as resolution of the vasogenic edema.

Typical

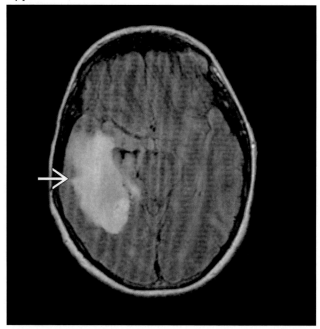 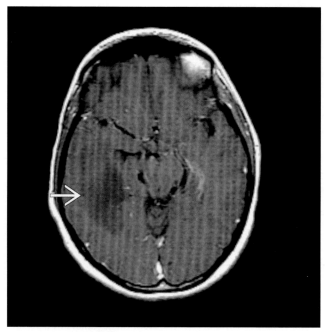

(Left) Axial FLAIR MR shows abnormal signal involving the majority of the right temporal lobe ➡ in this patient with a known low grade glioma. *(Right)* Axial T1 C+ MR shows no evidence for enhancement within the right temporal lobe mass ➡. Most low grade glial tumors do not show enhancement on post-contrast MR images.

PRIMARY BRAIN NEOPLASMS

Typical

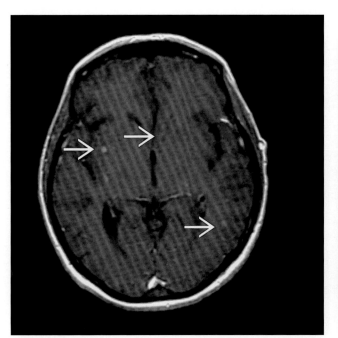 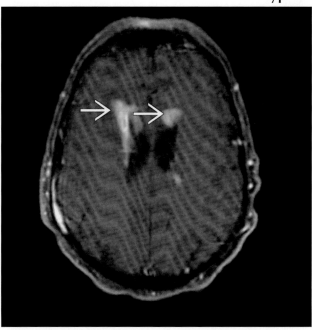

(Left) Axial T1 C+ MR shows innumerable bilateral subcentimeter enhancing lesions ➡ in this patient with extensive melanoma metastases. The majority of these lesions would not be visible on FDG PET using a whole-body protocol. *(Right)* Axial FLAIR MR shows abnormal subependymal signal adjacent to the lateral ventricles and extending across the corpus callosum ➡. The top differential diagnosis for this finding is lymphoma vs. glioblastoma multiform.

Typical

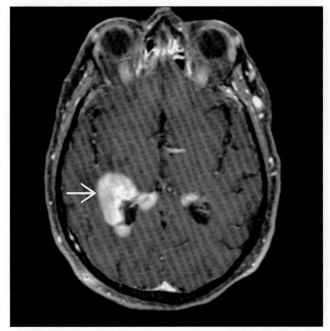 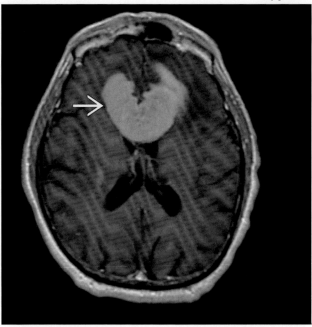

(Left) Axial T1 C+ MR shows an enhancing tumor in a subependymal location ➡, compatible with subependymal spread of tumor. *(Right)* Axial T1 C+ MR shows abnormal enhancements along the corpus callosum ➡ in a butterfly-wing distribution in this patient with primary CNS lymphoma.

PRIMARY BRAIN NEOPLASMS

Typical

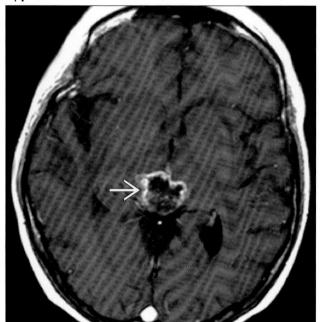
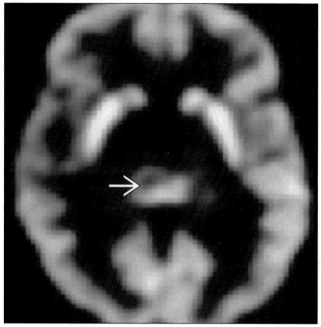

(Left) Axial T1 C+ MR shows enhancement and central necrosis ➔ following radiation therapy. Differential diagnosis includes radiation necrosis vs. tumor. *(Right)* Axial PET in the same patient following radiation therapy shows focal intense FDG activity ➔ that correlates with the enhancing lesion on MR, compatible with residual/recurrent tumor.

Typical

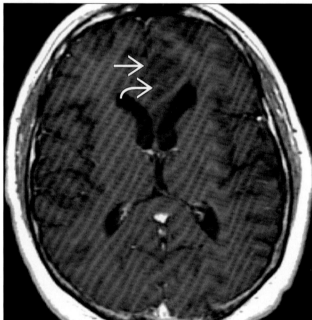
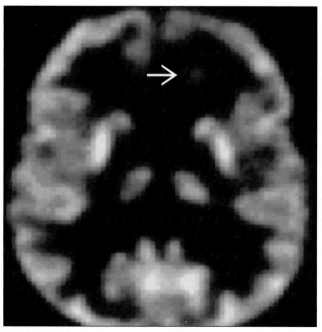

(Left) Axial post-gadolinium T1 weighted MR shows a left frontal lesion ➔ with minimal posterior enhancement ➔ following radiation treatment for a WHO grade III lesion equivocal for residual tumor. *(Right)* Axial PET shows moderate FDG activity ➔ correlating with the lesion on MR (previous image). The FDG uptake is fairly intense, compared to that of normal white matter, compatible with a low grade tumor.

PRIMARY BRAIN NEOPLASMS

Typical

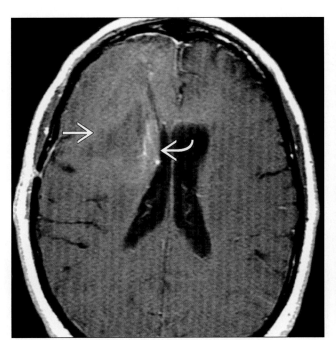
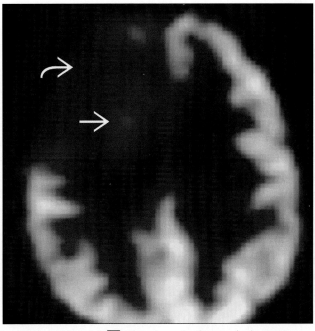

(Left) Axial T1 C+ MR shows a right frontal mass ➡ with mass effect on the right lateral ventricle ➡. There is no significant enhancement in this patient with a WHO grade I glioma after radiotherapy. *(Right)* Axial PET shows diffuse hypometabolism in the right frontal lobe ➡, compatible with post-radiotherapy changes, and mild FDG uptake ➡ in the right frontal tumor, compatible with residual low grade tumor.

Typical

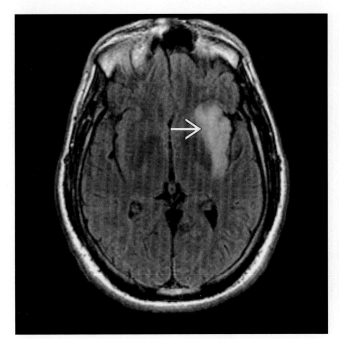
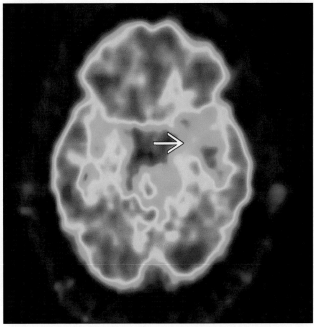

(Left) Axial FLAIR MR shows abnormal signal ➡ involving the insular cortex on the left in this patient with a WHO grade II glial lesion. Post-contrast images (not shown) revealed no abnormal enhancement in the area of signal abnormality. *(Right)* Axial PET shows relative hypometabolism on the left ➡, corresponding to the abnormal signal on the previous FLAIR MR image.

PRIMARY BRAIN NEOPLASMS

Typical

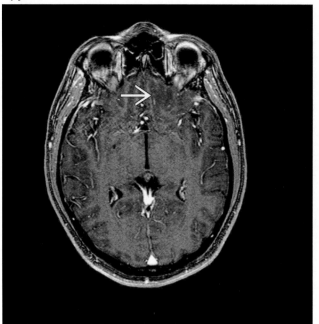 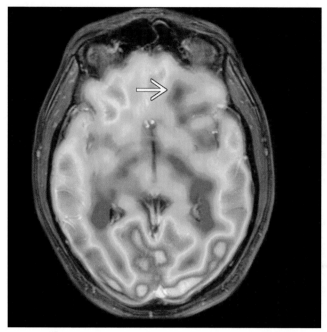

(Left) *Axial T1 C+ MR shows an area of low signal without abnormal enhancement* ➡ *in this patient with a low grade glioma being evaluated for radiation therapy planning.* *(Right)* *Axial fused PET/CT shows relative decreased hypometabolism in the left frontal lobe lesion* ➡*, a characteristic finding seen with lower grade gliomas.*

Typical

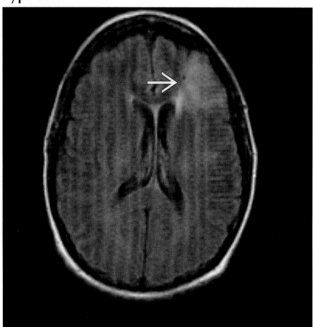 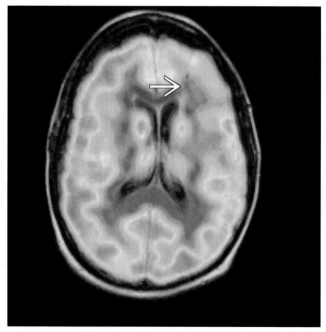

(Left) *Axial FLAIR MR shows abnormal signal in the left frontal lobe gray and white matter* ➡ *in this patient with a WHO grade II lesion. No abnormal enhancement was present on the post-contrast images.* *(Right)* *Axial fused PET/CT shows relative hypometabolism* ➡ *correlating with the lesion. This degree of FDG activity is compatible with a WHO grade II lesion.*

PRIMARY BRAIN NEOPLASMS

Typical

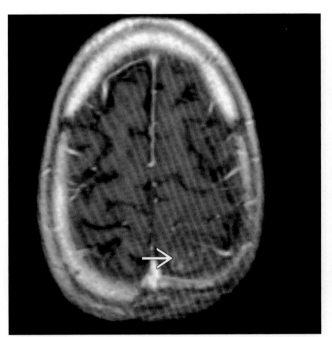
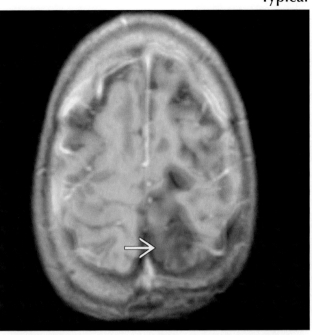

(Left) Axial T1 C+ MR shows minimal abnormal enhancement corresponding to a posterior left parietal lesion ➡ in this patient with a newly diagnosed WHO grade II glioma. *(Right)* Axial fused PET/MR shows relative hypometabolism that corresponds to the posterior left parietal lesion ➡, characteristic of a WHO grade II lesion.

Typical

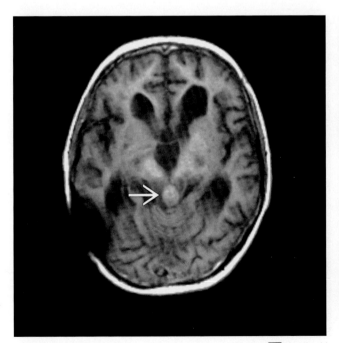
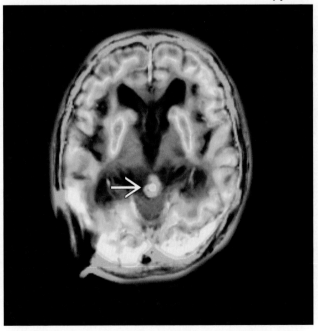

(Left) Axial T1WI MR shows a WHO grade I tectal lesion ➡ that had been stable for several years and showed no increased metabolic activity on the original PET scan. A follow-up PET scan was ordered due to new worsening clinical symptoms. *(Right)* Axial fused PET/MR shows a new focus of moderately increased FDG activity correlating to the center of the tectal mass ➡, suggestive of high grade transformation of this previously low grade glioma.

PRIMARY BRAIN NEOPLASMS

Typical

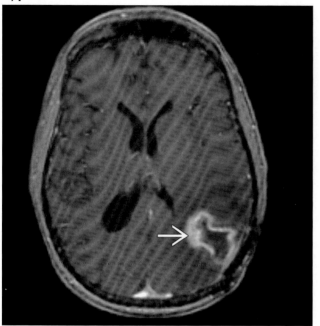 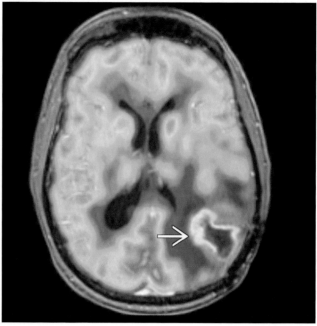

(Left) Axial T1 C+ MR in this patient with a history of prior glioblastoma status post resection and radiation shows extensive rim enhancement ➡, worrisome for possible recurrent tumor. *(Right)* Axial fused PET/MR shows no increased metabolic activity in the area of abnormal enhancement ➡, compatible with radiation necrosis. Both radiation necrosis and residual/recurrent tumor may have abnormal enhancement on MR, and PET can often be used to distinguish between the two diagnoses.

Typical

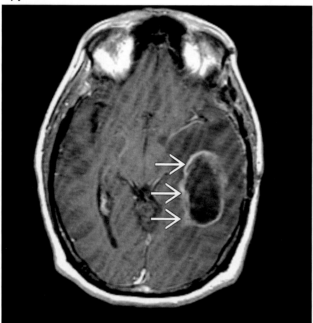 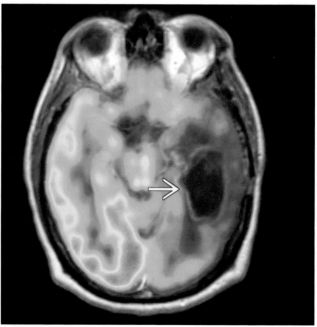

(Left) Axial T1 C+ MR was performed in this patient after resection and radiation therapy to a left temporal glioblastoma. The patient was referred for rim enhancement ➡, interpreted as either residual tumor or post-treatment changes. *(Right)* Axial fused PET/MR shows abnormal FDG activity correlating with the abnormal enhancement in the left temporal lobe post-surgical cavity ➡, compatible with post-treatment changes.

PRIMARY BRAIN NEOPLASMS

Typical

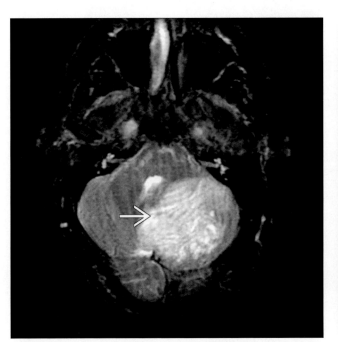
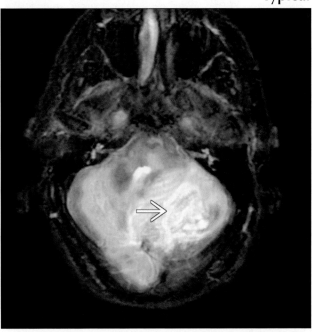

(Left) Axial FLAIR MR shows abnormal signal ➡ involving the majority of the left cerebellum. *(Right)* Axial fused PET/MR shows areas of focal intense FDG activity ➡ corresponding to the cerebellar mass. Biopsy showed cerebellar dysplastic gangliocytoma, a rare primary brain neoplasm.

Typical

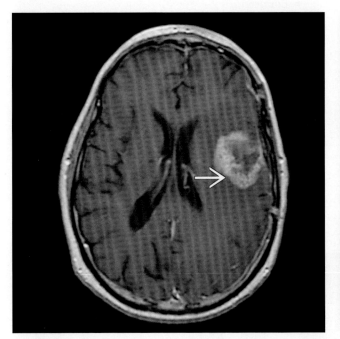
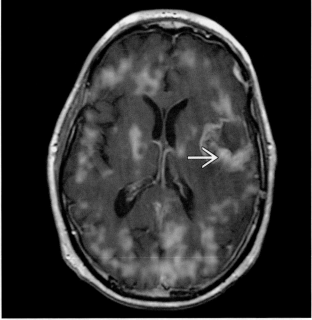

(Left) Axial T1 C+ MR shows ring enhancement with a thicker rind of enhancement more posteriorly ➡ in this patient with a history of glioblastoma multiforme status post radiation. *(Right)* Axial PET/MR with suboptimal coregistration shows focal areas of increased activity ➡ posteriorly along the radiation bed, compatible with residual/recurrent tumor.

BRAIN METASTASES

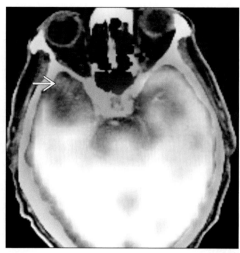

Axial fused PET/CT shows diffuse hypometabolism ➜ corresponding to the right temporal lobe.

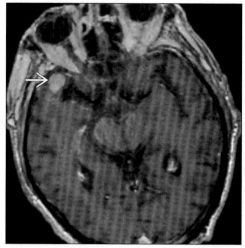

Axial T1 C+ MR shows an abnormally focal enhancing lesion in the right temporal lobe ➜, compatible with a metastatic lesion from lung cancer.

TERMINOLOGY

Abbreviations and Synonyms
- Central nervous system (CNS) metastases, brain metastases

Definitions
- Secondary tumors in brain or spinal cord originating from primary extracranial or CNS malignancy

IMAGING FINDINGS

General Features
- Best diagnostic clue: Focal hypermetabolic activity in the brain or spinal cord
- Location
  - **Classic**
    - Cerebral hemispheres (80%)
    - Cerebellum (15%)
    - Basal ganglia (3%)
  - **Less common**
    - Choroid plexus
    - Ventricular ependyma
    - Pituitary gland
    - Pineal gland
    - Leptomeninges
  - **Uncommon**
    - Diffusely infiltrating tumors (carcinomatous encephalitis)
    - Perivascular
    - Perineural
  - **Rare**
    - Brainstem
- Size: Microscopic to several cm
- Morphology
  - Usually discrete, spherical
  - Infiltrating
  - Along vascular or neural structures
- Number of lesions
  - One (50%)
  - Two (20%)
  - ≥ Three (30%)

Imaging Recommendations
- Best imaging tool
  - FDG PET
    - Improved resolution over SPECT

DDx: Enhancing Lesions on MR

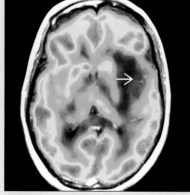

Low Grade Glioma

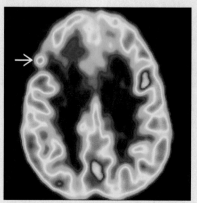

Glioblastoma Multiforme

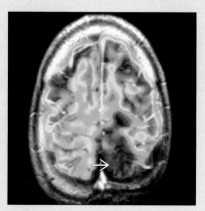

Radiation Necrosis

BRAIN METASTASES

Key Facts

Imaging Findings

- Focal hypermetabolic activity in the brain or spinal cord
- Can detect ≈ 1.5 cm metastases
- Cannot rule out small metastases with PET (C+ MR gold standard)
- Normal brain metabolism of FDG (glucose) can hide small metastases
- To increase sensitivity, re-window image to make normal brain activity less intense
- CECT
  ○ Ring enhancement
- FDG PET
  ○ Activity in CNS metastases depends on tumor histology

○ Sensitivity 79-82% specificity, 94% for detection of primary origin
○ Early studies showed 81-86% sensitivity and 40-94% specificity for distinguishing between radiation necrosis and tumor

Top Differential Diagnoses

- Abscess
  ○ Central hypometabolism signifies necrosis
- Cerebrovascular Accident
- Primary Brain Tumor
- Post-Treatment Effects

Diagnostic Checklist

- Cases have been described in which primary lung tumors showed hypermetabolic foci, but brain lesions are photopenic

---

  ■ Can detect ≈ 1.5 cm metastases
  ■ Cannot rule out small metastases with PET (C+ MR gold standard)
- Protocol advice
  ○ Normal brain metabolism of FDG (glucose) can hide small metastases
  ○ To increase sensitivity, re-window image to make normal brain activity less intense
  ○ Review 3D and tomographic images
  ○ Glucose loading can enhance detection of brain tumors, with 27% increase in FDG uptake ratio of tumor to normal gray matter
    ■ Difficult to perform clinically; requires IV glucose infusion and blood glucose monitoring
    ■ 10% glucose 50 mL for 5 minutes IV
  ○ FDG imaging 3-8 hours after injection can improve distinction between tumor and normal gray matter

CT Findings

- NECT
  ○ Iso- or hypodense mass
  ○ Peritumoral edema: None to striking
  ○ Intracranial hemorrhage (ICH) variable
    ■ Mets may cause "spontaneous" ICH in elderly
- CECT
  ○ Enhancement patterns
    ■ Intense
    ■ Punctate
    ■ Nodular
    ■ Ring enhancement
- Metastases frequently multiple, seen at the junction of gray and white matter; usually with significant surrounding edema
  ○ On noncontrast CT, metastatic lesions may be of a density less than, equal to, or greater than adjacent brain parenchyma
    ■ Most of the patterns are variable and nondiagnostic
  ○ Noncontrast CT is performed to detect hemorrhage into metastases
    ■ Hyperdensity in a metastasis is more likely to be hemorrhage than calcification

○ Most metastases enhance after a standard dose of IV contrast
○ Detecting additional metastases has important diagnostic implications
  ■ If a solitary lesion is found on routine enhanced CT, an additional lesion may suggest a metastatic process
  ■ Particularly true in a patient with no known primary cancer (if the solitary lesion was believed to be a primary lesion)
  ■ Detection of an additional lesion may modify or change treatment
- Contrast-enhanced CT is effective in detecting major leptomeningeal spread
  ○ Contrast-enhancing subdural or epidural metastases may be seen, usually secondary to calvarial lesions
  ○ Of breast, lung, prostate, and renal cell neoplasms, 5% metastasize to the calvarium and 15% of these extend into the subdural space
- Multiple enhancing solid lesions at the gray-white matter junction and prominent surrounding edema
  ○ Can be diagnosed confidently as metastases in a patient with known primary cancer
- ≈ 90% of patients with a history of cancer who present with a single supratentorial lesion have brain metastases
- Patients with multiple lesions are even more likely to have metastatic disease
  ○ Prior to definitive therapy, patients with a single metastasis by contrast-enhanced CT should undergo a contrasted MR examination
- Contrast-enhanced CT is useful and perhaps the best method to identify calvarial metastases
  ○ ≈ 20% of patients who demonstrate a single lesion on contrast-enhanced CT may demonstrate multiple lesions on contrast-enhanced MR
  ○ Lesions missed on CECT are mostly smaller (< 2 cm in diameter), located next to the bone, & in a frontotemporal location
  ○ Dural-based metastases may mimic meningioma

BRAIN METASTASES

Nuclear Medicine Findings

- **PET**
  - FDG PET
    - Activity in CNS metastases depends on tumor histology
    - Classically hypermetabolic on FDG PET: Lung, breast, colorectal, head and neck, melanoma, thyroid
    - Classically hypometabolic on FDG PET: Mucinous adenocarcinoma, renal cell carcinoma
    - Variable uptake on FDG PET: Gliomas, lymphoma
    - Central hypometabolism suggests necrosis
  - 18-F choline allows differentiation among benign lesions, metastatic tumors, and high grade glial tumors
    - Metastatic lesions generally show significantly higher fluorocholine uptake than high grade gliomas
- FDG PET sensitivity 79-82%, specificity 94% for detecting origin of primary
- FDG PET detected few primaries not already detected in standard workup, including CXR or chest CT
  - Primary benefit: Detection of nodal involvement and extent of metastases to other regions for staging and therapeutic decisions
- Uptake in low grade tumors is usually similar to normal white matter
- In area of interest, any FDG uptake higher than expected background level in adjacent brain tissue should be considered recurrent tumor
  - Even if it is same or less than cortical uptake
- Early studies showed 81-86% sensitivity and 40-94% specificity for distinguishing between radiation necrosis and tumor
  - Recurring tumor can occur along same time lines as necrosis
  - Optimal time for performing FDG PET after radiotherapy is not known
    - For purpose of evaluating tumor growth, at least 6 weeks should elapse prior to imaging
- Discovery of extrathoracic metastases is contraindication for surgery except in specialized circumstances
  - e.g., solitary brain metastasis
- Unsuspected brain metastases in patients with non-CNS cancer found in only 0.4% of patients who had already been worked up w/conventional imaging
- Cytotoxic edema that frequently surrounds metastatic deposits shows relatively low FDG accumulation
  - May decrease conspicuity of lesions through volume-average effects
- **SPECT**
  - Tl-201, Tc-99m sestamibi, Tc-99m tetrofosmin
  - Focal increased activity suggests metastasis

DIFFERENTIAL DIAGNOSIS

Abscess
- Usually hypermetabolic
- Central hypometabolism signifies necrosis

Cerebrovascular Accident
- Hyper- or hypometabolic

Primary Brain Tumor
- Anaplastic astrocytoma/oligodendroglioma, glioblastoma multiforme (GBM)
- Lymphoma

Meningioma
- Hypometabolic

Post-Treatment Effects
- Hypermetabolic activity in the acute period (surgery, radiotherapy)
- Hypometabolic regions correspond to treated tumor
- Necrosis from stereotactic radiotherapy may mimic tumor recurrence several months post treatment

Epilepsy
- Seizure activity after FDG injection can cause focal hypermetabolic activity

PATHOLOGY

General Features
- Etiology
  - Hematogenous spread
    - Most common primary tumors are lung, colorectal, melanoma, and breast
    - Receptor-mediated attachment of circulating tumor cells in CNS
    - 10% unknown source
  - Local extension
    - Extension to dura from calvarium
    - Through skull base or via foramina, fissures
    - Perineural
    - Perivascular
    - Cerebrospinal fluid
  - Regional metastasis from CNS primary (e.g., GBM, lymphoma)
- Epidemiology
  - Patients with CNS metastases diagnosed annually in USA: 100,000-500,000
  - Metastases account for ≈ 50% of cerebral tumors
  - 20-40% of patients with systemic cancer have brain metastases; incidence is increasing
  - Primary remains undiscovered in 16-35% of patients with metastatic brain tumors presenting with CNS symptoms
  - Approximately 80% of primary tumors are lung cancer
  - More than 100,000 people per year die with intracranial metastases
  - Frequency of brain mets with NSCLC at time of diagnosis is 10%
- Associated abnormalities
  - Extracranial metastases
    - 90% of patients with CNS metastases have metastases in other organs

Gross Pathologic & Surgical Features
- Round, confluent tan or gray-white mass

BRAIN METASTASES

- Edema
- Local mass effect
- Hemorrhage (common in melanoma, choriocarcinoma, lung and renal cell carcinomas)

Microscopic Features
- Usually similar to primary
- Usually displaces brain parenchyma
- Necrosis common
- Neovascularity common
- Marked mitotic figures

CLINICAL ISSUES

Presentation
- Most common signs/symptoms
  - Neurological
    - Headache
    - Seizure
    - Mental status changes: Confusion, obtundation
    - Ataxia
    - Nausea and vomiting
    - Vision problems
    - Papilledema
  - 10% of patients with CNS metastases asymptomatic

Demographics
- Age
  - Incidence increases with age
    - Rare in children (skull/dura more common site than parenchyma)
    - Peak prevalence over 65 years
- Gender: Slight male predominance

Natural History & Prognosis
- Progressive increase in size and number of metastases
- No treatment: ~ 1 month survival
- With treatment: Median survival improved but < 1 year
- Significant differences in survival times among different primary tumors
- Most patients with brain metastases die from systemic disease

Treatment
- Medical management
  - Corticosteroids: Diminish effects of edema
  - Anticonvulsants: Seizure prophylaxis
  - Hyperosmolar agents: Decrease intracranial pressure
- Whole brain external beam radiotherapy
  - Traditional treatment due to high frequency of multiple lesions
  - Prolong survival, improve neurological function
  - Improved survival when surgery also performed
- Stereotactic radiotherapy (masses < 3 cm)
  - Prolong survival, minimally invasive, symptom palliation slower than with surgery
  - Necrosis: Complication that may occur several months later and mimic tumor recurrence
- Surgical resection
  - Indicated in patients with relatively good performance status or large solitary lesions with significant mass effect
  - Prolong survival, symptom palliation, histopathologic tissue sample

DIAGNOSTIC CHECKLIST

Consider
- Cases have been described in which primary lung tumors showed hypermetabolic foci but brain lesions were photopenic
  - Possibly due to mucin producing nature or necrosis

SELECTED REFERENCES

1. Bading JR et al: Imaging of cell proliferation: status and prospects. J Nucl Med. 49 Suppl 2:64S-80S, 2008
2. Kosaka N et al: 18F-FDG PET of common enhancing malignant brain tumors. AJR Am J Roentgenol. 190(6):W365-9, 2008
3. Lee HY et al: Comparison of FDG-PET findings of brain metastasis from non-small-cell lung cancer and small-cell lung cancer. Ann Nucl Med. 22(4):281-6, 2008
4. Liu Y: Metastatic brain lesions may demonstrate photopenia on FDG-PET. Clin Nucl Med. 33(4):255-7, 2008
5. Terakawa Y et al: Diagnostic accuracy of 11C-methionine PET for differentiation of recurrent brain tumors from radiation necrosis after radiotherapy. J Nucl Med. 49(5):694-9, 2008
6. Bedre G et al: Cerebellar, pancreatic, and paraspinal metastases in soft tissue sarcomas: unusual sites or changing patterns? JOP. 8(4):444-9, 2007
7. Orts Giménez D et al: Positron emission tomography: a false negative result in cystic encephalic metastases from a small cell bronchial carcinoma. Clin Transl Oncol. 8(8):618-20, 2006
8. Chernov M et al: Differentiation of the radiation-induced necrosis and tumor recurrence after gamma knife radiosurgery for brain metastases: importance of multi-voxel proton MRS. Minim Invasive Neurosurg. 48(4):228-34, 2005
9. Ghosh L et al: Management of patients with metastatic cancer of unknown primary. Curr Probl Surg. 42(1):12-66, 2005
10. Young RJ et al: Neuroimaging of metastatic brain disease. Neurosurgery. 57(5 Suppl):S10-23; discusssion S1-4, 2005
11. Lippitz BE et al: Gamma knife radiosurgery for patients with multiple cerebral metastases. Acta Neurochir Suppl. 91:79-87, 2004
12. Pirotte B et al: Combined use of 18F-fluorodeoxyglucose and 11C-methionine in 45 positron emission tomography-guided stereotactic brain biopsies. J Neurosurg. 101(3):476-83, 2004
13. Ludwig V et al: Cerebral lesions incidentally detected on 2-deoxy-2-[18F]fluoro-D-glucose positron emission tomography images of patients evaluated for body malignancies. Mol Imaging Biol. 4(5):359-62, 2002

BRAIN METASTASES

Typical

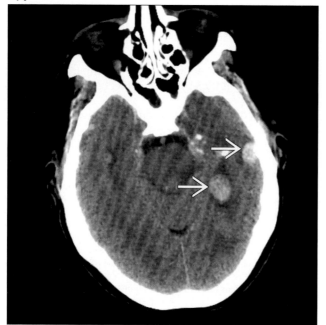 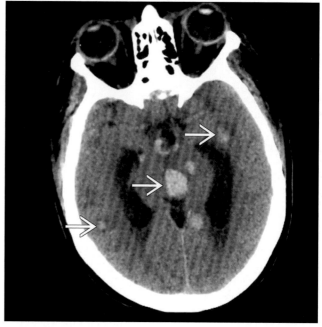

(Left) Axial NECT shows multiple hyperdense metastatic brain lesions ➔, compatible with the patient's known history of metastatic melanoma. *(Right)* Axial CECT shows extensive hyperdense metastatic brain lesions ➔ in this patient with a history of melanoma.

Typical

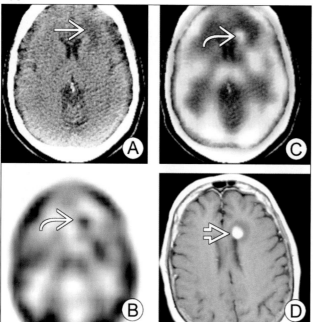 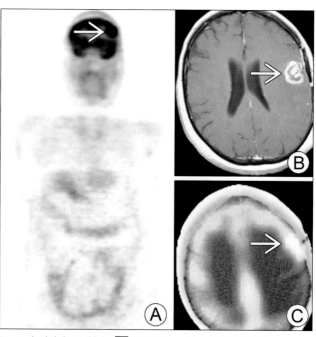

(Left) In a patient with lung cancer, NECT (A) shows a low attenuation lesion in the left frontal lobe ➔, PET (B) and fused PET/CT (C) demonstrates focal intense activity ➔, and post-contrast T1WI MR (D) shows the enhancing lesion ➔, compatible with metastatic disease. *(Right)* Coronal PET (A), axial T1 MR (B) and fused PET/CT (C) show a metastatic lesion in the left frontal lobe ➔ from melanoma. Melanoma metastases are almost always FDG avid.

BRAIN METASTASES

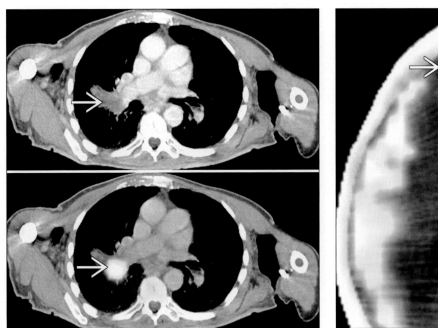
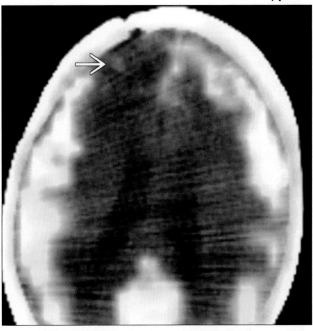

(Left) Axial CT (top) and fused PET/CT (bottom) demonstrate focal intense activity ➡ that corresponds with a mass in the right lung, compatible with primary squamous cell carcinoma of the lung. *(Right)* Axial fused PET/CT shows hypometabolism in the right frontal lobe ➡, correlating with a metastatic lesion from a primary lung carcinoma.

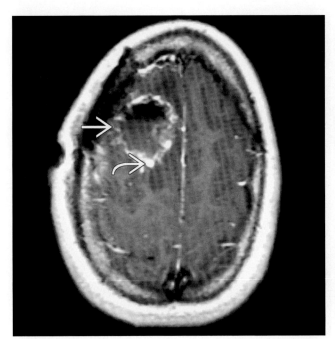
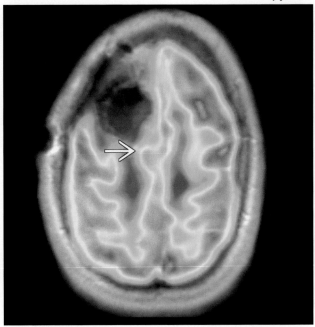

(Left) Axial T1 C+ MR shows a resection bed from a metastatic lesion ➡ with a small focus of enhancement posteriorly ➢ compared to the nonenhanced axial T1WI MR image (not shown). *(Right)* Axial fused PET/MR image shows focal intense FDG activity correlating with the area of enhancement ➡, compatible with residual/recurrent tumor.

BRAIN METASTASES

Typical

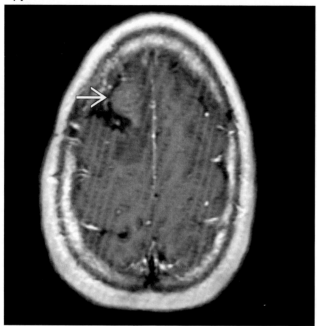 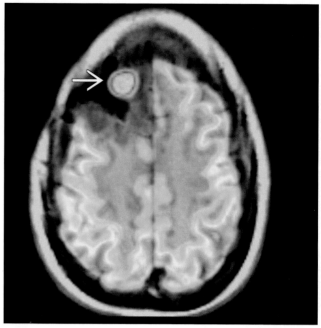

(Left) Axial T1WI MR shows a new nodular area medially in a resection bed ➡ status post resection for a metastatic lesion and worrisome for residual/recurrent tumor. *(Right)* Axial fused PET/MR shows focal intense FDG activity correlating with the nodular area medially ➡, compatible with residual/recurrent malignancy.

Typical

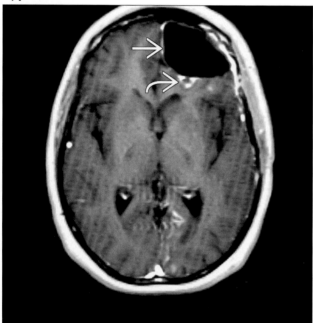 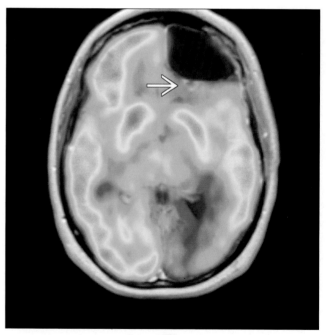

(Left) Axial T1 C+ MR shows expected post-operative appearance of a resection cavity in the left frontal area ➡ after resection of a metastatic lesion with a new subtle area of enhancement posteriorly ➡. *(Right)* Axial fused PET/MR shows no increased activity correlating with the abnormal area of enhancement ➡, suggesting post-operative changes. Continued follow-up is warranted, since a small percentage of metastatic lesions may not be FDG avid in the brain.

BRAIN METASTASES

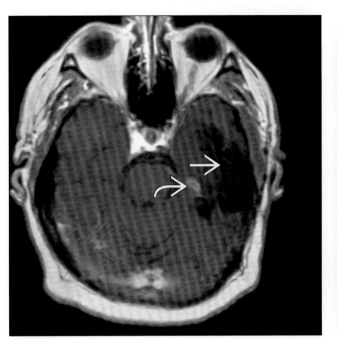 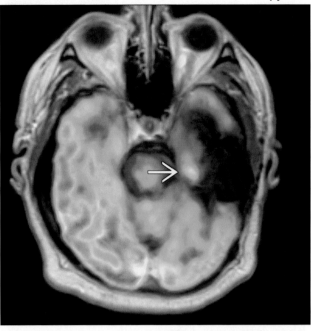

(Left) Axial T1 C+ MR shows expected appearance after resection of a metastatic lesion in the left temporal lobe ➡. A new area of enhancement is noted medially ➡, suggestive of tumor recurrence. *(Right)* Axial fused PET/MR demonstrates focal moderately increased FDG activity immediately correlating with the area of abnormal enhancement ➡, compatible with recurrent malignancy.

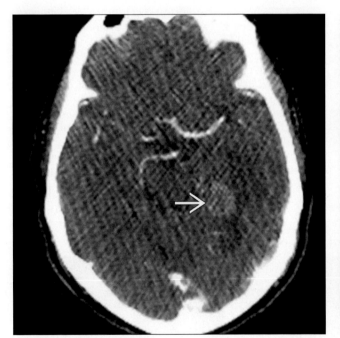 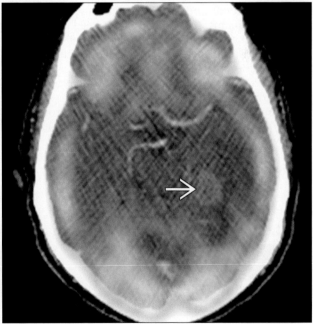

(Left) Axial CECT shows an enhancing mass in the medial aspect of the left temporal lobe ➡ in this patient with lung cancer. *(Right)* Axial fused PET/CT shows minimal background activity ➡ in the enhancing lesion shown on the previous image. Overall, up to 20% of brain metastases may be hypometabolic, despite having hypermetabolic primary lesions.

HEAD AND NECK CANCER, SQUAMOUS

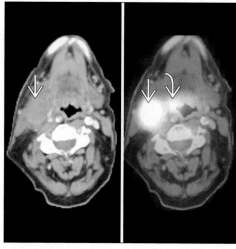

Axial CT (left) and fused PET/CT (right) show a right parapharyngeal space mass ➡ and a mucosal lesion only identified on the fused PET/CT ➘.

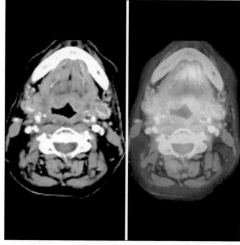

Follow-up axial CT (left) and fused PET/CT (right) after surgery demonstrate no residual or recurrent tumor.

TERMINOLOGY

Abbreviations and Synonyms
- Squamous cell carcinoma of the head and neck (SCCHN)
- Squamous cell carcinoma (SCCA) nodes
- Unknown mucosal primary
- Therapeutic assessment/restaging

Definitions
- Primary, regional, and distant malignancy from tumors of squamous cell origin in the head and neck
- Primary unknown: Metastatic squamous cell carcinoma of the neck without an identifiable mucosal primary lesion
  - Undetectable mucosal lesions by clinical exam or
  - Negative anatomical imaging
- Head and neck cancers include those arising from the lip, oral cavity, nasal cavity, paranasal sinuses, pharynx, and larynx
  - 90-95% are squamous cell carcinomas arising from mucosal linings of upper aerodigestive tract

IMAGING FINDINGS

General Features
- Best diagnostic clue
  - Intensely FDG-avid nodes in the neck on PET or PET/CT
  - Enlarged or necrotic lymph nodes in the neck ± enhancement on CT
  - Primary unknown
    - PET shows asymmetrical focal fluorodeoxyglucose (FDG) uptake, with or without an identifiable abnormality on CT
    - Sensitivity for PET and PET/CT is 26-43% in cases where primary has eluded diagnosis
    - Fused PET/CT images often helpful for determining whether potential FDG abnormalities are mucosal lesions
    - Helpful for directing clinicians to areas for directed biopsies
  - Intense FDG activity in or around treated primary tumor with corresponding CT evidence of residual tumor
- Location

DDx: Asymmetrical FDG Activity in a Patient with Newly Diagnosed SCCHN

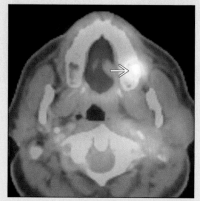

Dental Abscess

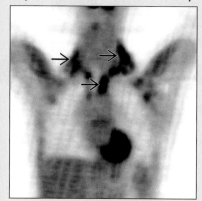

Muscle/Brown Fat

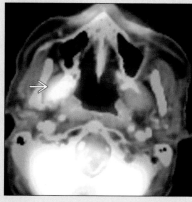

Muscle

HEAD AND NECK CANCER, SQUAMOUS

Key Facts

Terminology
- Squamous cell carcinoma of the head and neck (SCCHN), squamous cell carcinoma (SCCA) nodes

Imaging Findings
- Intensely FDG-avid nodes in the neck on PET or PET/CT
- Enlarged or necrotic lymph nodes in the neck ± enhancement on CT
- PET/CT key for several clinical scenarios
  - Delineate extent of regional lymph node involvement
  - Detect distant metastases
  - Identify unknown primary tumor
  - Detect occasional synchronous primary

- Combined PET/CT may offer additional localization information and improve interpreting physician's confidence level
- Overall sensitivity and specificity of FDG PET and PET/CT > 90%; PET/CT sensitivity 96% and specificity 98%

Top Differential Diagnoses
- Abscess or Suppurative Nodes
- Lymphoma
- Physiologic Activity
- Reactive Nodes

Diagnostic Checklist
- Consider PET/CT in patients with primary tumors that are prone to bilateral metastases, which are often less conspicuous on conventional imaging

---

- Primary squamous cell lesions may involve any mucosal surface
  - Commonly involve the base of tongue, tonsils, or adenoids
  - Mucosal surfaces of the oropharynx, nasopharynx, and hypopharynx
- Lymph node metastases involve neck nodes in expected drainage pattern based on primary tumor
- SCCHN has high propensity to harbor malignancy in small lymph nodes
- Most common metastatic sites: Lung, liver, skeletal system
- Size
  - Early primary SCCHN may be undetectable (unknown primary SCCHN)
  - Lymph node metastases may range in size from normal (< 1 cm) to several centimeters
- Morphology
  - Mass effect, abnormal enhancement, or necrosis may exist in larger tumors
  - Fatty lymph node hilum usually denotes benign lesion on CT (may be positive on PET if occult malignancy present)
  - Indistinct borders usually denote extranodal spread

Imaging Recommendations
- Best imaging tool
  - PET/CT key for several clinical scenarios
    - Delineate extent of regional lymph node involvement
    - Detect distant metastases
    - Further evaluate potentially abnormal findings on another exam, such as mediastinal adenopathy detected by chest CT
    - Identify unknown primary tumor
    - Detect occasional synchronous primary
    - Monitor treatment response to select appropriate patients for salvage surgery
    - Conduct long-term surveillance for recurrence and metastases
    - Check any patient who presents with clinical evidence of recurrent disease

- TNM staging
  - MR better than CT for specific questions such as presence of perineural spread or invasion of bone marrow
- N stage
  - CT generally superior to MR for detection of regional lymph node metastases
- M stage
  - Only patients at substantial risk of nodal or hematogenous metastases, T3 or T4, should undergo routine PET/CT for staging
- Combined PET/CT may offer additional localization information and improve interpreting physician's confidence level
  - Overall sensitivity and specificity of FDG PET and PET/CT > 90%; PET/CT sensitivity 96% and specificity 98%
  - PET/CT more helpful for radiation therapy planning; can lead to changes in gross tumor volume
  - Extended field FDG PET staging may detect disease outside of the head and neck in up to 21% of patients with head and neck cancer
  - Sensitivity for PET and PET/CT 26-43% in which primary has eluded diagnosis
  - Sensitivity for PET/CT better for accurate localization of lesion and directed biopsy recommendations
- MR typically initial imaging study of choice for staging
  - Compared to noncontrast PET/CT, more accurate delineation of tumor extent, perineural involvement, and intracranial extent
  - Nearly comparable in accuracy in detecting regional LN metastases
- Contrast-enhanced CT used only in laryngeal cancer; PET/CECT may be better for this indication than MR or CECT alone
- Restaging: Combined PET/CT is more sensitive and specific than CT alone
- Protocol advice

HEAD AND NECK CANCER, SQUAMOUS

- o High resolution PET/CT from top of head to carina using standard head and neck protocol (especially for unknown primary)
- o Scan with arms down on PET/CT to avoid beam hardening artifact
  - Whole-body scan performed with arms above head and shorter acquisition time
  - Use neck immobilization device
- o Scan in mask for radiation planning PET/CT
  - Display images with PET intensity kept low-moderate (avoid "blooming")
- o Pre-treatment with benzodiazepines in patients with excessive muscular FDG uptake on FDG PET
- o Warm patients before and after injection of FDG to reduce brown fat FDG uptake
- o Restaging
  - Scan with arms down, CECT, and neck immobilization device
  - Consider dual-time point imaging to help differentiate between inflammatory and neoplastic FDG activity

CT Findings

- **CECT**: Early enhancement, rim enhancement, central necrosis, indistinct borders
- Post-therapy neck difficult to interpret
  - o Accuracy of CT ranges from 50-70%
  - o Loss of fat planes and extensive post-surgical changes reduce the specificity of CT
  - o Distortion of normal anatomy can be due to bony-cartilaginous necrosis, edema, and desmoplastic changes
  - o CT may show enhancement, necrosis, or mass effect with residual/recurrent tumor
  - o Best method of detection using CECT is serial examination
- CT and MR may be negative for unknown primary if
  - o Tumor is subtle or difficult to separate from adjacent normal structures (as with lingual tonsillar tissue)
  - o Primary is superficial or very small
  - o Scan is limited by motion or streak artifact
- Abnormal size criteria for CT: ≥ 1 cm for most nodes; ≥ 1.5 cm for level I-II nodes; ≥ 8 mm for retropharyngeal nodes
  - o FDG PET can detect smaller positive nodes (limited by spatial resolution)
- Central necrosis specific for malignancy, but it is a late marker of metastatic adenopathy
  - o Usually seen only in nodes ≥ 20 mm, which is beyond the typical cutoff of 10 mm for suspicion of malignancy
- Contrast enhancement generally improves detection of malignancy
- Round morphology more suspicious than reniform

Nuclear Medicine Findings

- PET/CT is more accurate than PET and CT separately; PET is more accurate than CT alone
  - o FDG PET sensitivity and specificity for residual disease 90% and 83%, respectively
  - o PET/CT sensitivity, specificity, and accuracy 98%, 92%, and 94%, respectively

- o PET/CT decreases number of equivocal lesions by ~ 50% and provides improved biopsy localization information
- o 74% better localization with PET/CT compared to PET in regions previously treated; 58% for untreated regions
- **Initial diagnosis**
  - o Squamous cell carcinoma almost always FDG avid
  - o Look for primary lesion along the mucosal surfaces
  - o Unknown primary: FDG PET typically shows focal asymmetrical FDG uptake in the mucosal primary
    - 5-10% of cases involve primary that cannot be found by physical exam, panendoscopy, or conventional radiographic imaging
    - PET/CT has been shown to find primary in 40% of patients whose primary was not identified in office or with surgical panendoscopy
    - False negatives with PET/CT means that this modality is a supplement to, but not a substitute for, endoscopy and biopsy with unknown primary
  - o FDG PET shows no advantage over traditional techniques for identification and characterization of primary head/neck tumors for stage I/II lesions
    - Rarely adds information regarding initial T staging of primary
    - Exception is unknown primary
- **Staging**
  - o Screening for distant metastases advised for patients who have
    - Four or more lymph node metastases
    - Bilateral positive nodes
    - Nodes greater than 6 cm
    - Zone 4 nodes
    - Recurrent SCCHN
    - Second primary tumor
  - o In one study, 24% of patients newly diagnosed with SCCA of the oral cavity had distant metastases picked up by PET/CT
    - However, PET/CT cannot preclude neck dissection in patients with advanced primaries but clinically node-negative necks
  - o PET/CT may alter TNM score in 30-35% of patients by identifying nodal disease not apparent on CT, MR, or clinical exam
  - o PET/CT has advantage in identifying distant disease because it can detect occult metastatic disease (e.g., subtle bone metastases)
    - Present in as many as 10% of patients with advanced local-regional disease
  - o PET may alter treatment in many patients, decreasing toxic wide-field radiotherapy
  - o Unclear whether PET/CT useful in identification of nodal metastases in patients with SCCHN and N0 necks on exam
  - o Stage III/IV patients have high risk of distant metastases, creating a greater role for FDG PET
    - PET has a distinct advantage over CT/bronchoscopy, especially in the lung
  - o Target volumes for IMRT and stereotactic radiosurgery may be modified in as many as 20% of cases with PET/CT vs. CT alone

HEAD AND NECK CANCER, SQUAMOUS

- PET/CT used primarily to include normal-sized lymph nodes with increased metabolic activity as part of high dose target volume
- Helpful for contouring primary tumors whose borders are difficult to distinguish by anatomic imaging alone, as with some tongue-based tumors
  - PET/CT limited in staging local lymph node involvement if patient's disease is clinically stage N0 after physical examination and anatomic imaging
    - Due to limited spatial resolution
    - Selective neck dissection or sentinal lymph node biopsy is more definitive
    - However, even in stage N0 disease PET/CT may be useful
    - Serves as a baseline to differentiate incidental physiologic FDG-avid foci from malignant foci on subsequent post-treatment exams
    - Otherwise a significant interpretive challenge if comparison images are not available
- **Restaging**
  - Following surgery, no detectable tumor should be present
    - Variable amounts of post-surgical change expected
  - Post-surgery: Usually wait 4-6 weeks after to reevaluate with PET and PET/CT to avoid false positive studies due to inflammation
    - Reevaluation following surgery may be particularly helpful in cases where surgical margins are positive
  - Post-radiation
    - Positive PET one month after XRT has a positive predictive value of ~ 100%
    - Negative PET one month after XRT has a lower negative predictive value (14%) early; fewer false negatives with longer follow-up period
- **Response to therapy**
  - Following chemoradiation, metabolic response may precede reductions in tumor volume
  - Post-chemotherapy (approximately 1 month after completion): Sensitivity and specificity of FDG PET 90% and 83%
    - Little data evaluating early response to chemotherapy
    - Inflammatory changes seen with radiotherapy are not seen, and PET can be performed at earlier time point, such as 4-8 weeks
  - Post-chemoradiation
    - PET/CT has high negative predictive value and allows confident exclusion of residual cancer, thereby deferring planned neck dissection
  - Pitfalls and limitations
    - Several structures in the neck with variable physiologic FDG activity
    - Common muscles with asymmetrical FDG activity: Pterygoids, sternocleidomastoid, strap muscles, and mylohyoid
    - Glands: Salivary glands (submandibular and parotid); can have intense FDG activity following some chemo regimens
    - Lymphoid tissue: Lingual tonsils, palatine tonsils, and adenoids (Waldeyer ring)

- Brown fat: Can be symmetrical or asymmetrical, can be focal anywhere in the neck
- FDG PET may not detect small areas of residual/ recurrent disease, leading to early false negative exams after therapy
- PET frequently fails to identify hypermetabolism in areas of marrow space infiltration and perineural extension
- Cartilage necrosis may be FDG avid indefinitely
- Cricoarytenoids typically FDG avid and often asymmetric

DIFFERENTIAL DIAGNOSIS

Metastatic Disease from Thyroid or Melanoma
- May look identical to squamous cell carcinoma

Abscess or Suppurative Nodes
- Usually has central necrosis; identical in appearance to necrotic lymph node
- FDG PET not helpful for differentiation; biopsy required
- Often indistinguishable from tumor; correlate clinically

Lymphoma
- Difficult to differentiate from SCCHN based on imaging; associated mucosal lesion favors SCCHN
- NHL: May mimic tonsillar inflammatory disease

Residual/Recurrent Malignancy
- Often indistinguishable from abscess/inflammation
- Short-term serial evaluation very helpful
- CT may show asymmetrical mass effect

Radiation-Induced Inflammation
- FDG uptake from inflammation usually present for 4-8 weeks following therapy
- Osteoradionecrosis can cause false positive early (before frank necrosis causes negative PET)
- Dual-time point PET imaging at 1 hour and 3 hour post FDG injection may be helpful in differentiating tumor vs. inflammation
  - FDG uptake from 1-3 hours: Tumor may increase; inflammation may plateau or decrease

Physiologic Activity
- Benign tonsil FDG uptake typically will be symmetrical but can be intense
- Muscle activity may be focal and asymmetrical
  - Correlate PET with CT; pre-treatment with benzodiazepines may reduce muscle uptake
- Measure Hounsfield units (HU); -50 to -150 compatible with brown fat
  - Warm patient before FDG injection to reduce brown fat uptake of FDG

Reactive Nodes
- Tend to be normal to minimally enlarged, symmetrical, low level FDG uptake
- May be associated with diffuse tonsillar uptake if recent upper respiratory or viral infection

HEAD AND NECK CANCER, SQUAMOUS

- Careful history for recent upper respiratory infection is advisable

PATHOLOGY

General Features
- General path comments
  - Nodal level classification scheme
  - American Joint Committee on Cancer (AJCC) and American Academy of Otolaryngology-Head and Neck Surgery (AAO-HNS)
    - Level IA: Submental nodes between anterior digastrics
    - Level IB: Submandibular, lateral to IA anterior to the posterior margin of submandibular gland (SMG)
    - Level IIA: Upper internal jugular nodes; anterior, lateral, or posterior and touching the jugular vein
    - Level IIB: Posterior, not touching jugular
    - Level III: Mid-internal jugular nodes, extend from inferior hyoid to cricoid arch
    - Level IV: Low internal jugular nodes, extend from cricoid arch to the level of the clavicle
    - Level V: Spinal accessory group, nodes in the posterior triangle; level VA: Above cricoid; level VB: Below inferior cricoid border
    - Level VI: Upper visceral nodes; between the carotid arteries from bottom of the hyoid to the top of the manubrium
    - Level VII: Superior mediastinal nodes; between the carotid arteries from below the top of the manubrium above the innominate vein
    - Supraclavicular nodes: At or caudal to the level of the clavicle and lateral to the carotid artery
    - Retropharyngeal nodes: Within 2 cm of the skull base medial to the carotid arteries
    - Parotid: Nodes within the parotid gland
  - Initial workup with physical exam, office endoscopy, and MR/CT
    - If definitive for nodal disease, PET/CT is appropriate for accurate evaluation of nodal metastases
    - Suggestive PET/CT findings should prompt fine needle aspiration (FNA)
    - If FNA is negative, definitive treatment is pursued and PET/CT is optional, to serve as baseline prior to therapy
  - If a focus of unknown primary is suspected on metabolic imaging
    - Panendoscopy and frozen section biopsy
    - Panendoscopy includes oropharynx, hypopharynx, nasopharynx, larynx, and upper esophagus
  - If negative, further biopsy specimens may be obtained from most common sites for primary tumors
    - Base of tongue
    - Nasopharynx
    - Contralateral tonsillar fossa
    - Pyriform sinus
    - Ipsilateral tonsillar fossa
  - Reassessment

- Biopsy areas that appear suspicious on PET or PET/CT
- Alternatively, short-term interval follow-up PET or PET/CT
- Etiology: Smoking, chewing tobacco, alcohol abuse
- Epidemiology
  - SCCHN newly diagnosed in 40,000 patients annually in United States
  - Mortality is 23%
  - Average 5 year survival 56%
- Associated abnormalities: Risk factors also predispose to esophageal and lung cancer

Staging, Grading, or Classification Criteria
- T stage: Assessment requires knowledge of size of primary lesions, depth of invasion, and involvement of surrounding structures
- N stage: AJCC characteristics include number of nodes involved, size of nodes, location (laterality and level), and morphology
- Staging of SCCHN requires
  - Complete history and physical
  - Histologic confirmation
  - Characterization of primary
  - Recognition of local/regional nodal disease
  - Identification of distant metastatic disease

CLINICAL ISSUES

Presentation
- Most common signs/symptoms
  - May present with pain associated with primary mass or neck mass
  - Symptoms of residual/recurrent tumor overlap with post-treatment complications; pain is most common
- Other signs/symptoms: Mass on clinical exam

Demographics
- Age: Generally > 40-45 years
- Gender: M > F

Natural History & Prognosis
- Nodal metastasis is most accurate prognostic factor for SCCHN
  - Unilateral nodal involvement indicates 50% reduction in expected lifespan; bilateral nodal involvement indicates 75% reduction
  - 10 year survival drops from 85% to 10-40% in patients with positive nodes
  - Carotid artery involvement or encasement portends dismal prognosis with 100% mortality
  - Majority of patients do not have metastatic disease within cervical nodes at presentation
    - 20% risk of occult metastasis in patients with clinically node-negative necks
- 10-15% of patients with SCCHN will present with distant metastases
- Unknown primary
  - PET and PET/CT can help direct biopsy
  - 2-9% of SCCHN patients present with cervical lymph node metastases without clear evidence of primary site

HEAD AND NECK CANCER, SQUAMOUS

- If imaging is negative, patients are usually followed with serial imaging evaluation
- FDG PET has prognostic implications for SCCHN
  - SUV > 9 = poorer prognosis for initial staging (22% three year survival vs. 73% for SUV ≤ 9)
  - In one study, reevaluation with FDG PET in the early phase of treatment was associated with tumor response, survival, and local control
- Most recurrence appears within 24 months of initial definitive therapy
  - PET should be performed no sooner than 2-3 months after surgery ± chemoradiation to decrease false positives
  - Recurrence rates as high as 50% with advanced stage SCCA
  - Primary SCCHN patients are more likely than any other group of cancer patients to develop second primary
    - Due to widespread toxic effects from tobacco and alcohol
- In most patients, distant metastases will be clinically silent
- SUV has potential to predict malignant potential and outcome in patients with SCCHN, but no strict reliance can currently be recommended

Treatment

- Over 80% of early stage tumors are cured
- Nearly half of patients have advanced local disease at presentation
- Radical, modified radical, or selective neck dissection
  - Radical neck dissection: Excision of levels I-V lymph nodes, sternocleidomastoid muscle (SCM), internal jugular vein (IJV), and cranial nerve XI
  - Modified radical neck dissection: Excision of levels I-V lymph nodes ± cranial nerve XI
  - Selective neck dissection: Excision of selected nodal groups
- Radiation therapy ± chemotherapy
  - Commonly includes cisplatin-based chemotherapy and intensity-modulated radiation therapy (IMRT)
  - Non-surgical route may be chosen for organ preservation
    - In patients with laryngeal/tongue cancer
    - In scenarios in which non-surgical treatment proven equal to surgical protocols
  - Radiation of entire upper aerodigestive tract, as with unidentified primary, can lead to xerostomia and fibrosis

DIAGNOSTIC CHECKLIST

Consider

- Consider PET/CT in patients with primary tumors that are prone to bilateral metastases, which are often less conspicuous on conventional imaging
  - Primary tumors of the nasopharynx, tongue base, and supraglottis
- Consider PET or PET/CT for patients at substantial risk of metastatic disease, both nodal and hematogenous
  - Patients with T3 or T4 lesions of the oral cavity, oropharynx, or larynx

- PET or PET/CT evaluation recommended after negative exam prior to random biopsies
- MR may provide additional information for unknown primary
- Reassessment
  - General scanning guidelines
    - Wait at least 3-5 weeks following surgery
    - Wait 6-12 weeks following radiation therapy; fewer false positives and false negatives with later follow-up periods
    - Wait one month after chemo

Image Interpretation Pearls

- Know physiologic FDG uptake patterns in the neck to avoid misinterpretation
- When in doubt determining post-therapy FDG uptake vs. tumor, perform short-term follow-up
  - Post-treatment inflammation almost always resolves on short-term follow-up exam
  - Also consider dual-time point PET exam

SELECTED REFERENCES

1. Gourin CG et al: Identification of distant metastases with positron-emission tomography-computed tomography in patients with previously untreated head and neck cancer. Laryngoscope. 118(4):671-5, 2008
2. Horiuchi C et al: Early assessment of clinical response to concurrent chemoradiotherapy in head and neck carcinoma using fluoro-2-deoxy-d-glucose positron emission tomography. Auris Nasus Larynx. 35(1):103-8, 2008
3. Kyzas PA et al: 18F-fluorodeoxyglucose positron emission tomography to evaluate cervical node metastases in patients with head and neck squamous cell carcinoma: a meta-analysis. J Natl Cancer Inst. 100(10):712-20, 2008
4. Linecker A et al: Uptake of (18)F-FLT and (18)F-FDG in primary head and neck cancer correlates with survival. Nuklearmedizin. 47(2):80-5; quiz N12, 2008
5. Marur S et al: Head and neck cancer: changing epidemiology, diagnosis, and treatment. Mayo Clin Proc. 83(4):489-501, 2008
6. Miller FR et al: Management of the unknown primary carcinoma: long-term follow-up on a negative PET scan and negative panendoscopy. Head Neck. 30(1):28-34, 2008
7. Ong SC et al: Clinical utility of 18F-FDG PET/CT in assessing the neck after concurrent chemoradiotherapy for Locoregional advanced head and neck cancer. J Nucl Med. 49(4):532-40, 2008
8. Senft A et al: Screening for distant metastases in head and neck cancer patients by chest CT or whole body FDG-PET: a prospective multicenter trial. Radiother Oncol. 87(2):221-9, 2008
9. Shah GV et al: New directions in head and neck imaging. J Surg Oncol. 97(8):644-8, 2008
10. Shintani SA et al: Utility of PET/CT imaging performed early after surgical resection in the adjuvant treatment planning for head and neck cancer. Int J Radiat Oncol Biol Phys. 70(2):322-9, 2008
11. Vernon MR et al: Clinical outcomes of patients receiving integrated PET/CT-guided radiotherapy for head and neck carcinoma. Int J Radiat Oncol Biol Phys. 70(3):678-84, 2008
12. Wong RJ: Current status of FDG-PET for head and neck cancer. J Surg Oncol. 97(8):649-52, 2008

HEAD AND NECK CANCER, SQUAMOUS

Unknown Primary

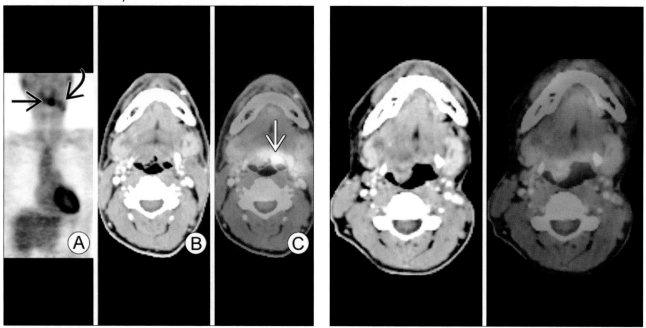

(Left) Coronal PET (A) demonstrates moderate linear activity in the left neck ⇗ following a recent excisional biopsy and a poorly localized medial focal area of intense activity ⇘. CECT (B) shows no definite correlative abnormality. Fused PET/CT (C) localizes the lesion to the left base of the tongue ➡, compatible with the primary mucosal lesion. *(Right)* Axial CT (left) and axial fused PET/CT from a follow-up examination 10 weeks after surgery and radiation demonstrates no residual or recurrent tumor.

Unknown Primary

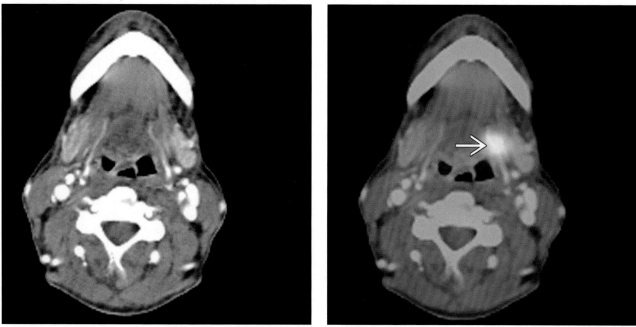

(Left) Axial CECT shows no definite abnormality in this patient with metastatic neck nodes positive for squamous cell carcinoma. *(Right)* Axial fused PET/CT shows focal intense activity just anterior to the left pyriform sinus ➡, compatible with the patient's primary malignancy.

HEAD AND NECK CANCER, SQUAMOUS

Unknown Primary

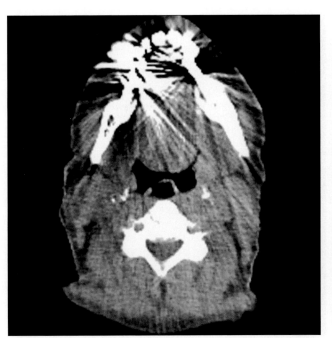 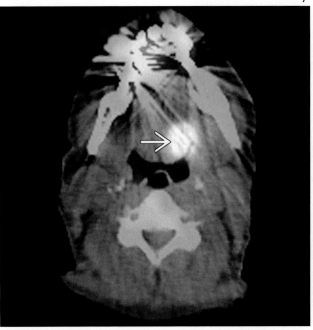

(Left) Axial NECT shows significant streak artifact without any identifiable mucosal primary lesion. *(Right)* Axial fused PET/CT shows focal intense asymmetrical activity ➡ in the left base of tongue, compatible with the patient's primary mucosal lesion. One of the benefits of combined PET/CT is the ability to detect and localize lesions in patients with significant artifacts on CT.

Unknown Primary

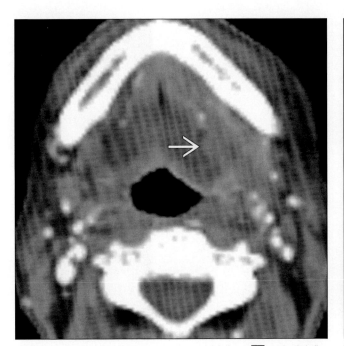 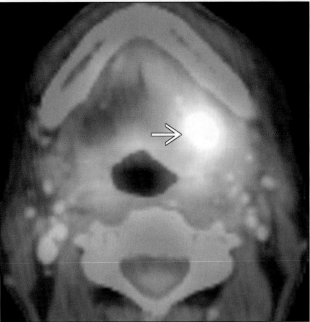

(Left) Axial CECT shows subtle asymmetrical fullness ➡ in the left floor of mouth. This patient was recently diagnosed with squamous cell carcinoma of the left neck without identifiable primary lesion. *(Right)* Axial fused PET/CT shows focal intense FDG activity ➡ in the area of questionable fullness on the CT portion of the exam, confirming the presence of malignancy.

HEAD AND NECK CANCER, SQUAMOUS

Unknown Primary

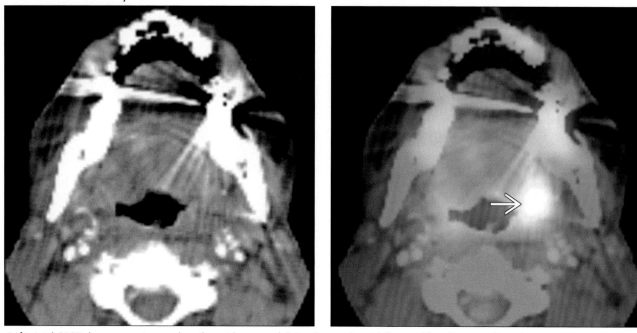

(Left) Axial CECT shows extensive streak artifact without any definite abnormality. *(Right)* Axial fused PET/CT shows focal intense asymmetrical activity ➡ in the left retromolar trigone, compatible with malignancy not otherwise visualized on the CT portion of the exam due to artifact.

Unknown Primary

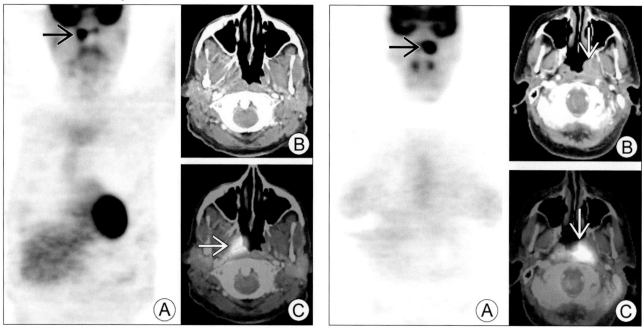

(Left) In this patient with newly diagnosed squamous cell carcinoma with an unknown primary, focal asymmetrical intense activity ➡ on coronal PET (A) is localized to the right nasopharynx ➡ on the fused PET/CT image (C). No definite correlative CT abnormality (B) is seen. *(Right)* In this patient recently diagnosed with nasopharyngeal carcinoma, focal intense FDG activity ➡ on coronal PET (A) correlates with an asymmetrical hypermetabolic mass ➡ in the left nasopharynx on axial CT (B) and fused PET/CT (C).

HEAD AND NECK CANCER, SQUAMOUS

Staging

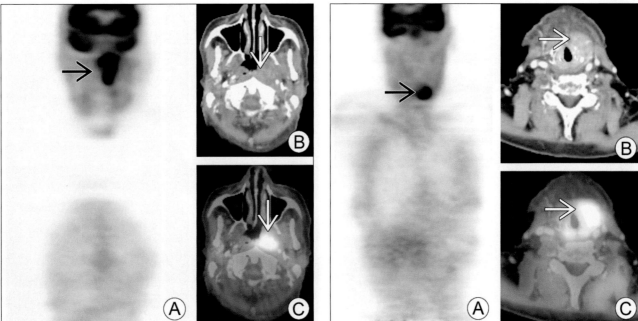

(Left) Coronal PET (A) demonstrates asymmetrical FDG activity in the left nasopharynx ➡, correlating with an asymmetrical metabolic mass in the left nasopharynx ➡ on axial CT (B) and fused PET/CT (C). These findings are compatible with squamous cell carcinoma. *(Right)* Coronal PET (A) demonstrates asymmetrical intense FDG activity to the left of midline ➡, corresponding to hypermetabolic primary laryngeal squamous cell carcinoma with involvement and erosion of the left thyroid cartilage ➡ on axial CT (B) and fused PET/CT (C).

Staging

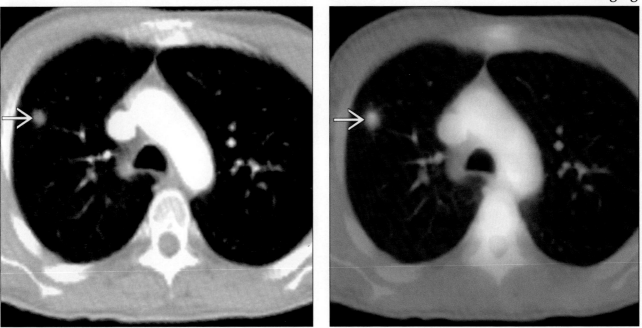

(Left) Axial CECT shows a 1 cm noncalcified pulmonary nodule ➡ in a patient with newly diagnosed laryngeal carcinoma. *(Right)* Axial fused PET/CT shows focal intense activity within the pulmonary nodule ➡, worrisome for metastatic disease. The nodule is well-circumscribed, making primary lung cancer less likely. However, approximately 6-15% of patients with newly diagnosed squamous cell carcinoma of the head and neck may have second primary malignancies, particularly in the lung.

HEAD AND NECK CANCER, SQUAMOUS

Staging

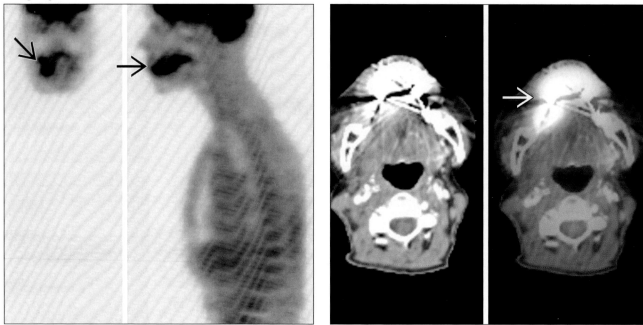

(Left) Coronal (left) and sagittal (right) images show intense FDG activity ➡ difficult to localize on PET alone. *(Right)* Axial CT (left) shows no obvious abnormalities due to extensive streak artifact. However, fused PET/CT image (right) shows asymmetrical intense FDG activity involving the right side of the mandible ➡, compatible with malignancy.

Staging

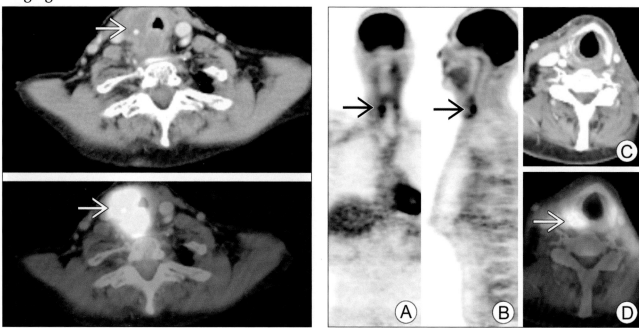

(Left) Axial CT (top) and fused PET/CT (bottom) show a bulky laryngeal tumor ➡ with intense FDG activity, compatible with primary squamous cell carcinoma of the larynx. *(Right)* Focal intense activity ➡ is identified to the right of midline on coronal (A) and sagittal (B) PET images. This patient underwent excisional biopsy of a metastatic lymph node in the right neck for squamous cell carcinoma without known mucosal primary. A lesion is confirmed in the posterior aspect of the larynx ➡ on fused PET/CT (D) without definite abnormality on CT (C).

HEAD AND NECK CANCER, SQUAMOUS

Staging

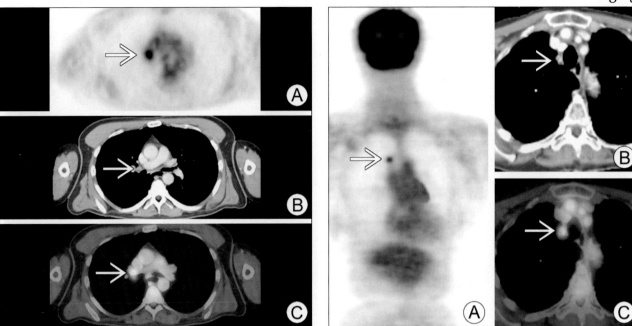

(Left) Axial PET (A), CECT (B), and PET/CT (C) images show a focal area of intense FDG activity ➡ in the right hilar area in this patient with newly diagnosed oropharyngeal carcinoma. Subsequent bronchoscopic evaluation demonstrated metastatic disease from the patient's primary head and neck malignancy. *(Right)* Coronal PET (A), axial CT (B) and fused PET/CT (C) show a focal area of moderate to intense FDG activity localized to a tiny right paratracheal lymph node ➡ in this patient with newly diagnosed solid carcinoma of the head and neck.

Staging

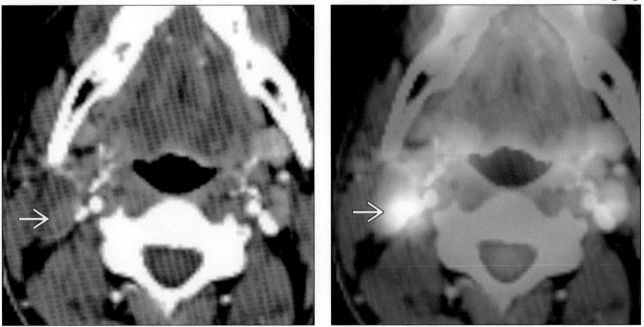

(Left) Axial CECT shows a large partially necrotic lymph node in the right neck ➡ on this staging PET/CT study. *(Right)* Axial fused PET/CT shows focal intense activity ➡ corresponding to the nodular portion of the large metastatic lymph node shown in the previous image. Partial or complete central necrosis is a finding occasionally identified on CT in patients with metastatic squamous cell carcinoma.

HEAD AND NECK CANCER, SQUAMOUS

Staging

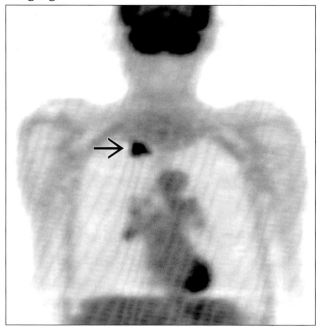 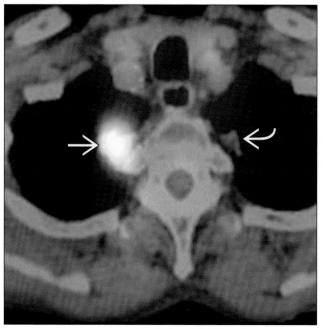

(Left) Coronal PET shows focal intense activity near the right apex ➡ in this patient with a newly diagnosed left oropharyngeal carcinoma. A recent CT scan of this patient was interpreted as negative for potential thoracic metastases and mentioned only bilateral apical scarring. *(Right)* Axial fused PET/CT shows focal intense activity corresponding to an area of soft tissue in the right apex ➡. Note a small amount of scarring ➡ in the left apex without increased metabolic activity. Subsequent biopsy of the right apical lesion confirmed a secondary lung adenocarcinoma.

Staging

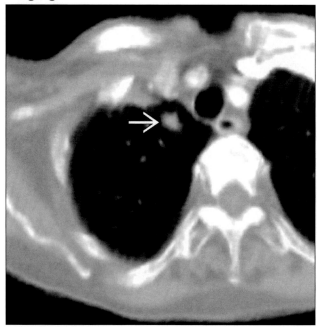 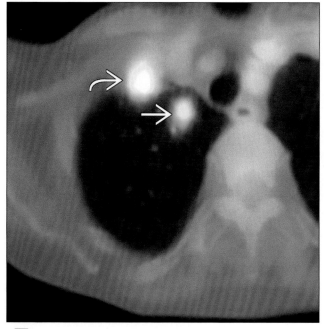

(Left) Axial CECT shows a slightly spiculated right apical pulmonary nodule ➡ in this patient with a diagnosis of carcinoma of the oropharynx. *(Right)* Axial fused PET/CT shows two foci of intense FDG activity, one correlating with the right upper lobe nodule ➡ and a second one correlating with a pleural-based lesion ➡. Subsequent biopsy showed a peripheral adenocarcinoma in this patient with a pleural metastasis.

HEAD AND NECK CANCER, SQUAMOUS

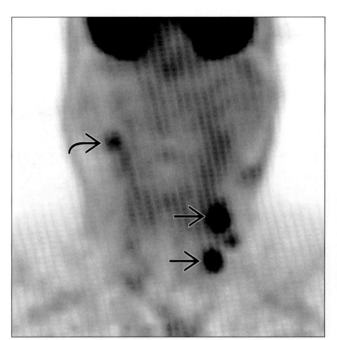
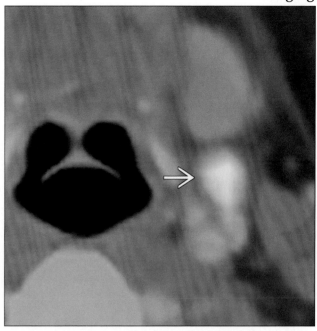

(Left) Coronal PET in this patient with newly diagnosed left-sided oropharyngeal carcinoma shows multiple left-sided enlarged hypermetabolic metastatic nodes ➡. Additionally, in the contralateral neck, there is a normal-sized single focal area of intense FDG activity ↗, suspicious for contralateral metastases. *(Right)* Axial fused PET/CT shows one of the enlarged hypermetabolic lymph nodes ➡ from the same patient, compatible with metastatic disease.

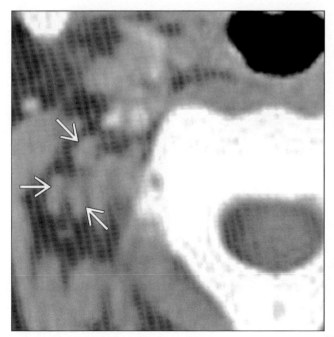
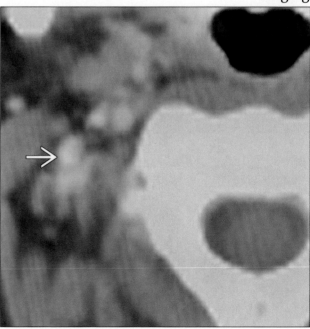

(Left) Axial CECT shows 3 normal-sized lymph nodes in the right neck ➡, which would not be suspicious for metastatic involvement. *(Right)* Axial fused PET/CT shows focal intense activity in the anterior lymph node ➡. Because of the node's small size, the amount of activity is likely underestimated due to partial volume averaging. Because of single contralateral nodal involvement, bilateral neck dissections were performed. Pathology revealed one 8 mm lymph node with metastatic involvement.

HEAD AND NECK CANCER, SQUAMOUS

Staging

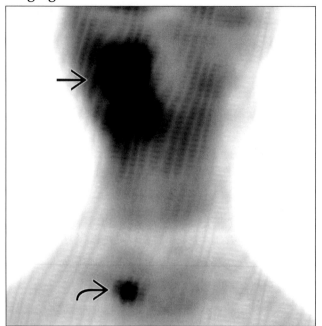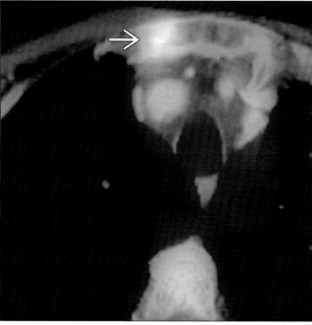

(Left) Coronal PET shows a large area of intense FDG activity ⇨ correlating with a large right-sided oropharyngeal carcinoma. An unsuspected second focus of intense FDG activity is present in the thorax ⇨, difficult to localize on PET imaging. *(Right)* Axial fused PET/CT shows a focal area of intense FDG activity in the right side of the sternum ⇨ without an abnormality on CT, compatible with metastatic disease.

Staging

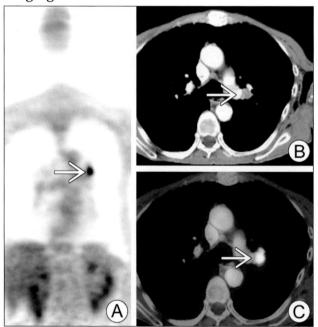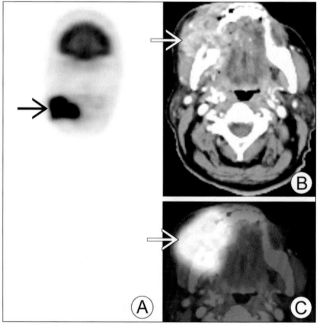

(Left) Coronal PET (A), axial CT (B) and fused PET/CT (C) in a patient recently diagnosed with left tonsillar squamous cell carcinoma show a focal area of intense FDG activity in the mediastinum, correlating with a small left hilar lymph node ⇨, compatible with metastatic disease. *(Right)* Coronal PET (A) demonstrates a large area of intense FDG activity ⇨, which correlates with a heterogeneously enhancing mass ⇨ on axial CT (B) and fused PET/CT (C), compatible with this patient's primary squamous cell carcinoma of the oropharynx.

HEAD AND NECK CANCER, SQUAMOUS

Staging

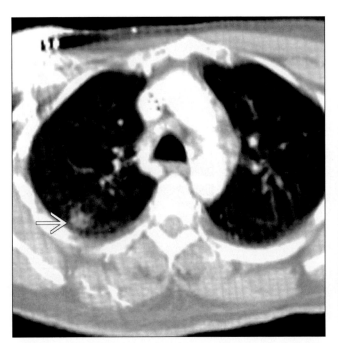 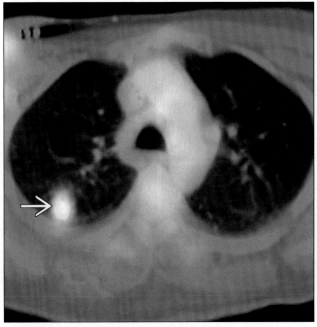

(Left) Axial CECT shows an incidental 1 cm right upper lobe pulmonary nodule ⮞ in a patient undergoing a staging PET/CT examination. *(Right)* Axial fused PET/CT shows focal intense FDG activity correlating with the right upper lobe pulmonary nodule ⮞, compatible with metastatic disease.

Restaging

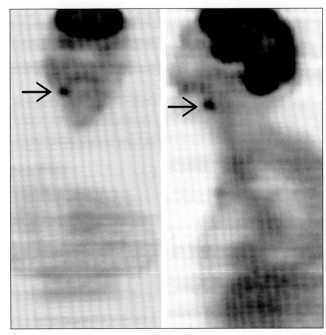 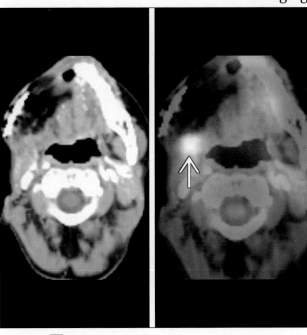

(Left) Coronal (left) and sagittal (right) PET images show a focal area of FDG activity ⮞ in this patient undergoing a restaging examination following a radical right neck dissection. *(Right)* Axial CT (left) shows extensive post-operative change without definite residual or recurrent tumor. Nevertheless, a focal area of intense FDG activity ⮞ is present along the posterior aspect of the resection margin on fused PET/CT (right). Subsequent biopsies proved residual disease approximately 10 weeks following surgery.

HEAD AND NECK CANCER, SQUAMOUS

Restaging

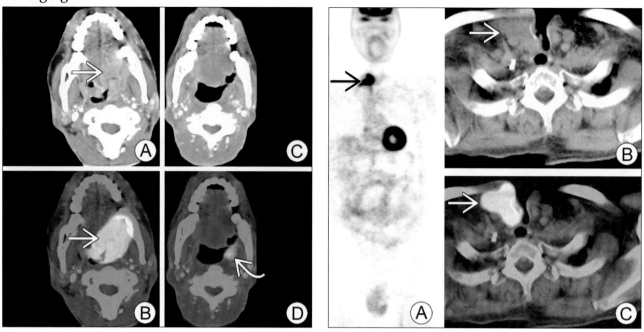

(Left) Compare the pre-treatment axial CT (A) and fused PET/CT (B) of a patient with left-sided oropharyngeal carcinoma ⮕ with the post-treatment axial CT (C) and fused PET/CT (D) following primary resection and radiation. The post-treatment images show no definite abnormality on CT. However, a small focus of moderate to intense FDG activity is present along the posterior resection bed ⮕, compatible with recurrent disease. *(Right)* Coronal PET (A) demonstrates a large area of intense FDG activity ⮕, correlating with recurrent disease around the tracheostomy tube on axial CT (B) and fused PET/CT (C) ⮕.

Restaging

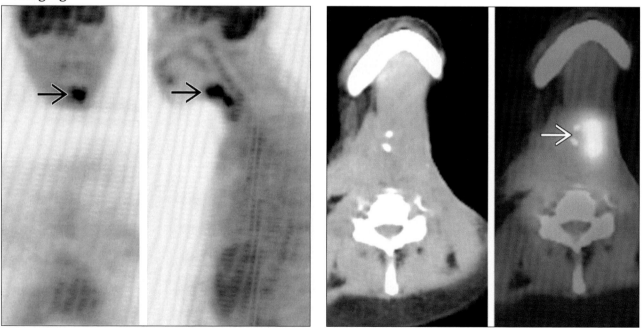

(Left) Coronal (left) and sagittal (right) PET images demonstrate abnormally increased FDG activity ⮕ in this patient who had a large left-sided squamous cell carcinoma of the oropharynx status post radical neck dissection. *(Right)* Axial NECT (left) shows no definite abnormality, although this is a suboptimal exam due to lack of intravenous contrast. A fused PET/CT (right) more accurately localizes the abnormal area of the FDG activity ⮕.

HEAD AND NECK CANCER, SQUAMOUS

Restaging

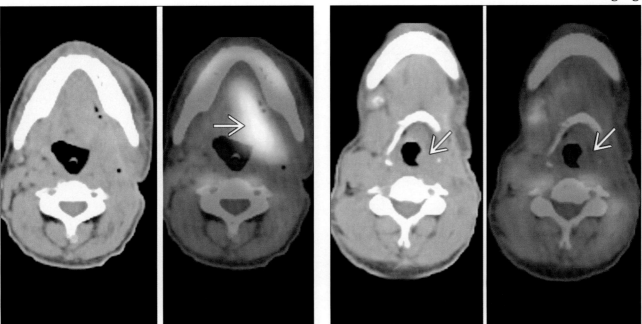

(Left) Axial CT (left) and fused PET/CT (right) imaging was performed to evaluate for possible resection of this patient's known left oral tongue squamous cell carcinoma ➡. However, a recent MR showed a questionable second lesion that would affect the surgical approach. *(Right)* Axial CT (left) and fused PET/CT (right) along the lateral pharyngeal border ➡, which was the questionable area on MR, shows no increased metabolic activity. Therefore, this likely represents prior post-treatment changes.

Restaging

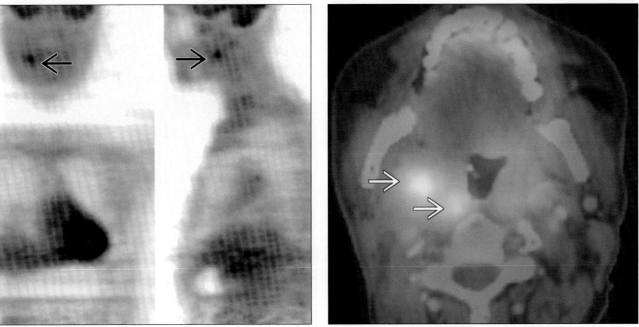

(Left) Coronal (left) and sagittal (right) PET demonstrate a focal area of increased metabolic activity ➡ in a patient with a history of squamous cell carcinoma status post resection and radiation therapy who underwent this PET/CT for restaging. *(Right)* Axial fused PET/CT shows two foci of increased metabolic activity ➡ without an abnormality on correlating CT, compatible with recurrent disease.

HEAD AND NECK CANCER, SQUAMOUS

Restaging

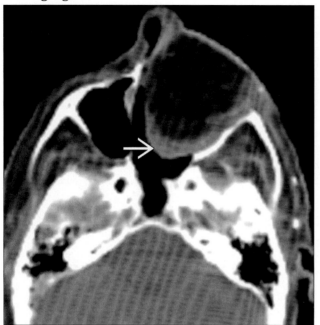 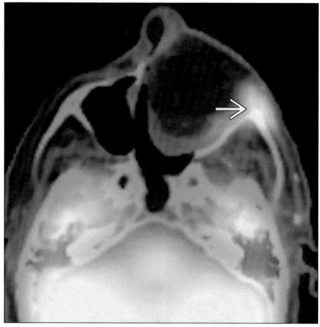

(Left) Axial NECT shows questionable thickening along the entire flap, particularly in the posterior aspect ➡, in this patient who is status post extensive surgery with positive surgical margins approximately 10 weeks prior to the imaging study. *(Right)* Axial fused PET/CT shows focal intense activity along the lateral flap border ➡, compatible with residual tumor.

Restaging

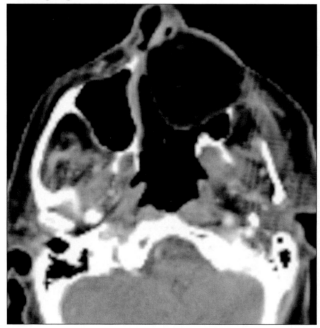 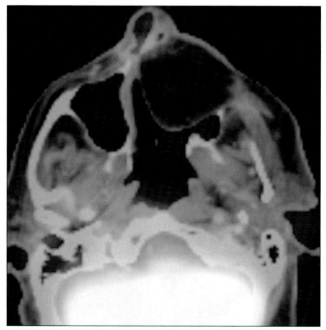

(Left) Axial CECT, performed 6 weeks following revision of flap and resection of the residual tumor, demonstrates no definite abnormality. *(Right)* Axial fused PET/CT shows no increased metabolic activity approximately 6 weeks after surgery. In this case, a PET/CT helped localize residual/recurrent tumor more precisely than CT approximately 10 weeks after surgery.

HEAD AND NECK CANCER, SQUAMOUS

Response to Therapy

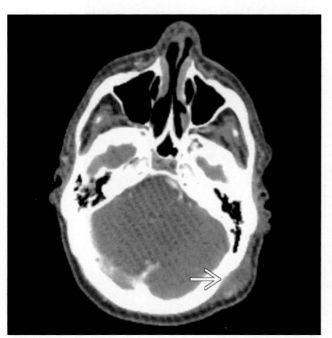 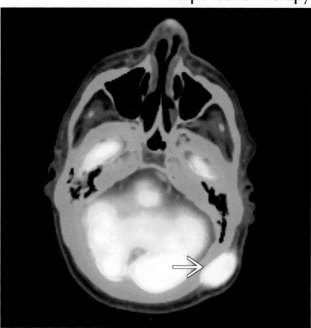

(Left) Axial CECT shows a crescent-shaped, minimally enhancing lesion ➡ in this patient with squamous cell carcinoma of the scalp. *(Right)* Axial fused PET/CT shows diffuse intense FDG activity ➡ correlating with the scalp mass, compatible with malignancy.

Response to Therapy

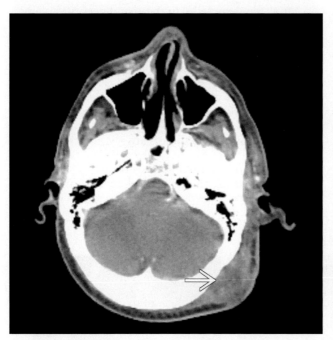 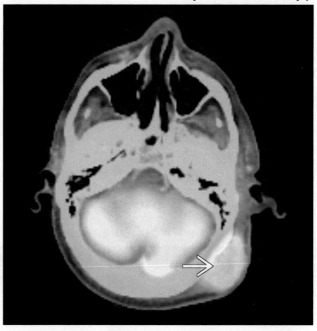

(Left) Axial CECT in the same patient after 6 cycles of chemotherapy shows no interval response ➡ and slight interval increase in size, compatible with a poor therapeutic response. *(Right)* Axial fused PET/CT shows slight interval increase in size and metabolic activity of the left scalp mass ➡.

HEAD AND NECK CANCER, NON-SQUAMOUS

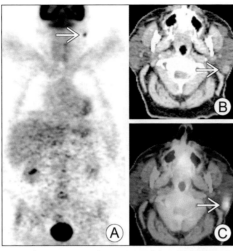

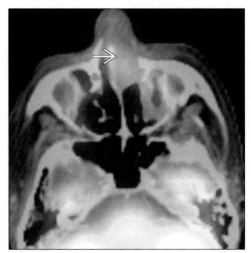

Coronal PET (A), axial CT (B) and fused PET/CT (C) demonstrate a focal area of intense activity in the left neck ➡, corresponding to a Warthin tumor in the posterior left parotid.

Axial fused PET/CT demonstrates a non-FDG-avid nasal neuroendocrine tumor ➡.

TERMINOLOGY

Abbreviations and Synonyms

- Non-squamous cell cancer of the head and neck (NSCCHN)
- Neuroendocrine tumors (NET), small cell undifferentiated carcinoma, Merkel cell carcinoma (MCC)
- Benign mixed tumors (BMT) or pleomorphic adenoma; Warthin tumor; parotid carcinoma (mucoepidermoid and adenoid cystic), primary lymphoma

Definitions

- Heterogeneous group of tumors of neuroendocrine origin
- Merkel cells first described by Frederick Merkel in 1875
  - Believed to be slow-acting mechanoreceptors in the basal layer of the epidermis
  - Provide information about touch and hair movement
- Tumors of the parotid and submandibular glands (salivary glands)

IMAGING FINDINGS

General Features

- Best diagnostic clue
  - **MCC**: Aggressive cutaneous mass
  - **NET**: Mass involving the structures listed below
  - **Salivary**: Negative Tc-99m pertechnetate and positive FDG PET
- Location
  - **MCC**: Sun-exposed skin (head and neck 50%), most common location periorbital area; about 40% occur along the extremities
    - MCC is thought to arise from hair follicles or dermal Merkel cells, although no definite evidence exists
  - **NET**: Salivary glands, larynx, sinonasal cavity, upper esophagus, and oral cavity for non-MCC NET tumors
  - Most salivary gland tumors arise within the parotid gland
  - Most parotid gland tumors are benign
- Size: Range in size from a few millimeters to several centimeters; average size < 2 cm

DDx: Cutaneous or Subcutaneous Hypermetabolic Mass

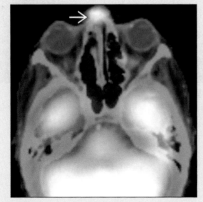

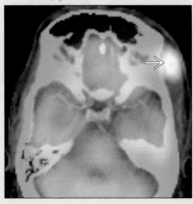

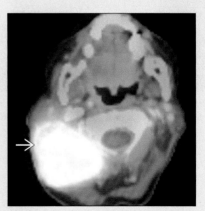

Nasal Melanoma

Squamous Cell Carcinoma

Lymphoma

HEAD AND NECK CANCER, NON-SQUAMOUS

Key Facts

Terminology
- Neuroendocrine tumors (NET), small cell undifferentiated carcinoma, Merkel cell carcinoma (MCC)
- Benign mixed tumors (BMT) or pleomorphic adenoma; Warthin tumor; parotid carcinoma (mucoepidermoid and adenoid cystic), primary lymphoma

Imaging Findings
- FDG PET overall sensitivity for all NET approximately 76%
- **MCC**
  - FDG PET usually shows intense uptake within primary and metastatic lesions for MCC
- For non-MCC NET, FDG may show variability

- Some head and neck NET may show very little FDG activity
- **Salivary**
  - PET: Sensitivity and specificity 75% and 67%
  - 30% false positive rate for malignancy (mostly due to Warthin tumor)
- PET/CT may be used to find primary in NSCCHN metastases

Top Differential Diagnoses
- Metastatic Disease from Small Cell Carcinoma of the Lung
- Benign Mixed Tumor or Pleomorphic Adenoma
- Warthin Tumor
- Parotid Metastases

- Morphology: **MCC**: Firm violaceous or reddish nodular papule or plaque ± ulceration

Imaging Recommendations
- Best imaging tool
  - CT scan with contrast or PET/CT with contrast
  - FDG PET likely helpful in MCC; other head and neck NET may have less FDG activity
  - FDG PET overall sensitivity for all NET approximately 76%
  - FDG PET may influence management in up to 25% of patients
  - Salivary: Combination FDG PET or PET/CT and salivary gland scintigraphy with Tc-99m pertechnetate
- Protocol advice: IV contrast for CT; arms down for PET or PET/CT
- Additional nuclear medicine imaging options
  - Radiolabeled octreotide not well-evaluated for NET tumors of the head and neck; better for evaluation of NET outside the head and neck
- Correlative imaging features
  - CT findings
    - Primary lesion may show necrosis, enhancement, or mass effect for both MCC and non-MCC NET
    - Lymphadenopathy range 1.2-11 cm; mean 4.2 cm

Nuclear Medicine Findings
- **MCC**
  - FDG PET usually shows intense uptake within primary and metastatic lesions for MCC
    - Average SUV max in one study 10.4
    - Several case studies and small series showing most MCC to be intensely FDG avid; occasional false negative
    - PET useful for staging, assessing tumor response, and surveillance
  - For non-MCC NET, FDG may show variability
    - Some head and neck NET may show very little FDG activity
    - Metastatic lesions may show photopenia compared to background normal activity

- **Salivary**
  - PET: Sensitivity and specificity 75% and 67%
    - 30% false positive rate for malignancy (mostly due to Warthin tumor)
    - High grade salivary tumors have been described as having wide range of maximum SUV values
    - In general, high grade salivary tumors have SUV greater than 5.0
    - Exception is adenoid cystic carcinoma, whose low SUV is attributed to slow growth
    - Normal salivary glands may have minimal to moderate uptake and diffuse asymmetric uptake
    - Mean SUV of normal parotid in one study was 1.9 ± 0.68
    - 76% of patients in one study had asymmetric uptake, attributed to normal variance or inflammation
    - Some asymmetric appearances may be due to artifact secondary to head movement between emission and transmission scans
    - Tilted head position can also create appearance of asymmetry
    - PET and PET/CT show low accuracy for distinguishing between benign and malignant tumors due to high uptake of benign tumors
    - Inability to distinguish low grade malignant tumors from benign disease may have little clinical impact
    - Patients with low grade salivary cancer appear to show good prognosis after conservative treatment, similar to patients with benign salivary tumors
  - Overall major impact in clinical treatment planning is seen in 40% of patients
- **Staging**
  - PET/CT may be used to find primary in NSCCHN metastases
    - Most primaries are located in thorax, head/neck, abdomen
  - In patients with high grade salivary cancer, PET/CT has been shown to

HEAD AND NECK CANCER, NON-SQUAMOUS

- Significantly improve diagnostic accuracy for evaluating extent of tumor and tumor stages compared with CT alone
  - o Superior for detection of cervical lymph node mets, distant mets, and second primaries
  - o PET has been shown to have significant impact on management of patients with salivary gland cancers for initial staging and restaging
  - o PET/CT provided correct staging in 85% of cases vs. 62% with CT
  - o Whole-body scan superior to conventional imaging for detection of distant mets
- **Additional nuclear medicine options**
  - o MCC: Octreotide scan using somatostatin analog tagged with indium-111 as tracer used to detect metastases
    - Limited in assessing uptake in organs with physiologic uptake of octreotide such as liver, kidneys, spleen
    - Liver is one of the main sites of metastasis for MCC
  - o Ga-67 scintigraphy: Sensitivity and specificity for differentiation of benign from malignant parotid masses 58% and 72% respectively
  - o F-DOPA PET also shows some variability in the uptake

CT Findings
- Criteria for malignant cervical lymph nodes
  - o Presence of necrosis
  - o Peripheral fatty hilum
- Morphologic imaging generally poor for differentiating benign from malignant parotid tumors
  - o Characteristics such as irregular margins and infiltration into parenchyma useful but not reliable

DIFFERENTIAL DIAGNOSIS

Melanoma
- Primary MCC usually more red in color
- Immunohistochemically positive for S100 protein and thyroid transcription factor-1

Cutaneous Lymphoma
- B or T cell origin
- May be localized or involve other organs and sites

Squamous Cell Carcinoma
- Usually mucosal surface involved

Benign Mixed Tumor or Pleomorphic Adenoma
- Can be positive or negative on FDG PET; tends to be less FDG avid than primary parotid malignancies and Warthin tumor

Warthin Tumor
- Tend to be positive on both FDG PET and Tc-99m pertechnetate

Primary Parotid Carcinoma (Adenoid Cystic or Mucoepidermoid)
- Almost always FDG avid

Non-Hodgkin Lymphoma
- Higher grade tumors more FDG avid

Parotid Metastases
- FDG avidity will depend on the primary lesion

Metastatic Disease from Small Cell Carcinoma of the Lung
- Non-MCC NET may be indistinguishable by imaging
- Look for primary lung lesions

PATHOLOGY

General Features
- General path comments
  - o MCC
    - Diagnosis relies exclusively on pathologic findings such as immunohistochemistry and electron microscopy
- Genetics
  - o MCC
    - Chromosomal rearrangements on chromosomes 1, 3, and 5 for MCC
    - Loss of more than one tumor suppressor gene
- Etiology
  - o MCC
    - Idiopathic or iatrogenic immunosuppression has been implicated
    - Sunlight (UVB index correlated to the incidence of MCC)
    - Exposure to arsenic and methoxsalen and UV treatment for psoriasis also implicated
    - Also documented in patients with congenital ectodermal dysplasia, Cowden disease, and Hodgkin
- Epidemiology
  - o **MCC** annual incidence 0.42 per 100,000 for Caucasian populations; about 1/20th this figure for African-American populations
    - 400 new cases/year in USA
    - Mortality 25%
  - o **Salivary gland malignancies** account for 5% of head and neck cancers
    - Mucoepidermoid tumors are most common malignant tumor of salivary gland
    - Adenoid cystic carcinoma accounts for 15% of parotid malignant neoplasms
- Associated abnormalities: Possible association between squamous cell and basal cell carcinoma

Gross Pathologic & Surgical Features
- Reddish papule or plaque that often demonstrates dermal invasion
- Can present with multiple satellite lesions from spread through the dermal lymphatics

Microscopic Features
- MCC
  - o Sheets, ribbons, or nests of small round blue cells
  - o Neurosecretory granules can be demonstrated in most lesions

HEAD AND NECK CANCER, NON-SQUAMOUS

- o Immunohistochemistry helpful for differentiation from lymphoma, Ewing sarcoma, melanoma, and basal cell carcinoma
    - ▪ Positive for cytokeratin 20, neurofilaments, chromogranin, CAM 5.2, and synaptophysin
    - ▪ Negative for S100 and leukocyte common antigen
    - ▪ KIT receptor tyrosine kinase (CD117) expressed in 95% of MCCs
- • Salivary
    - o Histopathologic features that indicate high grade behavior in mucoepidermoid tumors
        - ▪ Intracystic component of less than 20%
        - ▪ Four or more mitotic figures per ten high power fields
        - ▪ Neural invasion
        - ▪ Necrosis
        - ▪ Cellular anaplasia

Staging, Grading, or Classification Criteria

- • Staging for MCC
    - o IA disease confined to skin < 2 cm in diameter
    - o IB disease confined to skin > 2 cm in diameter
    - o Involvement in regional lymph nodes
    - o Metastatic disease

CLINICAL ISSUES

Presentation

- • Most common signs/symptoms
    - o MCC
        - ▪ Usually painless reddish ulcerated plaque on the skin near the orbits
        - ▪ May also have shiny surface, often with telangiectasia
        - ▪ Can be mistaken for basal cell carcinoma, amelanotic melanoma, squamous cell carcinoma, and cutaneous lymphoma
    - o Salivary
        - ▪ Cheek mass ± pain
        - ▪ Occasional VII nerve paralysis
- • Other signs/symptoms: Pain may be secondary symptom

Demographics

- • Age
    - o MCC: Most common between the ages of 69 and 82; only 5% of cases occur before age 50
    - o Salivary: BMT > 35
- • Gender
    - o MCC: M:F = 1.5:1
    - o Salivary: BMT M:F = 1:2
- • Ethnicity: MCC rarely seen in non-Caucasian patients

Natural History & Prognosis

- • MCC
    - o 30-60% mortality rate in patients with MCC in most studies
        - ▪ 5 year outcomes for MCC: Local control 94%, locoregional control 80%, and survival 37%
        - ▪ 70-80% have localized disease at initial presentation, 10-30% have regional mets, and 1-4% have distant mets

---

- ▪ 50% of patients who have undergone neck dissections have been found to have microscopic disease in surgical specimens
- • Salivary gland tumors
    - o Two most significant prognostic factors are histologic grade and clinical stage at presentation
    - o 54% occurrence of distant metastases in patients with high grade salivary cancer
    - o 5 year survival for small cell arising from the major salivary glands is 46%

Treatment

- • Salivary
    - o Treatment decisions depend on knowledge of local invasion, regional lymph node mets, and distant spread
- • Surgical treatment is only potentially curative option
    - o Radio-/chemotherapy has only adjuvant or palliative use
- • Depends on cell type
- • Resection or preservation of facial nerve
- • Extended radiation or superficial parotidectomy
- • Additional radical neck dissection in some cases

DIAGNOSTIC CHECKLIST

Consider

- • Contrast-enhanced CT or FDG PET/CT (particularly in MCC)
- • FNA may be most cost effective approach; sensitivity 64-92% and specificity 75-100%
    - o May increase risk of recurrence secondary to "spillage"

Image Interpretation Pearls

- • Primary parotid carcinoma almost always positive on FDG PET; Warthin tumor commonly positive on FDG PET; BMT occasionally positive on FDG PET

SELECTED REFERENCES

1. Gomes M et al: High-grade mucoepidermoid carcinoma of the accessory parotid gland with distant metastases identified by 18F-FDG PET-CT. Pediatr Blood Cancer. 50(2):395-7, 2008
2. Bhagat N et al: Detection of recurrent adenoid cystic carcinoma with PET-CT. Clin Nucl Med. 32(7):574-7, 2007
3. Shah VN et al: Oncocytoma of the parotid gland: a potential false-positive finding on 18F-FDG PET. AJR Am J Roentgenol. 189(4):W212-4, 2007
4. Yamada H et al: Epithelial-myoepithelial carcinoma of the submandibular gland with a high uptake of 18F-FDG: a case report and image diagnosis. Oral Surg Oral Med Oral Pathol Oral Radiol Endod. 104(2):243-8, 2007
5. Hagino K et al: Oncocytoma in the parotid gland presenting a remarkable increase in fluorodeoxyglucose uptake on positron emission tomography. Otolaryngol Head Neck Surg. 134(4):708-9, 2006
6. Ozawa N et al: Retrospective review: usefulness of a number of imaging modalities including CT, MRI, technetium-99m pertechnetate scintigraphy, gallium-67 scintigraphy and F-18-FDG PET in the differentiation of benign from malignant parotid masses. Radiat Med. 24(1):41-9, 2006

HEAD AND NECK CANCER, NON-SQUAMOUS

PET/CT: Neuroendocrine

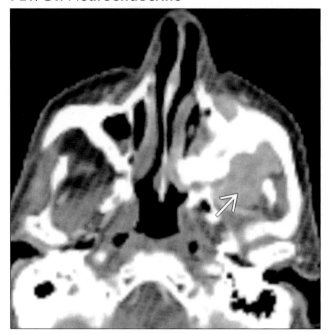
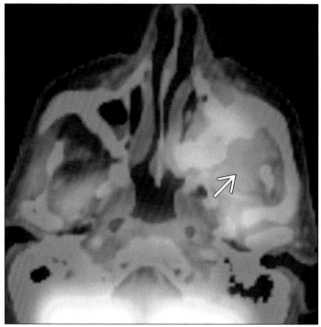

(Left) Axial CECT shows a large partially enhancing mass ➡ due to a neuroendocrine tumor. *(Right)* Axial fused PET/CT shows minimal FDG activity in the area of the enhancing mass ➡. Many neuroendocrine tumors, such as this, are poorly FDG avid.

PET/CT: Neuroendocrine

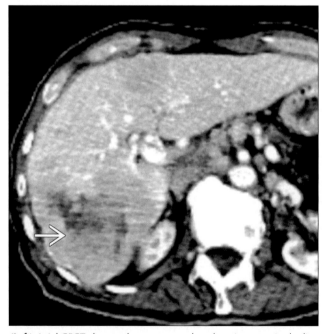
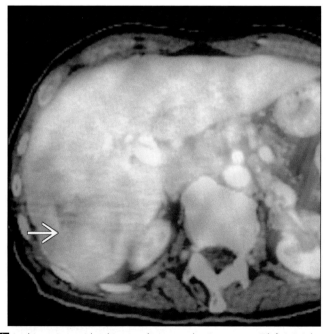

(Left) Axial CECT shows a heterogeneously enhancing mass in the liver ➡ in this patient with a history of neuroendocrine tumor. *(Right)* Axial fused PET/CT shows decreased metabolic activity in the area of the enhancing mass ➡ compared to physiologic FDG in the liver, typical of many metastatic neuroendocrine tumors.

HEAD AND NECK CANCER, NON-SQUAMOUS

PET/CT: Neuroendocrine

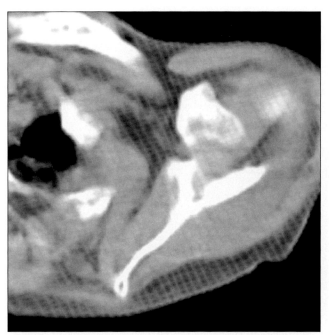 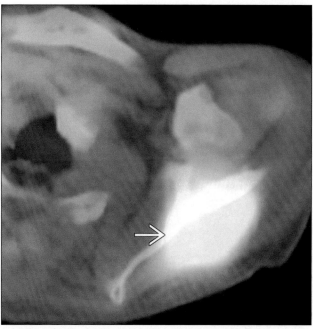

(Left) Axial NECT shows no definite abnormality in this patient with known metastatic neuroendocrine tumor. *(Right)* Axial fused PET/CT shows chest metabolic activity that correlates with the left suprascapular muscle ➡ with questionable bony invasion. Biopsy showed metastatic neuroendocrine tumor from a primary head and neck lesion.

PET/CT: Neuroendocrine

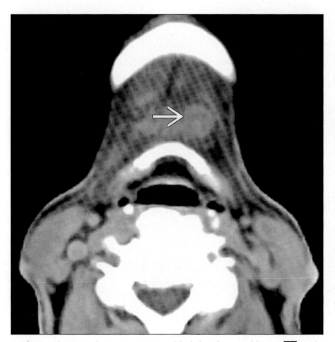 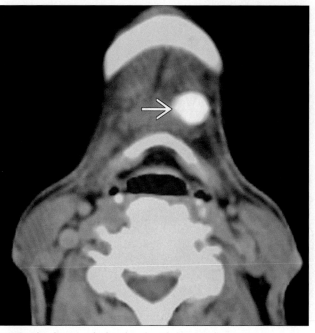

(Left) Axial NECT shows a questionable left submental lesion ➡ in this patient with a history of a head and neck neuroendocrine tumor. *(Right)* Axial fused PET/CT shows focal intense metabolic activity corresponding to the left submental lesion ➡, compatible with malignancy.

HEAD AND NECK CANCER, NON-SQUAMOUS

PET/CT: Neuroendocrine

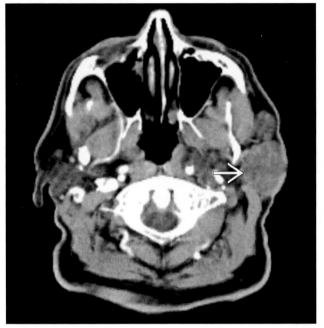 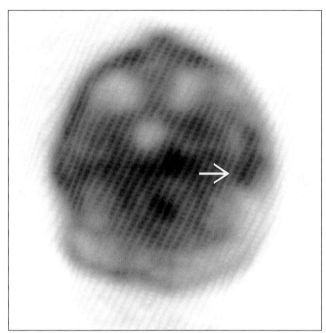

(Left) Axial CECT shows a relatively homogeneous left neck lesion ➡ in a patient with known metastatic neuroendocrine tumor. This mass was proven after biopsy to be a metastatic neuroendocrine tumor, but it demonstrated only minimally increased FDG activity. *(Right)* Axial PET in the same patient shows minimally increased FDG activity correlating with the left neck mass ➡.

PET/CT: Warthin Tumor

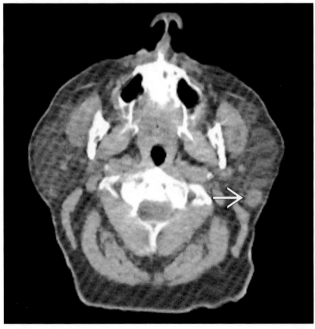 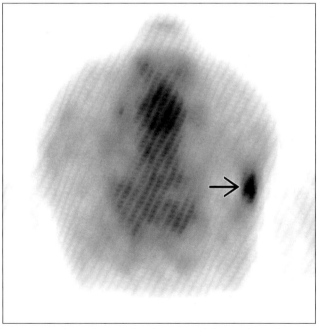

(Left) Axial NECT shows a focal left intraparotid soft tissue nodule ➡ in this patient without a history of malignancy. *(Right)* Axial PET shows focal intense FDG activity correlating with the left intraparotid node ➡. Subsequent biopsy showed Warthin tumor.

HEAD AND NECK CANCER, NON-SQUAMOUS

PET/CT: Pleomorphic Adenoma

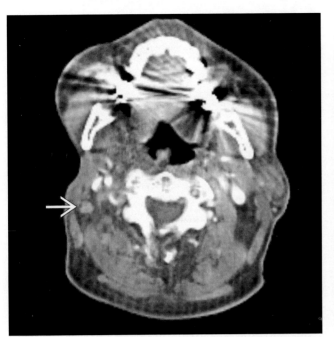
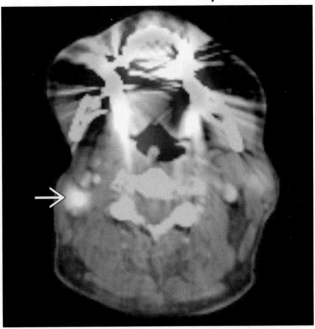

(Left) Axial CECT shows an enhancing right-sided soft tissue lesion adjacent to the right parotid gland ➡ in this patient being evaluated on PET/CT for pulmonary nodule. *(Right)* Axial fused PET/CT shows focal moderately increased FDG activity correlating with the lesion in the right neck ➡. Subsequent resection showed pleomorphic adenoma.

PET/CT: Pleomorphic Adenoma

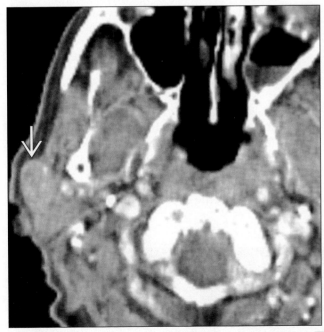
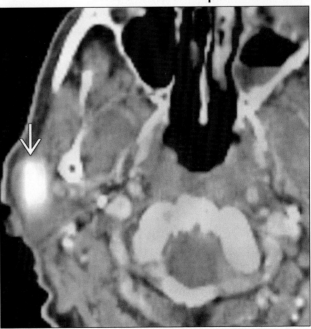

(Left) Axial CECT shows an enhancing right-sided intraparotid lesion ➡ in this patient being evaluated on PET/CT for lymphoma. *(Right)* Axial fused PET/CT shows focal intense FDG activity correlating with the right intraparotid lesion ➡. Subsequent resection showed pleomorphic adenoma.

THYROID CANCER

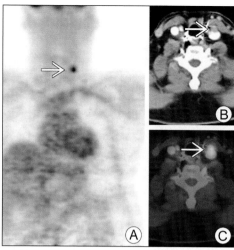

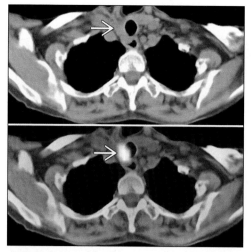

Coronal PET (A), axial CT (B) and fused PET/CT (C) show a subtle recurrent thyroid carcinoma ➜ in a patient with rising thyroglobulin levels and a negative iodine study.

Axial CT (top) and fused PET/CT (bottom) show focal thyroid cancer recurrence in the thyroidectomy bed ➜.

TERMINOLOGY

Abbreviations and Synonyms

- Well-differentiated thyroid cancer (WDTC)
- Medullary thyroid carcinoma (MTC)
- Anaplastic thyroid carcinoma

Definitions

- **WDTC:** Carcinoma of the thyroid arising from papillary &/or follicular cell origin
- **MTC:** Uncommon malignant neuroendocrine neoplasm arising from thyroid parafollicular "C cells"
- **Anaplastic:** Aggressive form of mostly undifferentiated cells

IMAGING FINDINGS

General Features

- Best diagnostic clue
  - **WDTC**
    - Non-physiologic, focal, asymmetric uptake of FDG
    - However, many WDTC may not be FDG avid when iodine avid
  - **MTC**
    - Solid, low attenuating, discrete thyroid masses with punctate calcification and nodal mets
  - **Anaplastic**
    - Diffuse, intense FDG activity correlating with an infiltrative thyroid mass
- Location
  - **WDTC**
    - Primary and recurrent disease arise mostly in the parenchyma and bed of the thyroid gland
    - Metastatic disease travels to cervical/mediastinal lymph nodes and then to bone, lungs, and mediastinum
    - Papillary: Lymphatic invasion and spread to multifocal nodal regions
    - Follicular: Hematogenous spread to lung and bone
  - **MTC**
    - Intraglandular
    - Often multifocal and bilateral (2/3 sporadic, almost 100% familial)
    - Lymph nodes: Level VI and superior mediastinal; also retropharyngeal and levels III & IV
  - **Anaplastic**
    - May involve the entire thyroid gland

DDx: FDG Activity in Thyroid

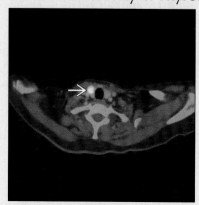

Adenoma

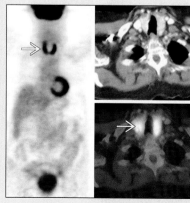

Physiologic

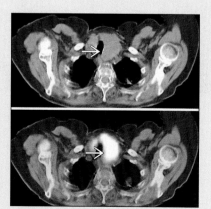

Multinodular Goiter

THYROID CANCER

Key Facts

Terminology
- Well-differentiated thyroid cancer (WDTC)
- Medullary thyroid carcinoma (MTC)
- Anaplastic thyroid carcinoma

Imaging Findings
- WDTC: Focal asymmetrically increased uptake on FDG PET (not due to normal structure or inflammatory condition)
- MTC: Solid lesions in thyroid gland with nodal metastases; ± calcifications
- I-123 or I-131 whole body scan when tumor is iodine avid
- FDG PET scan for non-iodine-avid tumor
- Considerations for IV contrast for PET/CT; need to know if patient will be treated with radioactive iodine

Top Differential Diagnoses
- Benign Thyroid Conditions
- Other Cancers of Head and Neck
- Normal/Benign Extrathyroidal Structures
- Multinodular Goiter (MNG)
- Follicular Adenoma
- Reactive Lymph Nodes
- Thyroid Non-Hodgkin Lymphoma (NHL)

Diagnostic Checklist
- Perform FDG PET and PET/CT in all patients with
  - History of WDTC
  - Status post thyroidectomy
  - Negative I-131 study
  - Rising thyroglobulin
- FDG uptake may be modest (SUV 2-3) in recurrent/residual thyroid cancer

---

- Early metastatic disease
- Size
  - **WDTC**
    - Often diffuse microscopic disease
    - Lymph node and pulmonary metastases may be below limits of detection
    - Metastases to bone, in contrast, may grow very large
  - **MTC**
    - Up to 2.5 cm
  - **Anaplastic**
    - Bulky
- Morphology
  - **WDTC**
    - Typical lymph node findings of roundedness and calcification may be absent
    - Differentiate from typical thymus morphology (variable by age)
    - Skeletal metastases typically lytic
  - **MTC**
    - Solid, nonencapsulated mass
    - Calcification in larger tumors
    - May be infiltrative in familial forms

Imaging Recommendations
- Best imaging tool
  - Ultrasound for initial evaluation of all thyroid masses with fine needle aspiration
  - **WDTC**
    - For iodine-avid disease: Diagnosis, staging, and follow-up best performed with I-123 or I-131 whole body scan
    - For non-iodine-avid tumor, FDG PET/CT is superior
  - **MTC**
    - Consider FDG PET/CT for staging and restaging
    - Current insurance coverage restrictions for MTC
  - **Anaplastic**
    - Most are intensely FDG avid, but there are current insurance coverage limitations
- Protocol advice
  - **General**

- Iodine scan: Withdrawal or thyrogen-stimulated
- Mediastinal lymph nodes near heart may be blurred due to motion, leading to false negatives
  - **FDG PET**
    - Thyroid-stimulating hormone (TSH) elevation/administration improves performance
    - Considerations for IV contrast for PET/CT; need to know if patient will be treated with radioactive iodine
    - Increased thyrocyte metabolism, glucose transport, hexokinase I levels, and overall glycolysis contribute to specific FDG uptake
    - Hormone withdrawal and administration of recombinant TSH (rhTSH = thyrogen)
    - Thyrogen dosage schedule not established, but Medicare pays for two injections
    - Recommended dosing: 0.9 g IM on day 1 and day 2, and FDG PET on day 3, 4, or 5
  - **Correlative tests**
    - Thyroglobulin measurement also best with elevated TSH
    - Serum thyroglobulin (Tg)
    - Correlate with radioiodine scan
    - Insensitive in presence of anti-Tg antibodies
    - Elevated levels post-therapy indicate residual thyroid tissue (> 2.0 ng/mL)

CT Findings
- WDTC
  - Normal thyroid findings include
    - Cystic changes (hypodense)
    - Calcifications (hyperdense)
    - Well-defined borders
  - Primary tumor
    - Typically highly variable morphology
    - May mimic normal gland
    - Low attenuation nodule within gland
    - May have dystrophic calcifications
  - Signs of more aggressive tumor
    - Large size
    - Diffuse infiltration
    - Ill-defined, heterogeneous morphology

THYROID CANCER

- Extension to surrounding tissues
  - Lymph node appearance also highly variable
    - Large to small (may appear as benign reactive nodes)
    - Solid to heterogeneous/hemorrhagic to cystic
    - Variable calcification
    - Isolated retropharyngeal nodal metastasis may occur
- **MTC**
  - Solid, low density, well-circumscribed mass in thyroid
  - Multifocality more common in familial types
  - Calcification in tumor and involved lymph nodes may be fine and punctate
  - Bone metastases typically lytic
- **Anaplastic**
  - Large infiltrative mass

Nuclear Medicine Findings

- **WDTC**
  - No current indication for pre-operative PET or PET/CT staging of WDTC
  - Consider in patients with anaplastic thyroid carcinoma for staging, although not covered by Medicare
  - Currently covered by Medicare for patients with
    - Documented history of follicular origin WDTC
    - Status post-thyroidectomy
    - Radioactive I-131 therapy
    - Current elevation in serum thyroglobulin
    - Negative I-131 whole-body scan
  - Consider performing FDG PET or PET/CT in all patients with these parameters
  - WDTC normally demonstrates mild to moderate FDG uptake (mean SUV ~ 2.5 at 60 min)
    - When iodine avid, may not have any FDG uptake
  - Elevated TSH may result in double the SUV of WDTC vs. suppressed state
    - Best with stimulated thyroglobulin > 10 mU/L
  - Invaluable for identifying recurrence and metastases in soft tissue, lymph nodes, liver, lungs, and bone
    - Many of these lesions not visible or detected prospectively by CT
  - FDG PET can follow a negative I-131 or I-123 whole-body scan in patients with elevated thyroglobulin (Tg)
    - 15-20% of patients with WDTC and high serum thyroglobulin have negative diagnostic I-131 whole-body scans
    - I-131 or I-123 whole-body scan should be performed prior to injection of FDG if both scans are performed on same day
    - Small deposits may produce false negatives on I-131 scan
    - Metastases tend to become more aggressive and FDG avid as they dedifferentiate and lose ability to concentrate I-131
    - 15% of these patients have persistent, recurrent, or metastatic disease
    - Generally 75% or better sensitivities for local recurrences and distant metastases
    - PET/CT imaging has diagnostic value regardless of thyroglobulin level

- Use of TSH to increase uptake by thyroid tissue is controversial, but has been shown to be effective in some studies
- Non-iodine-avid recurrence: FDG PET may help identify areas amenable to surgical removal
- **MTC**
  - MTC has low avidity for iodine, making radioiodine imaging and therapy ineffective
    - FDG PET effective for detection of disease
  - FDG PET improves detection of suspected recurrent disease undetectable by CT/MR
    - Elevated tumor markers, but no gross disease on cross-sectional imaging
    - Sensitivity 70-100%, specificity 79-90%
    - Poorer sensitivity for liver and lung foci, especially when < 1 cm
    - Controversy exists as to whether PET can reliably assess recurrent, persistent MTC
    - May be significant overlap of serum calcitonin levels between positive and negative FDG PET scans
    - Elevated calcitonin not specific; can be elevated in conditions such as CRI
    - I-123-PET/CT combined with FDG PET/CT allows localization of both foci of highly specific I-123 uptake and iodine-negative tumors

Other Modality Findings

- **I-123 or I-131 whole-body scan**
  - Tumors may become less well differentiated and lose iodine avidity
  - Whole-body scan may appear normal despite extensive metastatic disease
  - I-123 scans miss metastases in bone, lungs, and lymph nodes
- **I-131 scintigraphy and serial thyroglobulin measurements**
  - Used after near/total thyroidectomy and ablation
  - Standard method to detect differentiated thyroid cancer recurrence
  - Thyroglobulin threshold of 10 ng/mL commonly used as cutoff for suspicion of recurrence
    - Anti-thyroglobulin antibodies may lead to falsely low levels of measured serum thyroglobulin
- **Surveillance imaging following I-131 typically performed with high resolution US**
  - FNA can be performed at time of exam
  - FDG PET for suspicion of recurrence in sites inaccessible by US

DIFFERENTIAL DIAGNOSIS

Benign Thyroid Conditions

- 50% of FDG-avid nodules are benign (usually follicular adenoma [FA])
  - FA: Solitary mass without adenopathy or evidence of invasion
- Incidentally identified FDG-avid nodules should be biopsied, as 50% are malignant
- Multinodular goiter: Diffusely enlarged gland with multiple nodules and coarse calcifications

THYROID CANCER

Thyroid Non-Hodgkin Lymphoma (NHL)
- Infiltrating mass associated with diffuse enlargement of gland
- Calcification in mass or LN rare

Parathyroid Adenoma
- May present with similar features to thyroid carcinoma on FDG PET
- Usually extrathyroidal

Other Cancers of Head and Neck
- Anaplastic thyroid cancer
- Thyroid lymphoma
- Squamous cell carcinoma
- Neuroendocrine tumors
- Metastatic disease

Normal/Benign Extrathyroidal Structures
- Asymmetrical muscle uptake
  o Minimize activity and agitation (benzodiazepine useful)
  o Reschedule examination in hyperglycemic patients (> 200 mg/dL)
  o Provide comfortable support of head/neck
- Vocal cords and cricoarytenoids
  o Minimize talking, activity, and agitation during FDG uptake period
  o Unilateral vocal cord paralysis (surgery, invasion) can cause asymmetric uptake
- Tonsillar and adenoid tissue
  o FDG uptake observed due to inflammatory activity
  o Obtain careful history of recent illness and allergies
- Reactive lymph nodes
  o Correlate with presence of enhanced tonsillar FDG uptake, recent illness
- Salivary glands
  o Treatment with I-131 may lead to asymmetric salivary gland uptake
  o Accessory sites of salivary tissue may be difficult to distinguish from lymph nodes
- Cervical spine arthritis
  o Due to degeneration or rheumatic disease
  o Focal uptake in facet joints may mimic metastatic disease
- Tracheostomy sites

PATHOLOGY

General Features
- General path comments
  o WDTC
    ▪ Follicular thyroid cancer characterized by purely follicular or trabecular growth without papillary structures
    ▪ Has fibrous capsule, known to invade blood vessels (differentiating it from adenoma)
    ▪ Lymphatic spread less common but distant metastases more frequent
    ▪ Oncocytic thyroid cancer behaves as a slightly more aggressive form of follicular cancer
  o MTC

- ▪ Arises from calcitonin-secreting parafollicular "C cells" of thyroid
  o **Anaplastic**
    ▪ Generally found in elderly patients
    ▪ WDTC may dedifferentiate to become anaplastic
    ▪ Tumors usually fixed and difficult to delineate on physical exam
    ▪ Anaplastic thyroid cancer almost never iodine avid and uncommonly makes thyroglobulin
    ▪ Almost always FDG avid
- Genetics
  o WDTC
    ▪ Generally sporadic
    ▪ Higher incidence with family history and Gardner syndrome
  o MTC
    ▪ Most cases sporadic (85%)
    ▪ 15% of cases related to family history
    ▪ RET oncogene found in 100% of family and 50% of sporadic cases
  o **Multiple endocrine neoplasia (MEN)**
    ▪ Autosomal dominant
    ▪ Type 2A: Multifocal MTC, pheochromocytoma, parathyroid hyperplasia, hyperparathyroidism
    ▪ Type 2B: Multifocal MTC, pheochromocytoma, mucosal neuromas of lips, tongue, GI tract, conjunctiva (younger patients, more aggressive course)
  o **Familial medullary thyroid carcinoma (FMTC)**
    ▪ Autosomal dominant disease giving rise only to MTC
    ▪ Less aggressive and later onset than MEN syndromes
- Etiology
  o WDTC
    ▪ Relationship between high level of TSH and development of thyroid cancer not established
    ▪ Cancer commonly develops in goitrous thyroid
    ▪ Ionizing radiation results in 30% risk of thyroid cancer
    ▪ Iodine deficiency
  o MTC
    ▪ No external risk factors identified
    ▪ Unrelated to other thyroid conditions
  o **Anaplastic**
    ▪ Unknown
- Epidemiology
  o Frequency of thyroid cancer subtypes
    ▪ Papillary = 80% of all thyroid cancers
    ▪ Follicular = 12.6%
    ▪ Medullary = 3.6%
    ▪ Oncocytic (Hürthle cell) = 2.9%
    ▪ Anaplastic/undifferentiated = 1.7%
  o Papillary often presents after significant latency period (20-30 years)
  o 30,000 new cases of thyroid cancer diagnosed each year in USA
    ▪ Estimated 1,500 deaths per year
  o MTC
    ▪ Accounts for 5-10% of all thyroid cancer
    ▪ ~ 14% of all thyroid cancer death
    ▪ 10% pediatric thyroid malignancies (MEN 2)

THYROID CANCER

Gross Pathologic & Surgical Features
- Papillary: Firm, whitish, irregular mass that is not encapsulated
  - Ill-defined margins and absence of encapsulation
- Follicular: Brown, solitary, encapsulated mass
  - Often found in areas of fibrosis, hemorrhage, and cystic change
- MTC
  - Roughly textured, well-circumscribed, solid white/pink nodule
  - Nonencapsulated
  - Calcification, necrosis, hemorrhage in larger lesions

Microscopic Features
- Most thyroid cancer looks similar to normal thyroid histopathologically
  - May also trap iodine and secrete thyroglobulin
- Papillary
  - Multifocal
  - Complete or partial neoplastic epithelial papillae
  - Complex arborization into lymphatics
  - Empty ground-glass appearance of nuclei
- Follicular
  - Well-defined neoplastic follicles containing colloid
    - Difficult to distinguish from follicular adenoma
  - Identification of vascular invasion may require specialized stains
- MTC
  - Important diagnostic feature is strong staining for calcitonin in 80% of cases
  - No increased expression of GLUT 1-5, responsible for glucose/FDG uptake
  - Nests of atypical round or ovoid cells with granular cytoplasm
  - Fibrovascular stroma, hyalinized collagen, and amyloid separates cells

CLINICAL ISSUES

Presentation
- Most common signs/symptoms
  - Painless palpable mass at base of neck
    - Pain is an uncommon presenting symptom
- Other signs/symptoms
  - WDTC
    - Persistent cough or dyspnea
    - Hoarseness, dysphagia
    - Pain from bone metastases
    - Signs of venous obstruction
  - MTC
    - Similar to WDTC: Dysphagia, hoarseness, pain
    - Paraneoplastic syndromes (Cushing, carcinoid) may uncommonly present
    - Up to 75% have lymphadenopathy at presentation
  - Elevated serum calcitonin
    - Diarrhea is an associated symptom
    - Allow monitoring and estimation of disease extent
  - Bone pain and elevation in alkaline phosphatase should prompt bone scan
- Clinical profiles

- Patient with family history of MEN has tumor found on screening exam
- Middle-aged patient with lower neck mass

Demographics
- Age
  - WDTC
    - Papillary: Most common 30-40 years
    - Follicular: Most common 40-70 years
    - Occurs over wide age range, including pediatric population
    - Most common after age 30, and aggressiveness increases significantly in older patients
  - MTC
    - Sporadic cases occur at mean age of 50 years
    - Familial cases occur at a younger age; mean 30 years
    - Children may present with thyroid cancer, especially with MEN 2B
- Gender
  - WDTC
    - Female predominance: M:F = 1:3

Natural History & Prognosis
- WDTC
  - Worse prognosis
    - Patients with intense FDG activity have a poorer prognosis than those with more mild FDG uptake
    - Tumor size > 2.5 cm
    - Evidence of extension, invasion, and metastasis
    - Extracervical disease is rarely curable
    - Young or old age group (before 20, after 45)
    - 8% of patients with recurrence will die of the disease
  - Survival
    - 96% of patients are curable with current strategies
  - 10 year survival
    - 96% of papillary cases
    - 85% of follicular
    - 75% of Hürthle cell
    - 14% of anaplastic
- MTC
  - Overall 10 year survival: 56%
    - 90% when confined to gland
    - 70% when in cervical lymph nodes
    - 20% when in distant sites
    - Age younger than 40 years confers better prognosis
  - Overall 5 year survival: 72%
  - Sporadic and inherited forms have same outcome, except for MEN-2B, which has poorer prognosis
    - MEN-related MTC has higher incidence of recurrence
  - Better prognosis
    - Tumor < 10 cm, no nodes, early stage disease
    - Young age and female gender
    - FMTC and MEN 2A syndromes

Treatment
- WDTC
  - Primary < 2.5 cm has excellent prognosis
    - Controversial whether definitive surgery and radioiodine ablation is necessary

- Long-term thyroglobulin assessment is facilitated by ablation of remnant with ~ 30 mCi I-131
  - o Levothyroxine to suppress TSH below 0.01 mU/L
  - o Bone metastases treated with external beam radiation
  - o In 20% of cases, retinoids (Roaccutan)
    - Lead to redifferentiation in thyroid carcinomas
    - Re-induce radioiodine uptake in dedifferentiated tumor cells
    - Induce apoptosis and have growth-inhibiting effects
- MTC
  - o Complete resection of local and regional disease is current standard of care
    - MTC is not iodine avid and cannot be imaged or ablated with I-131
    - Total thyroidectomy with level VI nodal dissection ± superior mediastinal nodes
  - o Detection of familial RET mutation prompts prophylactic thyroidectomy
    - Age 5-6 for FMTC and MEN 2A
    - Infancy for MEN 2B
  - o Adjuvant radiation therapy
    - Radiotherapy has limited utility
    - Indicated for extensive soft tissue invasion or extracapsular nodal spread

DIAGNOSTIC CHECKLIST

Consider
- Perform FDG PET and PET/CT in all patients with
  - o History of WDTC
  - o Status post thyroidectomy
  - o Negative I-131 study
  - o Rising thyroglobulin
- Screen family members in thyroid cancer with suspected genetic association

Image Interpretation Pearls
- WDTC
  - o FDG uptake may be modest (SUV 2-3) in recurrent/residual thyroid cancer
  - o TSH stimulation may aid diagnosis
- MTC
  - o May be indistinguishable from WDTC on imaging
  - o PET/CT for detection of local/distant recurrence

SELECTED REFERENCES

1. Al-Nahhas A et al: Review. 18F-FDG PET in the diagnosis and follow-up of thyroid malignancy. In Vivo. 22(1):109-14, 2008
2. Alzahrani AS et al: The role of F-18-fluorodeoxyglucose positron emission tomography in the postoperative evaluation of differentiated thyroid cancer. Eur J Endocrinol. 158(5):683-9, 2008
3. Davison JM et al: The added benefit of a dedicated neck F-18 FDG PET-CT imaging protocol in patients with suspected recurrent differentiated thyroid carcinoma. Clin Nucl Med. 33(7):464-8, 2008
4. Freudenberg LS et al: Combined metabolic and morphologic imaging in thyroid carcinoma patients with elevated serum thyroglobulin and negative cervical ultrasonography: role of 124I-PET/CT and FDG-PET. Eur J Nucl Med Mol Imaging. 35(5):950-7, 2008
5. Grant CS et al: The value of positron emission tomography in the surgical management of recurrent papillary thyroid carcinoma. World J Surg. 32(5):708-15, 2008
6. Kloos RT: Approach to the patient with a positive serum thyroglobulin and a negative radioiodine scan after initial therapy for differentiated thyroid cancer. J Clin Endocrinol Metab. 93(5):1519-25, 2008
7. Palmedo H et al: PET and PET/CT in thyroid cancer. Recent Results Cancer Res. 170:59-70, 2008
8. Rubello D et al: The role of 18F-FDG PET/CT in detecting metastatic deposits of recurrent medullary thyroid carcinoma: a prospective study. Eur J Surg Oncol. 34(5):581-6, 2008
9. Rufini V et al: Role of PET in medullary thyroid carcinoma. Minerva Endocrinol. 33(2):67-73, 2008
10. Rutherford GC et al: Nuclear medicine in the assessment of differentiated thyroid cancer. Clin Radiol. 63(4):453-63, 2008
11. Smith RB et al: Preoperative FDG-PET imaging to assess the malignant potential of follicular neoplasms of the thyroid. Otolaryngol Head Neck Surg. 138(1):101-6, 2008
12. Zuijdwijk MD et al: Utility of fluorodeoxyglucose-PET in patients with differentiated thyroid carcinoma. Nucl Med Commun. 29(7):636-41, 2008
13. Are C et al: FDG-PET detected thyroid incidentalomas: need for further investigation? Ann Surg Oncol. 14(1):239-47, 2007
14. Freudenberg LS et al: Dual-modality FDG-PET/CT in follow-up of patients with recurrent iodine-negative differentiated thyroid cancer. Eur Radiol. 17(12):3139-47, 2007
15. Hall NC et al: PET imaging in differentiated thyroid cancer: where does it fit and how do we use it? Arq Bras Endocrinol Metabol. 51(5):793-805, 2007
16. Iagaru A et al: Detection of occult medullary thyroid cancer recurrence with 2-deoxy-2-[F-18]fluoro-D-glucose-PET and PET/CT. Mol Imaging Biol. 9(2):72-7, 2007
17. Mirallié E et al: Therapeutic impact of 18FDG-PET/CT in the management of iodine-negative recurrence of differentiated thyroid carcinoma. Surgery. 142(6):952-8; discussion 952-8, 2007
18. Toubert ME et al: Distant metastases of differentiated thyroid cancer: diagnosis, treatment and outcome. Nucl Med Rev Cent East Eur. 10(2):106-9, 2007
19. Gotthardt M et al: Improved tumour detection by gastrin receptor scintigraphy in patients with metastasised medullary thyroid carcinoma. Eur J Nucl Med Mol Imaging. 33(11):1273-9, 2006

THYROID CANCER

CT Findings: Thyroid Carcinoma

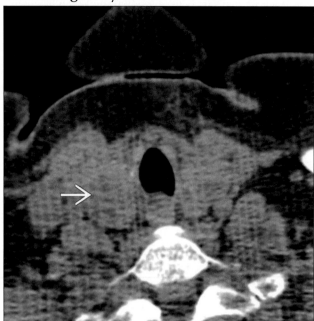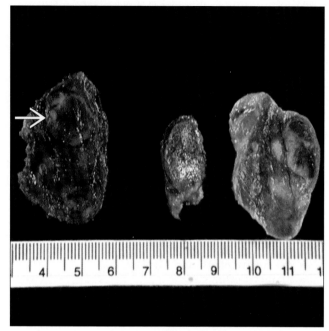

(Left) Axial NECT shows bilateral thyroid enlargement with a subtle low attenuation nodule in the right lobe ➡. Although the overall appearance is compatible with a multinodular goiter, a subsequent ultrasound and FNA revealed WDTC correlating with the right lobe nodule. *(Right)* Gross pathology surgical specimen shows multiple nodules within both thyroid lobes, as well as the right lobe nodule ➡ that was proven to be thyroid carcinoma.

PET/CT Findings: Incidental Thyroid Carcinoma

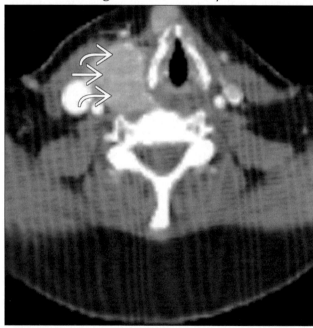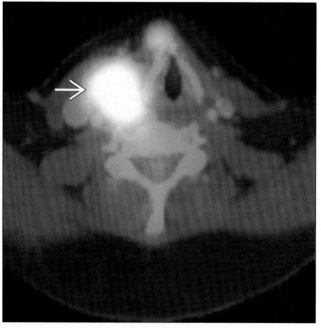

(Left) Axial CECT shows an enlarged right lobe of the thyroid ➡ with 2 subtle low attenuation masses ➡ in this patient who underwent PET/CT for solitary pulmonary nodule evaluation. A subsequent ultrasound-guided biopsy of the thyroid mass showed papillary carcinoma. *(Right)* Axial fused PET/CT shows diffusely increased FDG activity within the enlarged right lobe of the thyroid ➡, biopsy-proven to be thyroid carcinoma.

THYROID CANCER

PET/CT Findings: Incident Thyroid Carcinoma

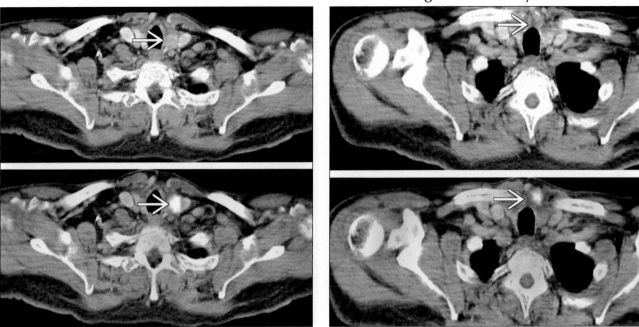

(Left) Axial CT (top) and fused PET/CT (bottom) show asymmetrical focal FDG activity within the left lobe of the thyroid ➡. Subsequent biopsy identified this as thyroid carcinoma. *(Right)* Axial CT (top) and fused PET/CT (bottom) show a focal area of increased metabolic activity anterior to the trachea ➡ in this patient with subsequently diagnosed thyroid cancer. This finding is compatible with nodal metastasis.

PET/CT Findings: Restaging Thyroid Carcinoma

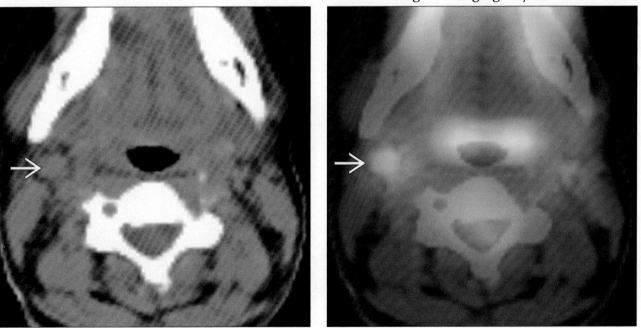

(Left) Axial NECT shows a borderline enlarged lymph node in the right neck ➡ in a patient with a history of well-differentiated primary carcinoma, status post thyroidectomy with rising thyroglobulin levels and a negative iodine study. *(Right)* Axial fused PET/CT in the same patient shows mildly increased FDG activity corresponding to the right neck node ➡. Subsequent resection revealed recurrent carcinoma.

THYROID CANCER

PET/CT Findings: Restaging Thyroid Carcinoma

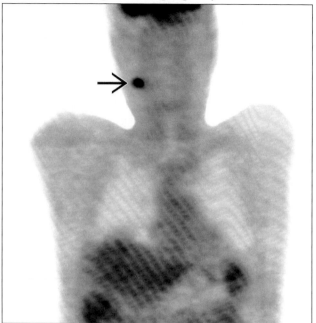
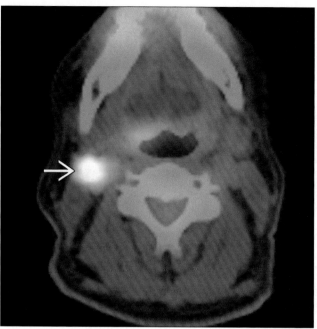

(Left) Coronal PET shows a focal area of intense FDG activity in the right neck ➡ in a patient with a history of thyroid carcinoma. *(Right)* Axial fused PET/CT shows intense FDG activity correlating to a borderline enlarged right neck node ➡, compatible with recurrent metastatic thyroid carcinoma.

PET/CT Findings: Restaging Thyroid Carcinoma

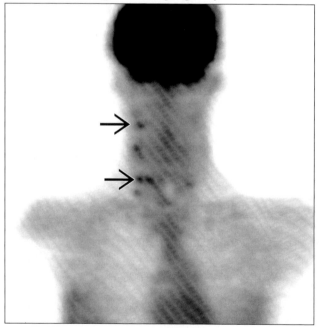
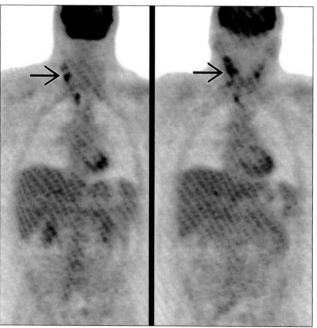

(Left) Coronal PET in a patient with a negative CT scan two weeks prior demonstrates multifocal areas of increased metabolic activity in the right neck ➡, compatible with recurrent thyroid carcinoma. *(Right)* Coronal PET shows multiple focal areas of intense metabolic activity within cervical lymph node chains bilaterally ➡ in this patient with a history of thyroid cancer and rising thyroglobulin level. The findings are compatible with recurrent malignancy.

THYROID CANCER

PET/CT Findings: Restaging Thyroid Carcinoma

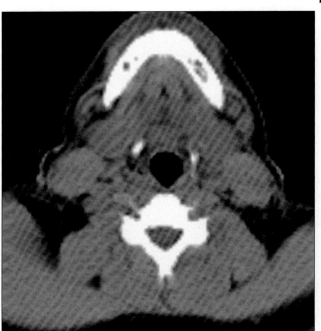 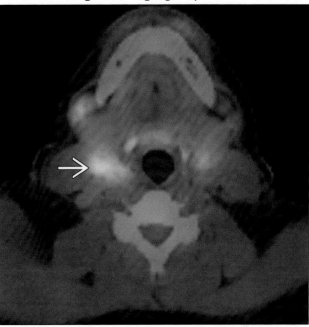

(Left) Axial NECT shows no definite evidence for malignancy. This image demonstrates a few nonenlarged bilateral cervical nodes. (Right) Axial fused PET/CT shows increased minimal activity within a right level 2 lymph node ➡, compatible with recurrent disease.

PET/CT Findings: Restaging Thyroid Carcinoma

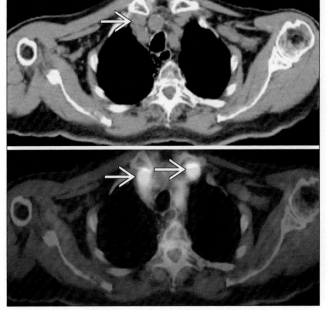 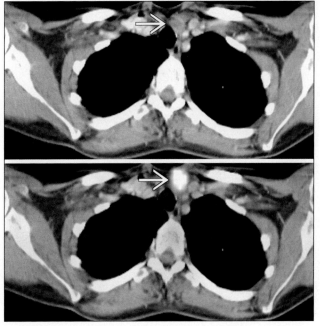

(Left) Axial CT (top) and fused PET/CT (bottom) show 2 focal areas of intense FDG activity posterior to the clavicular heads ➡ in a patient with a history of thyroid carcinoma, rising thyroglobulin levels, and a negative iodine study. These findings are compatible with recurrent thyroid carcinoma. (Right) Axial CT (top) and fused PET/CT (bottom) show a focal area of recurrent metastatic thyroid carcinoma to the left of the trachea in the thyroidectomy bed ➡ in this patient with a history of thyroid carcinoma and rising thyroglobulin levels.

THYROID CANCER

PET/CT Findings: Restaging Thyroid Carcinoma

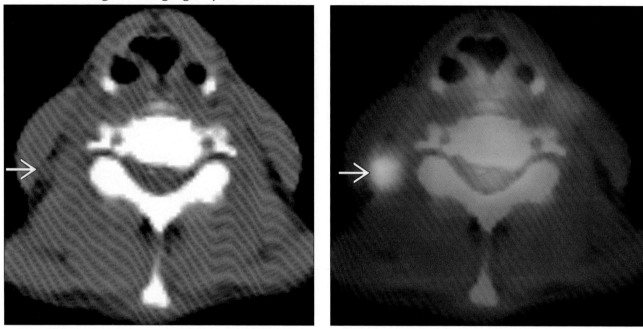

(Left) Axial NECT shows a normal-sized right neck node ➡ that was not prospectively identified as suspicious for malignancy. *(Right)* Axial fused PET/CT shows moderately increased FDG activity corresponding to the normal-sized right neck node ➡, compatible with recurrent disease.

PET/CT Findings: Restaging Thyroid Carcinoma

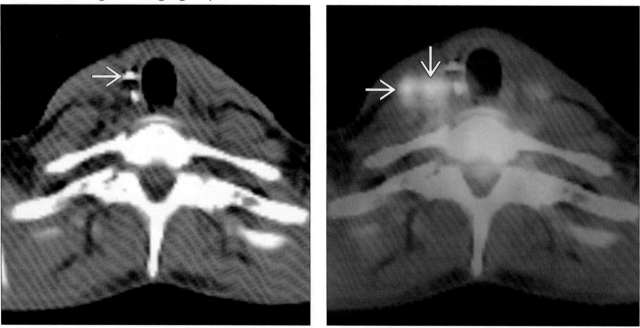

(Left) Axial NECT shows post-operative changes compatible with a prior thyroidectomy ➡ and small scattered lymph nodes, none of which are suspicious by CT criteria. *(Right)* Axial fused PET/CT shows multiple foci of increased metabolic activity corresponding to the small normal-sized right cervical lymph nodes ➡, compatible with recurrent malignancy.

THYROID CANCER

PET/CT Findings: Restaging Thyroid Carcinoma

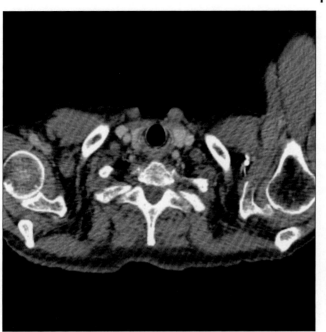 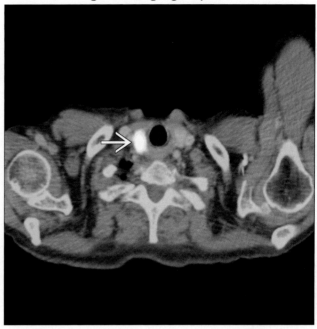

(Left) Axial CECT shows no definite abnormality. *(Right)* Combined PET/CT through the same level shows FDG hypermetabolism ⮕ in the right thyroid lobe.

PET/CT Findings: Restaging Thyroid Carcinoma

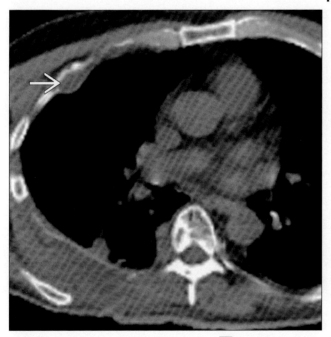 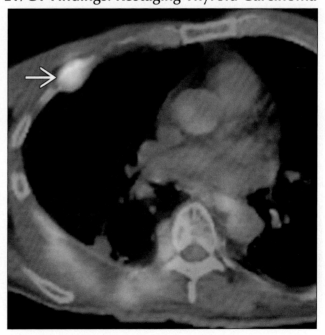

(Left) Axial NECT shows a pleural-based lesion ⮕ in this patient with a history of thyroid carcinoma, worrisome for metastatic disease. *(Right)* Axial fused PET/CT shows focally increased overall activity within the pleural-based lesion ⮕, compatible with recurrent thyroid carcinoma.

THYROID CANCER

PET/CT Findings: Restaging Thyroid Carcinoma

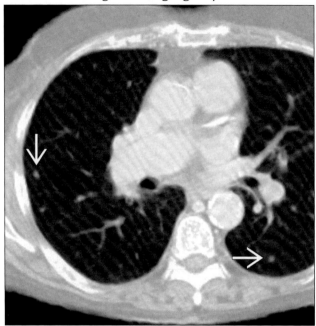 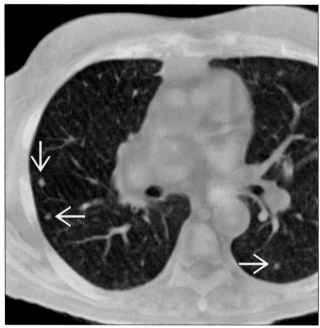

(Left) Axial CECT shows multiple subcentimeter pulmonary nodules ➡ that were not present on a CT scan 3 months earlier. This patient has a history of thyroid carcinoma and rising thyroglobulin levels, but negative iodine scan. *(Right)* Axial fused PET/CT shows no definite increased metabolic activity corresponding to the small pulmonary nodules ➡. Because all of the nodules are below the level of resolution of the PET camera, they should nonetheless be viewed with suspicion.

PET/CT Findings: Restaging Thyroid Carcinoma

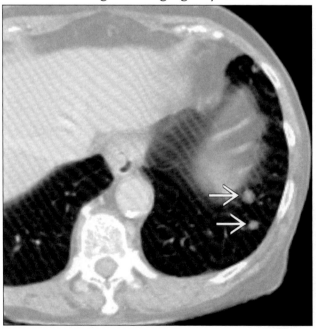 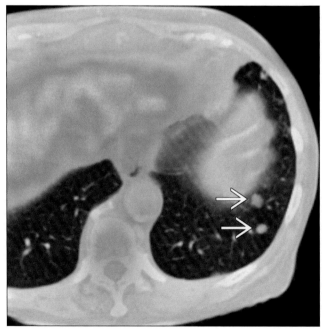

(Left) Axial CECT shows 2 left lower lobe pulmonary nodules ➡, approximately 1 cm each, in a patient with history of thyroid carcinoma and rising thyroglobulin levels. *(Right)* Axial fused PET/CT shows minimally increased FDG activity within the left lower lobe pulmonary nodules ➡, subsequently proven via biopsy to be metastatic thyroid carcinoma.

THYROID CANCER

PET/CT Findings: Anaplastic Thyroid Carcinoma

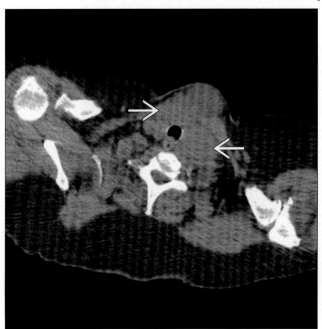 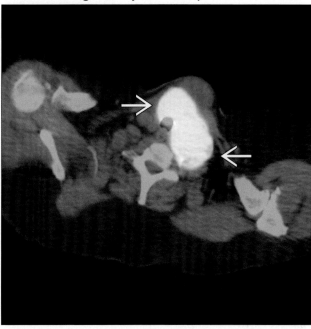

(Left) Axial NECT shows an enlarged thyroid anterior to the trachea ➡. *(Right)* Axial fused PET/CT shows that the enlarged thyroid has intense, diffuse FDG uptake ➡. Subsequent biopsy revealed anaplastic thyroid carcinoma.

PET/CT Findings: Anaplastic Thyroid Carcinoma

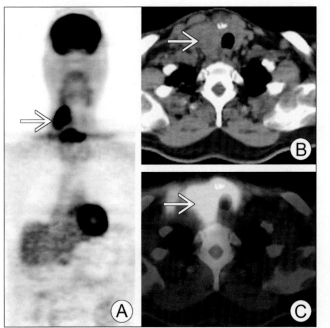 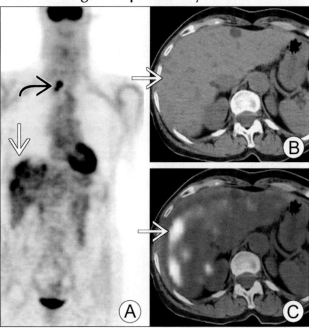

(Left) Coronal PET (A), axial CT (B) and fused PET/CT (C) demonstrate markedly increased FDG activity throughout the thyroid gland ➡. Subsequent biopsy demonstrated anaplastic thyroid carcinoma. *(Right)* Coronal PET (A), axial CT (B) and fused PET/CT (C) in a patient with a history of anaplastic thyroid carcinoma show disease in the thyroidectomy bed ➡ as well as multiple hepatic lesions ➡ with increased metabolic activity, compatible with hepatic metastases.

SOLITARY PULMONARY NODULES

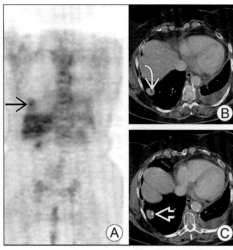

Coronal PET (A) shows increased FDG activity in a right lower lobe pulmonary nodule ➡ with areas of fat ➡ and calcification ➡ on axial CT (B, C), compatible with a hamartoma.

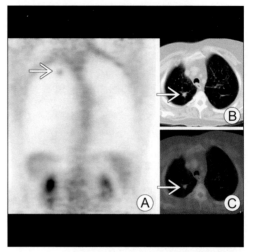

Axial CECT (B) shows an 8 mm spiculated adenocarcinoma ➡, which demonstrates only mildly increased FDG activity on coronal PET (A) and axial fused PET/CT (C).

TERMINOLOGY

Abbreviations and Synonyms
- Solitary pulmonary nodule (SPN)
- Bronchioloalveolar carcinoma (BAC)

Definitions
- Opacity in the lung parenchyma measuring up to 3 cm
  - Usually no associated mediastinal adenopathy or atelectasis

IMAGING FINDINGS

General Features
- Best diagnostic clue
  - **High suspicion for malignancy**
    - Any detectable FDG activity higher than background (> mediastinal blood pool) for SPN < 1.5 cm
    - SUV > 2.5 in any nodule
    - Spiculated morphology, particularly with a history of smoking
  - **Low suspicion for malignancy**
    - Round nodule with dense calcification and uniform morphology
    - FDG uptake equal to background activity
- Location
  - No regional pattern for benign nodules
  - 2/3 of primary lung tumors arise in upper lobes
  - SPN from extrapulmonary primary most often located in outer 1/3 of lower lobes
- Size
  - Definition: Nodule < 3.0 cm < mass
  - Larger SPN more likely malignant
    - Over 85% are cancer when larger than 2.0 cm
  - Growth rate
    - 26% increase in diameter corresponds to a doubling of the nodule's volume
    - Time to 26% increase in diameter = one doubling time
    - Most cancer doubling times: ~ 30-200 day range
    - Nodule dimension stability: > 2 years highly suggestive that nodule is benign
    - Increase in size seen within 30 days suggestive of infection, infarction, lymphoma, fast-growing metastases

DDx: FDG Avid Solitary Pulmonary Nodule

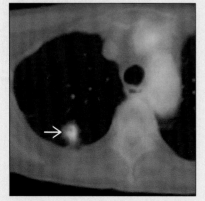

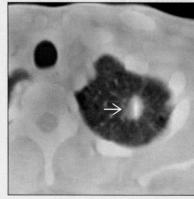

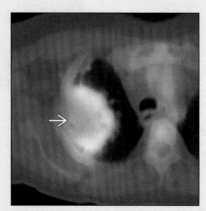

| *Infection: Tuberculosis* | *Malignancy: Metastasis* | *Inflammation: Pseudotumor* |

SOLITARY PULMONARY NODULES

Key Facts

Terminology
- Solitary pulmonary nodule (SPN)
  - Opacity in the lung parenchyma measuring up to 3 cm with no associated mediastinal adenopathy or atelectasis

Imaging Findings
- Risk of malignancy highest when nodule has SUV > 2.5 and spiculated morphology
- PET/CT superior to CT or PET alone for overall accuracy
- Nodules with internal calcifications generally benign
- Central calcification is characteristic of benign nodules
- Dual-time point imaging may be helpful in differentiating benign from malignant pulmonary nodules

Top Differential Diagnoses
- Metastasis
- Infection
- Granulomatous Disease
- Benign Lesions
- Pulmonary Infarct

Pathology
- Granuloma is the most common entity accounting for SPN

Diagnostic Checklist
- Continued CT follow-up in PET-negative SPN
- If nodule has features of BAC, a negative PET does not rule out malignancy
- Predictive value of stability in size over time of a SPN is only 65%

- Morphology
  - **Benign characteristics**
    - Margin: Well-circumscribed with smooth borders
    - Density: Fat or water density
    - Calcification: Common
    - Cavitation: Wall thickness < 5 mm
    - Enhancement: Usually minimal
    - Ground-glass opacity (suggests inflammation)
    - Air-fluid level (abscess)
    - Satellite nodules: Common in granulomatous lesions
  - **Malignant characteristics**
    - Margin: Irregular, lobulated, ill-defined with spiculated borders
    - Density: Soft tissue density
    - Calcification: 10% demonstrate calcification that is usually peripheral and stippled
    - Cavitation: Present in 80% of cavitary lung cancers (e.g., squamous cell carcinoma)
    - BAC may appear entirely as ground-glass opacity
    - Enhancement: More prominent
    - Spiculation highly specific for malignancy
    - Up to 20% of smooth nodules with sharp margins are malignant (e.g., carcinoid)
    - Air bronchogram: Present in 25-65% of cancers
    - Pseudocavitation: Common to malignancies such as BAC
    - Wall thickness > 1.5 cm strongly suggestive of malignancy

Imaging Recommendations
- Best imaging tool: PET/CT demonstrates superior accuracy to CT or PET alone
- Protocol advice
  - Dual-time point imaging may be helpful in differentiating benign from malignant pulmonary nodules
    - Malignant nodules gain intensity between hour 1 and hour 2
    - Benign nodules decrease in intensity

Radiographic Findings
- Chest X-rays (CXR) helpful for determining time course of nodule development
  - Little change over 2 years or longer is strongly suggestive of a benign process
- 1-2 SPN detected per 1,000 CXR, routine screening radiographs
  - CXR has low sensitivity for detection of subcentimeter noncalcified nodules

CT Findings
- **Indications**
  - Accurate localization of nodule (intra-/extrapulmonary)
  - Detection of additional unsuspected nodules
  - Characterization of margin, density, and calcification patterns
  - Assessment of extrapulmonary involvement (lymph nodes, pleura, chest wall, liver, adrenals, etc.)
- **Malignant morphology**
  - CT may misclassify 25-40% of nodules as benign based on morphologic characteristics
    - BAC and lymphoma, for example, often appear benign
  - Coarse spiculation and bronchovascular bundle thickening around tumor
    - More common in presence of vessel invasion &/or lymph node metastasis
  - Heterogeneous internal composition
  - Hazy or indistinct margins
  - Peripheral spiculation with halo
  - Pleural retraction adjacent to tumor
  - Necrosis
  - Extension to bronchi or pulmonary veins
- **SPN calcification characteristics**
  - Malignant
    - Generally not calcified
    - Nodules with eccentric calcification cannot be classified as benign
    - Bone cancer, soft tissue sarcoma, and mucinous adenocarcinoma metastases may calcify

SOLITARY PULMONARY NODULES

- 1/3 of carcinoid tumors calcify
- Colon and ovarian metastases may show psammomatous calcification
- Internal hemorrhage may simulate calcification (melanoma and choriocarcinoma)
  o Benign
    - Central, laminated, popcorn, diffuse
    - Diffuse calcifications > 300 HU through nodule
    - > 1/2 granulomas are calcified
    - 1/3 of hamartomas have popcorn calcification
- **Ground-glass opacity (GGO)**
  o GGO nodules are lower density than solid nodules and do not obscure lung parenchyma
  o 20% of lung nodules demonstrate this density
    - 34% of these are malignant
  o More difficult to distinguish malignant from benign disease based on morphology
    - Much higher incidence of malignancy among ground-glass and mixed opacity nodules
  o Bronchoalveolar carcinoma often demonstrates this density
    - Also adenocarcinoma with BAC features
  o Adenocarcinoma > 2 cm with > 50% GGO has low risk of lymph node metastasis and vessel invasion
- **Enhancement**
  o Malignant nodules often hypervascular and highly enhancing
  o Generally, > 25 HU = malignant, and < 15 HU = benign
  o Insensitive for subcentimeter, cavitary, or necrotic nodules
- **Fat**
  o Malignant: Liposarcoma, renal cell carcinoma metastases (uncommon)
  o Benign: Hamartoma, lipoid pneumonia
- **Air bronchograms**
  o Caused by small airway distortion
  o More typical of malignant than benign nodules
    - Seen in 30% of malignant nodules and 6% of benign nodules
  o As much as 55% of BAC shows bubble-like lucencies = pseudocavitation

Nuclear Medicine Findings
- PET
  o Significant overlap in FDG activity between benign and malignant nodules
  o SUV > 2.5 has sensitivity/specificity 90-100%, 69-95% for detection of malignancy
  o Detection depends largely on size
    - Lower resolution limit 6-8 mm
    - Partial volume averaging of small nodules can produce falsely low SUV
  o Bronchioloalveolar carcinoma has multifocal form that is often detected with FDG PET
    - Overall, BAC tends to have lower FDG uptake than other pulmonary malignancies
  o **False positives**
    - Focal hypermetabolic uptake unrelated to malignancy
    - Most common include infection, inflammatory reaction, granulomata, hamartoma
  o **False negatives**

- Malignant subcentimeter nodules may not be detected on FDG PET
- Hypometabolic tumors: BAC, carcinoid
- Temporary decrease in FDG uptake of active lesions post-therapy ("stunned tumor")
- Ground-glass nodules often false negative due to size and association with BAC
  o PET provides prognostic information for malignant nodules
    - May be more accurate than pathology in predicting recurrence-free survival
    - Low stage tumor with high SUV often has poor prognosis
    - Max SUV ≥ 9: 68% 2 year survival
    - Max SUV ≤ 9: 96% 2 year survival

DIFFERENTIAL DIAGNOSIS

Metastasis
- Variable FDG according to primary
- Often located in outer 1/3 of lower lobes
- SPN is most often primary bronchogenic carcinoma in the setting of another primary
- Multiple well circumscribed lower lobe nodules are most often metastases

Infection
- Includes TB, fungal or viral infections
- Consider TB with a posteriorly located upper lobe/superior segment lower lobe cavitary lesion
- Look for resolution following treatment to rule out underlying malignancy

Inflammation
- Inhalational: Silicosis, lipoid pneumonia
- Rheumatoid, Wegener, sarcoidosis

Granulomatous Disease
- May have associated calcifications

Benign Lesions
- Hamartoma, bronchogenic cyst, pleural plaque
- Presence of macroscopic fat essentially diagnostic of hamartoma

Pulmonary Infarct
- Associated with pulmonary emboli, which may be small
- Typically resolves over time

PATHOLOGY

General Features
- General path comments: Prevalence of nodal metastases in patients with peripheral T1 lung cancer presenting as SPN is considered low
- Etiology
  o Granuloma is the most common entity accounting for SPN
    - In order of descending frequency: Granuloma, bronchogenic carcinoma, hamartoma, solitary metastasis, and carcinoid

SOLITARY PULMONARY NODULES

- Epidemiology
  - Noted on 1/500 chest radiographs
  - Malignancy most often detected in those at highest risk for pulmonary malignancy (smokers, asbestos exposure, etc.)
  - Risk of malignancy by age
    - < 39: ≤ 3%
    - 40-49: 15%
    - 50-59: 43%
    - 60+: > 50%
  - SPN found in the setting of another primary (e.g., breast, head & neck, colon, etc.)
    - Most often a primary bronchogenic carcinoma
  - Multiple lower lobe well-circumscribed nodules in the presence of a known primary
    - Usually represents metastatic disease

Microscopic Features
- Most common malignant SPN is adenocarcinoma

CLINICAL ISSUES

Presentation
- Most common signs/symptoms
  - Early stage malignant SPN generally has few signs and symptoms
  - Detected incidentally
- Other signs/symptoms
  - Cough
  - Hemoptysis

Demographics
- Age
  - 1/3 of SPN are malignant in patients over 35 years of age
  - Benign nodules may be seen from neonates to elderly
  - HIV patients may present at younger age
- Gender: Slight male predominance

Natural History & Prognosis
- Determination of risk status must be made
  - Consider risk factors, clinical history, prior imaging
- Standard of care for low risk individuals is to prove stability over 2 year period with follow-up imaging
  - Over 50% of radiographically indeterminate nodules resected at thoracoscopy are benign
  - Predictive value of stability in size over time of a SPN is only 65%
- High risk individuals may undergo follow-up imaging with biopsy, bronchoscopy, VATS, and resection
  - 5 year survival following resection of stage IA solitary bronchogenic carcinoma is 80-90%

Treatment
- After biopsy confirms primary lung malignancy, surgical resection is primary treatment
- Patients with significant comorbidities may be treated with radiofrequency ablation

DIAGNOSTIC CHECKLIST

Consider
- For nodules with features of BAC, a negative PET scan does not rule out malignancy
  - Follow-up imaging should be performed with CT

Image Interpretation Pearls
- Nodules adjacent to heart and in lung bases may be obscured due to motion on PET imaging

SELECTED REFERENCES

1. Alkhawaldeh K et al: Impact of dual-time-point (18)F-FDG PET imaging and partial volume correction in the assessment of solitary pulmonary nodules. Eur J Nucl Med Mol Imaging. 35(2):246-52, 2008
2. Cronin P et al: Solitary pulmonary nodules and masses: a meta-analysis of the diagnostic utility of alternative imaging tests. Eur Radiol. 18(9):1840-56, 2008
3. Cronin P et al: Solitary pulmonary nodules: meta-analytic comparison of cross-sectional imaging modalities for diagnosis of malignancy. Radiology. 246(3):772-82, 2008
4. Fletcher JW et al: A comparison of the diagnostic accuracy of 18F-FDG PET and CT in the characterization of solitary pulmonary nodules. J Nucl Med. 49(2):179-85, 2008
5. Jeong SY et al: Efficacy of PET/CT in the characterization of solid or partly solid solitary pulmonary nodules. Lung Cancer. 61(2):186-94, 2008
6. Kim SC et al: Fluoro-deoxy-glucose positron emission tomography for evaluation of indeterminate lung nodules: assigning a probability of malignancy may be preferable to binary readings. Ann Nucl Med. 22(3):165-70, 2008
7. Klein JS et al: Imaging evaluation of the solitary pulmonary nodule. Clin Chest Med. 29(1):15-38, v, 2008
8. Tian J et al: A multicenter clinical trial on the diagnostic value of dual-tracer PET/CT in pulmonary lesions using 3'-deoxy-3'-18F-fluorothymidine and 18F-FDG. J Nucl Med. 49(2):186-94, 2008
9. Beigelman-Aubry C et al: Management of an incidentally discovered pulmonary nodule. Eur Radiol. 17(2):449-66, 2007
10. De Wever W et al: Additional value of integrated PET-CT in the detection and characterization of lung metastases: correlation with CT alone and PET alone. Eur Radiol. 17(2):467-73, 2007
11. Gould MK et al: A clinical model to estimate the pretest probability of lung cancer in patients with solitary pulmonary nodules. Chest. 131(2):383-8, 2007
12. Ireland JC et al: Solitary pulmonary nodule. Mo Med. 104(3):243-5, 2007
13. Kim SK et al: Accuracy of PET/CT in characterization of solitary pulmonary lesions. J Nucl Med. 48(2):214-20, 2007
14. Miller JC et al: Evaluating pulmonary nodules. J Am Coll Radiol. 4(6):422-6, 2007
15. O JH et al: Clinical significance of small pulmonary nodules with little or no 18F-FDG uptake on PET/CT images of patients with nonthoracic malignancies. J Nucl Med. 48(1):15-21, 2007
16. Ung YC et al: 18Fluorodeoxyglucose positron emission tomography in the diagnosis and staging of lung cancer: a systematic review. J Natl Cancer Inst. 99(23):1753-67, 2007
17. Xiu Y et al: Dual-time point FDG PET imaging in the evaluation of pulmonary nodules with minimally increased metabolic activity. Clin Nucl Med. 32(2):101-5, 2007

SOLITARY PULMONARY NODULES

CT Findings: Benign vs. Malignant SPN

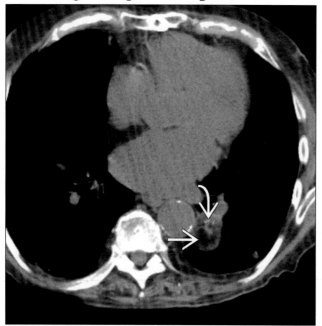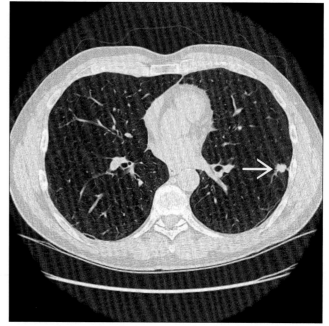

(Left) Axial NECT shows a solid mass with areas of fat attenuation ➡ and punctate calcifications ➘, compatible with a hamartoma. The presence of fat within a pulmonary nodule is pathognomonic for a hamartoma. Hamartomas may have increased FDG activity. *(Right)* Axial NECT shows a left lower lobe spiculated nodule ➡, biopsy-proven to be an adenocarcinoma. A peripheral spiculated nodule is highly suspicious for adenocarcinoma.

PET/CT Findings: SPN

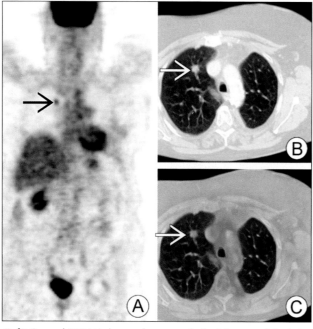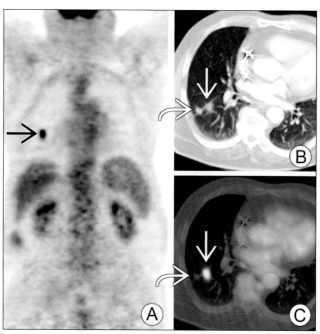

(Left) Coronal PET (A) shows a hypermetabolic right upper lobe lesion ➡ correlating with the spiculated 8 mm upper lobe lesion ➡ seen on axial CT (B) and PET/CT (C) images, compatible with adenocarcinoma. *(Right)* Coronal PET (A) demonstrates a focal lesion with FDG activity in the right mid-lung zone ➡. Axial CT (B) and PET/CT (C) show two pulmonary nodules, one with intense FDG activity ➡ (adenocarcinoma) and one with no activity ➘, later proven to be a focal infarct.

SOLITARY PULMONARY NODULES

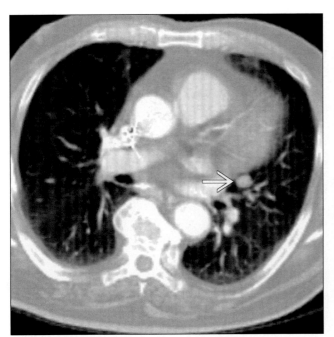
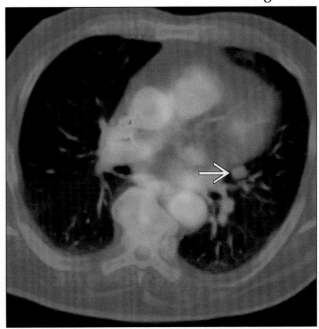

(Left) Axial CECT shows a well-rounded approximately 1 cm left upper lobe pulmonary nodule ➡ interpreted as indeterminate on CT. *(Right)* Axial fused PET/CT shows mildly increased FDG activity within the pulmonary nodule ➡, suggestive of a benign lesion. Subsequent wedge resection showed this to be a hamartoma.

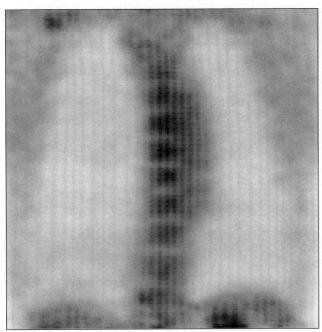
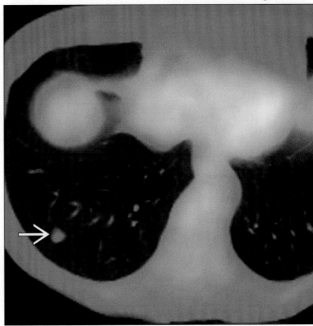

(Left) Coronal PET shows no abnormal areas of increased activity in this patient with a 1.5 cm right lower lobe pulmonary nodule. *(Right)* Axial fused PET/CT shows no increased metabolic activity within this right lower lobe pulmonary nodule ➡, suggesting a benign lesion. However, subsequent follow-up CT showed increased interval growth, and a biopsy demonstrated bronchoalveolar carcinoma.

SOLITARY PULMONARY NODULES

PET/CT Findings: SPN

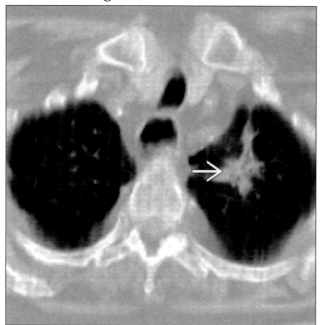 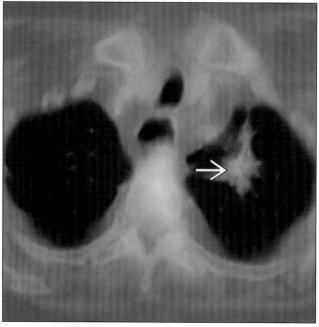

(Left) Axial NECT shows a spiculated left upper lobe mass ➡ in a patient with a remote history of tuberculosis and a recent indeterminate CT scan. (Right) Axial fused PET/CT shows minimal background activity within the left upper lobe mass ➡, suggestive of a benign lesion. Subsequent biopsy identified this as scarring with minimal inflammatory cells.

PET/CT Findings: SPN

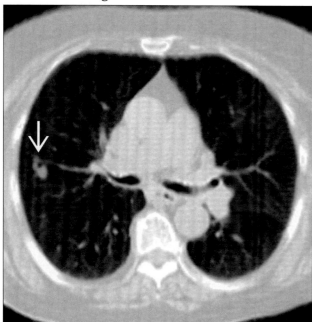 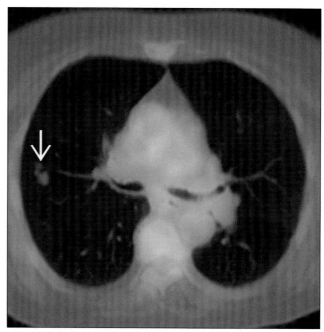

(Left) Axial CECT shows a 1 cm well-rounded pulmonary nodule ➡ in the right mid-lung zone, interpreted as indeterminate on CT. (Right) Axial fused PET/CT shows no increased metabolic activity within the nodule ➡ shown on the previous image, suggesting a benign process. Subsequent follow-up CT over two years showed no interval growth.

SOLITARY PULMONARY NODULES

PET/CT Findings: SPN

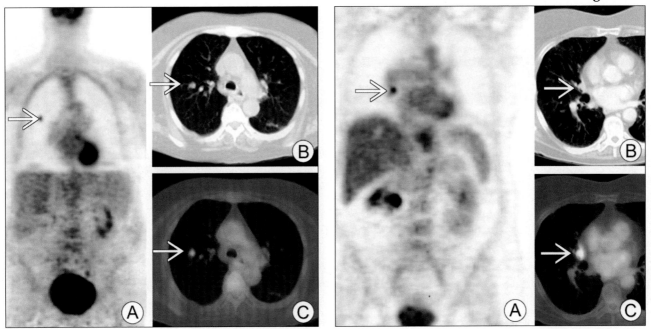

(Left) Coronal PET (A), axial CT (B) and fused PET/CT (C) show a 7 mm hypermetabolic adenocarcinoma in the right lung ➡. (Right) Coronal PET (A) shows intense FDG activity. It correlates with a subtle ill-defined pulmonary nodule ➡ adjacent to the right mediastinal border, seen on axial CT (B) and fused PET/CT (C). At resection, the nodule proved to be adenocarcinoma.

PET/CT Findings: SPN

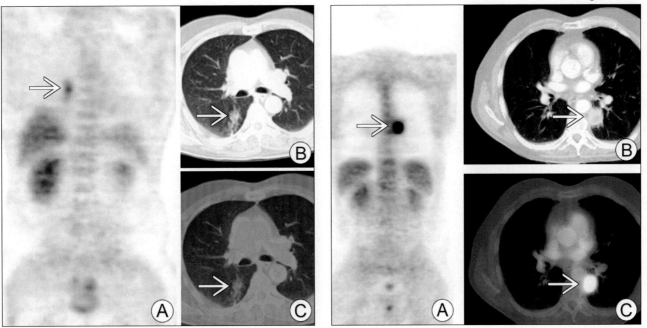

(Left) PET/CT evaluation of a patient referred for a solitary pulmonary nodule shows a ground-glass opacity lesion ➡ in the superior segment of the right lower lobe on axial CT (B). There is mildly increased FDG activity ➡ on coronal PET (A) and fused PET/CT (C). The lesion was subsequently proven to be bronchoalveolar carcinoma. (Right) Coronal PET (A), axial CT (B) and fused PET/CT (C) show a hypermetabolic mass in the left lower lobe medial segment ➡, subsequently proven to be squamous cell carcinoma.

SOLITARY PULMONARY NODULES

PET/CT Findings: SPN

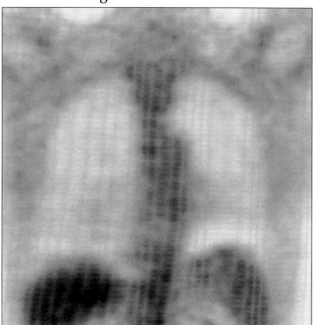
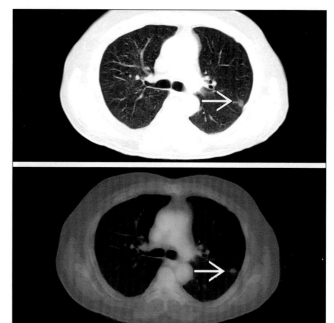

(Left) Coronal PET shows no abnormal areas of increased activity in the thorax of this patient with a left lower lobe pulmonary nodule. *(Right)* Axial CT (top) and fused PET/CT (bottom) show no increased metabolic activity in the nodule ➡, although the activity is likely underestimated due to the small size and effects of partial volume averaging. Wedge resection revealed adenocarcinoma.

PET/CT Findings: SPN

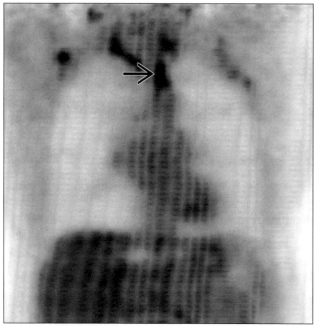
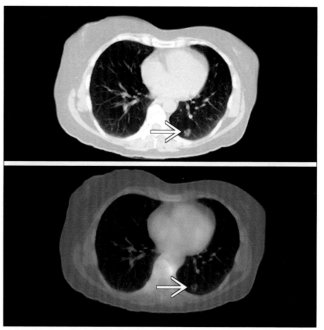

(Left) Coronal PET shows no abnormal areas of increased metabolic activity within the lung parenchyma. Incidental FDG activity was noted in the left paratracheal ➡ and supraclavicular areas, compatible with brown fat. *(Right)* Axial CT (top) and fused PET/CT (bottom) show no increased metabolic activity in the left lower lobe pulmonary nodule ➡, subsequently biopsy-proven to be bronchioloalveolar carcinoma.

SOLITARY PULMONARY NODULES

PET/CT Findings: SPN

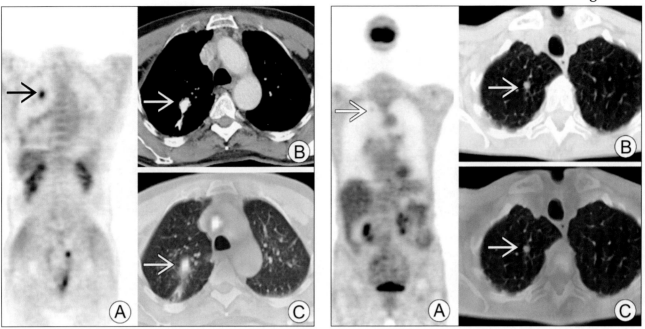

(Left) Coronal PET (A) in a patient with silicosis shows a hypermetabolic lesion ⇨ in the right upper lung zone. It correlates with a calcified mass in the right upper lobe ⇨ seen on axial CT (B) and PET/CT (C), compatible with progressive massive fibrosis. *(Right)* Coronal PET (A), axial CT (B) and PET/CT (C) show mildly increased metabolic activity ⇨ within a 6-7 mm well-circumscribed right upper lobe adenocarcinoma.

PET/CT Findings: SPN

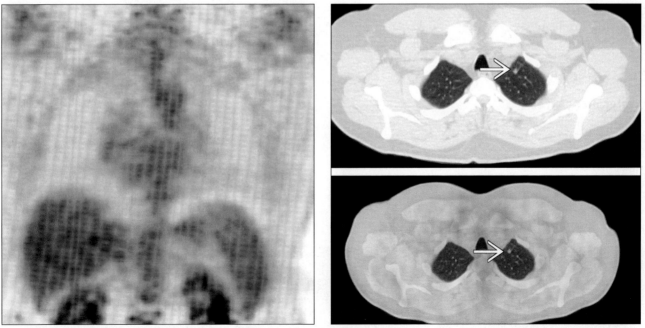

(Left) Coronal PET demonstrates no abnormal FDG activity in the thorax in a patient referred for a pulmonary nodule, which was well below the limits of resolution of the camera. *(Right)* Axial CT (top) and fused PET/CT (bottom) show a 4 mm left upper lobe pulmonary nodule without increased metabolic activity ⇨. The nodule remains indeterminate, as the amount of FDG activity cannot be accurately determined due to the nodule's small size. PET should not be ordered for nodules < 6 mm.

LUNG CANCER

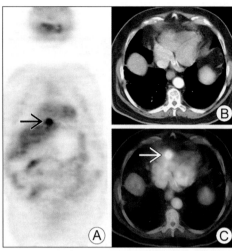

One week after discharge status post right lower lobectomy for NSCLC, coronal PET (A) shows focal FDG activity ➡. PET/CT (C) localizes the lesion ➡ to the pericardium, without obvious abnormality on the CECT (B). Autopsy confirmed a pericardial metastasis.

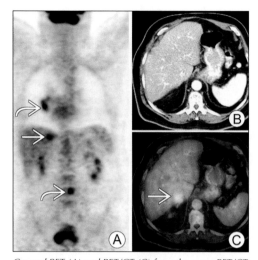

Coronal PET (A) and PET/CT (C) from the same PET/CT exam as the previous image show a hepatic lesion ➡ not detected on axial CECT (B). Unsuspected additional lesions were also present ➡.

TERMINOLOGY

Abbreviations and Synonyms
- Non-small cell lung cancer (NSCLC)
- Adenocarcinoma
- Bronchogenic carcinoma
- Squamous cell carcinoma (SCCA)
- Bronchoalveolar carcinoma (BAC)
- Large cell carcinoma (LCCA)

Definitions
- Glandular carcinomas of varying histology arising in lung parenchyma

IMAGING FINDINGS

General Features
- Best diagnostic clue
  - Peripheral irregular spiculated pulmonary nodule in a smoker
    - Malignant in > 90% of patients
  - Hilar and mediastinal lymphadenopathy
  - Bronchial stenosis and associated atelectasis

- Location
  - Adenocarcinoma: Periphery of upper lobe
  - SCCA: Central
- Size
  - By time of detection
    - At screening: 8-15 mm
    - Symptomatic: 25 mm
  - Size is not a reliable indicator of nodal involvement
    - 21% of subcentimeter nodes = malignant
    - 40% of nodes > 1 cm = benign
  - LCCA: > 4 cm at diagnosis
- Morphology
  - Spiculated irregular ill-defined nodule is specific for malignancy
    - Borders may also be lobulated or smooth

Imaging Recommendations
- Best imaging tool
  - CT for delineating extent of disease
  - PET/CT for prognosis and staging
  - MR for diagnosing neural invasion
    - CNS, Pancoast invasion of brachial plexus
  - No imaging tool is specific enough to defer lymph node biopsy if required for treatment planning

DDx: Focal FDG Activity in the Lung

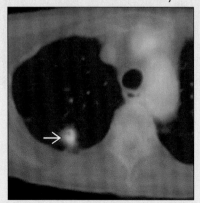

Infection

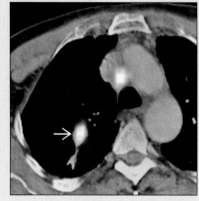

Progressive Massive Fibrosis

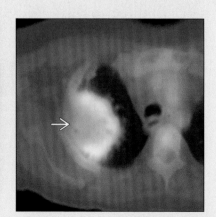

Inflammatory Pseudotumor

LUNG CANCER

Key Facts

Terminology
- Non-small cell lung cancer (NSCLC), bronchogenic carcinoma (CA), adenocarcinoma (adenocarcinoma), squamous cell carcinoma (SCCA), large cell carcinoma (LCCA), bronchoalveolar carcinoma (BAC)

Imaging Findings
- Spiculated pulmonary nodule in a smoker
- Hilar and mediastinal lymphadenopathy
- Whole body PET/CT is superior to CT or PET alone
- PET/CT currently best technique for imaging diagnosis of nodal staging in NSCLC
- PET can identify metastases that would have been occult on conventional workup (e.g., adrenal metastases)
- Prognostic information from FDG PET: Max SUV > 5.0 suggests aggressive neoplasm, poorer prognosis

Top Differential Diagnoses
- Pulmonary Infarct, Infection
- Granulomatous Disease
- Mediastinal Mass
- Hamartoma
- Infection

Pathology
- > 85% smoke; 50% in former smokers

Diagnostic Checklist
- Consider PET/CT for **all** patients with newly diagnosed NSCLC
- Suspicious FDG PET findings should be biopsied/removed without following growth on CT
- Suspicious CT morphology should be biopsied even with negative PET

- o Mediastinoscopy most common method for assessing mediastinal lymph nodes
- Protocol advice
  - o **CT**
    - To include adrenals, image caudally from thoracic inlet to inferior edge of liver
    - Pleural and diaphragmatic tumor spread best imaged with multiplanar reformatting
    - Screening CT studies should be performed without contrast and with the lowest possible mAs
  - o **FDG PET**
    - Serum glucose < 150 mg/dL (reschedule hyperglycemic patients)
    - 90 minute uptake period
  - o **PET/CT**
    - Modified breath-hold techniques employed to reduce misregistration artifact
    - Sensitivity in lower lobes may be minimized without maximal inspiration

CT Findings
- **General findings**
  - o Current CT does not provide adequate anatomic detail to separate invasion from simple contact between tumor and adjacent organ
  - o NECT adequate for evaluation of primary tumor, but less sensitive for vascular invasion and liver metastases
  - o CECT can reveal small endobronchial lesions and better elicit small mediastinal nodes
    - Particularly hilar nodes that may otherwise missed due to proximity to vessels
  - o Bronchial obstruction with lobar collapse or post-obstructive pneumonitis
  - o Peripheral lesions
    - SCCA more likely to demonstrate cavitation
    - Peripheral adenocarcinoma may be solid, mixed solid/ground-glass, or ground-glass
- **Staging**
  - o CT has not demonstrated improved staging accuracy with the advent of multislice detectors

- o Malignant potential and degree of contrast enhancement may be related due to increased vascularity of lung cancer lesions
- **Lymph nodes**
  - o Upper size limits for suspicion of malignancy
    - > 5 mm hilum and > 10 mm mediastinum
  - o Size criteria are insensitive, as normal-sized nodes often harbor malignancy
    - Sensitivity 41-54%
    - Combined PET/CT may correct 81% of false negatives on CT
  - o Measurement errors inherent with borderline node size of 5 mm
  - o Mediastinal and hilar nodal metastasis is not predicted by characteristics of primary tumor
    - Size, margins, necrosis, bronchovascular thickening
  - o Best predictor of mediastinal nodal metastasis is peak enhancement of malignant lung nodules
    - > 100 HU or > 60 HU of net enhancement in stage T1 NSCLC
    - Mediastinoscopic biopsy recommended in the setting of these findings whether FDG PET is positive or not
  - o Supraclavicular nodal sensitivity of 67-85%
    - Area often obscured by beam-hardening artifacts
    - Delayed scans may improve detection
    - Transverse scan may not accurately depict short-axis measurement of nodes
  - o Normal structures that mimic lymph nodes
    - External/internal jugular veins
    - Vertebral veins
    - Common carotids
    - Scalene and longus colli muscles
- **Metastatic disease**
  - o High resolution CT to detect lymphangitic carcinomatosis
  - o Look for metastasis to non-tumor lobe
  - o CECT can demonstrate pleural metastases in pleural effusion
  - o Adrenal evaluation complicated by insensitivity of morphologic criteria for presence of malignancy

2

LUNG CANCER

- May be evaluated with NECT
- 17% of normal-appearing adrenals may harbor malignancy
- Overall, fewer than half of adrenal masses in patients with lung cancer will be due to metastasis

Nuclear Medicine Findings
- **PET/CT**
  - Central to initial and post-treatment evaluation and management of NSCLC
  - Depicts response to treatment accurately and predicts prognosis
  - Influences management by demonstrating occult disease
  - Provides high contrast between tumor and adjacent structures like mediastinum, chest wall, atelectasis
  - Helps determine cause of pleural effusion
- **Normal uptake**
  - Low level in thyroid, breast, and mediastinal blood pool
  - Talking can cause laryngeal uptake
  - Anxiety may be manifested as uptake in the SCM
  - Brown fat in neck, paravertebral, mediastinal, and axillary regions
  - Also seen in esophagus, spleen, liver, and bowel
- **Initial diagnosis**
- FDG PET criteria for malignancy (less specific than sensitive)
  - FDG uptake > background mediastinal uptake
  - Max SUV ≥ 2.5; however wide overlap of SUVs between benign and malignant processes
  - Any activity above background levels in lesion < 1-1.5 cm
- For SPN larger than 1.0 cm, PET has sensitivity and specificity of 95-98% and 73-85% respectively
  - Same predictive value as observation of nodule growth on CT
- Nodules < 2.5 cm may be misinterpreted as non-FDG-avid due to partial volume averaging on PET
  - Recovery coefficient helps correct SUV in smaller nodules for purposes of quantitative determinations
- Tumor with low metabolic rate (low grade adenocarcinoma, BAC, carcinoid)
- Subtypes may show low FDG uptake despite aggressiveness
  - BAC, carcinoid, low grade adenocarcinoma
- **Staging**
- Detection of disease
  - PET can identify metastases that would be occult on conventional workup (e.g., adrenal metastases)
  - Detects bone metastases with equal sensitivity to and greater specificity than bone scintigraphy
  - False positives with benign inflammatory disease > 1.0 cm
  - False negatives in subcentimeter lesion with limited cancer invasion
  - Low sensitivity of 47% for stage T1 NSCLC
  - 100% PPV and high NPV for mediastinal nodal metastasis
  - Brain metastases may be overlooked due to high background FDG avidity

- Necrotic metastases may be negative (e.g., adrenal masses)
- Influence on management
  - PET more sensitive than clinical exam for supraclavicular lymphadenopathy
    - Significant indicator of inoperable disease
    - Confirmation by histopathology is mandatory when positive PET/CT would deny patient chance for potentially curative treatment
  - High NPV of 93% helps avoid invasive procedures like fine needle aspiration (FNA) when there is no FDG uptake
    - Microscopic disease may be present, and mediastinal surgical staging may still be indicated
  - Thoracotomy
    - PET has greater than 90% NPV for nodal disease
    - Patients with negative mediastinal nodes may proceed directly to thoracotomy without need for mediastinoscopy
    - PET may also avoid non-therapeutic thoracotomy in 20% by detecting previously occult distant disease
  - PET/CT may alter 50% of radiotherapy gross tumor volume estimation compared to targeting with CT alone
    - Clinical impact yet to be determined
    - Gross tumor volume (GTV) shown to include all pathologically involved mediastinal lymph nodes
    - More positive lymph nodes are detected by PET/CT compared to CT alone
- Prognosis
  - FDG PET may provide information on prognosis independent from standard staging algorithms
  - Primary tumor with SUV ≥ 5.0
    - Associated with significant increase in post-operative relapse in early stage lung cancer
  - Intense uptake in bone marrow also associated with poorer outcome
- **Response to treatment**
- Decrease in FDG avidity of malignant lesion by 60% following 2-3 cycles of chemotherapy
  - May indicate good response and be predictive of improved survival
- Some tumors may show falsely decreased SUV post-therapy ("stunned") but still represent threat of recurrence
- **False positives**
  - Nonmalignant metabolically active conditions
    - Active inflammation, infection, granulomatous disease
  - Pattern of physiologic muscle uptake typically
    - Bilateral, symmetric, fusiform, or elongated; seldom confused with presence of malignancy
    - Asymmetric uptake can occur
  - Increased glycolysis in leukocytes, lymphocytes, macrophages
    - Produce uptake in areas of infection, inflammation
  - **Examples of benign processes that may mimic malignancy**
    - Atherosclerotic plaque
    - Reflux esophagitis

LUNG CANCER

- Tuberculous caseating granuloma
- Sarcoidosis
- Wegener granulomatosis
- Amyloidosis
- Pulmonary infarction
- Pulmonary embolus
- Pulmonary hamartomas
- Needle biopsy site
- Mediastinoscopy
- Talc pleurodesis, which may remain FDG positive for several years
- Empyema
- Pneumonias usually produce low grade uptake but avid uptake can occur
- Organizing pneumonia as a single focus of consolidation can mimic lung cancer
- Patients with false positives on PET/CT often have comorbid pulmonary complications, such as
  - Obstructive pneumonia
  - Chronic bronchitis
  - Interstitial pneumonia
  - Bronchiectasis
  - Silicosis
  - Previous pulmonary tuberculosis

DIFFERENTIAL DIAGNOSIS

Metastases
- Usually less spiculated than primary pulmonary malignancies
- Variably FDG avid

Infection
- Pneumonia may show intense focal uptake and is easily mistaken for malignancy
- Repeat PET to rule out presence of underlying malignancy

Granulomatous Disease
- Mediastinal and hilar adenopathy generally symmetrical and FDG avid
- Predominantly in upper lobes
- Calcification is common

Pulmonary Infarct
- Early following infarct, may show intense FDG activity
- Usually becomes less intense over time
- Distribution of occluded artery

Hamartoma
- Generally noninflammatory with little FDG uptake
- "Popcorn" calcifications

PATHOLOGY

General Features
- General path comments: Sputum analysis is insensitive, with false negative in 40% of cases
- Genetics
  - NSCLC associated with amplification of oncogenes (e.g., ras family) in 30% of cases
    - Also inactivation of tumor suppression genes

- Portends worse prognosis
  - Genetic predisposition plays role in vulnerability to risk factors (e.g., smoking)
- Etiology
  - Tobacco is the cause of lung cancer in ~ 90% of cases
    - Disease was practically unknown prior to the rise of cigarette smoking in the 1920s
    - 15% of lung cancer in patients who do not smoke is caused by passive smoke
  - Asbestos exposure in a patient who smokes confers 80-90x increased risk of lung cancer
  - Radon accounts for 2-3% of lung cancer and is a byproduct of uranium decay (miners)
- Epidemiology
  - In USA: 170,000 new cases/year (90k in men and 80k in women); 150,000 deaths/year
  - Estimated 1 million new cases/year worldwide
  - NSCLC accounts for ~ 80% of all lung cancers
- Associated abnormalities: COPD

Gross Pathologic & Surgical Features
- Cavitation is common in SCCA

Microscopic Features
- Adenocarcinoma: Forms glands and produces mucin, which can be identified with mucicarmine or PAS staining
- SCCA: Large irregular nuclei, coarse nuclear chromatin, large nucleoli
  - Presence of intercellular bridging among cells arranged in sheets is pathognomonic
- LCCA: Large cells with prominent nucleoli in the absence of mucin production or intercellular bridging

Staging, Grading, or Classification Criteria
- Primary lesion (T)
  - Tx: Tumor cannot be assessed, + sputum/washings
  - T0: No evidence of primary tumor
  - Tis: Carcinoma in situ
  - T1: < 3 cm, completely surrounded by lung; no main bronchi invasion
  - T2: > 3 cm, involving main bronchus > 2 cm from the carina, visceral pleura; atelectasis/pneumonitis extending to hila
  - T3: Invading chest wall, diaphragm, mediastinal pleura, parietal pericardium, main bronchus < 2 cm from the carina
    - Total atelectasis of whole lung
  - T4: Invading the mediastinal structures, vertebrae, carina; separate tumor nodules in same lobe; malignant pleural effusion
- Mediastinal and hilar lymph nodes (N)
  - N1: Hilar lymph nodes at vessel branch point
  - N2: Ipsilateral to primary tumor (subcarinal lymph node is ipsilateral)
  - N3: Contralateral lymph node, supraclavicular fossa
- Stages
  - 0 (TisN0M0)
  - 1A (T1N0M0)
  - IB (T2N0M0)
  - IIA (T1N1M0)
  - IIB [(T2N1M0), (T3N0M0)]
  - IIIA [(T1-3 N2M0), (T3N1M0)]

LUNG CANCER

o IIIB [(any T, N3M0), (T4, any N, M0)]
o IV (any T, any N, M1)

o Some patients with inoperable NSCLC can be cured with radiotherapy

CLINICAL ISSUES

Presentation
- Most common signs/symptoms
  - Central primary tumor
    - Cough, dyspnea, wheezing, and hemoptysis
    - Atelectasis and post-obstructive pneumonia
  - Peripheral primary tumor may cause the above
    - ± Pleural effusion and pain related to pleural and chest wall invasion
  - Locoregional spread may cause SVC obstruction and nerve infiltration
    - Leads to hoarseness, diaphragm paralysis, and Horner syndrome, as well as brachial plexus neuropathy
  - Paraneoplastic symptoms may include hypercalcemia and PTHrP production
- Other signs/symptoms
  - Recurrent pneumonia in same lobe
  - Metastasis to supraclavicular lymph node
    - Indicator of inoperable disease
    - Palpation of supraclavicular lymph nodes is unreliable for detection

Demographics
- Age: > 50 years
- Gender
  - M:F approaching 1:1 in USA
  - M > F worldwide
  - Mortality higher in males, increasing in females
- Ethnicity: African-American:Caucasian:Native American = 1.5:1:0.2

Natural History & Prognosis
- Most patients present with advanced disease
- Adenocarcinoma has worse prognosis per stage than SCCA (except T1N0)
- Staging criteria include
  - Histologic type
  - Tumor size
  - Regional lymph node involvement
  - Presence of metastatic disease
- Mediastinal lymph node metastasis is found in 16-21% of patients with stage T1 NSCLC
- Metastatic relapse occurs in up to 20% of patients who have undergone surgery

Treatment
- Stages 1 & 2: Patients with no metastatic lymph nodes (N0 disease) or with only intrapulmonary or hilar lymph nodes (N1 disease)
  - Resection with adjuvant chemo in selected cases
- Stage 3A: Neoadjuvant chemoradiation, then surgery in selected
- Stage 3B: Chemoradiation, then surgery in selected T4N0
- Stage 4: Chemotherapy, palliative radiation in selected
  - Solitary brain mets: Resection of brain met and primary if possible
- Radiation or RFA: Symptomatic inoperable lesions

DIAGNOSTIC CHECKLIST

Consider
- Suspicious CT morphology should be biopsied even with negative PET
- Suspicious FDG PET findings should be biopsied/removed without following growth on CT
- Consider PET/CT for ALL patients with newly diagnosed NSCLC

SELECTED REFERENCES

1. Bryant AS et al: Differences in outcomes between younger and older patients with non-small cell lung cancer. Ann Thorac Surg. 85(5):1735-9; discussion 1739, 2008
2. Cerfolio RJ et al: Survival of patients with unsuspected N2 (stage IIIA) nonsmall-cell lung cancer. Ann Thorac Surg. 86(2):362-6; discussion 366-7, 2008
3. Decker RH et al: Advances in radiotherapy for lung cancer. Semin Respir Crit Care Med. 29(3):285-90, 2008
4. Hampton T: New studies target lung cancer prevention, imaging, and treatment. JAMA. 300(3):267-8, 2008
5. Hanin FX et al: Prognostic value of FDG uptake in early stage non-small cell lung cancer. Eur J Cardiothorac Surg. 33(5):819-23, 2008
6. Hart JP et al: Radiation pneumonitis: correlation of toxicity with pulmonary metabolic radiation response. Int J Radiat Oncol Biol Phys. 71(4):967-71, 2008
7. Higaki F et al: Preliminary retrospective investigation of FDG-PET/CT timing in follow-up of ablated lung tumor. Ann Nucl Med. 22(3):157-63, 2008
8. Kased N et al: Prognostic value of posttreatment [18F] fluorodeoxyglucose uptake of primary non-small cell lung carcinoma treated with radiation therapy with or without chemotherapy: a brief review. J Thorac Oncol. 3(5):534-8, 2008
9. Lima CG Jr et al: Is there a definitive answer to the question of involved-field radiotherapy for inoperable non-small-cell lung cancer? J Clin Oncol. 26(13):2235; author reply 2235-6, 2008
10. Ohno Y et al: Non-small cell lung cancer: whole-body MR examination for M-stage assessment--utility for whole-body diffusion-weighted imaging compared with integrated FDG PET/CT. Radiology. 248(2):643-54, 2008
11. Yi CA et al: Non-small cell lung cancer staging: efficacy comparison of integrated PET/CT versus 3.0-T whole-body MR imaging. Radiology. 248(2):632-42, 2008
12. Poettgen C et al: Correlation of PET/CT findings and histopathology after neoadjuvant therapy in non-small cell lung cancer. Oncology. 73(5-6):316-23, 2007
13. Decoster L et al: Complete metabolic tumour response, assessed by 18-fluorodeoxyglucose positron emission tomography ((18)FDG-PET), after induction chemotherapy predicts a favourable outcome in patients with locally advanced non-small-cell lung cancer (NSCLC). Lung Cancer. (In Press)
14. Wilson DO et al: The Pittsburgh Lung Screening Study (PLuSS): Outcomes within 3 years of a first CT Scan. Am J Respir Crit Care Med. (In Press)

LUNG CANCER

CT Findings: Primary

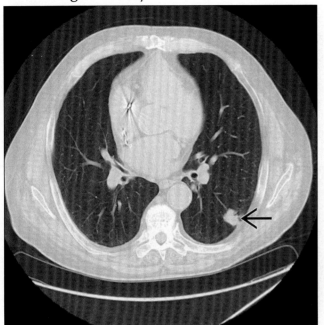 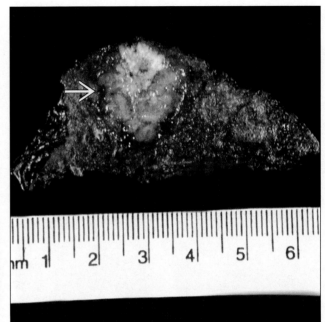

(Left) Axial CECT shows a subpleural, left lower lobe, lobulated lesion ➡. *(Right)* Gross surgical pathology shows the same lower lobe lesion ➡.

CT Findings: Primary

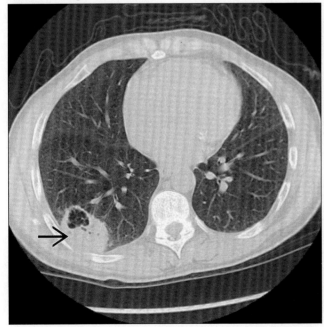 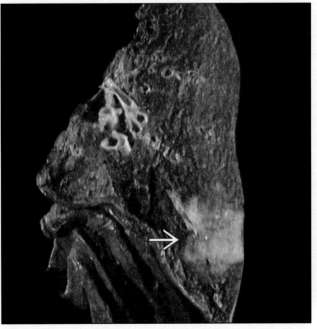

(Left) Axial NECT shows a right lower lobe lesion with apparent cavitation ➡ that was subsequently confirmed as bronchoalveolar carcinoma. *(Right)* Gross surgical pathology reveals the same right lower lobe subpleural lesion ➡.

LUNG CANCER

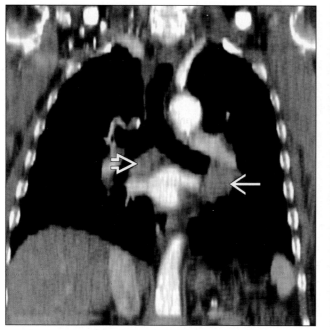
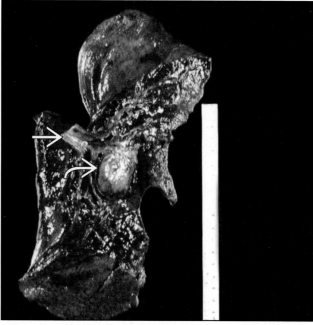

(Left) Coronal CECT shows subcarinal ⇨ and left hilar ➡ adenopathy. *(Right)* Gross pathology from the same patient as the previous image shows the left hilar mass ➡ and its relationship to the left main stem bronchus ➡. Final pathology revealed adenocarcinoma.

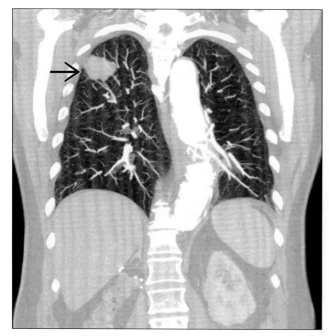
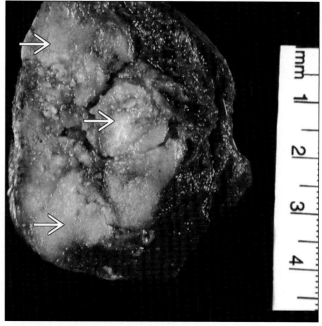

(Left) Coronal CECT reconstructed image shows a right upper lobe lesion ➡ in this patient with recently diagnosed NSCLC. *(Right)* Gross surgical pathology of the same right upper lobe lesion ➡ shows the typical tan nodular appearance of primary NSCLC.

LUNG CANCER

PET/CT Findings: Staging

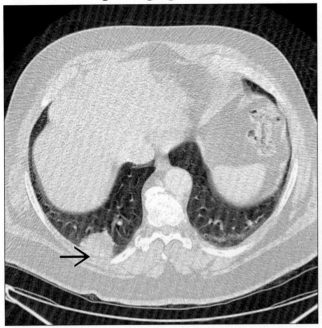 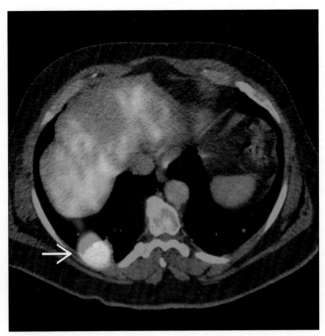

(Left) Axial CECT shows a peripherally based right lower lobe nodule ➡. *(Right)* Axial fused PET/CT shows the same lesion with intense FDG uptake ➡, compatible with a primary lung cancer.

PET/CT Findings: Staging

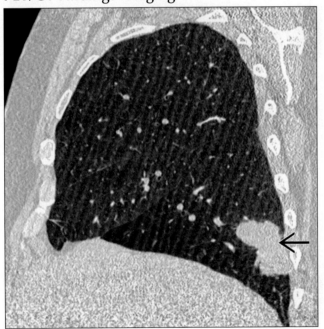 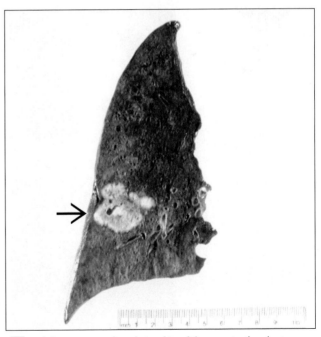

(Left) Sagittal CECT reconstructed image shows the same subpleural lesion ➡ and demonstrates the relationship of the mass to the chest wall. *(Right)* Gross surgical pathology shows the same right lower lobe lesion ➡. Chest wall invasion was not present.

LUNG CANCER

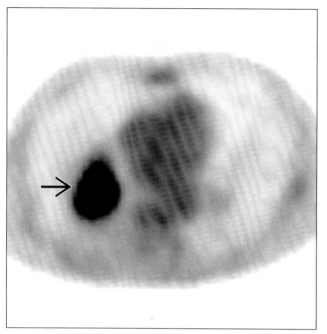 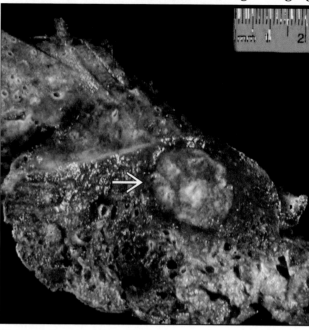

(Left) Axial PET shows a right lower lobe lesion with intense FDG uptake ➡. *(Right)* Gross pathological specimen from the same patient shows the large lesion ➡.

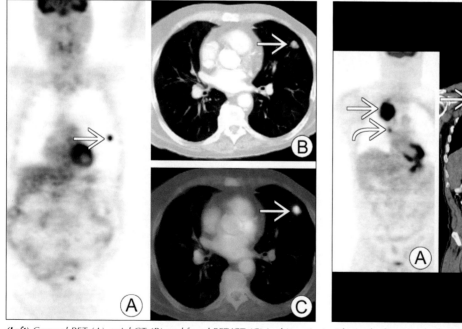 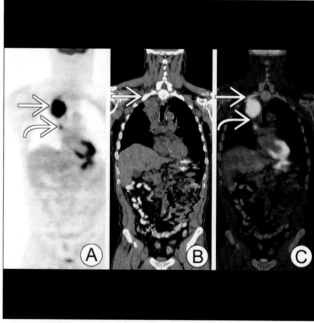

(Left) Coronal PET (A), axial CT (B) and fused PET/CT (C) in this patient with newly diagnosed adenocarcinoma show intense increased FDG activity in a left upper lobe mass ➡. Generally, well differentiated adenocarcinomas tend to have less FDG activity than poorly differentiated ones. *(Right)* Coronal PET (A), CT (B) and fused PET/CT (C) demonstrate a superior sulcus squamous cell carcinoma with diffusely increased metabolic activity ➡ and a small ipsilateral right paratracheal lymph node ➡.

LUNG CANCER

PET/CT Findings: Staging

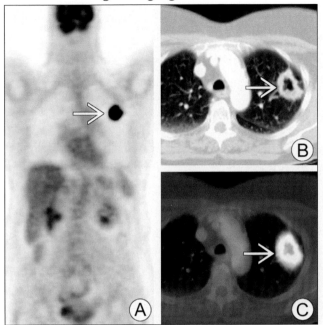 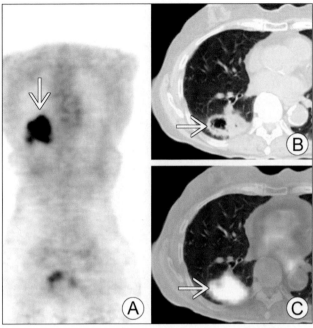

(Left) Coronal PET (A), axial CT (B) and fused PET/CT (C) show a large FDG-avid cavitary lesion in the left upper lobe ➡. This patient was newly diagnosed with squamous cell carcinoma, the most likely primary lung neoplasm to cavitate. *(Right)* Coronal PET (A), axial CT (B) and fused PET/CT (C) demonstrate a cavitary squamous cell carcinoma ➡ during a staging PET/CT.

PET/CT Findings: Staging

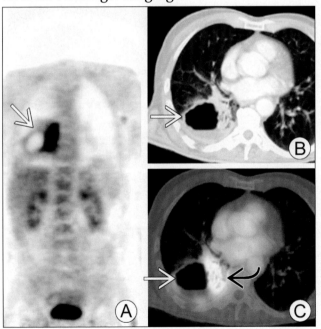 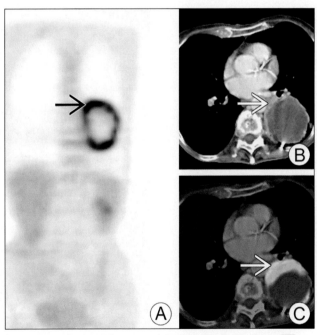

(Left) Coronal PET (A), axial CT (B) and fused PET/CT (C) demonstrate a large cavitary lesion with increased FDG activity at its margins ➡. PET/CT helped guide the biopsy to the metabolically active aspect ➾ of the lesion seen medially. *(Right)* Coronal PET (A) demonstrates a large mass in the left lower lobe with peripheral FDG activity ➡ and a large area of central photopenia, compatible with necrosis. Axial CT (B) and fused PET/CT (C) show the area targeted for biopsy ➡.

LUNG CANCER

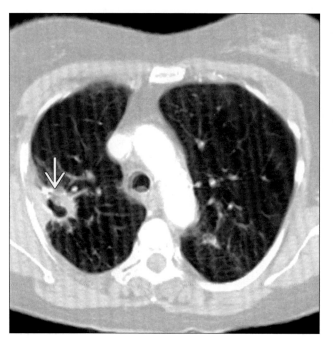 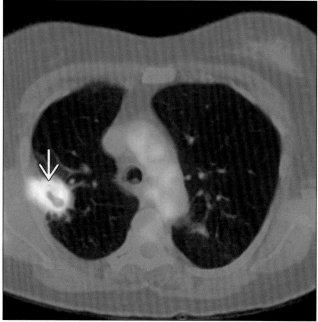

(Left) Axial CECT shows a large spiculated cavitary lesion in the right lung ➡, compatible with the patient's recent diagnosis of squamous cell carcinoma. *(Right)* Axial fused PET/CT shows intense metabolic activity in the walls of the right upper lobe cavitary lesion ➡.

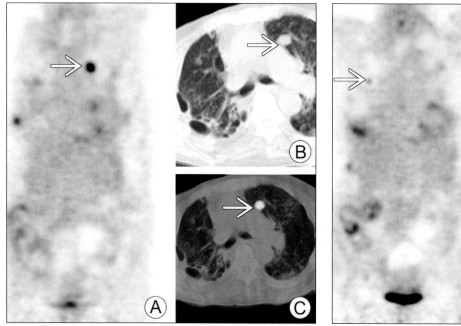 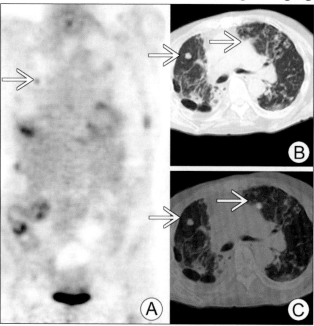

(Left) Coronal PET (A), axial CT (B) and fused PET/CT (C) reveal a left upper lobe FDG avid nodule ➡. *(Right)* Coronal PET (A), axial CT (B) and fused PET/CT (C) from the same patient show bilateral, noncalcified pulmonary nodules with variably increased FDG activity ➡. A biopsy of the contralateral right lung lesion confirmed metastatic adenocarcinoma.

LUNG CANCER

PET/CT Findings: Staging

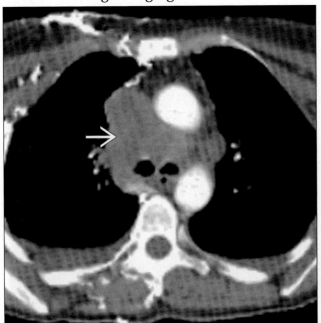 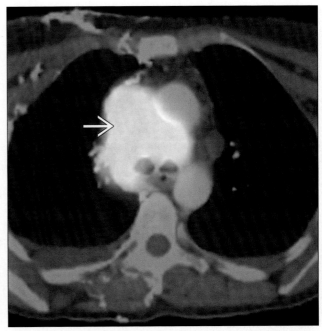

(Left) Axial CECT shows a large low attenuation mediastinal mass ➤ in this patient with recently diagnosed small cell carcinoma. *(Right)* Axial fused PET/CT shows intense diffusely increased FDG activity throughout the mediastinal mass ➤. In general, small cell carcinoma tends to be very FDG avid; however, it may occasionally be only mildly to moderately FDG avid.

PET/CT Findings: Staging

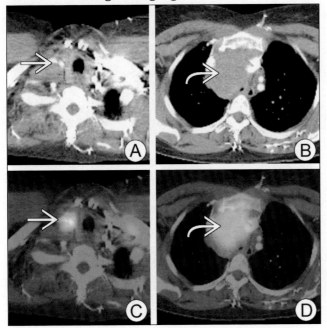 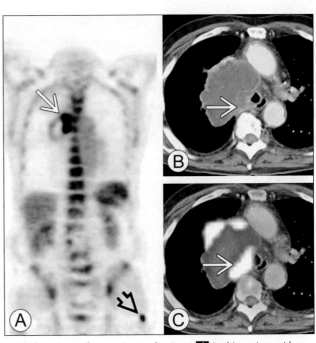

(Left) Axial CT (A, B) and fused PET/CT (C, D) show a moderately hypermetabolic mass in the anterior mediastinum ➤ in this patient with recently diagnosed small cell carcinoma. A small right supraclavicular lymph node ➤ is also identified. *(Right)* Coronal PET (A), axial CT (B) and fused PET/CT (C) show intense FDG activity along the medial margin of a large necrotic mass ➤, biopsy-proven to be small cell carcinoma. Additional findings include a focal metastasis to the left femur ➤.

LUNG CANCER

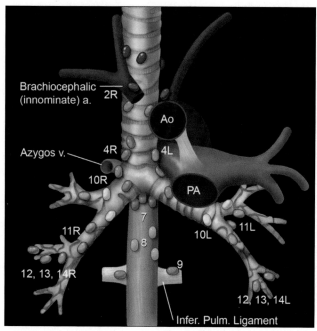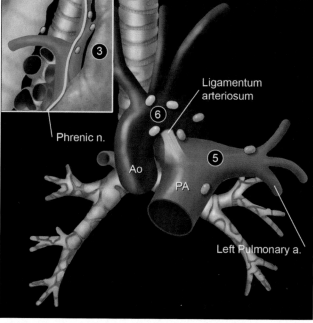

(Left) Graphic shows the American Thoracic Society (ATS) mediastinal nodal classifications. Many surgeons use this information for pre-operative planning, so it is important to include this material in a PET/CT report. *(Right)* Graphic shows additional ATS classifications for mediastinal nodes. These two graphics constitute a complete listing of ATS classifications.

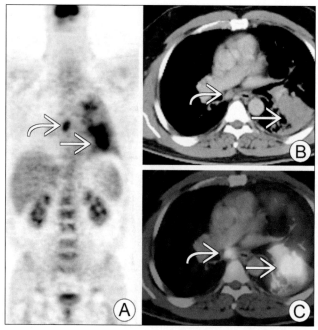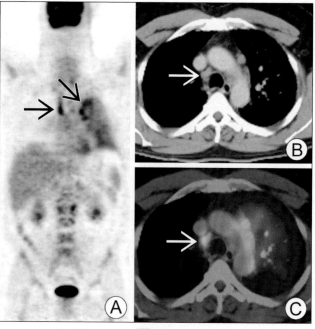

(Left) Coronal PET (A), axial CT (B) and fused PET/CT (C) demonstrate a hypermetabolic left lower lobe ➡ squamous cell carcinoma and a hypermetabolic subcarinal lymph node ➡ that was not enlarged. *(Right)* Coronal PET (A) of the same patient shows more hypermetabolic lymph nodes in the mediastinum ➡. The axial CT (B) and fused PET/CT images (C) show an abnormal but regular-sized contralateral lymph node ➡. Together, the findings classify this patient's disease as stage IIIB.

LUNG CANCER

PET/CT Findings: Staging

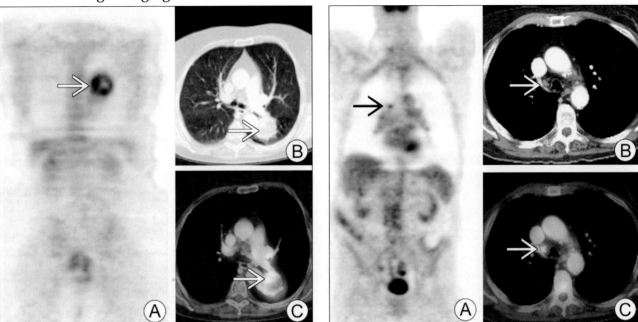

(Left) *Coronal PET (A), axial CT (B) and fused PET/CT (C) demonstrate a partially cavitary hypermetabolic mass in the left lower lobe ➡,* *compatible with a newly diagnosed squamous cell carcinoma.* *(Right)* *In this patient with newly diagnosed left-sided adenocarcinoma, coronal* *PET (A) reveals a tiny focus of moderately increased FDG activity in the right paratracheal area ➡, which corresponds to a 6 mm lymph node* *➡ visible on axial CT (B) and fused PET/CT (C).*

PET/CT Findings: Staging

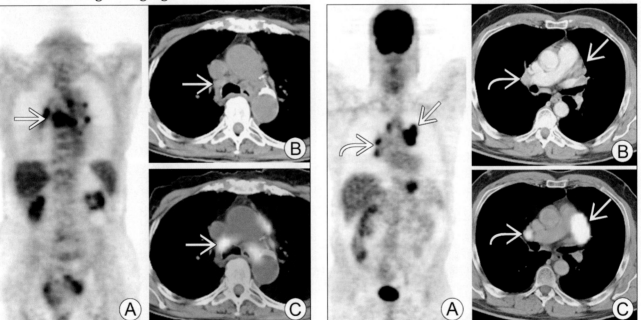

(Left) *Coronal PET (A), axial CT (B) and fused PET/CT (C) show multiple mediastinal lymph nodes ➡. Some are normal in size, while others* *are borderline enlarged, with intense metabolic activity. These findings are very suspicious for metastatic disease.* *(Right)* *Multiple images (A, B,* *C) from a staging PET/CT in a patient with a newly diagnosed left-sided non-small cell lung carcinoma ➡ show contralateral lymph nodes with* *intense metabolic activity ➡, worrisome for metastatic involvement.*

LUNG CANCER

PET/CT Findings: Staging

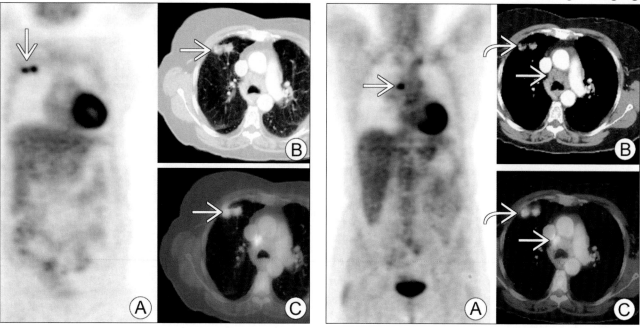

(Left) Coronal PET (A), axial CT (B) and fused PET/CT (C) demonstrate multifocal primary adenocarcinoma of the lung ➡. *(Right)* Axial CT (B) and fused PET/CT (C) show a primary adenocarcinoma ➡ of the right lung. In addition, there is a small 8 mm pretracheal lymph node ➡ with intense FDG activity on coronal PET (A) and on the PET/CT (C). Subsequent biopsy, via bronchoscopy, confirmed metastatic disease.

PET/CT Findings: Staging

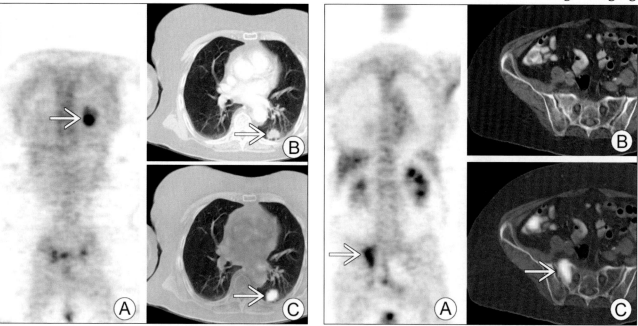

(Left) Coronal PET (A), axial CT (B) and fused PET/CT (C) demonstrate a left lower lobe adenocarcinoma with intense FDG activity ➡. *(Right)* Coronal PET (A) and fused PET/CT (C) in the same patient show linear intense FDG activity within the right hemisacrum ➡. If malignant, this finding would make the patient's disease stage IV. However, an MR demonstrated a linear fracture line not seen on axial CT (B), compatible with an insufficiency fracture, not metastatic disease.

LUNG CANCER

PET/CT Findings: Staging

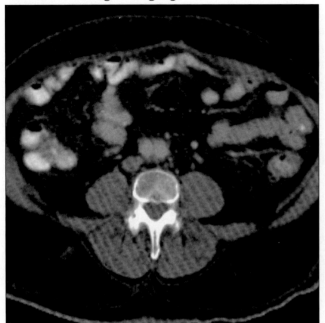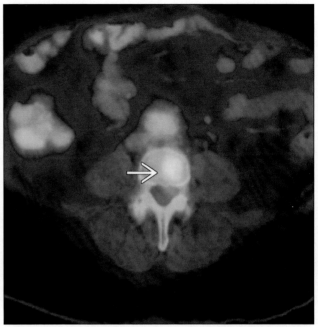

(Left) Axial CECT shows no definite abnormality in this patient with a history of NSCLC. *(Right)* Axial fused PET/CT shows focal intense activity in the left side of the L4 vertebral body ➡, compatible with unsuspected metastatic disease. This patient had a total of 3 metastatic lesions, which were identified just after the patient had been discharged following a right lower lobectomy.

PET/CT Findings: Staging

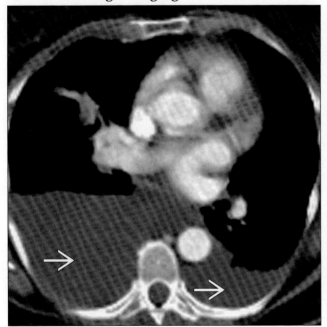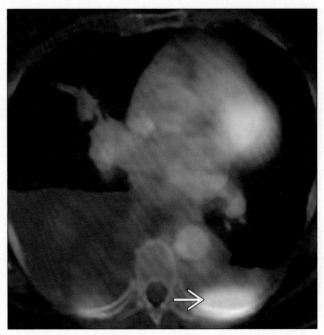

(Left) Axial CECT shows bilateral pleural effusions ➡ that are larger on the right than the left. *(Right)* Axial fused PET/CT shows intense metabolic activity in the posterior aspect of the left pleural effusion ➡. In general, it is difficult to diagnose malignant effusions, especially as many will not have increased metabolic activity. In this patient, however, the intense FDG activity suggested malignant pleural effusion. Subsequent thoracentesis proved the effusion to be malignant.

LUNG CANCER

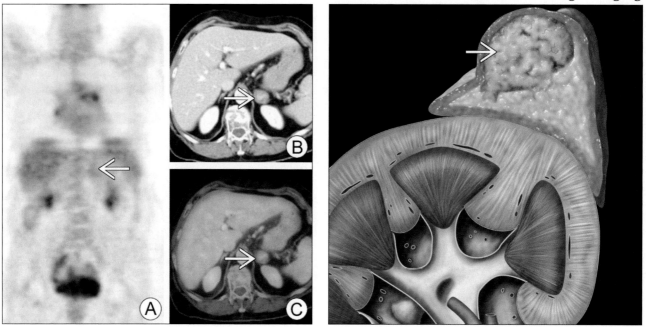

(Left) Coronal PET (A), axial CT (B) and fused PET/CT (C) show a left adrenal lesion ➡ in a patient with newly diagnosed squamous cell carcinoma of the lung. NECT demonstrated this to be 5 Hounsfield units, compatible with an adenoma. *(Right)* Graphic shows the typical appearance of an adrenal adenoma ➡ with lipid content.

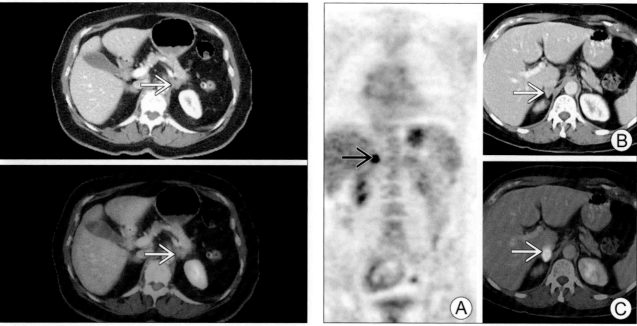

(Left) Axial CT (top) and fused PET/CT (bottom) show a nodular left adrenal lesion ➡ in a patient newly diagnosed with non-small cell lung cancer. Absence of increased metabolic activity favors an adenoma. *(Right)* Coronal PET (A) shows a focus of intense activity in the right suprarenal space ➡. Axial CT (B) and fused PET/CT (C) show a right adrenal lesion with intense FDG activity ➡. The metabolic activity observed is benign, and the malignant lesions overlap.

LUNG CANCER

PET/CT Findings: Staging

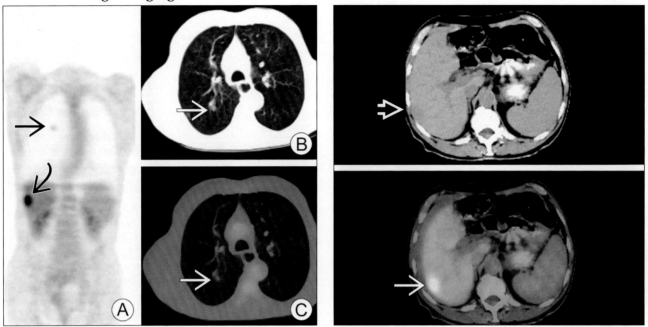

(Left) Coronal image (A) shows a faint focus of increased FDG activity in the right lung ➔ and a hepatic lesion with intense FDG activity ➔. Axial CT (B) and fused PET/CT (C) show a 6 mm pulmonary nodule with increased FDG activity ➔, worrisome for metastasis in this patient with right-sided non-small cell lung cancer. *(Right)* Axial CT (top) and fused PET/CT (bottom) both demonstrate a hepatic metastasis ➔. Note that the metastasis is not well seen on noncontrast CT ➔.

PET/CT Findings: Restaging

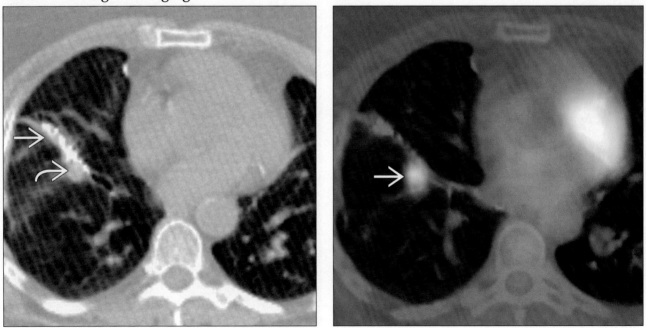

(Left) Axial CECT, performed in this patient who had a wedge resection, shows thickening along the resection margin ➔ with nodular thickening medially ➔, worrisome for malignancy. *(Right)* Axial fused PET/CT shows intense FDG activity along the medial resection margin ➔. Given a 6 month interval since surgery, the differential includes scarring vs. residual or recurrent malignancy. In general, scarring shows no increased FDG activity, which confirms this activity as malignant.

LUNG CANCER

PET/CT Findings: Restaging

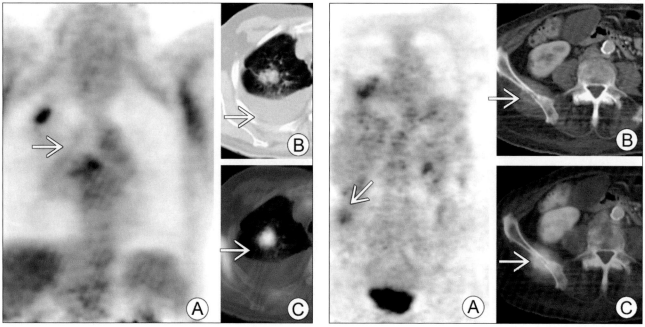

(Left) Coronal PET (A), axial CT (B) and fused PET/CT (C) demonstrate a right upper lobe mass with intense FDG activity ➡ in this patient with newly diagnosed adenocarcinoma of the lung. *(Right)* Coronal PET (A), axial CT (B) and fused PET/CT (C) in a patient recently diagnosed with adenocarcinoma show a lesion with moderately increased FDG activity in the right iliac bone ➡.

PET/CT Findings: Restaging

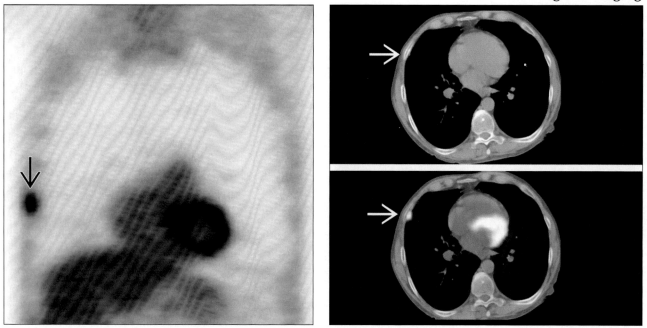

(Left) Coronal PET shows focal intense activity along the right chest wall ➡ in this patient with a history of squamous cell carcinoma of the lung. *(Right)* Axial CT (top) and fused PET/CT (bottom) localize the focal activity seen in the previous image to a right anterior rib ➡. The patient had no history of trauma, and there was no radiographic evidence of a fracture. This lesion is therefore very suspicious for metastatic disease.

LUNG CANCER

PET/CT Findings: Restaging

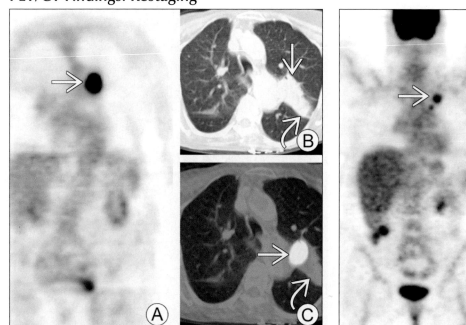

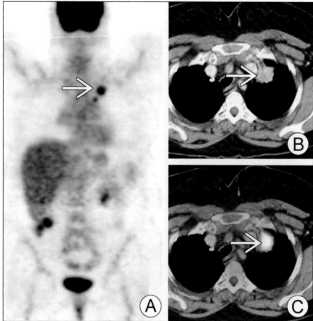

(Left) Coronal PET (A), axial CT (B) and fused PET/CT (C) show a left upper lobe mass with intense FDG activity ➡, compatible with recurrent lung cancer with post-obstructive atelectasis ➡. *(Right)* Coronal PET (A), axial CT (B) and fused PET/CT (C) demonstrate an FDG-avid mass at the left apex ➡. The scans were taken as part of radiation treatment planning in this patient with proven squamous cell carcinoma.

PET/CT Findings: Response to Therapy

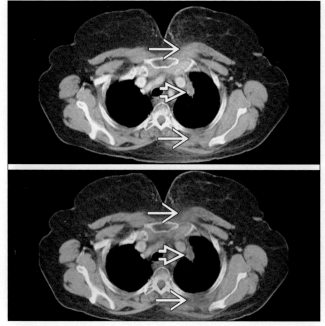

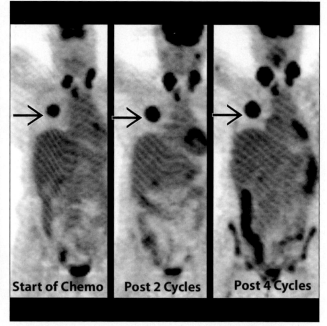

Start of Chemo   Post 2 Cycles   Post 4 Cycles

(Left) Axial CT (top) and fused PET/CT (bottom) of a patient 10 weeks post radiation treatment for a left upper lobe mass ➡ show only minimal FDG activity in the primary mass. Also note linear increased activity in the musculature in the anterior and posterior thorax ➡, secondary to radiation-induced myositis. *(Right)* Multiple coronal images from three PET scans show increased metabolic activity ➡ after two and four cycles of chemotherapy. This is typical of patients who are considered nonresponders.

LUNG CANCER

PET/CT Findings: Response to Therapy

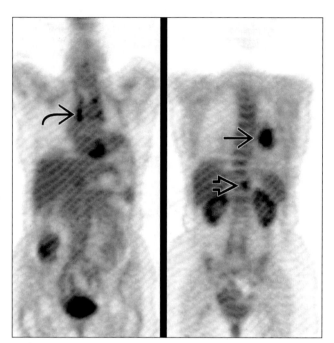

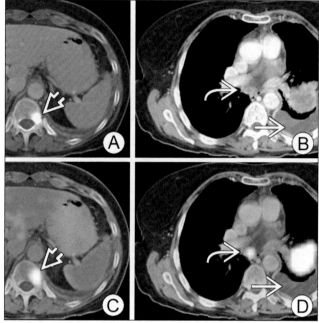

(Left) Coronal PET images demonstrate a primary left lung adenocarcinoma ⇒ with contralateral lymph node involvement ⇒ as well as a probable metastatic lesion to the mid-thoracic spine ⇒. *(Right)* Axial CT (A, B) and fused PET/CT (C, D) confirm a blastic lesion ⇒ in the thoracic vertebral body. Subcarinal adenopathy is detected ⇒, as is a small left-sided pleural effusion ⇒.

PET/CT Findings: Response to Therapy

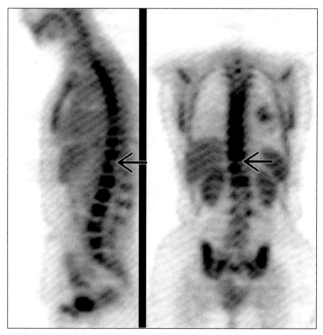

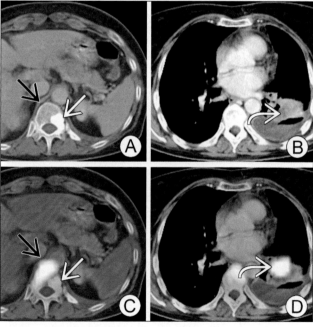

(Left) Sagittal (left) and coronal (right) PET show diffuse intense FDG activity throughout the osseous structures. This patient, also shown in the previous images, received chemotherapy and G-CSF support. Note the photopenic area where the primary blastic lesion has been treated ⇒. *(Right)* Axial CT (A, B) and fused PET/CT (C, D) show photopenia in the treated blastic vertebral metastasis ⇒ compared to the normal stimulated bone marrow ⇒. Persistent activity is identified in the primary lung carcinoma ⇒.

LUNG CANCER

PET/CT Pitfalls: Bronchioloalveolar Carcinoma

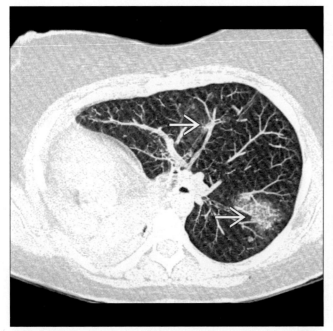
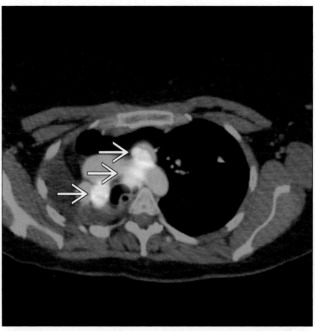

(Left) Axial CT shows two ground-glass opacities in the left lung ➔. The patient had a history of prior pneumonectomy for BAC on the right side. After a trial of antibiotics, the lesion did not resolve; subsequent biopsy showed BAC. *(Right)* Axial fused PET/CT shows multiple mediastinal nodes ➔ with intense FDG activity in the same patient. The patient was potentially eligible for lung transplantation if she had no evidence of tumor outside the lung.

PET/CT Pitfalls: Bronchioloalveolar Carcinoma

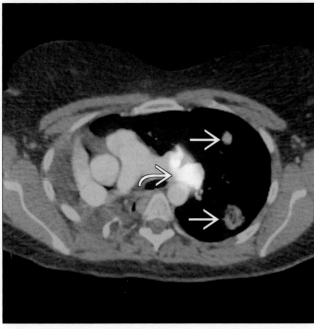
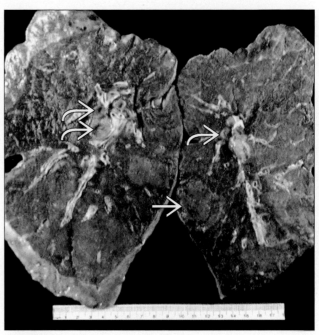

(Left) Axial fused PET/CT shows mild FDG activity in the known areas of BAC ➔. Mild FDG activity is characteristic of BAC. However, the nodes are very hypermetabolic ➔ and do not correlate with the FDG activity of the primary lesions. Bronchoscopic evaluation showed sarcoidosis. The patient became a transplant candidate and later recipient. *(Right)* Gross pathology from the same patient (previous 3 figures) shows primary BAC ➔ with non-caseating nodes ➔. The patient has continued to do well after transplantation.

LUNG CANCER

PET/CT Pitfalls: Bronchioloalveolar Carcinoma

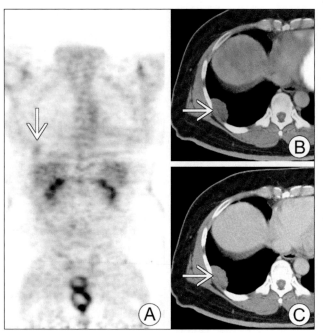

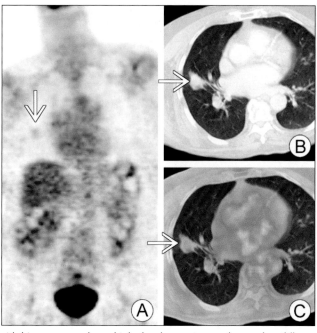

(Left) Coronal PET (A), axial CT (B) and fused PET/CT (C) in this patient with biopsy-proven bronchioloalveolar carcinoma show only mildly increased metabolic activity in the primary mass ➡. Bronchioalveolar carcinoma has variable FDG activity ranging from almost none to intense. (Right) Coronal PET (A), axial CT (B) and fused PET/CT (C) in a patient recently diagnosed with bronchioloalveolar carcinoma demonstrate only mildly increased metabolic activity ➡.

PET/CT Pitfalls: Bronchioloalveolar Carcinoma

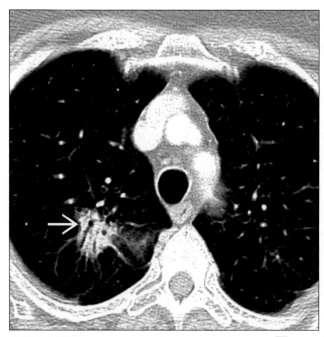

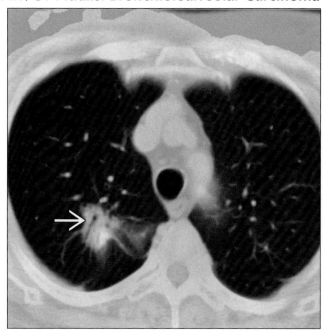

(Left) Axial CECT shows ground-glass right upper lobe mass ➡ that did not resolve with a course of antibiotics. (Right) Axial fused PET/CT shows only mildly increased FDG activity associated with the mass ➡, confirmed to be BAC.

LUNG CANCER

PET/CT Pitfalls: Bronchioloalveolar Carcinoma

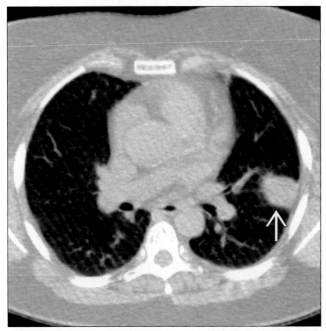 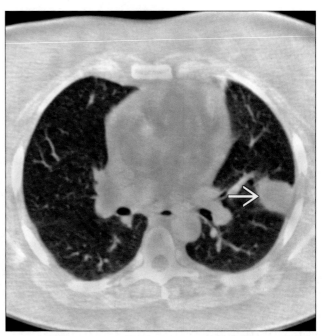

(Left) Axial CECT shows solid airspace lesion adjacent to the major fissure on the left ➔ that did not resolve over time. *(Right)* Axial fused PET/CT shows only mildly increased FDG activity associated with the mass ➔, confirmed to be BAC.

PET/CT Pitfalls: Bronchioloalveolar Carcinoma

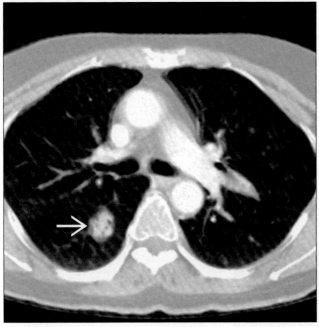 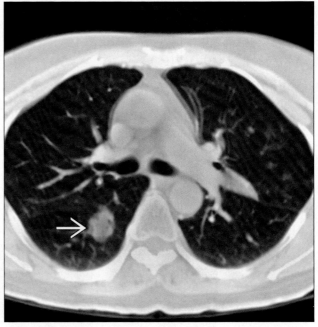

(Left) Axial CECT shows a "bubbly" lesion in the superior segment left lower lobe ➔, worrisome for BAC. *(Right)* Axial fused PET/CT shows only mildly increased FDG activity associated with the mass ➔, confirmed to be BAC.

BREAST CANCER

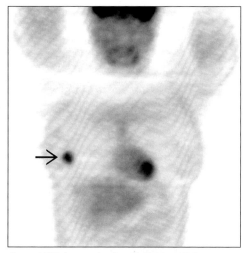

Coronal PET shows a focal area of intense FDG activity in the right breast ➡, which is compatible with this patient's known history of recently diagnosed breast cancer.

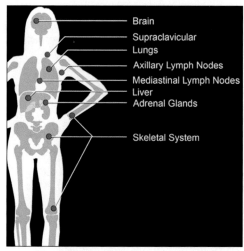

Graphic shows the most common areas of metastatic involvement from breast cancer.

TERMINOLOGY

Abbreviations and Synonyms
- Ductal carcinoma
- Lobular carcinoma
- Breast cancer
- Breast carcinoma
- Inflammatory breast cancer
- Paget disease

Definitions
- Primary malignancy of breast tissue

IMAGING FINDINGS

General Features
- Best diagnostic clue
  - **Primary**
    - Correspondence between suspicious lesion on mammography/ultrasound (US) and focal uptake on FDG PET
    - Incidental focal FDG activity on PET or PET/CT should be further evaluated with mammography/US and biopsy
  - **Metastasis**
    - Uptake and morphologic changes in axillary, internal mammary, and distant lymph nodes
    - Most common metastatic locations are bone, liver, and lung
- Location
  - **Primary**
    - Within breast parenchyma, sometimes including contiguous skin or intramammary lymph nodes
  - **Metastasis**
    - Location by relative frequency: Axillary lymph node (LN) > internal mammary LN > bone > liver
    - Metastases may be seen in any location, often unpredictable
- Size
  - Range from microscopic calcifications to large mass
  - Lesions may grow to several centimeters
  - Many smaller lesions not visible on CT or PET
- Morphology
  - Range of morphologies
    - Microcalcifications

DDx: Breast Mass on PET/CT

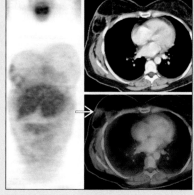

Post-Operative Changes

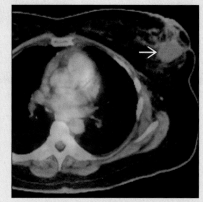

Seroma

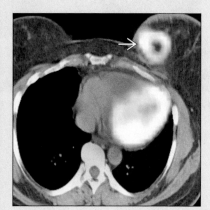

Abscess

BREAST CANCER

Key Facts

Imaging Findings

- Lesions < 1 cm difficult to detect on whole-body PET/CT or scintigraphy
- Primary lesion: Focal increased activity on PET/CT corresponding to suspicious mammographic lesion or lesion on ultrasound
- Metastatic disease: Axillary, internal mammary, and distant lymph nodes (LN); bone, liver, and lung most common metastatic locations
- PET/CT: Optimal detection of distant metastases in high risk patients; more sensitive for detecting osteolytic bone metastases
- Recent evidence suggests can proceed to full axillary lymph node dissection when multiple nodes positive in the axilla

- Refinement of locoregional assessment and detection of occult distant metastases in stage II/III disease
- Dual time point imaging not universally accepted or used but may be helpful in certain patient populations

Top Differential Diagnoses

- Infection/Inflammation
- Trauma and Surgery
- Lactating Breast
- Nonmalignant Tumors

Diagnostic Checklist

- PET/CT excellent for staging patients with potentially aggressive breast cancers and for monitoring response to treatment
- PET/CT demonstration of osseous metastases usually precludes need for bone scan

---

- Spiculated mass
- Ill-defined mass
- Well-circumscribed mass (less common)

Imaging Recommendations

- Best imaging tool
  - **Mammography**
    - Still the gold standard for screening
    - Most cases of breast cancer detected on screening exam are stage I; therefore, PET/CT is not cost effective in this group
    - For patients with suspected advanced disease or otherwise deemed "high risk", consider PET/CT for overall staging evaluation
  - **Ultrasound (US)**
    - Preferred modality for determining cystic vs. solid nature of suspicious lesions found on mammography
  - **Image-guided biopsy**
    - US, stereotactic devices, and MR are employed to sample tissue for pathologic evaluation
  - **CT**
    - Dynamic contrast-enhanced CT for detection of intraductal extension of breast cancer
    - Generally more useful for assessment of spread than for imaging of the primary lesion
    - 3D CT imaging can provide useful information for surgical planning
  - **PET/CT: Lymph nodes**
    - Twice the sensitivity of CT for abnormal nodal findings in internal mammary and mediastinal regions
    - Improved detection of disease in internal mammary, sub- and interpectoral, supra- and infraclavicular, and Berg level III nodes
    - Although its sensitivity is lower, the PPV of PET is nearly 100% for detecting malignant nodes
    - When axillary lymph nodes are positive on PET/CT, may obviate the need for sentinel lymph node scintigraphy
  - **PET/CT: Locoregional disease**
    - May help detect multiple primary tumor sites

- Location of primary in patients with breast cancer metastases and indeterminate mammography
- Replaces biopsy in patients for whom this is undesirable
- Increases confidence of locoregional assessment in stage II/III disease
  - **PET/CT: Distant disease**
    - Whole-body staging is improved, helping to avoid unnecessary surgery
    - Early detection of bony involvement to help avoid fracture
    - Best for detection of osteolytic bone mets (bone scan preferred for detection of osteoblastic mets)
  - **PET/CT: Treatment monitoring**
    - Baseline tumor SUV can be established for accurate assessment of therapy response
  - **MR**
    - Modality of choice to evaluate for brain metastases and confirmation of hepatic metastases
    - Also used in some patients to look at bilateral breast involvement in high risk patients
    - Used as a problem solving tool in other patients with dense breasts or other processes in which mammography is less sensitive
- Protocol advice
  - 10-15 mCi (370-550 MBq) F18-FDG IV
  - Supine whole-body PET/CT, usually with arms up
  - Prone imaging
    - May increase sensitivity when performed following supine study
    - Improved sensitivity for evaluation of breast, axilla, and mediastinum
  - Time point of imaging is controversial
    - Standard is 30-60 minutes after FDG injection
    - Inflammatory lesions can take up FDG more quickly and intensely than tumor, obscuring evaluation of malignant foci
    - Increased uptake of tumor over 1-3 hours
    - Decreasing nonmalignant tissue uptake at these time points
    - Dual-time point imaging may help avoid inaccuracies imposed by several factors

BREAST CANCER

- Serum glucose, insulin, injection-acquisition interval variability, and partial volume effects may all affect image quality and FDG uptake by cells
- Use of dual-time point imaging recommended for patients whose breast masses show mild uptake on initial PET images
- Dual-time point imaging not routinely used

CT Findings
- **NECT**
  o Useful for lung & pleural metastases
  o Can also detect lymphangitic spread
  o Suboptimal for organ evaluation
- **CECT**
  o Useful for evaluating mediastinal & organ metastases, particularly in the liver
  o Lesions appear attenuating compared with fatty background
  o May show early enhancement on arterial phase on dynamic contrast-enhanced CT
  o Tumors appear as dense lesions on CT and usually show early contrast enhancement similar to that seen with dynamic MR
  o **CT performance parameters**
    - Sensitivity, specificity, and accuracy in detecting intraductal spread or DCIS: 71.9%, 83.3%, and 76.0%
    - Sensitivity, specificity, and accuracy for diagnosing muscular invasion: 100%, 99%, and 99%
    - Sensitivity, specificity, and accuracy in diagnosing skin invasion: 84%, 93%, and 91%
    - Sensitivity rate for microcalcifications: 59%
    - 3D CT shown to depict and define extent of nearly all tumors in most patients

Nuclear Medicine Findings
- **PET/CT: General**
  o Sensitivities for PET and PET/CT range from 80-90% for evaluation of primary tumors
    - Lower sensitivity for smaller primary lesions
    - 60-80% sensitivity for lesions ≥ 2 mm
    - Prone PET/CT may allow detection of smaller lesions (5-7 mm)
  o Superior resolution may be afforded by positron emission mammography (PEM), which can detect lesions as small as 2 cm
    - Sensitivity 90% and specificity 86%
    - Still investigational
  o High lesion SUV seen in
    - Larger invasive tumor
    - Higher histologic grade, mitotic counts, and nuclear atypia
    - Absence of hormone receptors
    - Presence of c-erbB-2 expression
    - Metastasis to lymph nodes
    - Infiltrating ductal type (vs. infiltrating lobular type)
- **Initial Diagnosis**
  o PET/CT is not recommended for initial diagnosis but may be helpful in select patient populations or when standard modalities are ineffective
    - Consider for occasional use in patients with implants

- Dense breast tissue can render mammography nondiagnostic
- Cross-sectional morphologic imaging may be equivocal
  o Lower FDG uptake seen in well differentiated and lobular carcinomas compared to other breast cancers
    - Normal-range SUV in these malignancies can lead to false negatives
    - If CT shows a spiculated enhancing mass with low level FDG activity, may represent non-FDG-avid malignancy
  o Tubular cancer may also have have low FDG uptake
  o High grade DCIS may be positive on PET if > 1.5-2.0 cm
  o Tumors with higher tendency to relapse often have SUV above 3.3-4.0
- **Staging**
  o Overall, whole-body PET/CT limited in detection of < 8 mm lesions
  o Although not currently recommended for axillary nodal evaluation, positive axillary lymph node on PET/CT has high PPV for malignancy
  o Characterization of axillary metastases depends on several factors
    - Size and number of lymph nodes
    - PET/CT has lower sensitivity of 60-80% for axillary mets
    - FDG PET can provide resolution only to level of 6-8 mm lesions
    - Optimal axillary staging depends on sentinal LN biopsy
  o Evaluation of internal mammary and mediastinal lymph nodes
    - PET/CT superior for detection and localization (vs. CT and MR)
    - Accurate staging of these lymph node stations is crucial for prognosis and therapy
  o PET/CT has 80-95% sensitivity for detecting distant metastases at the time of initial diagnosis
    - NPV > 70-90%
    - PPV lower due to confounding factors such as infection, inflammation, etc.
    - NPV and PPV both benefit from combined modality PET/CT or MR fusion
  o Detection of hepatic metastases
    - Combination of low density lesion on CT and increased uptake on FDG PET is highly suggestive of malignancy
    - MR can clarify cases with positive FDG PET and negative CT
    - False negatives may be seen with subcentimeter lesions and low density lesions with nonelevated FDG uptake
    - False positives most often due to infection/inflammation or interposed colon
    - Occasionally seen incidentally on bone scan
  o Detection of osseous metastases
    - Consideration should be given to performing both bone scan and FDG PET/CT at initial staging in high risk patients
    - Information complementary in breast cancer osseous metastatic assessment

BREAST CANCER

- Lytic and trabecular metastases are detected with high sensitivity > 90% on FDG PET
- Blastic lesions poorly seen on PET but can be detected on CT
- Bone scan is preferred for detection of cortical blastic metastases but has poor sensitivity for lytic or trabecular metastases (75-80% and < 50%)
  - Effect on management: FDG PET or PET/CT may change patient management up to 51% of the time
  - PET/CT plays an increasingly important role in radiation therapy planning
    - Pre-treatment planning or follow-up with PET/CT benefits 40-60% of patients in multiple studies
- **Restaging**
  - Overall, FDG PET has equal or better accuracy for restaging compared to conventional imaging
  - Combined PET/CT offers higher sensitivity and specificity than PET alone
  - False positives due to prior lymphadenectomy
    - Surgical site may remain positive for 3-12 months
    - Inflammation may persist surrounding clips or sutures
  - FDG PET is superior to conventional imaging for diagnosis of metastatic disease (87-90% vs. 50-78%)
    - In patients with rising serum tumor markers and asymptomatic breast cancer
- **Response to Therapy**
  - SUV response has proven an accurate indicator of treatment response
  - Major criterion for good treatment response is approximately 50-60% reduction in SUV following 2 cycles of chemotherapy
    - > 55% reduction after 1 cycle portends good clinical response
    - Increase in SUV 7-10 days after antiestrogen therapy may occur due to a metabolic flare
    - Typically associated with good response
  - Detection of poor response is equally valuable
    - Early institution of alternate therapy
    - Side effects are minimized from inadequate treatments

Other Modality Findings
- Positron emission mammography (PEM)
  - Investigational modality
  - F-18 used as radiotracer
  - Improves accuracy for primary lesion detection
- F-18 fluoride PET/CT
  - Superior to traditional bone imaging agents (Tc-99m MDP)
  - Pending resolution of reimbursement and FDA issues
- F-18 estradiol compounds demonstrate whether malignant lesions are estrogen receptor (ER) positive (investigational)
- F-18 L-thymidine demonstrates tissue with high DNA turnover (investigational)

DIFFERENTIAL DIAGNOSIS

Infection/Inflammation
- Generally lower SUV-to-background ratio than equal-sized tumors
- Granuloma-producing disease (e.g., sarcoidosis)
- Soft tissue infection (e.g., esophagitis, abscess)
- Atherosclerosis
- Sites of surgical intervention (e.g., resection, ostomy sites)
- Intramuscular injection sites
- Degenerative bone disease
- Non-puerperal mastitis

Trauma and Surgery
- Inflammatory uptake related to surgical procedures last 3-6 months
- Uptake can be due to hematoma
- Scar tissue may demonstrate uptake indefinitely
- Traumatic fracture and soft tissue injuries (e.g., lytic bone metastases)

Fibrocystic Disease
- Low level FDG uptake may be seen in multiple focal sites

Nonmalignant Tumors
- Fibroadenoma, papilloma, and others
- Characterized by low level FDG uptake
  - Hypercellular benign tumors may show increased uptake

Lactating Breast
- Glandular tissue may show intense FDG uptake
- May see patchy areas of intense FDG activity
- History is critical to reduce misinterpretation

Normal Breast
- FDG uptake more intense with increasing breast density

Other Malignancy
- Second primary neoplasm (e.g., thyroid, lung, colon, etc.)
- Primary breast lymphoma

Implants
- Inflammatory response to silicone or saline leakage can produce positive PET
  - Silicone > saline
- Calcifications can produce inflammatory uptake or AC artifact (in the case of bulky calcification)

PATHOLOGY

General Features
- General path comments: Higher SUV correlates with higher density of viable cancer cells
- Genetics
  - Increased incidence with close family history (e.g., mother, sister)
  - > 80-85% breast cancer occurs in absence of family history

BREAST CANCER

- o BRCA-1, BRCA-2
  - Genetic mutations present in ~ 0.5% of population
  - Confer 3-7x risk of developing breast cancer compared to women without these mutations
  - BRCA-2 may increase breast cancer risk in men
- Etiology
  - o Risk factors
    - Age
    - Family history
    - Personal history
    - Early menarche
    - Late menopause
    - Postmenopausal obesity
    - Radiation exposure (greatest risk with external beam)
    - Alcohol ingestion
    - Hormone replacement therapy
  - o Full-term pregnancy at early age reduces risk
- Epidemiology
  - o Most common cancer in women
    - Second to lung as most common cause of cancer death
  - o Lifetime risk in women for breast cancer: 13.2%
    - With BRCA mutation: Up to 85%

Microscopic Features

- Ductal cancers (arising from ductal cells)
  - o In situ: Ducts containing tumor cells with no stromal invasion
  - o Invasive: Tumor penetrates ductal epithelium and invades stroma
- Lobular cancers (arising from lobule cells)
  - o In situ: Lobules containing tumor cells with no lobule wall penetration
  - o Invasive: Stromal invasion by tumor cells

Staging, Grading, or Classification Criteria

- Tumor (T) staging for primary breast cancer
  - o TX: Primary tumor cannot be assessed
  - o T0: No evidence of primary tumor
  - o Tis: Carcinoma in situ
    - Tis (DCIS): Intraductal carcinoma in situ
    - Tis (LCIS): Lobular carcinoma in situ
    - Tis (Paget): Paget disease of nipple with no tumor;
    - Tumor-associated Paget disease classified according to primary tumor size
  - o T1: Tumor ≤ 2 cm in greatest dimension
    - T1mic: Microinvasion ≤ 0.1 cm in greatest dimension
    - T1a: 0.1 cm < tumor ≤ 0.5 cm in greatest dimension
    - T1b: 0.5 cm < tumor ≤ 1 cm in greatest dimension
    - T1c: 1 cm < tumor ≤ 2 cm in greatest dimension
  - o T2: 2 cm < tumor ≤ 5 cm in greatest dimension
  - o T3: Tumor > 5 cm in greatest dimension
  - o T4: Tumor of any size with direct extension to (a) chest wall or (b) skin
    - T4a: Extension to chest wall
    - T4b: Edema (including peau d'orange) or ulceration of breast skin, or satellite skin nodules confined to same breast
    - T4c: Both T4a and T4b

- T4d: Inflammatory carcinoma
  - o Stage I: Tumor < 2 cm
  - o Stage II: Tumor < 2 cm, 1-3 positive axillary LN; tumor 2-5 cm, negative LN or 1-3 positive LN; tumor > 5 cm, negative LN
  - o Stage III: Tumor < 5 cm with 4-9 positive axillary LN or positive internal mammary LN
    - Tumor > 5 cm, positive axillary/internal mammary LN; tumor invades chest wall, ± axillary/internal mammary LN
  - o Stage IV: Distant metastases

CLINICAL ISSUES

Presentation

- Most common signs/symptoms
  - o Breast mass discovered by self-examination or routine screening mammography
  - o Higher PPV for malignancy with unilateral nipple discharge or nipple inversion/retraction
  - o Organ specific findings
  - o Brain
    - Neurological dysfunction
  - o Bone
    - Most are asymptomatic (50-60% of patients with bone mets on FDG PET area have no pain)
    - Not uncommon though for patients to have bone pain
  - o Liver
    - Most are asymptomatic
    - May advance to cause abdominal pain or liver failure
  - o Axilla
    - Mass
    - Arm swelling
  - o Many asymptomatic

Demographics

- Age: Predominantly occurs in women over age 50 (80% of cases)
- Gender: Male breast cancer occurs about 1/55 as frequently as female breast cancer
- Ethnicity: Mortality rate: African-Americans > Caucasians

Natural History & Prognosis

- **Survival**
  - o Overall about 2/3
  - o Early stage disease: 98%
  - o Disease with distant metastases
    - Remission rare at 10-20%, and cure is extremely rare
    - Average survival 1-2 years
  - o Recurrence: Most patients die of recurrent disease
    - 75% of recurrent disease occurs within 5 years of initial diagnosis
- **Prognosis**
  - o More than 4 positive axillary lymph nodes indicates high risk of recurrence
  - o Correlates with size of primary
  - o Higher risk with C-erbB-2 status

BREAST CANCER

o Correlates with estrogen and progesterone receptor status

Treatment

- Mastectomy extremely successful in cure of all types of DCIS
  o Recurrence 1-2%
- Lumpectomy with radiotherapy less effective
  o Local recurrence rates of 7-14%
  o Recurrence 27-43% with lumpectomy only
- Tamoxifen remains the mainstay of hormonal therapy
  o 44% and 52% decrease in recurrence in ipsilateral and contralateral breast
  o 50% decrease in risk of recurrence
  o 28% decrease in mortality
- Ovarian ablation has similar benefit to some chemotherapies
- Radiotherapy follows lumpectomy
  o Depends on site of lymphadenopathy
  o Used for treatment and palliation of metastatic disease

DIAGNOSTIC CHECKLIST

Consider

- PET/CT excellent for staging patients with potentially aggressive breast cancers and for monitoring response to treatment
- PET/CT demonstration of osseous metastases usually precludes need for bone scan but may miss osteoblastic lesions

Image Interpretation Pearls

- Multifocal breast cancer is not uncommon
  o Both breasts should be evaluated routinely
- Be aware of potential pitfalls and artifacts with PET/CT, including motion and misregistration
- Evaluate study quality prior to interpretation
  o Insulin effect due to poor dietary preparation may produce false negative study
  o Adequate time following injection (~ 60 minutes)
  o Optimization of scan time and FDG dose for quality
- Be aware of pertinent history, physical and other imaging findings prior to final interpretation
- False negatives in primary lesion with lobular, mucinous, tubular, and small-sized lesions

SELECTED REFERENCES

1. Castell F et al: Quantitative techniques in 18FDG PET scanning in oncology. Br J Cancer. 98(10):1597-601, 2008
2. Ford EC et al: Comparison of FDG-PET/CT and CT for delineation of lumpectomy cavity for partial breast irradiation. Int J Radiat Oncol Biol Phys. 71(2):595-602, 2008
3. Groheux D et al: Effect of (18)F-FDG PET/CT imaging in patients with clinical Stage II and III breast cancer. Int J Radiat Oncol Biol Phys. 71(3):695-704, 2008
4. Haug A et al: FDG-PET and FDG-PET/CT in breast cancer. Recent Results Cancer Res. 170:125-40, 2008
5. Hayashi M et al: PET/CT supports breast cancer diagnosis and treatment. Breast Cancer. 15(3):224-30, 2008
6. Heusner TA et al: Breast Cancer Staging in a Single Session: Whole-Body PET/CT Mammography. J Nucl Med. 49(8):1215-1222, 2008
7. Hodgson NC et al: Is there a role for positron emission tomography in breast cancer staging? J Clin Oncol. 26(5):712-20, 2008
8. Konecky SD et al: Comparison of diffuse optical tomography of human breast with whole-body and breast-only positron emission tomography. Med Phys. 35(2):446-55, 2008
9. Le-Petross CH et al: Evolving role of imaging modalities in inflammatory breast cancer. Semin Oncol. 35(1):51-63, 2008
10. Mahner S et al: Comparison between positron emission tomography using 2-[fluorine-18]fluoro-2-deoxy-D-glucose, conventional imaging and computed tomography for staging of breast cancer. Ann Oncol. 19(7):1249-54, 2008
11. Shie P et al: Meta-analysis: comparison of F-18 Fluorodeoxyglucose-positron emission tomography and bone scintigraphy in the detection of bone metastases in patients with breast cancer. Clin Nucl Med. 33(2):97-101, 2008
12. Tafra L: Positron emission mammography: a new breast imaging device. J Surg Oncol. 97(5):372-3, 2008
13. Tateishi U et al: Bone metastases in patients with metastatic breast cancer: morphologic and metabolic monitoring of response to systemic therapy with integrated PET/CT. Radiology. 247(1):189-96, 2008
14. Ueda S et al: Utility of 18F-fluoro-deoxyglucose emission tomography/computed tomography fusion imaging (18F-FDG PET/CT) in combination with ultrasonography for axillary staging in primary breast cancer. BMC Cancer. 8:165, 2008
15. Chen YW et al: Discordant findings of skeletal metastasis between tc 99M MDP bone scans and F18 FDG PET/CT imaging for advanced breast and lung cancers--two case reports and literature review. Kaohsiung J Med Sci. 23(12):639-46, 2007
16. Du Y et al: Fusion of metabolic function and morphology: sequential [18F]fluorodeoxyglucose positron-emission tomography/computed tomography studies yield new insights into the natural history of bone metastases in breast cancer. J Clin Oncol. 25(23):3440-7, 2007
17. Ikenaga N et al: Standardized uptake values for breast carcinomas assessed by fluorodeoxyglucose-positron emission tomography correlate with prognostic factors. Am Surg. 73(11):1151-7, 2007
18. Lim HS et al: FDG PET/CT for the detection and evaluation of breast diseases: usefulness and limitations. Radiographics. 27 Suppl 1:S197-213, 2007
19. Rosen EL et al: FDG PET, PET/CT, and breast cancer imaging. Radiographics. 27 Suppl 1:S215-29, 2007
20. Kumar R et al: Clinicopathologic factors associated with false negative FDG-PET in primary breast cancer. Breast Cancer Res Treat. 98(3):267-74, 2006
21. Kumar R et al: FDG PET positive lymph nodes are highly predictive of metastasis in breast cancer. Nucl Med Commun. 27(3):231-6, 2006
22. Radan L et al: The role of FDG-PET/CT in suspected recurrence of breast cancer. Cancer. 107(11):2545-51, 2006
23. Avril NE et al: Monitoring response to treatment in patients utilizing PET. Radiol Clin North Am. 43(1):189-204, 2005
24. Dose Schwarz J et al: Early prediction of response to chemotherapy in metastatic breast cancer using sequential 18F-FDG PET. J Nucl Med. 46(7):1144-50, 2005
25. Esserman L: Integration of imaging in the management of breast cancer. J Clin Oncol. 23(8):1601-2, 2005

BREAST CANCER

Initial Diagnosis

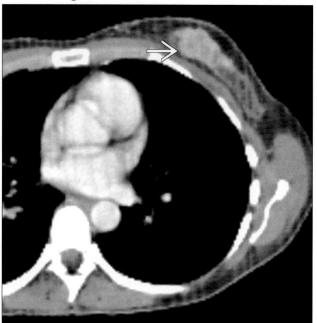 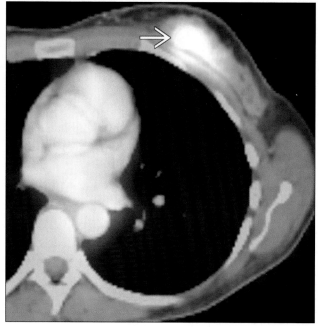

(Left) Axial CECT shows a heterogeneously enhancing mass in the left breast ➡ that is compatible with breast cancer. *(Right)* Axial fused PET/CT shows focal intense FDG activity ➡ that correlates with the enhancing mass in the left breast, compatible with primary breast carcinoma.

Initial Diagnosis

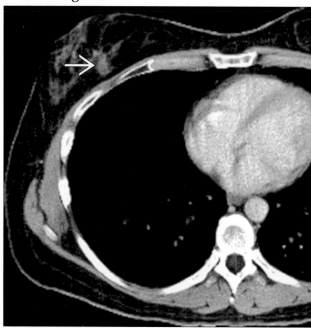 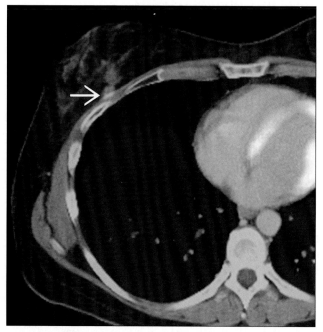

(Left) Axial CECT shows a nonspecific small mass-like area in the posterior right breast ➡ in this patient with recently diagnosed ductal carcinoma. *(Right)* Axial fused PET/CT shows focal intense activity posterior to the mass in the posterior right breast ➡. The activity is slightly misregistered due to differences in respiratory positioning during acquisition of the CT portions of the exam.

BREAST CANCER

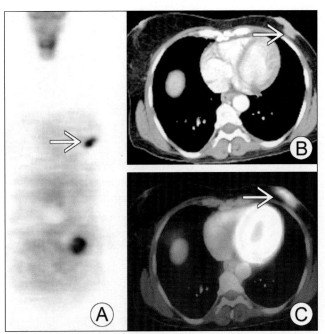 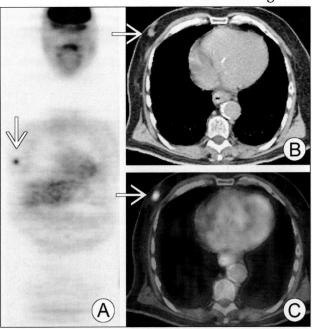

(Left) Coronal PET (A), axial CT (B) and fused PET/CT (C) demonstrate a focus of FDG activity in the left breast, correlating with a mass just posterior to the left nipple ➡️ and compatible with primary breast cancer. *(Right)* Coronal PET (A), axial CT (B) and fused PET/CT (C) demonstrate a focal area of intense FDG activity present in the right breast ➡️ in this man with newly diagnosed breast cancer.

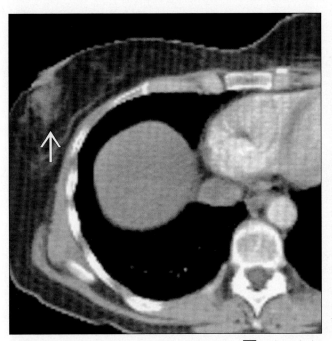 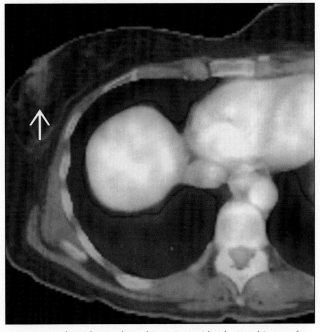

(Left) Axial CECT shows nonspecific mass-like tissue ➡️ in the right breast posterior to the right nipple in this patient with a known history of lobular carcinoma. *(Right)* Axial fused PET/CT shows minimally increased FDG activity within the mass ➡️, a common finding in patients with lobular carcinoma. This mild degree of FDG activity is characteristic of lobular carcinoma, with 65% being false negative on FDG PET.

BREAST CANCER

Initial Diagnosis

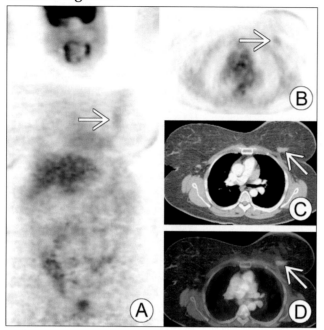

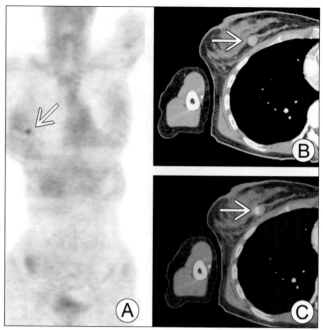

(Left) Coronal PET (A), axial PET (B), CECT (C), and fused PET/CT (D) show only minimally increased FDG activity correlating with the mass in the left breast ➡ in this patient with newly diagnosed breast cancer. (Right) Coronal PET (A), axial CT (B) and fused PET/CT (C) demonstrate focal, moderately increased FDG activity in the right breast correlating with a small but abnormally enhancing mass in posterior right breast ➡, compatible with breast cancer.

Staging

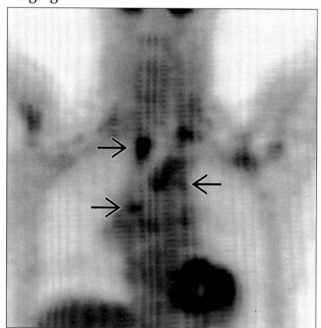

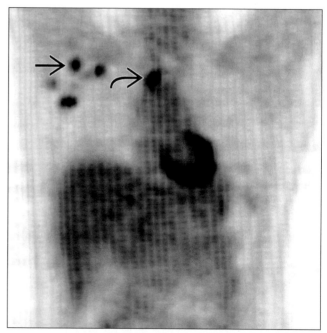

(Left) Coronal PET shows multiple abnormal foci of FDG activity ➡ in the mediastinum, compatible with metastatic disease. (Right) Coronal PET shows multiple foci of intense FDG activity in the right axilla ➡, compatible with metastatic disease. In addition, there is a focal area of activity along the right internal mammary nodal chain ➘.

BREAST CANCER

Staging

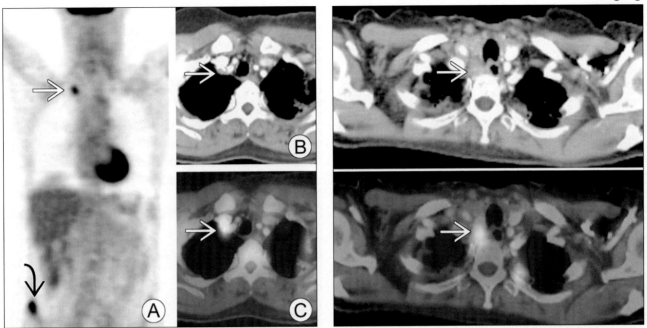

(Left) Coronal PET (A), axial CT (B) and fused PET/CT (C) demonstrate a focal area of intense FDG activity corresponding to a small soft tissue lesion just posterior to the right subclavian vein ➔. An additional metastasis is present in the right iliac bone ➔. *(Right)* Axial CT (top) and fused PET/CT (bottom) demonstrate focal intense activity corresponding to the subtle soft tissue attenuation lesion ➔ adjacent to the esophagus and posterior to the trachea.

Staging

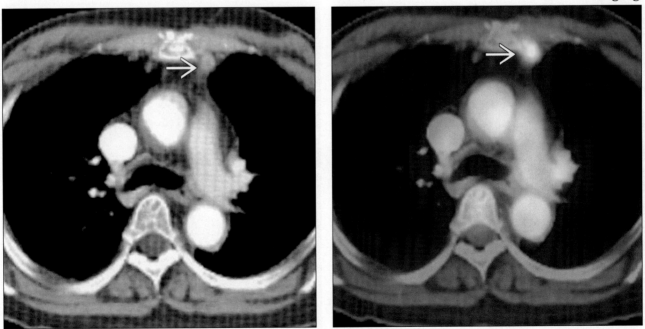

(Left) Axial CECT shows a borderline enlarged left internal mammary lymph node ➔ in this patient with a history of left-sided breast carcinoma. *(Right)* Axial fused PET/CT shows moderate to intense FDG activity within the borderline enlarged left internal mammary lymph node ➔, compatible with malignancy. PET/CT is superior to CT alone in the evaluation of internal mammary nodal involvement.

BREAST CANCER

Staging

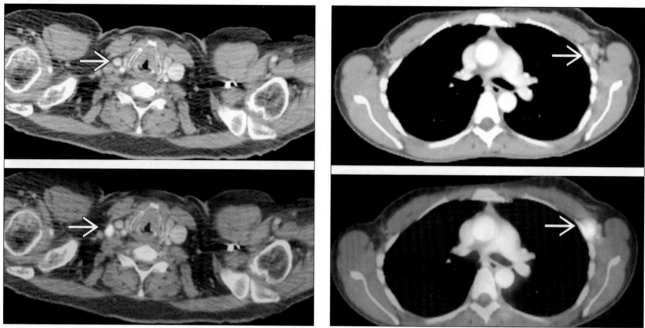

(Left) Axial CT (top) and fused PET/CT (bottom) demonstrate focal intense activity in a normal-sized but abnormally enhancing right supraclavicular lymph node ➡, compatible with malignancy. *(Right)* Axial CT (top) and fused PET/CT (bottom) demonstrate focal intense activity within the left axillary lymph node ➡, which is mildly enlarged on the CT and is compatible with regional metastatic disease. This patient was newly diagnosed with breast cancer.

Staging

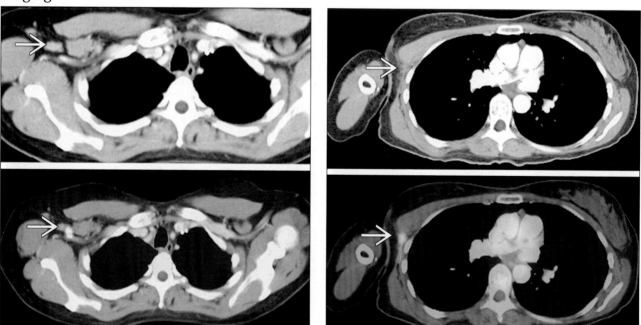

(Left) Axial CT (top) and fused PET/CT (bottom) demonstrate focal intense activity in a normal-sized but malignant lymph node in the right superior axilla ➡. *(Right)* Axial CT (top) and fused PET/CT (bottom) demonstrate moderate linear activity within the right axilla ➡ in this patient who underwent right axillary nodal dissection approximately 8 weeks prior to this scan. Subsequent follow-up scan demonstrated no abnormal activity, compatible with resolution of inflammatory uptake.

BREAST CANCER

Staging

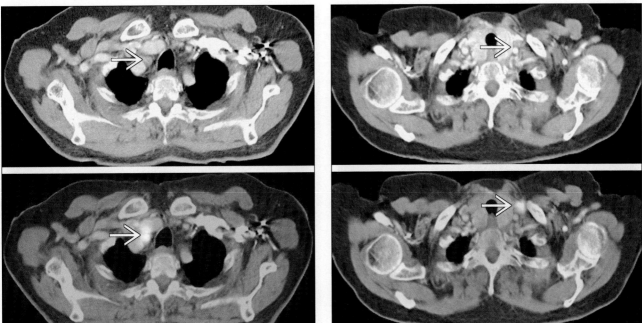

(Left) Axial CT (top) and fused PET/CT (bottom) demonstrate a normal-sized lymph node in the right supraclavicular area ➔, corresponding to a malignant lymph node. *(Right)* Axial CT (top) and fused PET/CT (bottom) show focal intense FDG activity in the left supra-clavicular area correlating with small, normal-sized lymph nodes ➔.

Staging

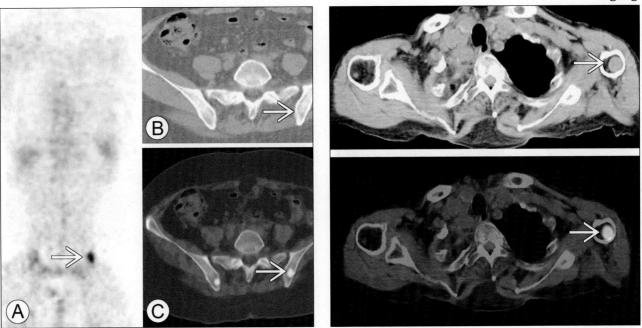

(Left) Coronal PET (A), axial CT (B) and fused PET/CT (C) demonstrate focal intense activity bilaterally in the iliac bones ➔, compatible with osseous metastases. Lesions are not clearly visible on the CT portion of the exam, which is not unusual for early osteolytic lesions in breast cancer. *(Right)* Axial CT (top) and fused PET/CT (bottom) show a sclerotic lesion of the left proximal humerus inferior to the left humeral head ➔, compatible with blastic metastases. Focal moderate to intense FDG activity is present within this lesion.

BREAST CANCER

Staging

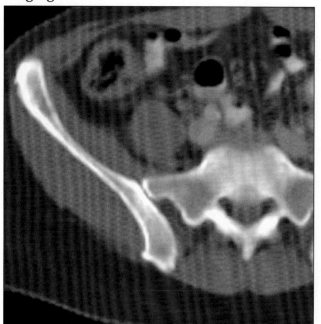 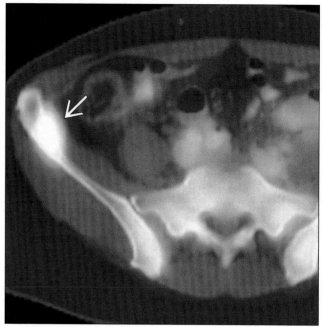

(Left) Axial CECT shows no definite abnormality within the osseous structures. *(Right)* Axial fused PET/CT shows focal intense FDG activity correlating with the right iliac wing ➡, compatible with an osteolytic lesion in this patient with a history of breast cancer. FDG PET is superior to bone scans for detection of osteolytic lesions.

Restaging

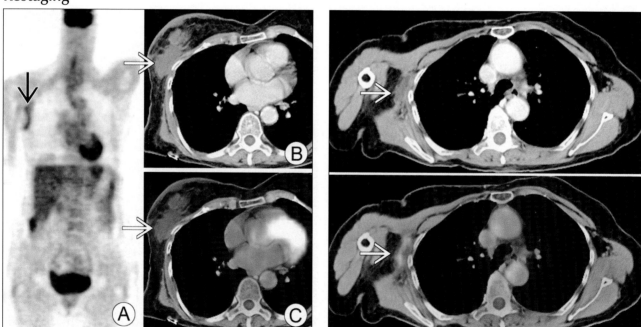

(Left) Coronal PET (A), axial CT (B) and fused PET/CT (C) demonstrate abnormal FDG activity in the right axilla ➡ and water attenuation mass in the right breast ➡. These findings are compatible with a seroma in this patient who underwent a lumpectomy and axillary lymph node dissection 2 months prior to this examination. *(Right)* Axial CT (top) and fused PET/CT (bottom) demonstrate linear activity in the right axilla ➡ secondary to inflammation in this patient with a recent right axillary node dissection.

BREAST CANCER

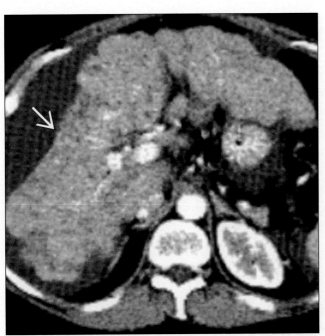 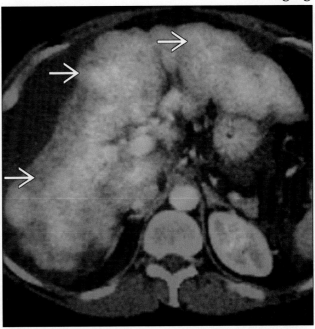

(Left) Axial CECT shows end-stage cirrhotic morphology ➡ in this patient who had a normal-appearing liver on ultrasound approximately 9 months before this examination. (Right) Axial fused PET/CT shows mild heterogeneous activity throughout the liver ➡ without any focal areas of intense activity of uncertain clinical significance. Subsequent autopsy showed pseudocirrhosis, secondary to diffuse metastases and subsequent diffuse shrinkage of liver parenchyma after initiation of chemotherapy.

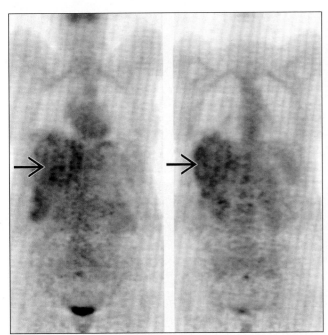 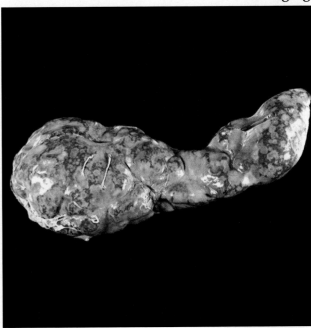

(Left) Coronal PET shows mild heterogeneous activity throughout the liver ➡ in this patient with new onset rapid cirrhosis of the liver. Of note, the patient had a history of metastatic disease to the liver and was recently started on chemotherapy. (Right) Autopsy specimen demonstrates diffuse metastatic disease throughout the liver. The overall appearance is compatible with pseudocirrhosis, as described in the previous three image captions.

BREAST CANCER

Restaging

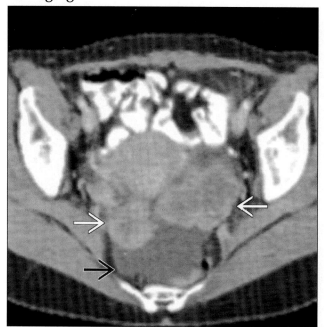 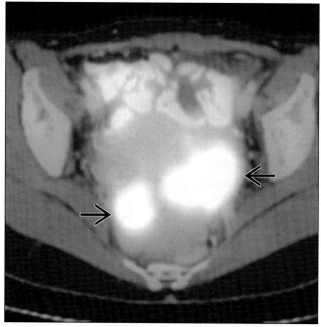

(Left) Axial CECT shows bilateral ovarian masses ➡, compatible with Krukenberg tumors with accompanying pelvic ascites ➡. *(Right)* Axial fused PET/CT shows intense FDG activity ➡ correlating with the ovarian metastases in this patient with breast cancer.

Restaging

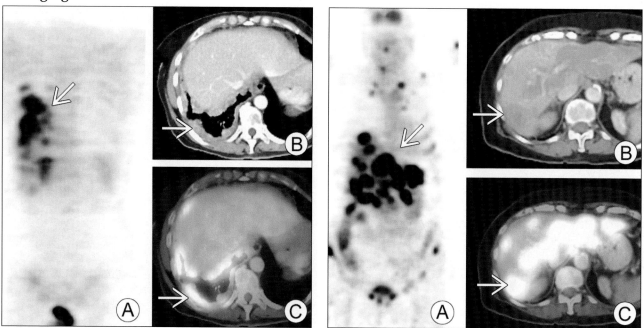

(Left) Coronal PET (A), axial CT (B) and fused PET/CT (C) demonstrate multifocal intense FDG activity correlating with nodular thickening along the pleura and compatible with pleural metastases ➡ in this patient with breast cancer. *(Right)* Coronal PET (A), axial CT (B) and fused PET/CT (C) demonstrate extensive bilobar hepatic disease ➡ in this patient with a history of stage IV breast cancer.

BREAST CANCER

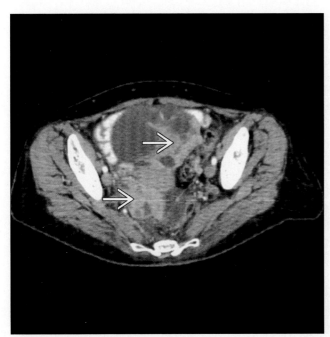 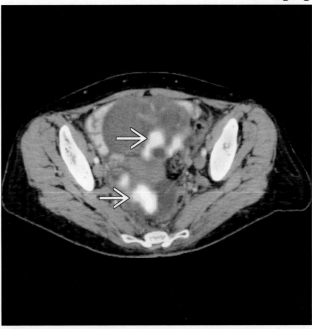

(Left) Axial CECT shows extensive nodular thickening along the peritoneal surfaces in the pelvis ➡, compatible with peritoneal drop metastases. *(Right)* Axial fused PET/CT shows areas of intense FDG activity ➡, corresponding to the nodular areas of peritoneal drop metastases.

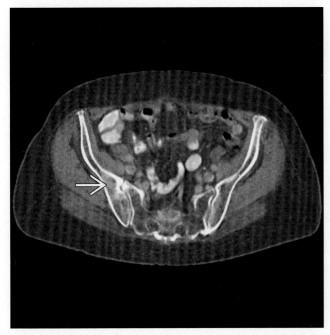 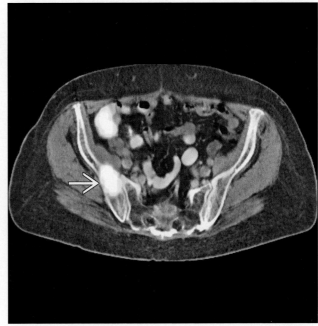

(Left) Axial NECT shows subtle equivocal sclerotic change involving the right iliac bone ➡. *(Right)* Axial fused PET/CT shows intense FDG activity ➡ correlating with the questionable sclerotic change with metastatic disease.

BREAST CANCER

Restaging

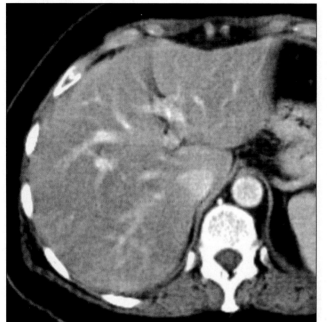 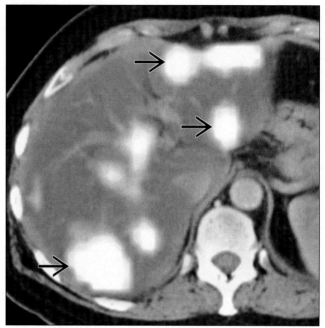

(Left) Axial CECT shows no evidence of metastatic disease in the liver of this patient with a rising tumor marker. *(Right)* Axial fused PET/CT shows extensive bilobar hepatic metastases ⮕ that were not visualized on the contrast-enhanced CT portion of the exam.

Restaging

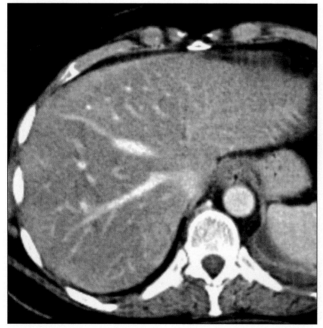 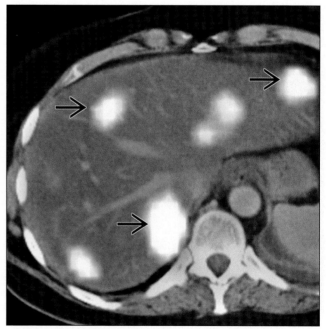

(Left) Axial CECT shows no evidence of metastatic disease in the liver, despite good contrast enhancement. *(Right)* Axial fused PET/CT shows extensive bilobar hepatic metastases ⮕ that were not visualized on the contrast-enhanced CT portion of the exam.

BREAST CANCER

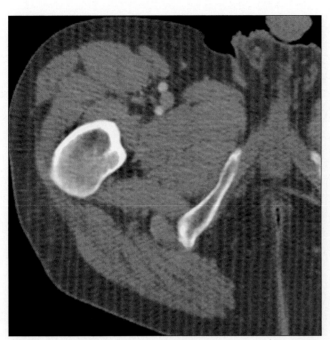 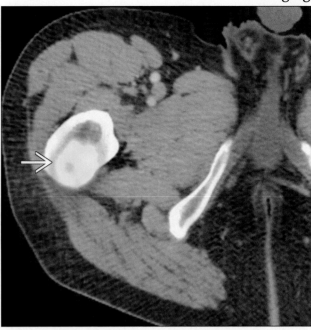

(Left) Axial CECT shows no obvious abnormalities in this patient with rising CA 27-29. *(Right)* Axial fused PET/CT shows intense FDG activity in the proximal right femur ➡, compatible with metastatic disease.

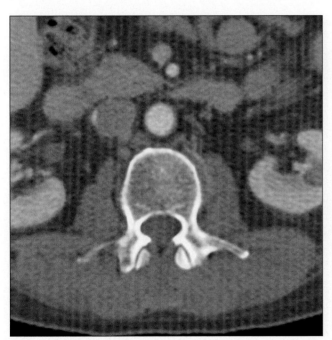 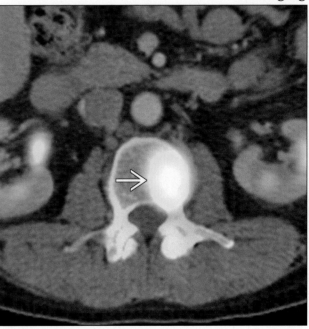

(Left) Axial CECT shows no obvious abnormalities within this vertebral body in this patient with a history of breast cancer and rising tumor markers. *(Right)* Axial fused PET/CT shows focal intense FDG activity in the left side of the vertebral body ➡, indicating metastatic disease. Early lytic lesions are often not visible by CT and are detected much more commonly with PET/CT.

BREAST CANCER

Typical

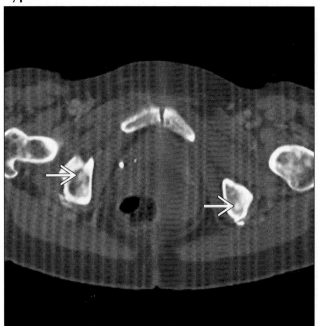 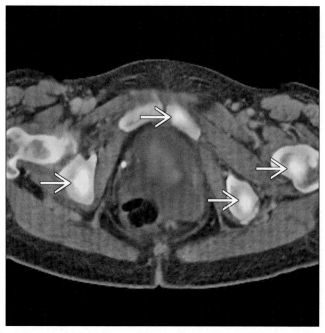

(Left) Axial NECT shows multiple mixed sclerotic and lytic lesions ➡ *in this patient with breast cancer who was being treated with chemotherapy. (Right) Axial fused PET/CT shows multiple foci of intense FDG activity correlating with the mixed sclerotic and lytic lesions* ➡ *visible in the previous image.*

Typical

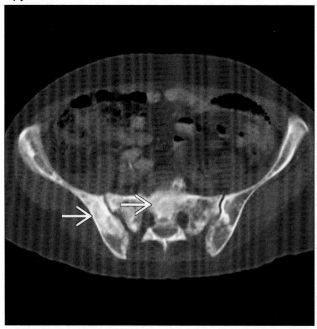 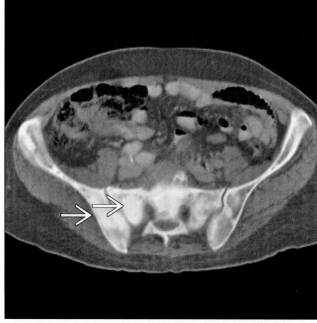

(Left) Axial CECT shows multiple mixed sclerotic and lytic lesions ➡ *in this patient with breast cancer treated with chemotherapy. (Right) Axial fused PET/CT shows multiple foci of intense FDG activity corresponding to the mixed sclerotic and lytic lesions* ➡ *in the previous image, compatible with active metastatic disease.*

BREAST CANCER

Response to Therapy

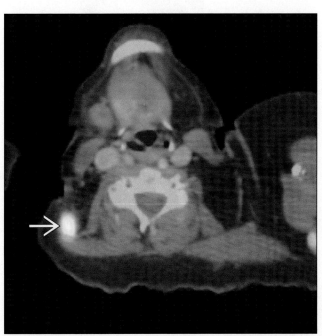 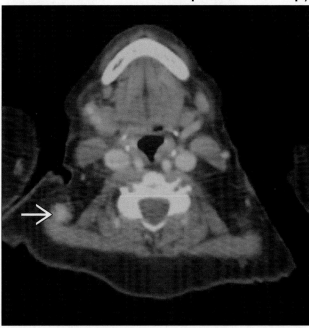

(Left) Axial fused PET/CT shows focal intense FDG activity corresponding to a mildly enlarged right supraclavicular node ➡ in this patient with newly diagnosed breast carcinoma, compatible with metastatic disease. *(Right)* Axial fused PET/CT in the same patient as the previous image shows interval decrease in FDG activity ➡ (reduction of SUV from 9.8 to 3.3), compatible with a good response to therapy.

Typical

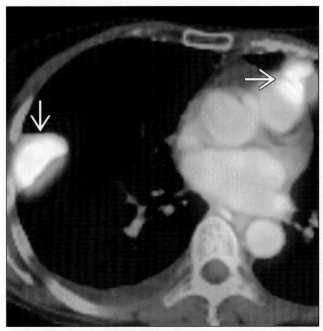 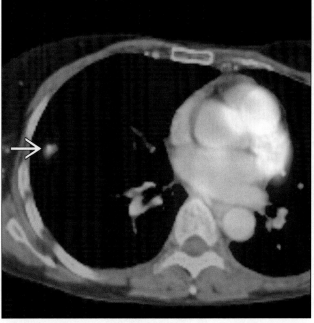

(Left) Axial fused PET/CT in a patient with metastatic breast cancer shows two metastatic lesions with intense FDG activity in the lungs ➡. *(Right)* Axial fused PET/CT performed after 4 cycles of chemotherapy shows marked interval decrease in size and metabolic activity ➡, compatible with a good response to therapy.

ESOPHAGEAL CANCER

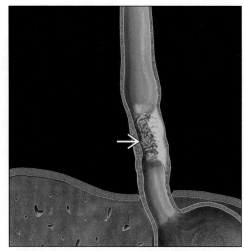

Graphic shows a distal esophageal mass ➔ that causes narrowing of the esophageal lumen, compatible with esophageal cancer.

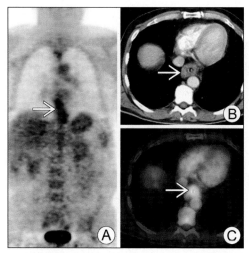

Coronal PET (A) and axial CT (B) & PET/CT (C) show a distal esophageal mass with intense FDG activity ➔, compatible with malignancy.

TERMINOLOGY

Abbreviations and Synonyms
- Esophageal cancer or carcinoma (EC)

Definitions
- Squamous cell carcinoma (SCCA): Malignant transformation of squamous epithelium
- Adenocarcinoma (ACA): Malignant dysplasia in columnar metaplasia (Barrett mucosa)

IMAGING FINDINGS

General Features
- Best diagnostic clue
  - Thickening and irregularity of esophageal lumen on CT
  - FDG uptake in primary esophageal lesion, lymph nodes, and metastases
- Location
  - Arises in mucosa of esophagus
  - Commonly invades submucosa/muscularis with extension to tracheobronchial tree, aorta, and recurrent laryngeal nerve
  - Metastasis often to periesophageal lymph nodes (LN)
  - Distant metastasis to liver and lungs
  - Primary location: Middle 3rd (50%), lower 3rd (30%), upper 3rd (20%) of esophagus
- Size
  - Variable; size criterion for advanced EC is primary lesion > 3.5 cm
  - No significant correlation between lymph node size and frequency of nodal metastis
    - Average size of nonmalignant lymph node similar to average size of metastic lymph node
    - Only %12 of metastic nodes in one study were larger than the common cutoff of 10 mm
- Morphology
  - Primary tumor may have infiltrating, polypoid, ulcerative, or varicoid morphology
  - Morphology is unpredictable following treatment, as tissue is often distorted by edema, fibrosis, and scar formation

DDx: FDG Activity in Esophagus/Proximal Stomach

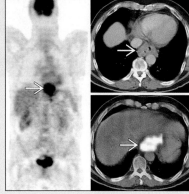

Hiatal Hernia

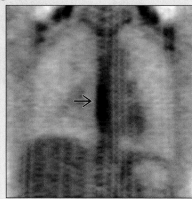

Reflux Esophagitis

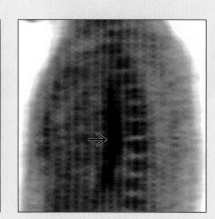

Radiation Esophagitis

ESOPHAGEAL CANCER

Key Facts

Imaging Findings

- Absence of a fat plane between the airway and the esophageal mass cannot be used as an indication of invasion
- FDG PET: Hypermetabolic esophageal mass, lymphadenopathy, distant metastases
- Endoscopic ultrasound (EUS) for most accurate T and N staging
- PET indicated for initial staging and to identify surgical candidates
- PET/CT used to
  - Determine precise location of pathological uptake near primary tumor
  - Identify distant metastases

  - Avoid unnecessary surgery in up to 38% of patients who were initially considered eligible for curative resection with conventional methods
  - PE/CT highly sensitive and accurate for detection of recurrent esophageal squamous cell carcinoma (93-96%)

Top Differential Diagnoses

- Inflammatory Esophagitis
- Intramural Primary Esophageal Tumor
- Other Thoracic Malignancy
- Normal Variants (FDG PET)

Diagnostic Checklist

- Overlap of imaging findings with inflammatory causes of hypermetabolic esophageal lesions

---

  - Elongated morphology with involvement of sections of the esophagus > 3.5 cm carries worse prognosis

Imaging Recommendations

- Best imaging tool
  - Accurate T and N staging best achieved with endoscopic ultrasound (EUS)
    - Ineffective for nonregional disease
    - Esophageal stricture may make passage of scope impossible
    - Combination with CT provides staging accuracy of 50-70%
  - CT useful for detecting locoregional LN metastases
  - **PET/CT used to**
    - Determine precise location of pathological uptake near primary tumor
    - Identify distant metastases
    - Exclude malignancy at sites of physiologic or benign tracer uptake
    - Avoid unnecessary surgery in up to 38% of patients who were initially considered eligible for curative resection with conventional methods
    - Characterize morphologically equivocal hepatic lesions
    - Reduce false positives on CT/EUS by ~ 50%
- Protocol advice
  - PET/CT should be scheduled long enough after therapy to minimize false positives
    - FDG uptake may be seen following invasive procedures such as esophageal dilation

CT Findings

- **General**
  - Wall thickening > 5 mm (eccentric or circumferential)
  - Fat stranding and soft tissue may be demonstrated in the periesophageal area
  - Esophageal dilation with fluid/debris contents will reveal distal obstructing lesion
- **Lymph node involvement**
  - Size criterion for malignancy is short-axis diameter (> 1 cm)

  - Subcarinal nodes are abnormal > 1.4 cm
  - Sensitivity for LN metastasis is 60-80%, and specificity is 90%
  - Lymph node enlargement may be due to inflammation or other benign cause
- **Tracheobronchial findings**
  - Airway may be displaced or impinged upon by esophageal mass
    - Posterior tracheal bowing may be due to tumor impingement
    - Posterior tracheal wall may normally bow anteriorly at end expiration; thus CT images acquired at full-inspiration are essential
  - Fat plane
    - Invasion is not necessarily indicated by absence of fat plane between airway and esophageal mass
    - In patients without disease, fat plane between esophagus and left mainstem bronchus usually is not evident
- **Other organs**
  - Aorta
    - Picus method: Tumor contact with aorta over < 45° suggests no invasion; contact > 90° predicts invasion of aortic wall
    - Alternatively, obliteration of triangular fat space that lies amid aorta, esophagus, and spine predicts aortic invasion
  - Solid organs
    - Lesions identified on CT generally require biopsy to determine malignancy
- **Guidelines for CT staging**
  - **Stage I**: Localized wall thickening of 3-5 mm or intraluminal tumor
    - CT less accurate than EUS
    - CT is not a reliable index of resectability
  - **Stage II**: Localized wall thickening > 5 mm without mediastinal extension
  - **Stage III**: Invasion through esophagus into mediastinum
    - Invasion of tracheobronchial tree: Indentation of posterior wall, compression or displacement of trachea/bronchus, lobar collapse

ESOPHAGEAL CANCER

- Invasion of aorta: Rare (2% prevalence)
- Invasion of pericardium: Mass effect &/or obliteration of fat plane are typical findings
- Adenopathy: Involved mediastinal lymph nodes may be separate from or continuous with primary tumor
  - Stage IV: Involvement of mediastinum and distant sites
    - Common sites include liver, lungs, pleura, adrenals, kidneys, lymph nodes
    - Adenopathy involving the subdiaphragmatic region is common, occurring in > 2/3 of distal cancers

Nuclear Medicine Findings
- **General**
  - 67% of false negatives and 37.5% of false positives on FDG PET were corrected by dual-modality PET/CT
  - FDG uptake is affected by numerous variables
    - Body fat and surface area
    - Serum glucose
    - Blood supply of target organ
    - Method used to draw outline of region of interest
- **Initial diagnosis**
  - Adenocarcinoma and SCCA are highly and almost equally FDG avid
  - Dual-modality PET/CT has no advantage in detection of primary tumor over FDG PET alone, which is highly sensitive
  - Intensity of FDG uptake is correlated with
    - Depth of tumor invasion
    - Likelihood of lymph node metastases
    - Lymphatic invasion
    - Overall prognosis
- **Staging**
  - Allows accurate staging for determination of surgical candidacy
  - Compared to FDG PET alone, locoregional lymph node metastasis is better evaluated with CT and EUS
    - Primary lesion uptake is often intense enough to obscure local nodal disease
    - FDG PET is limited by 6-8 mm resolution minimum
    - PET/CT highly valuable for depiction of local anatomy
  - Detection of locoregional lymph node disease depends on
    - Degree of nodal infiltration and background activity
  - Stage IV disease is better evaluated with FDG PET (sensitivity 69%, specificity 93%)
- **Restaging**
  - PET/CT
    - Highly sensitive and accurate for detection of recurrent esophageal squamous cell carcinoma (93-96%)
    - High incidence of false positive findings reduce specificity at local sites to ~ 50%
    - Accurately co-localized morphologic data allows superior assessment of cervical, abdominopelvic sites & anatomy distorted by operative procedures
- **Response to therapy**

- PET/CT is effective in assessing response to therapy
- Caution must be exercised in interpretation of irradiated lesions
  - Reduction in metabolic activity is common
  - Irradiated disease foci still represent threat of recurrence
- Substantial discordance in gross tumor volume may be found between standard CT/EUS and FDG PET imaging
  - Metabolic response more sensitive for early response assessment but more prone to false positives
  - Size criteria less sensitive but valuable for avoiding false positives
  - Relevant to issues of radiotherapy planning
- **False positives**
  - Infectious esophagitis
  - Reflux esophagitis
  - Barrett without malignancy
  - Post-procedural reactive inflammatory changes from
    - Balloon dilation of anastomotic stricture
    - Esophagogastric anastomosis
    - Gastric pull-up site
  - Lymph nodes in the following regions
    - Supraclavicular
    - Hilar (e.g., chronic respiratory tract disease, heavy smoking, radiation-induced pneumonitis)
    - Subcarinal
    - Paraesophageal
  - False positives may be minimized by
    - Thorough inquiry of the medical record
    - Careful physical examination
    - Repeated review of previous imaging results
    - Close communication between clinicians and radiologists/nuclear physicians
- **False negatives**
  - GI motion and physiologic uptake around stomach and GE junction may obscure true lesions
  - Head/neck anatomic complexity can add difficulty to lesion determination
  - Small lymph nodes in mobile organs are prone to blurring → false negative read

DIFFERENTIAL DIAGNOSIS

Inflammatory Esophagitis
- Radiation-induced
  - Vertebral bodies in radiation port may be photopenic
- Reflux-related
- Infectious
  - Common agents include fungus (candida) and viruses (herpes, CMV, HIV)

Other Intramural Primary Esophageal Tumor
- Leiomyomata
- Fibrovascular polyp
- May shown variable FDG uptake

Other Thoracic Malignancy
- May compress esophagus from exterior

ESOPHAGEAL CANCER

- Mediastinal lymphadenopathy with variable FDG uptake (low in bronchoalveolar carcinoma)
- Lung cancer most common

Normal Variants
- Hiatal hernia
- Normal diffuse esophageal activity

PATHOLOGY

General Features
- General path comments
  - Less common cancers of the esophagus
    - Sarcoma
    - Primary melanoma
    - Oat cell carcinoma, also known as APUDoma
  - Hypermetabolic activity in tumor deposits relates to cancer cell uptake as well as by intratumoral macrophages and granulation tissue
- Genetics: Mutations in oncogenes have been isolated as possible genetic factors in the development of cancer from Barrett esophagus
- Etiology
  - SCCA
    - External: Smoking, alcohol, radiation, lye strictures, HPV (China & South Africa)
    - Illness: Achalasia, celiac disease, Plummer-Vinson syndrome, head and neck cancer
  - ACA
    - Barrett metaplasia confers 30-60x increased risk over general population for development of adenocarcinoma
    - GERD, reflux esophagitis, and motility disorders predispose to Barrett metaplasia
- Epidemiology
  - Most common tumor of esophagus
    - 4% of all digestive tract cancers
    - SCCA > adenocarcinoma in worldwide prevalence
    - Increased incidence in Middle East and Asia
  - 7th most common cause of cancer death in developed countries
  - Barrett-related adenocarcinoma is rising in incidence fastest among all GI cancers
    - Barrett histology causative in 90-100% of cases of adenocarcinoma of esophagus

Gross Pathologic & Surgical Features
- Infiltrating, polypoid, ulcerative, or varicoid lesions

Microscopic Features
- Squamous cell atypia
- Columnar glands
- ACA and SCCA components

Staging, Grading, or Classification Criteria
- TNM staging
  - Stage 0: Carcinoma in situ
  - Stage I: Lamina propria or submucosa
  - Stage IIA: Muscularis propria & adventitia
  - Stage IIB: Lamina propria, submucosa, muscularis propria, and regional LN
  - Stage III: Adventitia, adjacent structures, regional LN, and any other LN
  - Stage IV: All layers, adjacent structures, regional LN, any other LN, and distant metastases

CLINICAL ISSUES

Presentation
- Most common signs/symptoms
  - Dysphagia progressing from solids to liquids
  - Weight loss 2nd most common symptom, present in 50% of patients
  - Pain with swallowing or palpation
    - Bony pain is indicator of metastatic disease
  - Hoarseness indicates recurrent laryngeal nerve invasion and consequent unresectability
  - Hematemesis
- Clinical Profile: Elderly man with history of reflux presents with dysphagia and weight loss
- Lab data
  - Hypochromic microcytic anemia secondary to iron deficiency or chronic disease
  - Hemoccult positive stool
  - Decreased liver synthetic function
  - Hypercalcemia with SCCA

Demographics
- Age: Most common in 6th and 7th decades
- Gender: M:F = 4-7:1
- Ethnicity: African-Americans > Caucasians (2:1)

Natural History & Prognosis
- Most patients present with advanced, metastatic disease
- Poor prognosis attributed to high rate of recurrence
  - Often arises from operative fields, radiotherapeutic targets, and regional lymph nodes
- 2/3 of recurrence within 1 year; nearly all occur within 2 years of initial therapy
- Complications include fistula formation with tracheobronchial tree and pericardium
- Survival
  - Early presentation: 5 year survival ~ 90%
  - Advanced: 5 year survival < 10%
  - Overall treated 5 year survival rate of 15-40%
  - Lymph node involvement dramatically reduces cure rate

Treatment
- **Curative**
  - Surgery
    - Most common outcome is incomplete resection
    - Aggressive surgery is only therapy that provides chance of cure
  - Radiation (pre- & post-operative)
    - Radiation alone rarely provides cure
    - Accurate delineation of tumor length is vital to the success of radiotherapy
- **Palliative**
  - Debulking efforts include surgery, radiotherapy, chemotherapy
  - Laser treatment
  - Esophageal stent

ESOPHAGEAL CANCER

- Assessment of locoregional lymph node status is vital to selection of appropriate treatment and anticipation of disease progression

DIAGNOSTIC CHECKLIST

Consider

- Multiple causes of nonmalignant esophageal metabolic activity
  - Endoscopic biopsy often required

SELECTED REFERENCES

1. Cheze-Le Rest C et al: Prognostic value of initial fluorodeoxyglucose-PET in esophageal cancer: a prospective study. Nucl Med Commun. 29(7):628-35, 2008
2. Chung HW et al: Comparison of uptake characteristics and prognostic value of 201Tl and 18F-FDG in esophageal cancer. World J Surg. 32(1):69-75, 2008
3. Higuchi I et al: Lack of fludeoxyglucose F 18 uptake in posttreatment positron emission tomography as a significant predictor of survival after subsequent surgery in multimodality treatment for patients with locally advanced esophageal squamous cell carcinoma. J Thorac Cardiovasc Surg. 136(1):205-12, 212, 2008
4. Jamil LH et al: Staging and restaging of advanced esophageal cancer. Curr Opin Gastroenterol. 24(4):530-4, 2008
5. Li Y et al: The use of dynamic positron emission tomography imaging for evaluating the carcinogenic progression of intestinal metaplasia to esophageal adenocarcinoma. Cancer Invest. 26(3):278-85, 2008
6. McDonough PB et al: Does FDG-PET add information to EUS and CT in the initial management of esophageal cancer? A prospective single center study. Am J Gastroenterol. 103(3):570-4, 2008
7. Omloo JM et al: Importance of fluorodeoxyglucose-positron emission tomography (FDG-PET) and endoscopic ultrasonography parameters in predicting survival following surgery for esophageal cancer. Endoscopy. 40(6):464-71, 2008
8. Rembielak A et al: The role of PET in target localization for radiotherapy treatment planning. Onkologie. 31(1-2):57-62, 2008
9. Sandha GS et al: Is positron emission tomography useful in locoregional staging of esophageal cancer? Results of a multidisciplinary initiative comparing CT, positron emission tomography, and EUS. Gastrointest Endosc. 67(3):402-9, 2008
10. Schreurs LM et al: Better assessment of nodal metastases by PET/CT fusion compared to side-by-side PET/CT in oesophageal cancer. Anticancer Res. 28(3B):1867-73, 2008
11. Smithers BM et al: Positron emission tomography and pathological evidence of response to neoadjuvant therapy in adenocarcinoma of the esophagus. Dis Esophagus. 21(2):151-8, 2008
12. van Vliet EP et al: Staging investigations for oesophageal cancer: a meta-analysis. Br J Cancer. 98(3):547-57, 2008
13. Vinjamuri S et al: Added value of PET and PET-CT in oesophageal cancer: a review of current practice. Nucl Med Commun. 29(1):4-10, 2008
14. Wieder HA et al: Esophageal cancer. Recent Results Cancer Res. 170:71-9, 2008
15. Bruzzi JF et al: PET/CT of esophageal cancer: its role in clinical management. Radiographics. 27(6):1635-52, 2007
16. Iyer RB et al: PET/CT and hepatic radiation injury in esophageal cancer patients. Cancer Imaging. 7:189-94, 2007
17. Lorenzen S et al: Visualisation of metastatic oesophageal and gastric cancer and prediction of clinical response to palliative chemotherapy using 18FDG PET. Nuklearmedizin. 46(6):263-70, 2007
18. Mamede M et al: Pre-operative estimation of esophageal tumor metabolic length in FDG-PET images with surgical pathology confirmation. Ann Nucl Med. 21(10):553-62, 2007
19. Bombardieri E: The added value of metabolic imaging with FDG-PET in oesophageal cancer: prognostic role and prediction of response to treatment. Eur J Nucl Med Mol Imaging. 33(7):753-8, 2006
20. Cerfolio RJ et al: Maximum standardized uptake values on positron emission tomography of esophageal cancer predicts stage, tumor biology, and survival. Ann Thorac Surg. 82(2):391-4; discussion 394-5, 2006
21. Das A et al: Reassessment of patients with esophageal cancer after neoadjuvant therapy. Endoscopy. 38 Suppl 1:S13-7, 2006
22. Duong CP et al: FDG-PET status following chemoradiotherapy provides high management impact and powerful prognostic stratification in oesophageal cancer. Eur J Nucl Med Mol Imaging. 33(7):770-8, 2006
23. Duong CP et al: Significant clinical impact and prognostic stratification provided by FDG-PET in the staging of oesophageal cancer. Eur J Nucl Med Mol Imaging. 33(7):759-69, 2006
24. Everitt C et al: Influence of F-fluorodeoxyglucose-positron emission tomography on computed tomography-based radiation treatment planning for oesophageal cancer. Australas Radiol. 50(3):271-4, 2006
25. Fiore D et al: Multimodal imaging of esophagus and cardia cancer before and after treatment. Radiol Med (Torino). 111(6):804-17, 2006
26. Jadvar H et al: 2-deoxy-2-[F-18]fluoro-D-glucose-positron emission tomography/computed tomography imaging evaluation of esophageal cancer. Mol Imaging Biol. 8(3):193-200, 2006
27. Korst RJ et al: Downstaging of T or N predicts long-term survival after preoperative chemotherapy and radical resection for esophageal carcinoma. Ann Thorac Surg. 82(2):480-4; discussion 484-5, 2006
28. Leccisotti L: Positron emission tomography in the staging of esophageal cancer. Rays. 31(1):9-12, 2006
29. Leong T et al: A prospective study to evaluate the impact of FDG-PET on CT-based radiotherapy treatment planning for oesophageal cancer. Radiother Oncol. 78(3):254-61, 2006
30. Lerut T et al: Diagnosis and therapy in advanced cancer of the esophagus and the gastroesophageal junction. Curr Opin Gastroenterol. 22(4):437-41, 2006
31. Levine EA et al: Predictive value of 18-fluoro-deoxy-glucose-positron emission tomography (18F-FDG-PET) in the identification of responders to chemoradiation therapy for the treatment of locally advanced esophageal cancer. Ann Surg. 243(4):472-8, 2006
32. Meenan J: Staging stenotic oesophageal tumours: are CT and/or PET enough? Dilate or not? Endoscopy. 38 Suppl 1:S8-12, 2006
33. Minsky BD: Primary combined-modality therapy for esophageal cancer. Oncology (Williston Park). 20(5):497-505; discussion 505-6, 511-3, 2006
34. Munden RF et al: Esophageal cancer: the role of integrated CT-PET in initial staging and response assessment after preoperative therapy. J Thorac Imaging. 21(2):137-45, 2006
35. Ott K et al: Metabolic imaging predicts response, survival, and recurrence in adenocarcinomas of the esophagogastric junction. J Clin Oncol. 24(29):4692-8, 2006

ESOPHAGEAL CANCER

CT Findings: Primary

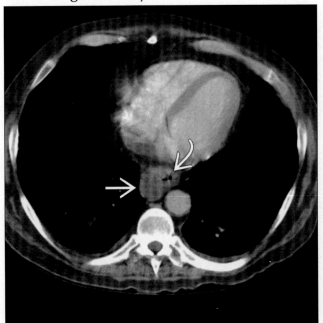 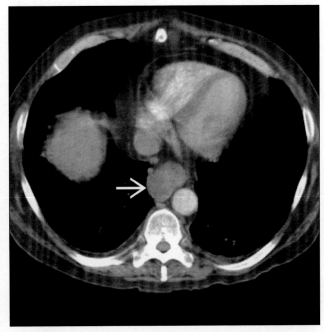

(Left) Axial CECT shows focal mass-like thickening involving the distal esophagus ➡, compatible with esophageal carcinoma. Note that the lumen ➡ of the esophagus is to the left of the mass. *(Right)* Axial CECT shows solid mass-like thickening of the distal esophagus ➡, compatible with esophageal carcinoma.

CT Findings: Metastases

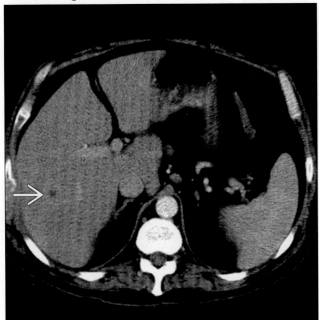 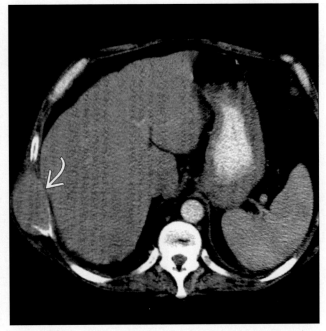

(Left) Axial CECT shows a low attenuation lesion with a subtle ring-enhancing rim ➡, compatible with metastatic disease, in this patient with newly diagnosed esophageal carcinoma. *(Right)* Axial CECT shows an expansile soft tissue attenuation lesion involving the right lateral chest wall ➡, compatible with metastatic disease.

ESOPHAGEAL CANCER

PET/CT Findings: Primary

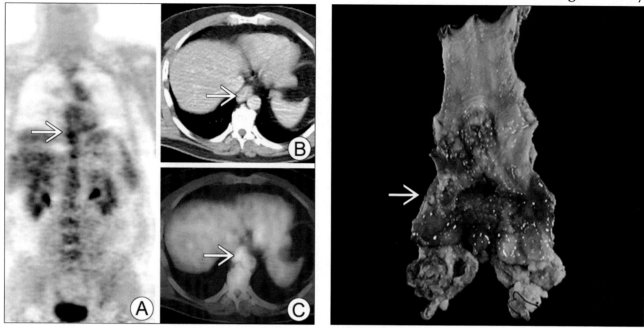

(Left) Coronal PET (A), axial CT (B) and fused PET/CT (C) show minimally increased FDG activity in the distal esophagus ➡ without any definite correlative CT abnormality. This patient was newly diagnosed with esophageal carcinoma. *(Right)* Specimen shows a distal esophageal mass with ulceration ➡, compatible with primary esophageal carcinoma.

PET/CT Findings: Primary with Metastases

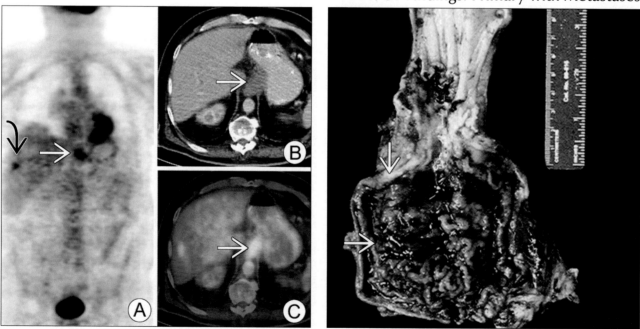

(Left) Coronal PET (A), axial CT (B) and fused PET/CT (C) demonstrate focal intense activity ➡ near the gastroesophageal junction, compatible with primary esophageal carcinoma. A focal area of intense activity ➡ is also present within the liver, compatible with a liver metastasis. *(Right)* Specimen shows a large mass involving the distal esophagus ➡, compatible with this patient's primary esophageal carcinoma.

ESOPHAGEAL CANCER

PET/CT Findings: Primary

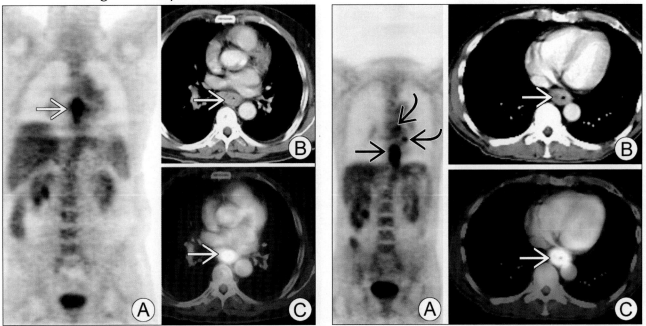

(Left) Coronal PET (A), axial CT (B) and fused PET/CT (C) demonstrate focal intense activity in the mid to distal esophagus ➡. This patient had an unknown primary and was subsequently diagnosed with poorly differentiated adenocarcinoma of the esophagus. *(Right)* Coronal PET (A) demonstrates intense activity in the distal esophagus ➡, compatible with poorly differentiated adenocarcinoma. Two small foci of FDG activity ➘ are present in the subcarinal area, compatible with small metastatic lymph nodes. Axial CT (B) and fused PET/CT (C) show focal thickening of the distal esophagus with intense FDG activity ➡.

PET/CT Findings: Primary

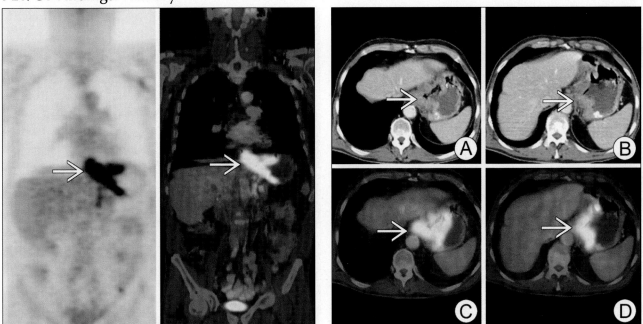

(Left) Coronal PET (left) and PET/CT(right) show diffuse intense FDG activity that involves the gastroesophageal junction and proximal stomach ➡. *(Right)* Axial CT (A, B) and fused PET/CT (C, D) demonstrate thickening of the proximal stomach with intense FDG activity ➡, as seen on the previous coronal images. These findings are compatible with the patient's history of recently diagnosed distal esophageal carcinoma with gastric involvement.

ESOPHAGEAL CANCER

PET/CT Findings: Primary

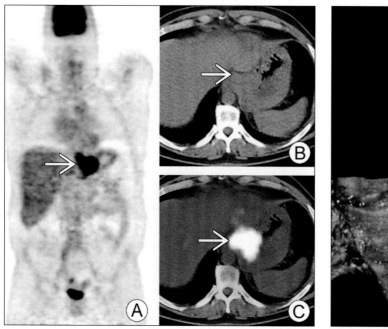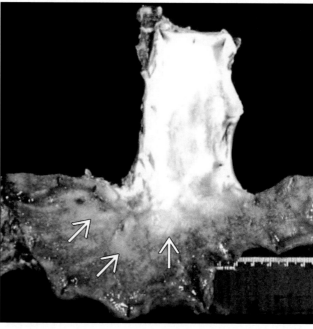

(Left) Coronal PET *(A)*, axial CT *(B)* and fused PET/CT *(C)* images demonstrate intense FDG activity along the gastroesophageal junction ➡ in this patient with newly diagnosed esophageal carcinoma. *(Right)* Specimen shows an infiltrative and nodular lesion at the gastroesophageal junction ➡, representing the patient's primary esophageal carcinoma.

PET/CT Findings: Primary

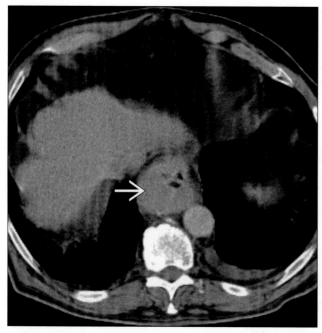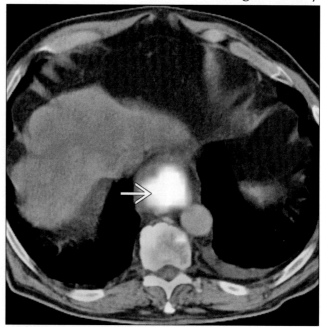

(Left) Axial CECT shows a mass in the distal esophagus ➡, representing this patient's primary poorly differentiated adenocarcinoma. *(Right)* Axial fused PET/CT shows intense activity correlating with the distal esophageal mass ➡. In general, poorly differentiated adenocarcinoma tends to be very FDG avid.

ESOPHAGEAL CANCER

PET/CT Findings: Primary

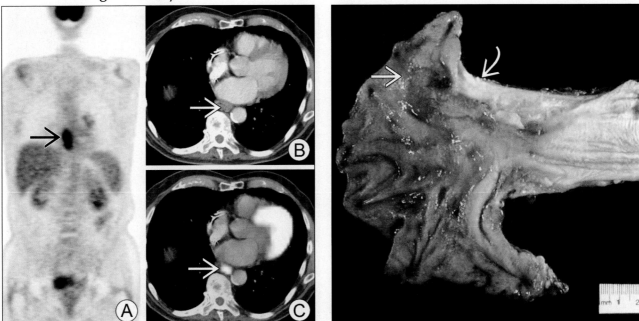

(Left) Coronal PET (A) shows a short segment area of intense FDG activity in the distal esophagus ➡. This corresponds to the subtle thickening of the esophagus ➡ seen on axial CT (B) and fused PET/CT (C). *(Right)* Specimen shows thickening of the wall of the distal esophagus ➡ and areas of mucosal ulceration near the gastroesophageal junction ➡, compatible with esophageal carcinoma.

PET/CT Findings: Primary

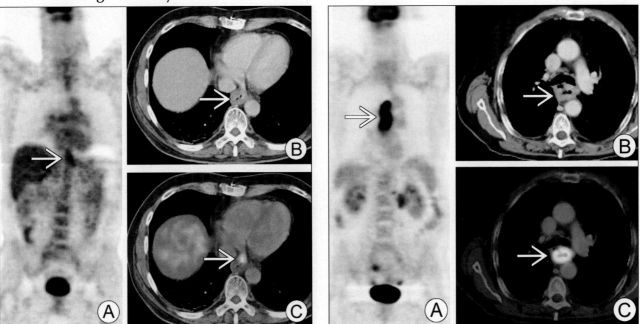

(Left) Coronal PET (A), axial CT (B) and fused PET/CT (C) show mild increased FDG activity in the distal esophagus ➡ in this patient with newly diagnosed, moderately differentiated adenocarcinoma of the esophagus. Approximately 25% of newly diagnosed adenocarcinoma primary lesions may not be visible on FDG PET. *(Right)* Coronal PET (A) demonstrates a short segment area of intense FDG activity in the mid-esophagus ➡, compatible with esophageal carcinoma. Axial CT (B) and fused PET/CT (C) demonstrate circumferential thickening of the esophagus ➡ in the correlative area.

ESOPHAGEAL CANCER

PET/CT Findings: Primary with Metastatic Nodes

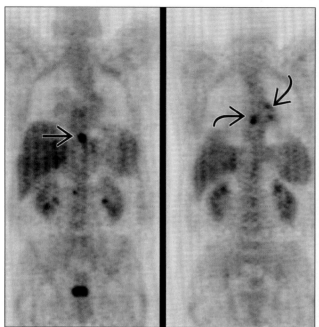 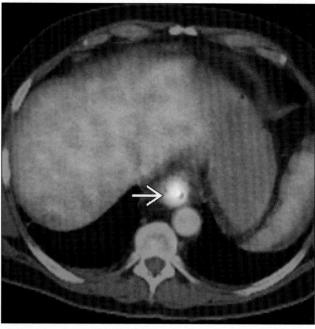

(Left) Coronal PET shows focal intense FDG activity in the distal esophagus ➡ in this patient with newly diagnosed, moderately differentiated adenocarcinoma of the esophagus. Several small foci of increased metabolic activity ➡ are also present in the mediastinum, which is suspicious for regional metastatic lymph nodes. *(Right)* Axial fused PET/CT shows focal intense FDG activity in the distal esophagus that corresponds to the lesion ➡ seen on the previous coronal PET images, a finding compatible with esophageal carcinoma.

PET/CT Findings: Primary with Metastatic Nodes

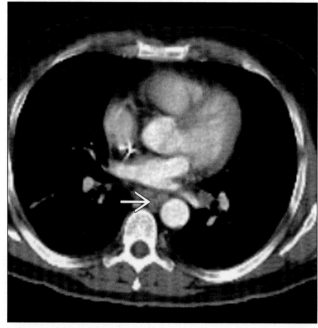 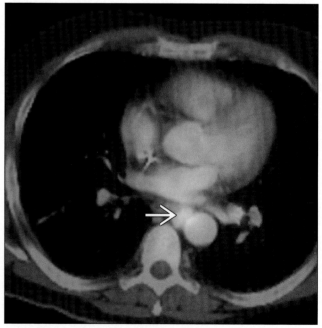

(Left) Axial CECT shows small left paraesophageal lymph nodes ➡ not identified on a recent CT scan. *(Right)* Axial fused PET/CT shows moderate FDG activity within the left paraesophageal lymph node ➡, compatible with metastatic disease.

ESOPHAGEAL CANCER

PET/CT Findings: Primary with Metastases

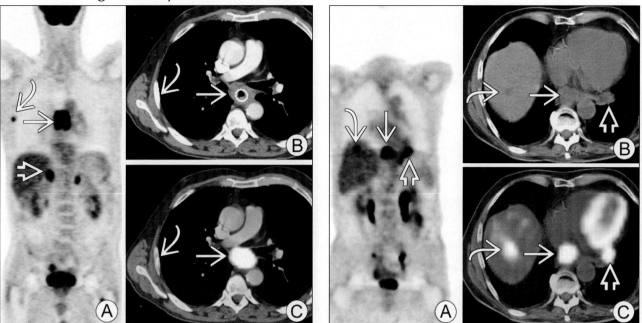

(Left) Coronal PET (A), axial CT (B) and fused PET/CT (C) of a patient with a newly diagnosed large esophageal carcinoma show the primary lesion in the mid-esophagus ➔, a metastasis to a right lateral rib ➔, and bilateral adrenal metastases ➔. *(Right)* This patient was recently diagnosed with esophageal mass at endoscopy. In this staging PET/CT, three foci of increased metabolic activity are identified on the coronal PET (A), axial CT (B) and fused PET/CT (C), involving the distal esophagus ➔, pericardiac region ➔, and the right lobe of the liver ➔. The 1 cm lesion in the liver is better characterized with FDG PET as malignant.

PET/CT Findings: Primary with Metastases

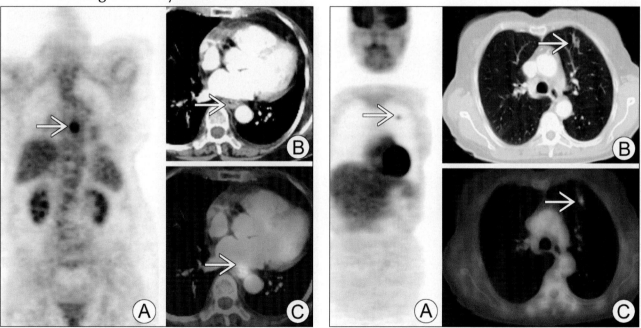

(Left) Coronal PET (A), axial CT (B) and fused PET/CT (C) demonstrate focal intense activity in the distal esophagus ➔, compatible with the patient's recently diagnosed esophageal carcinoma. *(Right)* Coronal PET (A), axial CT (B) and fused PET/CT (C) images show a focal area of moderate to intense FDG activity, corresponding to a left upper lobe pulmonary nodule ➔ adjacent to a small vessel. The findings of this staging PET/CT study are compatible with metastatic disease.

ESOPHAGEAL CANCER

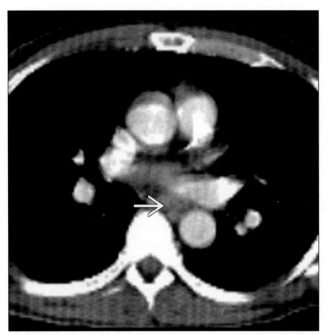 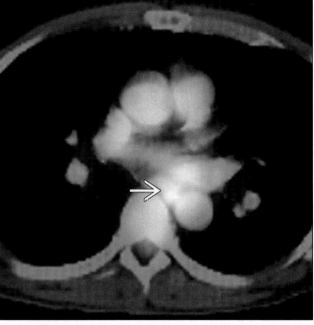

(Left) Axial CECT shows a subtle borderline enlarged paraesophageal lymph node ➔ of uncertain clinical significance. (Right) Axial fused PET/ CT shows focal intense activity in the questionable lymph node ➔, raising the suspicion for metastatic involvement.

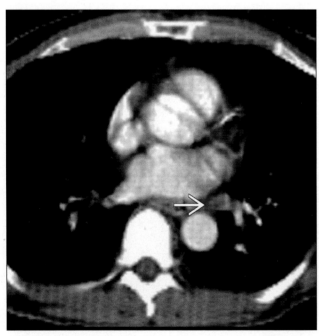 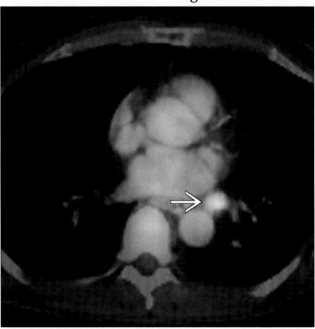

(Left) Axial CECT shows a small left infrahilar lymph node ➔ that was not prospectively identified as potential metastatic disease. (Right) Axial fused PET/CT shows focal intense activity within the left infrahilar lymph node ➔, compatible with metastatic disease.

ESOPHAGEAL CANCER

PET/CT: Regional Metastases

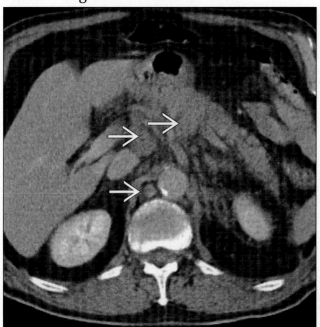 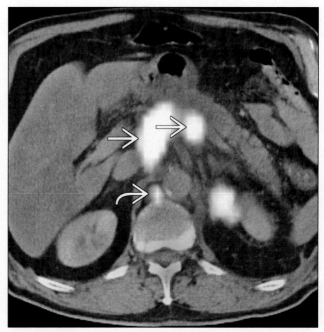

(Left) Axial CECT shows extensive abdominal and retroperitoneal lymphadenopathy ➡, compatible with metastatic disease. *(Right)* Axial fused PET/CT shows intense FDG activity within all of the enlarged lymph nodes ➡. Also note intense activity within a tiny right retrocrural lymph node ➡.

PET/CT Findings: Primary with Metastases

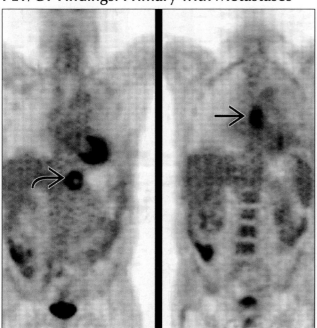 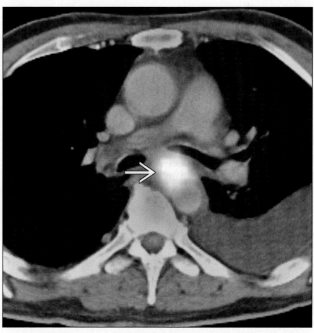

(Left) Coronal PET shows two areas of intense FDG activity, one below the diaphragm ➡ and one in the subcarinal area ➡, compatible with malignancy. *(Right)* Axial fused PET/CT shows focal intense FDG activity in the esophagus at the level of the carina ➡, compatible with the patient's known primary esophageal carcinoma.

ESOPHAGEAL CANCER

PET/CT Findings: Primary with Metastases

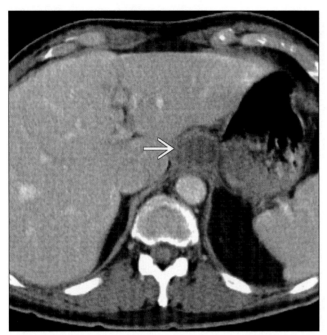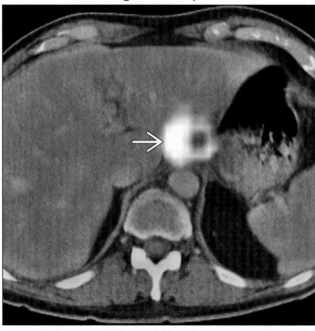

(Left) Axial CECT shows a large metastatic necrotic lymph node along the gastrohepatic ligament ➡ in this patient with newly diagnosed esophageal carcinoma. *(Right)* Axial fused PET/CT shows intense FDG activity ➡ corresponding to the metastatic adenopathy identified in the previous image. There is also a central area of photopenia that corresponds to regions of necrosis.

PET/CT Findings: Primary with Metastases

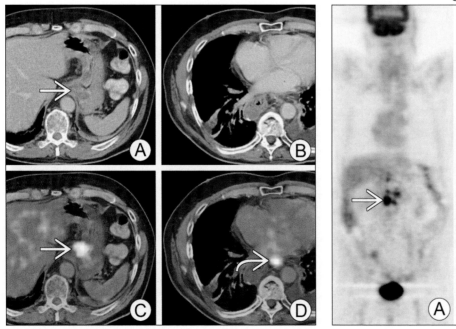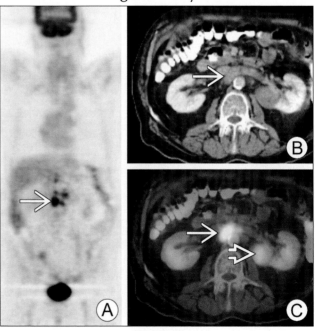

(Left) Axial CT (A, B) and fused PET/CT (C, D) show a focal area of intense FDG activity without a definite correlate to the CT abnormality at the gastroesophageal junction ➡, as well as a small, paraesophageal lymph node ➡ detected on PET/CT. *(Right)* Coronal PET (A), axial CT (B) and fused PET/CT (C) in a patient with a history of esophageal carcinoma show multiple foci of intense FDG activity in the retroperitoneal area ➡. An incidental mass with mild to moderate FDG activity ➡ is also present in the left kidney, compatible with a 2nd renal cell carcinoma with regional metastatic nodes.

ESOPHAGEAL CANCER

PET/CT Findings: Primary with Metastases

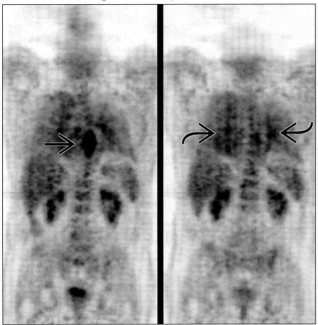 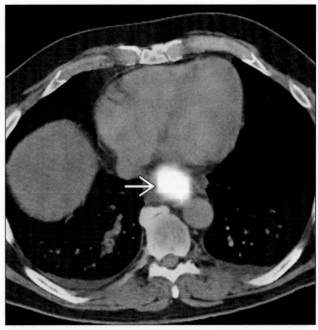

(Left) Coronal PET shows a short segment area of intense FDG activity near the distal esophagus ➡, compatible with the patient's known primary esophageal carcinoma. Note the increased haziness of both lower lung zones ➡. *(Right)* Axial fused PET/CT shows focal intense FDG activity ➡ corresponding to the previous PET images in this patient with newly diagnosed distal esophageal carcinoma.

PET/CT Findings: Primary with Metastases

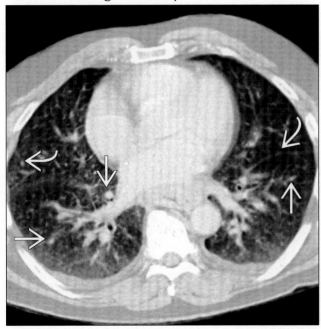 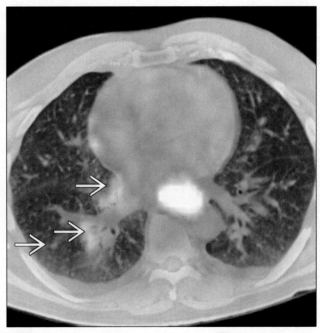

(Left) Axial CECT shows lower lungs with multiple small pulmonary nodules ➡ and subtle, interlobular septal thickening ➡, compatible with lymphangitic spread of tumor. *(Right)* Axial fused PET/CT shows areas of moderately increased FDG activity that correspond to the lymphangitic spread of tumor ➡, which accounts for the hazy appearance on the previous coronal PET images.

ESOPHAGEAL CANCER

PET/CT Findings: Lymph Node Metastases

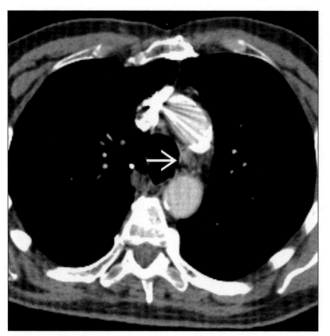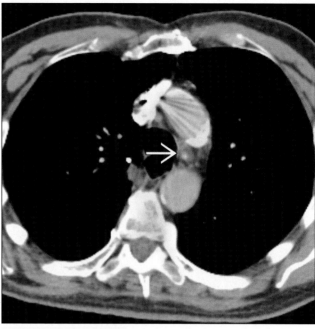

(Left) Axial CECT shows no definite suspicious lesions. However, a small AP window lymph node ➡ is present. *(Right)* Axial fused PET/CT shows focal intense FDG activity corresponding to the subcentimeter AP window lymph node ➡, compatible with metastatic disease.

PET/CT Findings: Lymph Node Metastases

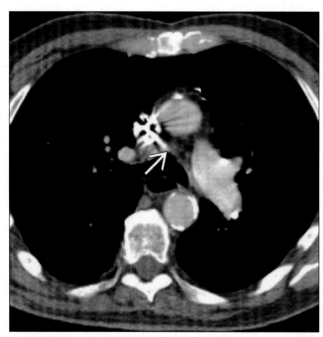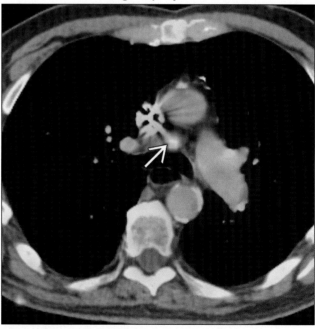

(Left) Axial CECT shows a subcentimeter pretracheal lymph node ➡ that does not have any worrisome features on CT. *(Right)* Axial fused PET/CT shows focal intense FDG activity corresponding to the subcentimeter pretracheal lymph node ➡, compatible with malignancy.

ESOPHAGEAL CANCER

PET/CT: Distant Metastases

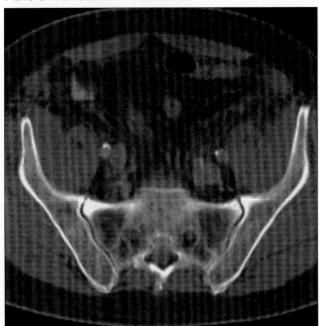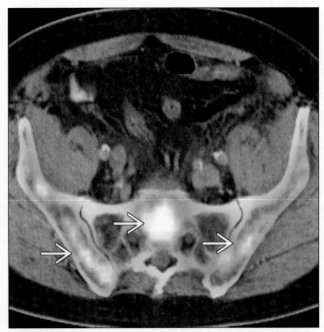

(Left) Axial NECT shows no definite evidence for osseous metastases. *(Right)* Axial fused PET/CT shows extensive metastatic involvement of the sacrum and, to a lesser extent, the iliac bones bilaterally ➡. FDG PET is more sensitive for osteolytic lesions than MDP bone scans but less sensitive for osteoblastic lesions.

PET/CT Findings: Restaging

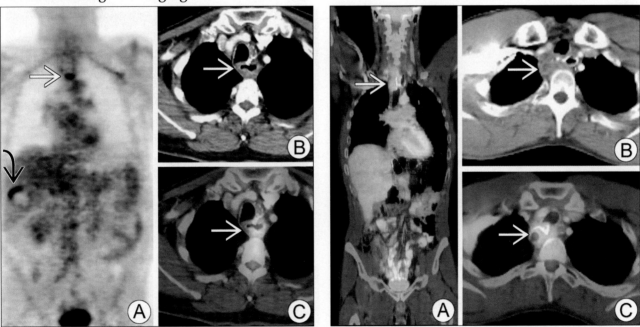

(Left) Coronal PET (A), axial CT (B) and fused PET/CT (C) show focal intense FDG activity near the proximal anastomosis ➡, compatible with recurrent esophageal carcinoma. Intense linear FDG activity is also present in the liver ➡, correlating to an area of recurrence status post radiofrequency ablation. *(Right)* Coronal fused PET/CT (A), axial CT (B) and fused PET/CT (C) demonstrate metastatic adenopathy ➡ at the thoracic inlet just posterior to the trachea and laterally to the esophagus on the right. The findings of this staging PET/CT study are compatible with metastatic lymphadenopathy.

ESOPHAGEAL CANCER

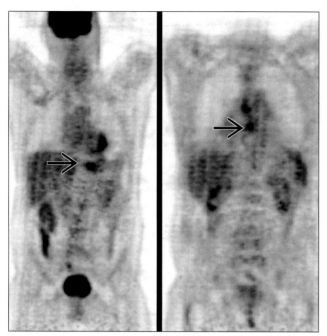 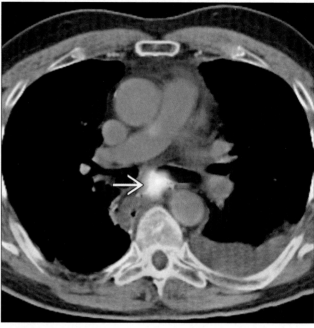

(Left) Coronal PET shows multiple abnormal foci of intense FDG activity ⇒ in this patient with a history of esophageal carcinoma status post esophagectomy. *(Right)* Axial fused PET/CT shows focal intense FDG activity ⇒ corresponding to surgical clips just posterior to the gastric pull-up at the level of the carina, compatible with recurrent disease.

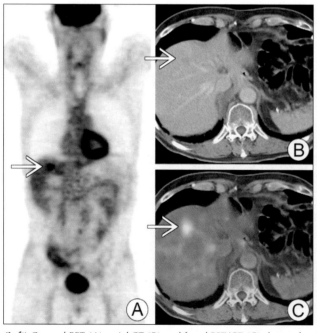 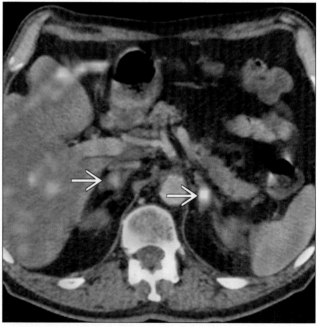

(Left) Coronal PET (A), axial CT (B) and fused PET/CT (C) show a focal area of intense FDG activity ⇒ corresponding to a subtle, approximately 1 cm, low attenuation lesion in the liver, compatible with metastatic disease. *(Right)* Axial fused PET/CT in the same patient shows bilateral adrenal metastases ⇒, with slightly increased metabolic activity in the left adrenal gland compared to the right.

ESOPHAGEAL CANCER

PET/CT Findings: Restaging

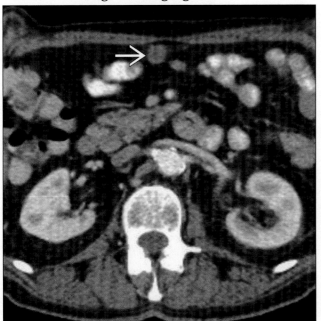 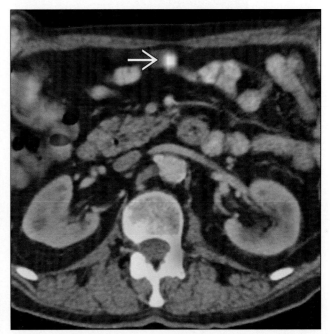

(Left) Axial CECT shows a soft tissue lesion in the omentum ➡, compatible with a metastasis in this patient with esophageal carcinoma. *(Right)* Axial fused PET/CT shows focal intense FDG activity correlating to the omental metastasis ➡. Consider performing the CT with oral contrast in patients with abdominal pelvic primary malignancies or those with primary neoplasms, which often metastasize below the diaphragm.

PET/CT Findings: Restaging

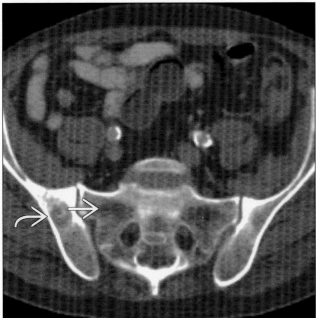 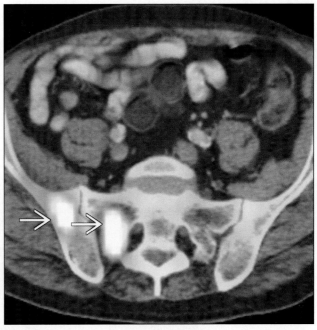

(Left) Axial CECT shows subtle increased lucency involving the right sacral ala ➡ as well as a more concerning lucent lesion in the right iliac bone ➡ in this patient with a history of esophageal carcinoma. *(Right)* Axial fused PET/CT demonstrates intense FDG activity within both of the questionable osseous lesions ➡ shown in the previous image, compatible with metastatic disease.

COLORECTAL CANCER

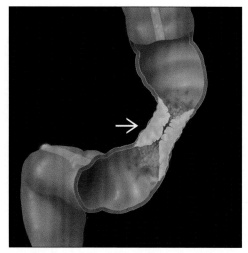

Graphic shows a circumferential mass in the sigmoid colon ➡ that causes marked narrowing of the colonic lumen. This appearance is often termed "apple core" lesion on barium enema.

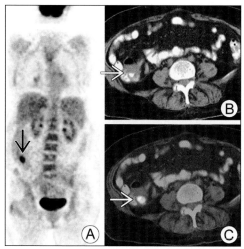

Coronal PET (A), axial CT (B) and fused PET/CT (C) show a focal area of intense FDG activity ➡, corresponding to primary colon carcinoma in the proximal ascending colon ➡.

TERMINOLOGY

Abbreviations and Synonyms
- Colorectal carcinoma (CRC), colon cancer, adenocarcinoma of the colon, rectal carcinoma

Definitions
- Malignancy of the colon &/or rectum

IMAGING FINDINGS

General Features
- Best diagnostic clue
  - **Initial diagnosis**: None, usually indicated in history, although incidental focal intense FDG activity may represent an incidental malignant lesion
  - **Staging**: PET/CT will often show additional lesions not seen on CT, particularly in the liver
  - **Restaging**: Combination of a rising CEA level and a focal abnormality on PET/CT, often without a correlative CT abnormality
- Location
  - **Initial diagnosis**: Colon/rectum

- **Staging**: Additional liver lesions will often affect patient management
- **Recurrence**: Surgical anastomosis, regional lymph nodes, presacral area
- Size: Variable, although PET has poor performance with small lesions including carcinomatosis
- CMS coverage 2009: Initial diagnosis, staging, restaging; response to therapy not currently covered

Nuclear Medicine Findings
- General
  - **Physiologic FDG activity**
    - Very common
    - Range from no activity to intense
    - Usually linear in appearance
    - Right colon and cecum more commonly demonstrate increased physiologic FDG activity
    - May be focal at ileocecal valve
    - Short segment or linear FDG activity in bowel without correlative CT abnormality almost always physiologic
    - Focal or short segment moderate to intense activity is also common at the anorectal junction

DDx: Focal FDG Uptake in Bowel

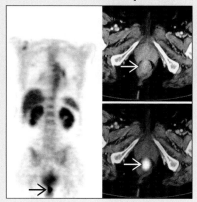

Physiologic Anorectal Junction

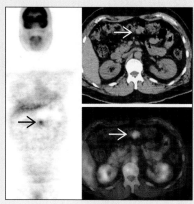

Polyp

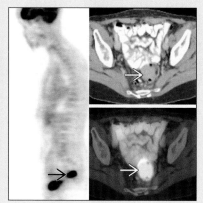

Villous Adenoma

COLORECTAL CANCER

Key Facts

Imaging Findings
- PET poorly sensitive for small (< 1 cm) lesions; high positive predictive value
- PET insensitive (29%) for small (< 1 cm) regional lymph nodes
- Clinical management: PET affects surgical planning in approximately 30% of colorectal cancer patients
- PET/CT more sensitive for regional/distant metastases than CT alone
- > 95% sensitivity and ~ 71% specificity for localization of relapse in patients with increased CEA
- Staging: PET/CT will often show additional lesions not seen on CT, particularly in the liver
- Restaging: Combination of a rising CEA level and a focal abnormality on PET/CT, often without a correlative CT abnormality

- May be focal at ileocecal valve

Top Differential Diagnoses
- Adenomas
- Abscess
- Physiologic FDG activity in bowel

Clinical Issues
- Recurrence: Rising CEA level, abdominal pain (obstruction)

Diagnostic Checklist
- Pre-treatment PET for staging, confirmation of FDG-avid disease
- Mucinous adenocarcinoma has variable PET activity
- Correlate focal increased activity in bowel on FDG PET with colonoscopy

---

- o PET poorly sensitive for small (< 1 cm) lesions; however, high positive predictive value
- o PET has limited sensitivity for peritoneal, omental metastases, highly mucinous tumors (may not be FDG avid)
- o Positive predictive value high for detection of omental or peritoneal disease, which may be difficult to detect with CT alone
- o Primary colon cancers may be incidentally identified with PET
  - ▪ Focal activity on FDG PET should be followed subsequently evaluated with colonoscopy
- o 1-3% of patients undergoing PET/CT will have incidental accumulation in GI tract
  - ▪ Associated with substantial risk of underlying cancer or pre-cancerous lesion
- **Initial diagnosis**
  - o Not recommended for screening, but PET/CT may play a role in screening patients with familial polyposis
  - o PET and PET/CT are CMS-covered but rarely used for initial diagnosis of colon cancer
  - o Colonoscopy is the preferred method for initial diagnosis
  - o Colonic adenoma and benign polyps can take up significant FDG and appear similar to carcinoma
  - o Not used for diagnosis of polyps &/or adenomas
    - ▪ However, FDG PET has 84% specificity for detecting colonic adenomas
    - ▪ Specificity improves with increasing size and grade of adenoma
- **Staging**
  - o Clinical management: PET affects surgical planning in approximately 30% of colorectal cancer patients
  - o Main indication for PET/CT in CRC is assessment for consideration for metastasectomy
    - ▪ Goal of avoiding major surgery in patients with undetected nodal/distant metastases
  - o Consider pre-treatment PET for staging of all high risk patients and confirmation of FDG-avid disease
  - o PET insensitive (29%) for small (< 1 cm) regional lymph nodes

- o Colon metastases most commonly go to liver
- o Accuracy of distant staging for colorectal cancer: PET 78%, PET/CT 89%
  - ▪ PET/CT more sensitive for regional/distant metastases than CT alone
- o Rectal metastases may bypass liver and metastasize to lung
  - ▪ Inspection of CT is pertinent to detect small pulmonary nodules that may be missed on PET
- o Mucinous adenocarcinoma metastases may show calcification on CT
  - ▪ May also be falsely negative on PET
- o Consider staging PET or PET/CT in any patient with a high risk primary lesion (> Dukes A lesion at surgery)
- **Restaging**
  - o Established role for PET/CT in patients with suspected recurrent disease, particularly in patients with rising CEA levels
  - o Restage to detect locally recurrent disease, isolated metastatic disease in liver/lung, diffuse metastases
  - o > 95% sensitivity and ~ 71% specificity for localization of relapse in patients with increased CEA
  - o PET to differentiate scar/fibrosis after surgery or radiation from tumor in rectal canal
  - o No evidence to support use of PET in routine surveillance following curative primary surgery
- **Response to chemotherapy**
  - o Not currently a CMS-covered indication
  - o Early, i.e., metabolic but not anatomic, response to therapy can be imaged with FDG PET
    - ▪ Also can identify those with biologically aggressive disease unsuitable for resection
    - ▪ Reduction in SUV after 1-3 cycles of chemotherapy may predict response and correlate with subsequent tumor shrinkage
    - ▪ Future chemotherapy that achieves cytostasis over cytotoxicity may benefit from PET imaging

COLORECTAL CANCER

CT Findings

- Localized tumor may be seen as intraluminal or intramural mass of soft tissue density adjacent to gas-filled or contrast-filled bowel lumen
  - No mural thickening or pericolic fat in stage A tumors
  - Some smaller primary tumors may not be visible on CT or PET
- More advanced tumors associated with > 6 mm thickening of bowel wall and infiltration of pericolic fat
- Annular carcinoma seen as a thickening of bowel wall and narrowing of lumen
  - Thickening is concentric given perpendicular scanning plane
- Extracolonic tumor spread indicated by loss of tissue fat planes between colon and surrounding structures
  - Invaded muscle may be enlarged
  - Colonic tumors may invade anterior abdominal wall, liver, pancreas, spleen, or stomach
- Intussuscepting tumor may have target-like appearance with alternating rings of soft tissue and fat on CT
  - Only seen if mesenteric fat is present between intussusceptum and intussuscipiens
- 60% of affected lymph nodes are detected by CT
- Rectosigmoid tumors may metastasize to external iliac nodes
- Liver is most common site of metastasis
  - CECT shows well-defined areas of low density (relative to normal parenchyma) in portal venous phase
  - In earlier arterial phase, hepatic mets may show rim enhancement or become hyper-/isodense to normal liver
  - Other common sites of metastasis are lungs, adrenal glands, peritoneum, and omentum
- Adrenal mets may be seen in as many as 14% of patients with CRC
  - Typical findings include enlargement (> 2 cm), asymmetry, and heterogeneity
- Bony and cerebral mets are uncommon

Imaging Recommendations

- Best imaging tool
  - PET/CT for initial staging and restaging
  - Other modalities: For detection of primary lesion
    - Colonoscopy, double contrast barium enema (low sensitivity for polyps < 1 cm), and virtual colonography (gaining acceptance)
  - Imaging of liver
    - PET/CT for high risk patients
    - Improves therapeutic management of patients with liver metastases
    - MR, US for indeterminate cases
  - Rectal cancer
    - PET/CT has significant impact on course of treatment through more accurate staging
    - MR is also established in staging by facilitating accurate assessment of mesorectal fascia
- Protocol advice

- PET/CT perform with diagnostic rather than noncontrast CT
  - Will help with abdominopelvic lesions adjacent to bowel and also increase confidence level for confirming hepatic lesions

DIFFERENTIAL DIAGNOSIS

Adenomas

- Variable PET activity
- Benign adenomas can show intense FDG activity and mimic carcinoma

Inflammatory Bowel Disease

- Ulcerative colitis, Crohn disease
- Increased activity often seen in affected bowel on PET

Infection

- Increased activity in affected segments of bowel
- Example: Pseudomembranous colitis

Abscess

- Abscess and tumor can both show increased FDG activity
- Increased FDG activity surrounding photopenic center = abscess, necrotic tumor
  - Time course, prior studies useful to differentiate
- Gas + fluid collection more specific for abscess

Physiologic FDG Activity in Bowel

- Diffuse activity in part of/or throughout bowel
- Usually linear
- No corresponding bowel thickening on CT

Seroma

- Photopenia on FDG PET; fluid density on CT

Post-Radiation Change

- Early: Often difficult to assess due to increased FDG activity secondary to inflammation
- Typically resolves in 2-6 months

Post-Surgical Scar/Fibrosis

- Mildly increased FDG activity with normal post-surgical healing
- Serial FDG PET: Scar/fibrosis has stable or decreased activity

PATHOLOGY

General Features

- General path comments
  - Colon polyps
    - 10% of all polyps are adenomatous
    - Increased incidence of carcinoma in villous tumors
- Genetics: Some genetic predisposition in familial polyposis syndromes
- Etiology
  - Arises from pre-existing adenomatous polyps in colonic or rectal mucosa

COLORECTAL CANCER

- Age, smoking, diet high in fat and cholesterol, inflammatory bowel disease (mostly ulcerative colitis), genetic predisposition
- Epidemiology
  - 3rd most common cancer in USA
  - 135,000 new cases per year in USA; 55,000 deaths per year
  - Lifetime risk in general population: 5.9%
  - 2/3 of colorectal cancers arise in colon, 1/3 in rectum

Staging, Grading, or Classification Criteria
- Modified Dukes staging system for colorectal cancer
  - Dukes A: Carcinoma in situ limited to mucosa or submucosa (T1N0M0)
  - Dukes B: Cancer that extends into the muscularis (B1), into or through the serosa (B2)
  - Dukes C: Cancer that extends to regional lymph nodes (T1-4, N1M0)
  - Dukes D: Modified classification; cancer that has metastasized to distant sites (T1-4, N1-3, M1)

CLINICAL ISSUES

Presentation
- Most common signs/symptoms
  - GI bleed, seen in 60% of patients presenting with colorectal carcinoma
  - Colonic adenoma presents: 50% with abdominal pain; 35% with bowel habit changes; 30% with occult bleeding
- Other signs/symptoms: Recurrence indicated by rising CEA level, abdominal pain (obstruction)

Demographics
- Age: Peak 7th decade; risk rises over age 40
- Gender: Male preponderance for colon polyps

Natural History & Prognosis
- Dukes A: 5 year > 90%
- Dukes B: 5 year > 70%
- Dukes C: 5 year < 60%
- Dukes D: 5 year ~ 5%
- Small studies have shown improved disease-free and overall survival in patients evaluated with FDG PET imaging prior to surgery
- Untreated patients with metastatic disease have life expectancy of 6-12 months
- > 20% of patients who present with hepatic metastases are resectable, but surgery remains only potentially curative therapy
- 5 year overall survival following complete resection of isolated liver metastasis is 30-40% with 10 year survival of ~ 25%
- 75% of patients who undergo liver metastasis resection experience relapse
  - Partly due to inaccurate staging with occult extrahepatic metastases that go undetected prior to surgery

Treatment
- Surgically curable if detected early

- Adjuvant chemotherapy to prolong survival with lymph node positive disease
- Rectal adenocarcinomas are sensitive to radiation
- Local recurrence: Surgery, chemo ± radiation
- Hepatic recurrence: Resection, radiofrequency ablation, hepatic arterial chemotherapy/radiotherapy
- Patients with unresectable disease have median survival up to 20 months with non-surgical therapy
- Estimation of gross tumor volume in reference to radiotherapy changed significantly in approximately 50% of patients when metabolic imaging was used

DIAGNOSTIC CHECKLIST

Consider
- PET/CT with diagnostic CT for staging and for restaging patients which elevated CEA levels
- Also consider PET/CT when the differential diagnosis is scar vs. residual or recurrent tumor

Image Interpretation Pearls
- Mucinous adenocarcinoma has variable PET activity
- Correlate focal increased activity in bowel on FDG PET with colonoscopy
- Rectal cancer: FDG PET to differentiate scar/fibrosis after surgery or radiation vs. tumor

SELECTED REFERENCES

1. de Geus-Oei LF et al: Chemotherapy response evaluation with FDG-PET in patients with colorectal cancer. Ann Oncol. 19(2):348-52, 2008
2. Dresel S et al: PET in colorectal cancer. Recent Results Cancer Res. 170:109-24, 2008
3. Fletcher JW et al: Recommendations on the use of 18F-FDG PET in oncology. J Nucl Med. 49(3):480-508, 2008
4. Geus-Oei LF et al: Predictive and prognostic value of FDG-PET. Cancer Imaging. 8:70-80, 2008
5. Inoue K et al: Diagnosis supporting algorithm for lymph node metastases from colorectal carcinoma on 18F-FDG PET/CT. Ann Nucl Med. 22(1):41-8, 2008
6. Kristiansen C et al: PET/CT and histopathologic response to preoperative chemoradiation therapy in locally advanced rectal cancer. Dis Colon Rectum. 51(1):21-5, 2008
7. Shin SS et al: Preoperative staging of colorectal cancer: CT vs. integrated FDG PET/CT. Abdom Imaging. 33(3):270-7, 2008
8. Sobhani I et al: Early detection of recurrence by 18FDG-PET in the follow-up of patients with colorectal cancer. Br J Cancer. 98(5):875-80, 2008
9. Soyka JD et al: Staging pathways in recurrent colorectal carcinoma: is contrast-enhanced 18F-FDG PET/CT the diagnostic tool of choice? J Nucl Med. 49(3):354-61, 2008
10. Tan MC et al: A prognostic system applicable to patients with resectable liver metastasis from colorectal carcinoma staged by positron emission tomography with [18F]fluoro-2-deoxy-D-glucose: role of primary tumor variables. J Am Coll Surg. 206(5):857-68; discussion 868-9, 2008
11. Tsunoda Y et al: Preoperative diagnosis of lymph node metastases of colorectal cancer by FDG-PET/CT. Jpn J Clin Oncol. 38(5):347-53, 2008

COLORECTAL CANCER

Typical Primary

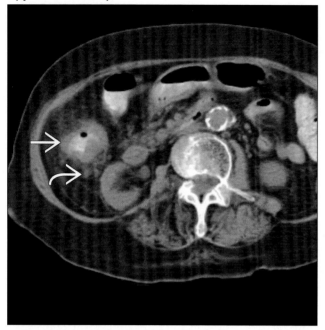 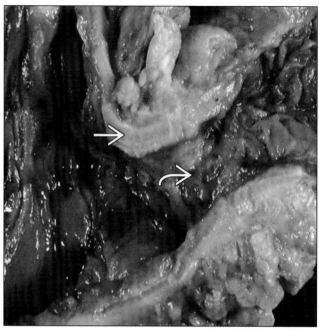

(Left) Axial CECT shows a short segment area of diffuse circumferential colonic mucosal thickening ➡ in this patient who underwent a recent colonoscopy with biopsy showing adenocarcinoma. Small pericolonic lymph nodes are present ➡; one adjacent to a colonic mass almost always represents metastatic regional nodes. *(Right)* Specimen from a partial colectomy shows mass-like diffuse circumferential colonic wall thickening ➡ and luminal narrowing ➡.

Typical Primary

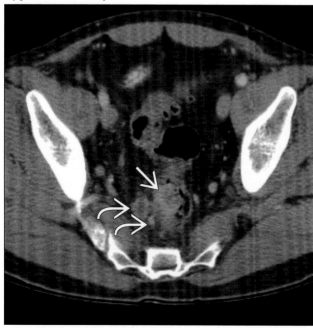 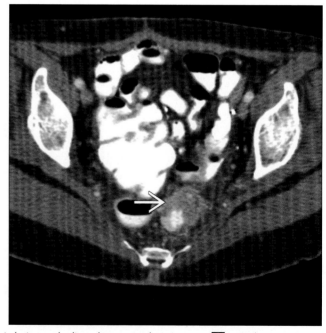

(Left) Axial CECT in the same patient with an unknown primary metastatic lesion to the liver shows an enhancing mass ➡ near the rectosigmoid junction with adjacent perirectal lymph nodes ➡. *(Right)* Axial CECT shows a mass in the distal sigmoid colon ➡ causing focal narrowing, compatible with colon carcinoma.

COLORECTAL CANCER

Typical Primary with Metastasis

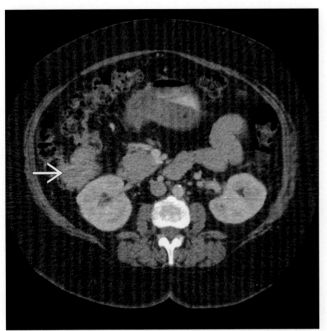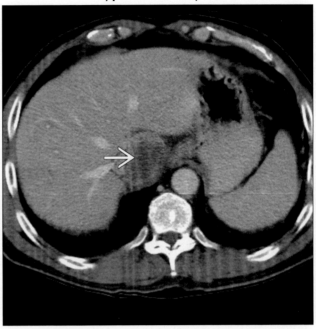

(Left) Axial CECT shows a short segment mass involving the proximal transverse colon ➡. Although a subtle finding, the patient was subsequently referred for colonoscopy, which proved a primary colonic adenocarcinoma. *(Right)* Axial CECT shows a low attenuation lesion within the caudate lobe of the liver ➡ in this patient without a history of malignancy or a known primary.

Initial Diagnosis

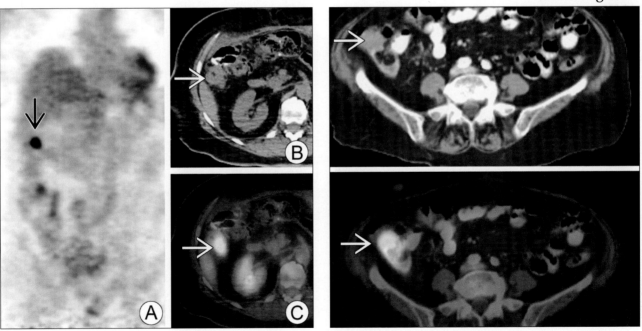

(Left) Coronal PET (A), axial CT (B) and fused PET/CT (C) show a focal area of intense FDG activity in the distal ascending colon ➡ that corresponds to an area of questionable thickening on the CT portion of the exam ➡. *(Right)* Axial CECT (top) and PET/CT (bottom) show intense FDG activity correlating with a focal mass within the lateral aspect of the proximal ascending colon ➡.

COLORECTAL CANCER

Inital Diagnosis Rectal Carcinoma

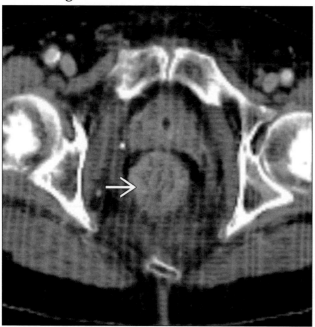
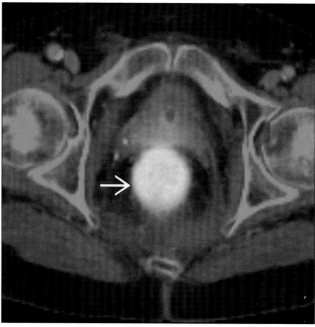

(Left) Axial CECT shows questionable diffuse rectal thickening ➡. The appearance is nonspecific on CT, but it may represent a primary rectal carcinoma, particularly in the presence of perirectal nodes. *(Right)* Axial fused PET/CT shows diffuse FDG activity in the area of rectal thickening ➡. This appearance in the presence of thickening on CT would be very suspicious for malignancy. However, focal intense FDG activity at the anorectal junction without thickening can be physiologic.

Initial Diagnosis

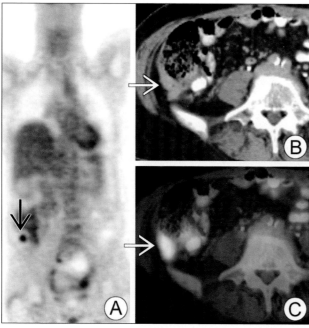
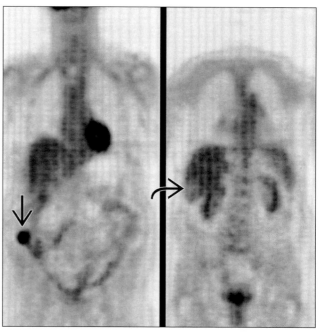

(Left) Focal intense FDG activity ➡ in the right lower quadrant on the coronal PET (A) is subsequently localized to the lateral aspect of the proximal descending colon corresponding to a focal area of thickening ➡ on axial CT (B) and fused PET/CT (C). Subsequent colonoscopy demonstrated colon carcinoma. *(Right)* Coronal PET images show focal intense colonic activity ➡ incidentally discovered on a PET/CT performed for pulmonary nodule evaluation. Subsequent colonoscopy confirmed adenocarcinoma. A subtle photopenic lesion is also present in the inferior liver ➘.

COLORECTAL CANCER

Variant: Benign Adenoma

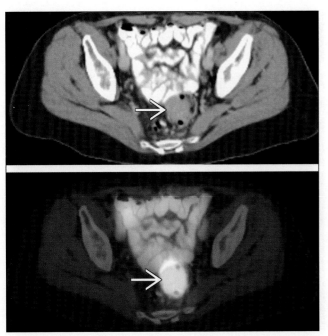

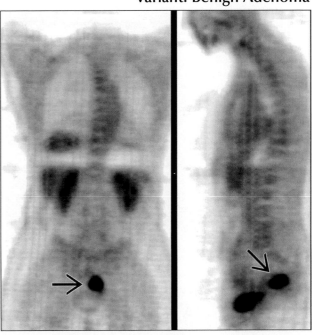

(Left) Axial CECT (top) and fused PET/CT (bottom) show a mass in the presacral area with intense FDG activity ➡. Subsequent colonoscopy and biopsy showed a large but benign villous adenoma. 50% of villous adenomas over 2 cm contain evidence of malignancy. This appearance on PET/CT usually indicates malignancy. *(Right)* Coronal (left) and sagittal (right) PET images of the same patient show a focal area of intense FDG activity in the presacral area ➡, suspicious for malignancy.

Rectal Carcinoma Staging

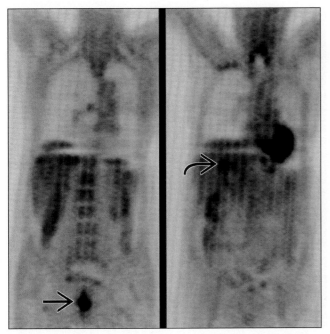

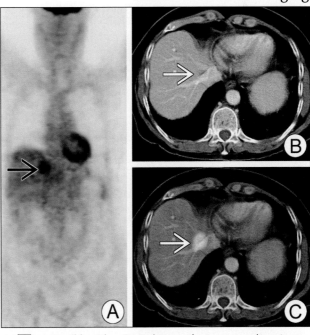

(Left) Coronal PET shows focal intense FDG activity in the area of the rectum ➡, compatible with patient's history of primary rectal carcinoma. In addition, there is a focal area of intense activity in the liver ➡ worrisome for a metastatic lesion. *(Right)* Coronal PET (A) demonstrates a focal area of intense FDG activity ➡ present in the medial aspect of the liver in this patient with newly diagnosed colonic carcinoma. Axial CT (B) and fused PET/CT (C) localize the activity to a very subtle lesion ➡ adjacent to the inferior vena cava, compatible with latency period.

COLORECTAL CANCER

Typical Staging

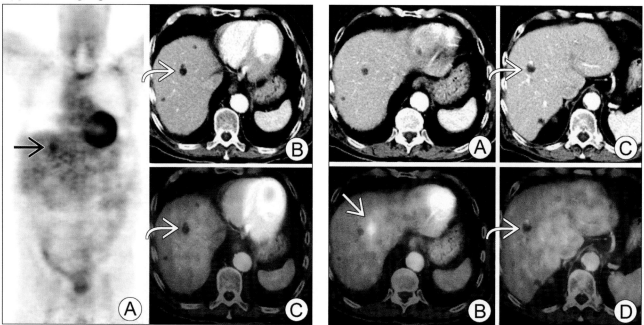

(Left) Coronal PET (A) shows focal moderate to intense FDG activity ➡ in the liver. Axial CT (B) and PET/CT (C) show lesions ➡ in the liver, compatible with cysts. *(Right)* Axial fused PET/CT (B) shows focal intense FDG activity ➡ without a correlative abnormality on CECT (A). Axial CT (C) and fused PET/CT (D) show more well-defined hepatic lesions ➡, compatible with benign cysts. Several studies in the literature have shown PET and PET/CT to be superior to CECT for staging patients with colon carcinoma.

Variant: Non-FDG-Avid Liver Metastasis

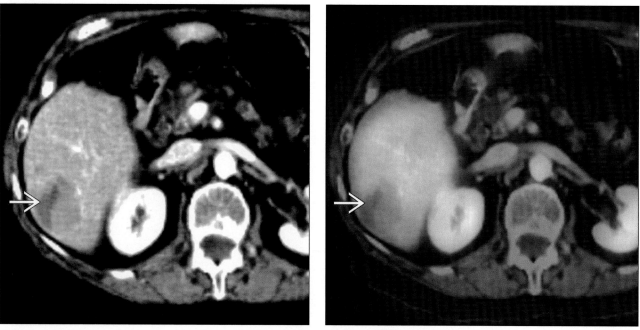

(Left) Axial CECT shows a heterogeneously enhancing lesion in segment 6 of the liver ➡ with an area of central necrosis, very worrisome for malignancy. *(Right)* Axial fused PET/CT shows relative photopenia ➡ compared to surrounding background liver. Despite the lack of increased metabolic activity, the appearance on CT remains suspicious for malignancy. A subsequent ultrasound-guided biopsy confirmed the diagnosis of hepatocellular carcinoma.

COLORECTAL CANCER

Variant: Non-FDG Avid Rectal Cancer Mets

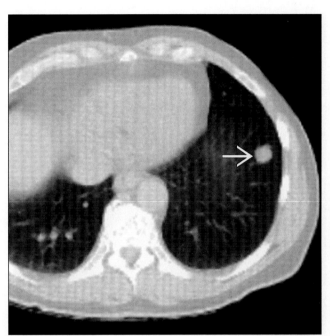
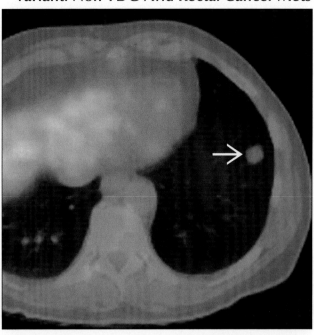

(Left) Axial CECT shows a well-rounded left lower lobe nodule ➡ in this patient with newly diagnosed rectal carcinoma. *(Right)* Axial fused PET/CT shows minimal FDG activity corresponding to the left lower pulmonary nodule ➡. Although the lack of FDG activity in a nodule over 1 cm has a high negative predictive value, a prior CT showed no pulmonary abnormalities, making this lesion worrisome for a relatively non-FDG-avid metastasis. Subsequent biopsy confirmed metastatic colon cancer.

Typical Staging

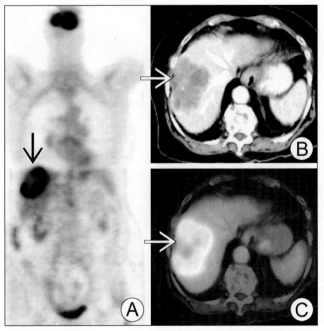
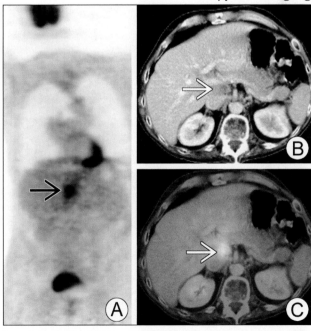

(Left) Coronal PET (A), axial CT (B) and fused PET/CT (C) demonstrate a large lesion in the right hepatic lobe ➡ with intense FDG activity ➡ and central photopenia, compatible with a central necrosis. *(Right)* Coronal PET (A) demonstrates focal intense activity ➡ in the area of the liver. Axial CT (B) and fused PET/CT (C) demonstrate a subtle lesion ➡ in the area of the caudate lobe of the liver.

COLORECTAL CANCER

Typical Staging with Atypical Metastasis

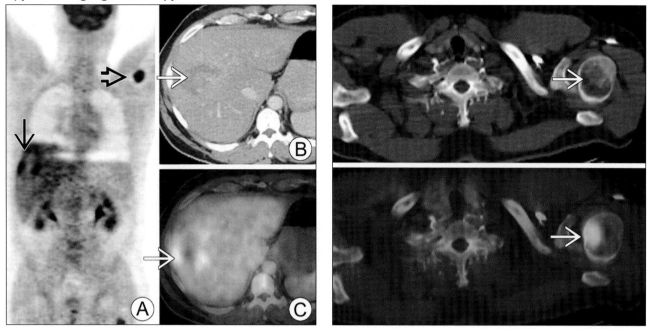

(Left) Coronal PET (A) demonstrates rim-enhancement-like FDG activity ➡ corresponding to a low attenuation lesion in the right hepatic lobe ➡ on axial CT (B) and fused PET/CT (C). An atypical metastatic lesion is also present in the left humeral head ➡. *(Right)* Axial CECT (top) and fused PET/CT (bottom) demonstrate a focal area of intense FDG activity ➡ in the medial aspect of the humeral head, corresponding to a metastatic lesion.

Typical Staging with Granulomatous Disease

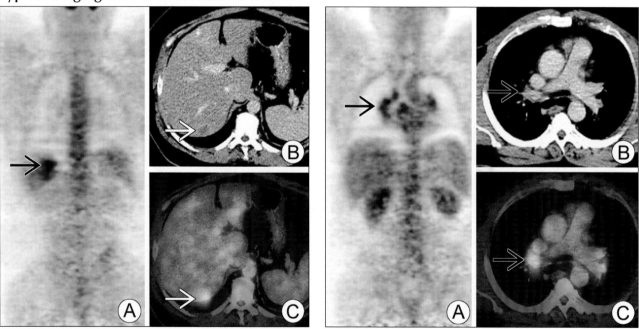

(Left) Coronal PET (A) shows a focal area of intense FDG activity in the posterior aspect of the liver ➡. Axial CT (B) and fused PET/CT (C) show the same activity to be within a ring-enhancing lesion in the posterior segment of the liver ➡, compatible with a metastatic lesion. *(Right)* Coronal PET (A), axial CT (B) and fused PET/CT (C) show bilateral hilar and right paratracheal areas ➡ of increased metabolic activity atypical for colon carcinoma metastases. Additional history reveals the patient had sarcoidosis for 5 years.

COLORECTAL CANCER

Typical Staging

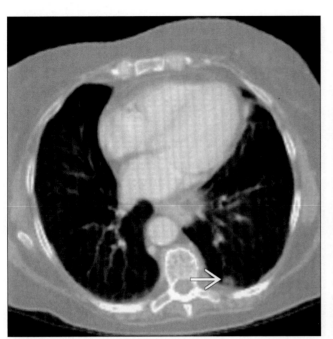 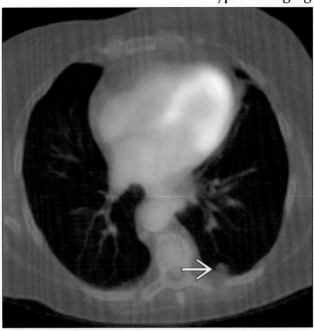

(Left) Axial CECT shows a subcentimeter pulmonary nodule ➡ in the posterior segment left lower lobe. *(Right)* Axial fused PET/CT shows no appreciably increased FDG activity within the left lower lobe pulmonary nodule ➡. The nodule is near the limits of resolution of the PET camera. Although there is no increased FDG activity, this lesion represented a metastatic lesion from rectal carcinoma.

Typical Staging

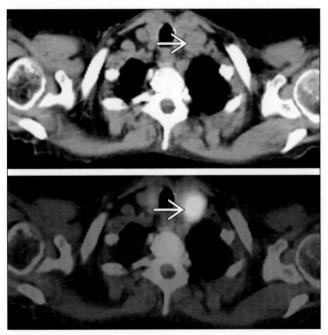 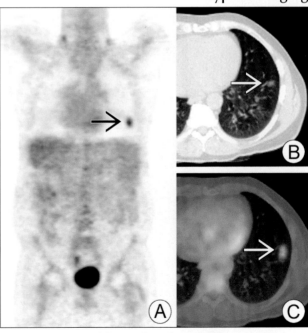

(Left) Axial CT (top) and fused PET/CT (bottom) show focal intense activity corresponding to a left supraclavicular node ➡ (Virchow node), compatible with a metastatic lesion from colon cancer. *(Right)* Coronal PET (A) shows focal intense FDG activity within the left hemithorax ➡, suspicious for metastatic disease. Axial CT (B) and fused PET/CT (C) demonstrate correlation of the increased metabolic activity to a subcentimeter pulmonary nodule ➡, compatible with metastatic rectal carcinoma.

COLORECTAL CANCER

Typical Restaging

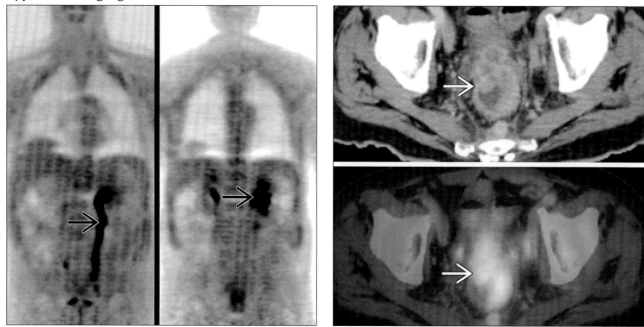

(Left) Coronal PET images show incidental left-sided hydronephrosis ⮕ secondary to shortening pelvic mass. *(Right)* Axial CECT (top) and fused PET/CT (bottom) demonstrate a heterogeneously enhancing pelvic mass ⮕ with areas of intense FDG activity, compatible with recurrent colorectal carcinoma.

Typical Restaging

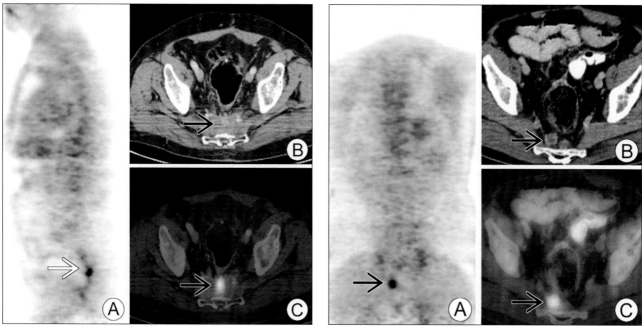

(Left) Sagittal PET (A) shows focal intense FDG activity in the presacral area ⮕ in this patient with a negative recent biopsy. Axial CT (B) and fused PET/CT (C) demonstrate focal FDG activity ⮕ within only the anterior medial aspect of the presacral soft tissue. Focused repeat biopsy based on PET/CT demonstrated recurrent adenocarcinoma. *(Right)* Coronal PET (A), axial CT (B) and fused PET/CT (C) show a focal area of intense activity in the presacral area ⮕. Focused biopsy of the metabolically active lesion showed recurrent adenocarcinoma.

COLORECTAL CANCER

Typical Restaging

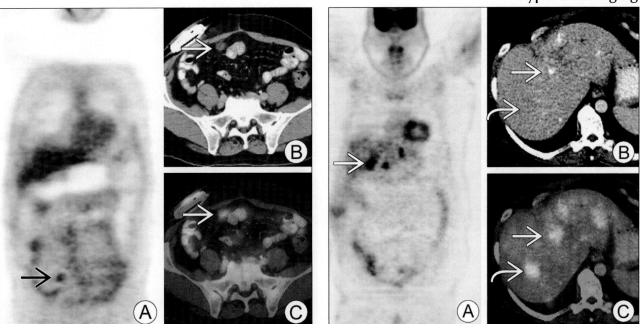

(Left) Selected images from a PET/CT study demonstrate mild FDG activity ⇒ on coronal PET (A). Axial CT (B) and fused PET/CT (C) localized the subtle abnormal FDG activity to an omental implant ⇒, compatible with metastatic disease. (Right) Coronal PET (A) shows multiple areas of focally increased FDG activity within the liver ⇒. Axial CT (B) and fused PET/CT (C) demonstrate several metastatic lesions ⇒, some of which are not apparent ⇒ even with a good contrast-enhanced CT examination.

Typical Restaging

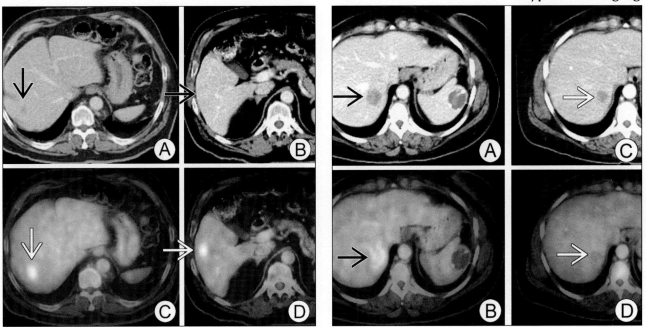

(Left) Selected axial CT (A, B) images demonstrate subtle subcentimeter low attenuation lesions ⇒ in the liver. Without the confirmation of focally increased FDG activity ⇒ on fused PET/CT (C, D), the lesions would be "too small to further characterize". (Right) Axial CECT and fused PET/CT (A, B) demonstrate a low attenuation lesion in the posterior segment of the liver ⇒ with intense FDG activity, compatible with malignancy. Axial CT and fused PET/CT (C, D) are from a follow-up PET/CT after 3 cycles of chemotherapy and show interval resolution of abnormal FDG activity ⇒.

COLORECTAL CANCER

Typical Restaging

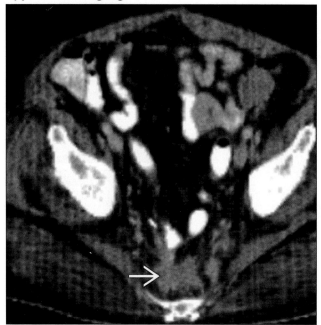 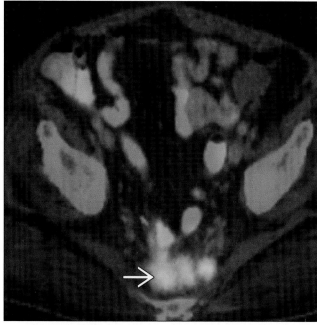

(Left) Axial CECT shows soft tissue change in the presacral area ➡ commonly seen after surgical intervention. The differential diagnosis includes post-operative change vs. residual or recurrent tumor. Combined PET/CT is the optimal test of choice for this type of evaluation. *(Right)* Axial fused PET/CT shows moderate to intense activity in the presacral area ➡, corresponding to the previously described soft tissue, most compatible with residual or recurrent malignancy.

Typical Restaging

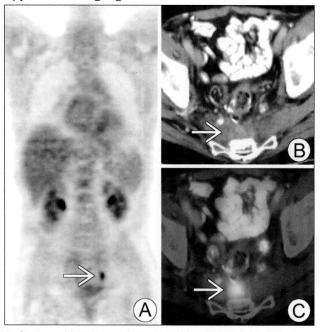 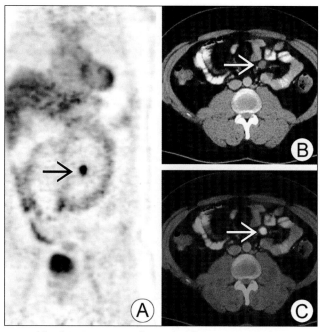

(Left) Coronal PET (A), axial CT (B) and fused PET/CT (C) demonstrate increased focal FDG activity in the presacral area, corresponding to the focal thickening on the CT portion of the exam ➡, compatible with malignancy. *(Right)* Coronal PET (A) demonstrates focal intense activity in the mid-abdomen ➡ in this patient with a rising CEA level. Axial CT (B) and fused PET/CT (C) localize the lesion to the mesentery ➡.

COLORECTAL CANCER

Variant Restaging

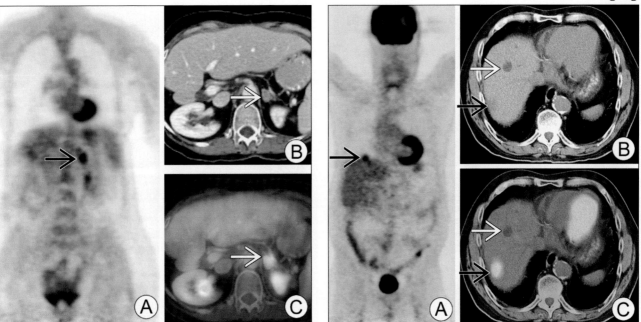

(Left) Coronal PET (A) demonstrates a focal area of increased metabolic activity superior to the left kidney ➡. Axial CT (B) and fused PET/CT (C) show the lesion to be an atypical metastatic lesion from colon cancer to the left adrenal gland ➡. *(Right)* Coronal PET (A), axial CT (B) and fused PET/CT (C) demonstrate a focal area of intense FDG activity near the dome of the liver ➡ without a definite correlate to a CT abnormality, compatible with a metastatic lesion from colon cancer. A small cyst is also present ➡ without increased metabolic activity.

Typical Restaging

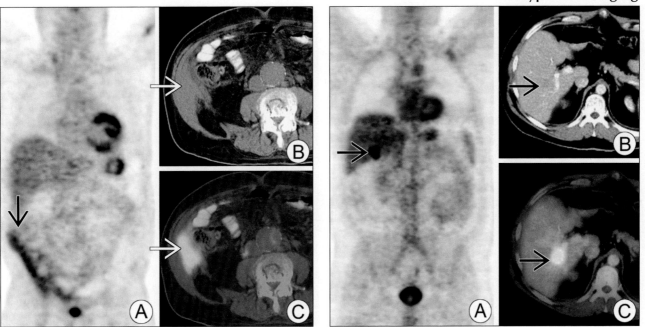

(Left) Diffuse linear activity ➡ identified on the coronal PET (A) has the appearance of physiologic FDG activity within bowel. Further evaluation on axial CT (B) and fused PET/CT (C) demonstrate pericolonic thickening ➡, compatible with malignancy. *(Right)* A restaging PET/CT in a patient with a rising CEA demonstrates a focal intense area of FDG activity in the inferior liver on coronal PET (A). Axial CT (B) and fused PET/CT (C) localize the lesion to a subtle low attenuation lesion in the right hepatic lobe ➡.

COLORECTAL CANCER

Typical Restaging

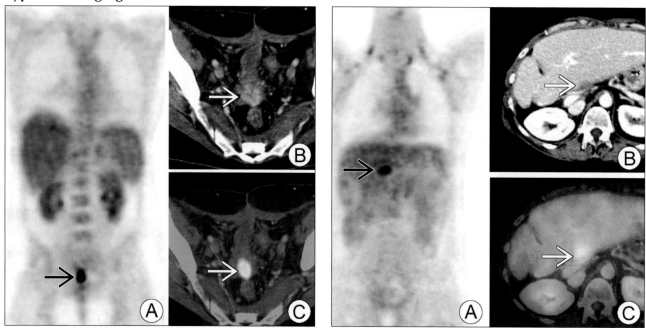

(Left) Focal area of intense FDG activity ➡ is present on the coronal PET (A). The abnormal FDG activity is localized to a lesion within the pelvis ➡ on axial CT (B) and fused PET/CT (C). The lesion demonstrates subtly increased enhancement near this patient's anastomosis, compatible with malignancy. *(Right)* Coronal PET (A) shows focal intense activity ➡ in the periportal area difficult to localize with PET. Axial CT (B) and fused PET/CT (C) show focal intense FDG activity corresponding to a subtle low attenuation lesion in the medial aspect of the liver ➡, compatible with malignancy.

Typical Restaging

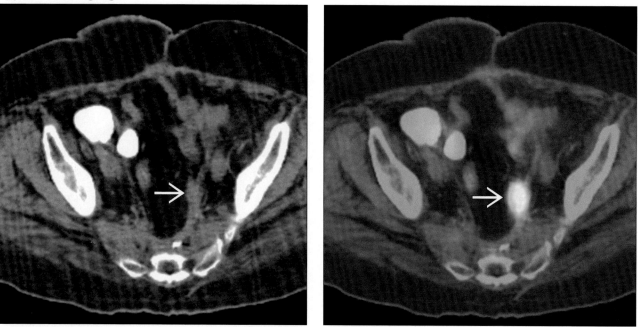

(Left) Axial NECT shows questionable subtle thickening ➡ near this patient's anastomosis in the left side of pelvis, equivocal for malignancy. *(Right)* Axial fused PET/CT shows focal intense activity ➡ corresponding to the questionable area of thickening, compatible with malignancy.

COLORECTAL CANCER

Typical Restaging

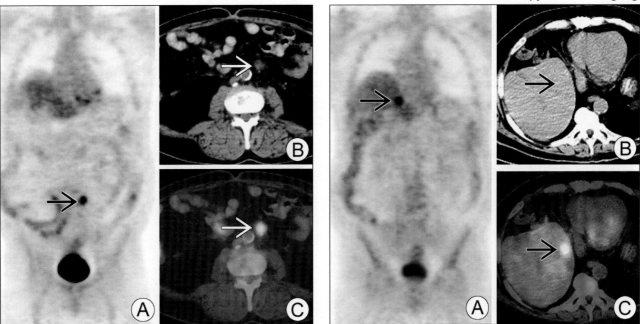

(Left) Coronal PET (A) demonstrates a focal area of intense activity ➡. Axial CT (B) and fused PET/CT (C) localize the activity to a subtle left periaortic lymph node ➡, compatible with malignancy. *(Right)* An additional lesion is present in the same patient without definite correlation to a CT abnormality ➡ on noncontrast CT exam.

Typical Restaging

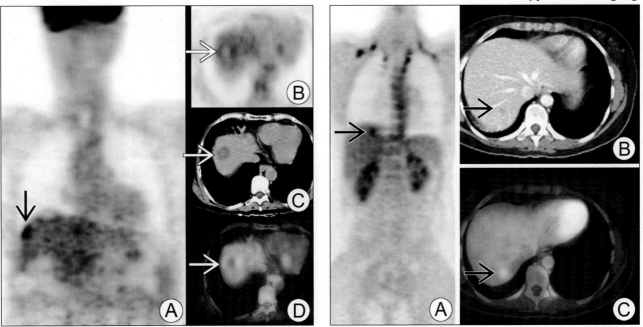

(Left) Coronal PET (A) shows an area of increased FDG activity in the liver ➡ in this patient who is status post radiofrequency ablation for a prior hepatic metastasis. Axial PET (B), CT (C), and PET/CT (D) demonstrate a photopenic area near the previously treated lesion ➡. *(Right)* A patient with colon carcinoma was sent for restaging PET/CT. CECT examination demonstrated a subcentimeter lesion in the posterior segment of the liver. Coronal PET (A) and axial CT (B) & PET/CT (C) show a focal area of increased FDG ➡ in the subtle low attenuation lesion, compatible with malignancy.

COLORECTAL CANCER

Typical Restaging

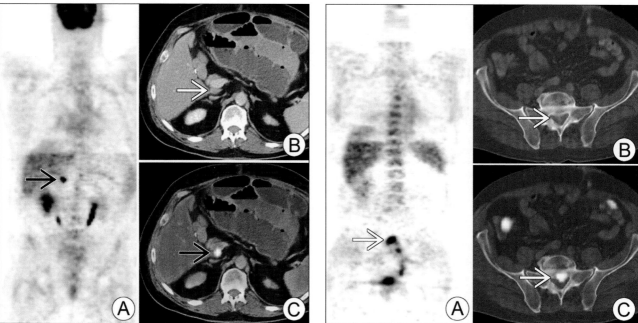

(Left) A normal-sized portacaval lymph node ➡️ is present on the contrast-enhanced CT examination (B). Focal intense activity ➡️ is present on the coronal PET (A) and fused PET/CT (C), confirming previously unsuspected metastatic disease. *(Right)* PET/CT performed in a patient with a rising CEA level demonstrates focal intense activity within the posterior aspect of the sacral vertebral body ➡️, worrisome for malignancy. A follow-up MR confirmed the presence of malignancy.

Typical Restaging

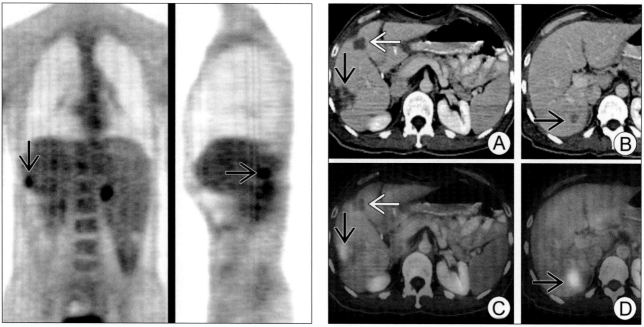

(Left) This patient underwent radiofrequency ablation of 3 hepatic lesions approximately 10 weeks before this study. Multiple foci of increased metabolic activity ➡️ are identified but difficult to localize on coronal (left) and sagittal (right) PET images. *(Right)* Correlated axial CT (A, B) and fused PET/CT (C, D) demonstrate two foci of increased metabolic activity ➡️ corresponding to failed ablation. One low attenuation lesion ➡️ without increased metabolic activity is present in a successful ablation.

COLORECTAL CANCER

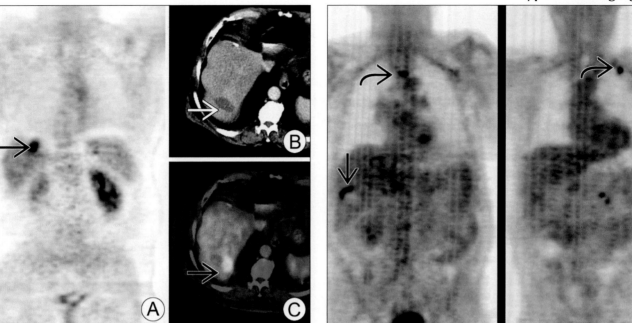

(Left) This patient underwent radiofrequency ablation 11 weeks prior to this PET/CT examination. Although the lesion ➡ has a typical appearance of post-ablation on CT (B), PET (A) and PET/CT (C) demonstrate intense activity along the medial aspect of the lesion, compatible with residual/recurrent disease ➡. *(Right)* This patient underwent radiofrequency ablation of a hepatic lesion 8 weeks before this study. Coronal PET images show that rim-enhancement-like activity is present along the superolateral aspect of the ablated lesion, compatible with residual tumor ➡. New lesions are also identified within the mediastinum and left supraclavicular area ➡.

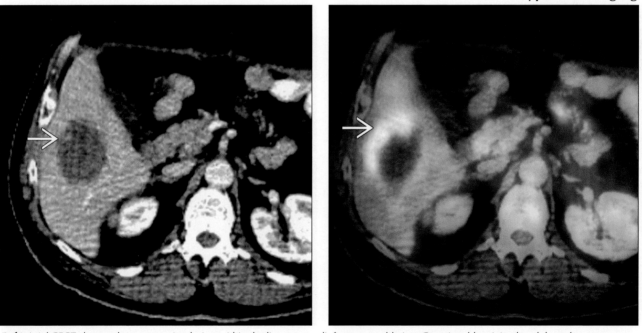

(Left) Axial CECT shows a low attenuation lesion within the liver post radiofrequency ablation. Questionable minimal nodular enhancement ➡ is present along the lateral border. *(Right)* Axial fused PET/CT shows intense metabolic activity ➡ along the anterior and lateral borders, confirming residual malignancy.

COLORECTAL CANCER

Typical Restaging

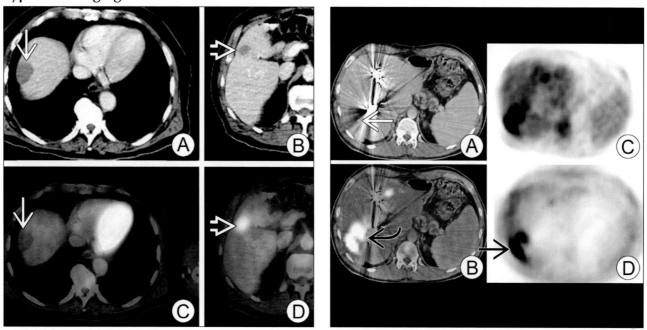

(Left) Axial CECT (A, B) and PET/CT (C, D) of a patient 10 weeks post radiofrequency ablation of a hepatic lesion demonstrate no increased activity in the successfully ablated lesion ➡ but also show an incidental new lesion more inferiorly ➡. *(Right)* This patient underwent hepatic chemoembolization for metastases 10 weeks prior to this exam. Extensive artifact ➡ from the embolization coils makes evaluation for residual/recurrent tumor difficult on axial CT (A). However, increased activity ➡ on the PET/CT (B) makes evaluation much easier. Activity ➡ on the non-attenuation corrected image (D) shows this is not an artifact.

Pitfall: Post-Operative Abscess

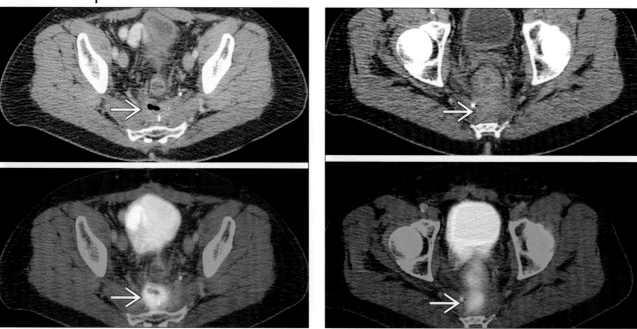

(Left) A PET/CT performed 2 weeks post-surgery demonstrates intense FDG activity ➡ correlating to a small amount of free air within extensive presacral post-operative changes, compatible with a small post-operative abscess. *(Right)* A subsequent PET/CT in the same patient performed 3 months after the original PET/CT shows resolution of the presacral free air and marked interval decrease of the FDG activity ➡, compatible with resolving inflammatory change.

COLORECTAL CANCER

Pitfalls

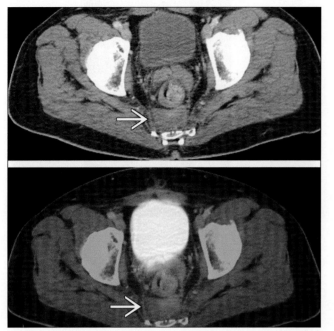

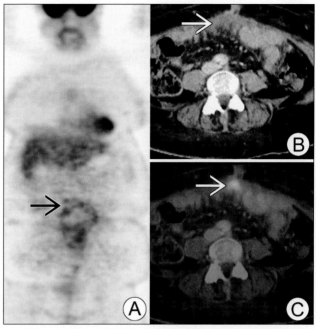

(Left) A PET/CT, performed approximately 6 months after the original post-operative head CT, demonstrates complete resolution of the abnormal FDG activity now with only non-FDG-avid presacral soft tissue, compatible with post-operative changes ➡. (Right) Restaging PET/ CT examination shows mild hazy increased metabolic activity ➡ on the coronal PET (A). However, subsequent evaluation of the axial CT (B) and fused PET/CT (C) demonstrates that diffuse omental metastases ➡ have only minimally increased FDG activity.

Response to Chemotherapy

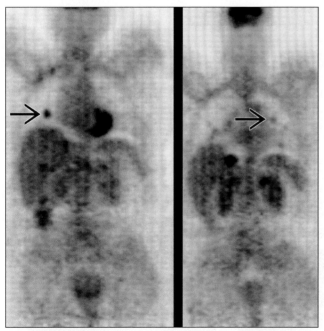

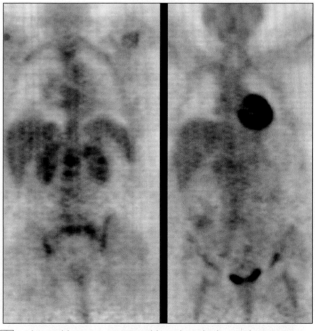

(Left) Coronal PET shows multiple areas of focally increased FDG uptake ➡ with variable activity, compatible with multiple rectal carcinoma metastases of varying size. (Right) Coronal PET in the same patient after receiving 3 cycles of chemotherapy shows complete resolution of the previously noted lesions, compatible with a good response to therapy.

HODGKIN LYMPHOMA

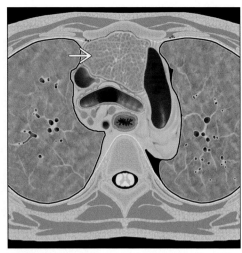

Graphic demonstrates a typical appearance of Hodgkin lymphoma in the anterior mediastinum as a fairly homogeneous mass ➡, typically with low attenuation on CT.

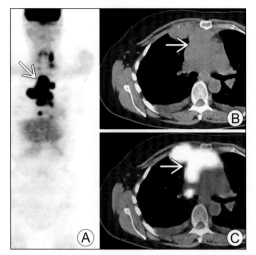

Coronal PET (A), axial CT (B) and fused PET/CT (C) demonstrate an anterior mediastinal mass ➡ with intense FDG activity, compatible with Hodgkin lymphoma.

TERMINOLOGY

Abbreviations and Synonyms
- Hodgkin lymphoma (HL)
- Hodgkin disease (HD)
- Lymph nodes (LN)

Definitions
- Malignant neoplasm arising from lymphocytes
- Rare variety is derived from histiocytes

IMAGING FINDINGS

General Features
- Best diagnostic clue
  - **FDG PET/CT**
    - Enlarged FDG-avid lymph nodes/conglomerate mass
    - In usual location: Anterior mediastinum with other nodal groups
  - **CT**
    - Mediastinal lymphadenopathy presenting as mediastinal mass

- ± Hepatomegaly, splenomegaly, lung nodules/ infiltrates, pleural effusions
- Location
  - Uncommon spread to extralymphatic locations
    - CNS, spine
  - Usual spread is to contiguous lymph nodes
    - Then to viscera or bone marrow
  - 30-40% of patients present with splenic involvement
  - 5-14% of patients have bone marrow involvement
  - Bone involvement
    - Primary bone invasion does not affect staging; rare (1-4%) at presentation
    - Hematogenous spread indicates stage IV disease
    - Stage IV occurs in 5-20% of patients during disease course
  - 6% of patients have chest wall involvement
    - Requires more aggressive therapy due to higher relapse rate
  - Thymic involvement considered "nodal"
    - Does not count as extranodal disease
    - Not associated with change in disease stage
    - Up to half of patients with thoracic HL may show enlarged thymus

DDx: Anterior Mediastinal Mass with Increased FDG Activity

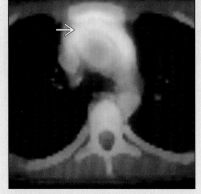

Normal Thymus in a Young Patient

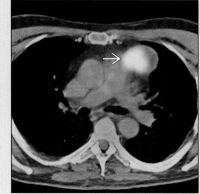

Invasive Thymoma

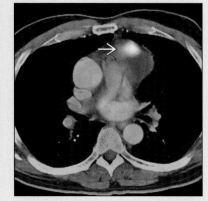

Cystic Teratoma

HODGKIN LYMPHOMA

Key Facts

Terminology
- Hodgkin lymphoma (HL); Hodgkin disease (HD)

Imaging Findings
- FDG PET/CT: Enlarged, hypermetabolic lymph nodes
- PET/CT or PET + CT (side-by-side) is superior to contrast CT or PET alone for staging HD
- Ga-67 inferior to FDG PET for initial staging
- CECT can help evaluate cortical bone involvement but has low sensitivity in detecting bone marrow disease
- Pooled true positive value of PET for HL 90% with upstaging rate ranging from 8-17% and downstaging rate from 2-23%
- PET has prognostic value after 1-3 cycles of chemotherapy

- After 2-3 cycles of chemo, PET-positive group had 39% 5 year survival vs. PET-negative group at 92%
- For tumor response to therapy, low-dose CT PET/CT may be enough
- PET has significant influence on staging of HL, upstaging 15-25% of patients with shift to more advanced treatment in 10% of patients
- SUV reduction of 60% is used as cutoff to separate treatment responders from nonresponders

Top Differential Diagnoses
- Granulomatous Process
- Infections
- Other Malignancy
- Normal Lymphoid Tissue
- Reactive Lymph Nodes

- - Present after successful treatment as a result of rebound thymic hyperplasia
  - Occasionally develop thymic cysts
  - Rare locations
    - Peritoneal and omental involvement found only in non-Hodgkin lymphoma
    - Renal parenchyma is rarely involved, although perirenal space may be invaded
    - GI tract uncommon and usually due to nodal extension
- Morphology
  - Rounded or bulky soft tissue mass due to nodal aggregation
  - Large masses may have areas of necrosis, hemorrhage, or cyst formation

Imaging Recommendations
- Best imaging tool
  - **PET/CT**
    - Best for staging HD (sensitivity 94-98% and specificity 95-100%)
  - **MR**
    - To delineate soft tissue margins and evaluate spinal cord impingement
- Protocol advice
  - Baseline FDG PET images should be obtained for initial staging
    - Prior to treatment
  - Patient should be kept warm and avoid activity prior to scan
    - Reduces physiologic uptake in muscle and fat
  - Low dose CT is acceptable for evaluating response to therapy

CT Findings
- CT has replaced more complicated invasive diagnostic procedures
  - Method of choice for identification of disease invisible on clinical exam
  - Rarely performed anymore: Laparotomy/ splenectomy, lymphangiography, and mediastinoscopy

- **Lymphadenopathy**
  - Lymph node enlargement and aggregation
    - Appearance of multiple round or bulky soft tissue masses
  - Large masses may develop necrosis, hemorrhage, or cyst formation (10-20%)
  - Minimal contrast enhancement
  - Calcification rare before treatment but 20% prevalence post-radiotherapy
    - Rim calcification
    - Multiple discrete deposits (mulberry)
  - CT useful for treatment/radiation planning
- **Extralymphatic involvement**
  - Mediastinal structures may show displacement, compression, or invasion
  - Cortical bone well evaluated with CT
  - Poor sensitivity for bone marrow disease
  - Invasion of gallbladder and pancreas usually from adjacent nodal disease
    - Absence of pancreatic capsule hinders diagnosis of invasion vs. contact
  - Thymic mass may be discrete or infiltrating
- **Therapy response**
  - Tumor masses have low density of malignant cells
  - Reduction in volume of lesion is an insensitive predictor of response

Nuclear Medicine Findings
- **Initial diagnosis**
  - Involved lymphoid tissue generally shows increased FDG uptake
    - No differentiation of subtypes by SUV has been demonstrated
  - Focal, super-physiologic uptake in nodal or extranodal tissue fairly specific indicator of disease
    - Diffuse uptake more difficult to interpret
    - Awareness of common FDG PET false positives is essential
  - Uptake may be seen in spleen and liver
    - Focal increased FDG activity generally indicative of malignant involvement
- **Staging**

HODGKIN LYMPHOMA

- o For organ staging, PET/CT seems to have no obvious advantage over FDG PET alone
  - Except in reducing false positives by better characterization of lesions using CT
- o Pooled true positive rate of FDG PET for HL: 90%
  - Upstaging rate: 8-25%
  - Shift to more advanced treatment: 10%
  - Downstaging: 2-23% (mean less than for upstaging)
- o FDG PET inclusion criteria are more accurate than CT inclusion criteria
  - Size is an insensitive indicator of malignancy
  - Enhancement characteristics are unreliable for inclusion
  - Combined PET/CT is superior for lesion delineation in radiotherapy planning
- o Bone marrow involvement
  - Diffuse marrow involvement may be intense
  - May also be indistinguishable from background
  - May be misinterpreted as negative for disease with diffuse marrow activity
  - Increased uptake can be iatrogenic
  - G-CSF, erythropoietin
  - Beta-thalassemia also increases uptake
  - Bone marrow biopsy (BMB) and PET/CT are complementary
  - Similar sensitivity/specificity but discordant findings
  - BMB more sensitive for detection of diffuse disease
  - PET/CT more likely to detect patchy disease
- o Spleen and liver
  - Full dose diagnostic CT necessary for adequate evaluation of liver and spleen
  - Splenic involvement may appear as diffusely increased uptake
  - Also seen in "reactive" spleen
  - Liver involvement may appear as diffuse uptake or patchy uptake in portal areas
  - Less commonly as large focal lesions
- **Response to therapy**
  - o SUV reduction of 60% is used as cutoff to separate treatment responders from nonresponders
  - o PET has prognostic value after chemotherapy: 5 year survival after 2-3 cycles of chemo
    - 92% for PET-negative group
    - 39% for PET-positive group
  - o 2 year progression-free survival after 2 cycles of ABVD-like chemo
    - 94% for PET-negative patients
    - 0-6% for early PET-positive patients
  - o Study showed no evidence that patients benefit from treatment alteration based on early PET
    - Patients with PET-negative residual mass after chemo who received radiotherapy to original bulky site had 2.5% relapse rate within 18 months vs. 14% relapse in non-radiotherapy arm
    - In contrast, the International Prognostic Index (IPS) poorly predicts improved survival

DIFFERENTIAL DIAGNOSIS

Granulomatous Process
- Active disease positive on FDG PET
- Infectious and non-infectious etiologies
- Will usually resolve over time
- More likely bilateral hilar and paratracheal distribution

Infections
- Pyogenic, fungal, parasitic, HIV-related, viral (e.g., varicella, zoster, HCV, CMV)
- Usually positive on FDG PET

Other Malignancy
- Variable enhancement and FDG uptake
- History is crucial

Normal Lymphoid Tissue
- Physiologic uptake common in Waldeyer ring, thymic tissue, cervical nodes
- Asymmetric uptake can occur normally and may be mistaken for malignancy

Reactive Lymph Nodes
- Usually much smaller than typical aggressive Hodgkin

PATHOLOGY

General Features
- Genetics
  - o 1% of patients with HD have family history of disease
  - o Sibling of affected individual has 3-7x increased risk
    - Higher in monozygotic twins
  - o HLA-DP alleles more common in HD
- Etiology
  - o Unknown
  - o Infection may be involved in pathogenesis, particularly Epstein-Barr virus (EBV)
    - Tumor cells are EBV-positive in ~ 50% of HD cases
    - Positivity higher in MCHD (60-70%) than in NSHD (15-30%)
    - ~ 100% of HIV-related HD are EBV-positive (though HD is not an AIDS-defining condition)
- Epidemiology
  - o 8,000 new cases and 1,000 deaths occur in the USA annually
  - o Incidence: 3-4/100,000 per year

Gross Pathologic & Surgical Features
- Cut surface white-gray and uniform
- Affected LN
  - o Usually enlarged
  - o Shape is preserved
  - o Capsule is not invaded
  - o Surface may be nodular in nodular sclerosis subtype

Microscopic Features
- Prominent lymphocytic infiltrate and Reed-Sternberg cells
  - o Reed-Sternberg cells: Large, binucleate, with characteristic CD15+, CD30+ immunophenotype
- Core biopsy preferred over fine needle aspiration

HODGKIN LYMPHOMA

- Malignant cells in HL make up only a very small, scattered proportion of the tumor volume
  - Subtyping requires core biopsy
  - Tumors pleomorphic
- Bone marrow disease is often patchy and focal resulting in low sensitivity of bone marrow biopsy
  - If positive on PET, directed biopsy of that area increases true positive yield

Staging, Grading, or Classification Criteria
- Staging criteria
  - Physical examination
  - Bloodwork
  - Bone marrow biopsy
  - CECT of neck, chest, abdomen, pelvis
  - MR in some cases
- WHO ICD10 classification of lymphoma
  - Nature of staging is shown by
    - Clinical stage as obtained by exam & tests
    - Pathological stage by exploratory laparotomy with splenectomy fallen out of favor
- Major categories of HL (preceded diagnosis by WHO classification)
  - Nodular lymphocyte predominance HL (NLPHL)
  - Classic Hodgkin lymphoma (CHL): Lymphocyte rich classic HL (LRCHL)
  - Nodular sclerosis HL (NSHL)
  - Mixed cellularity HL (MCHL)
  - Lymphocyte depletion HL (LDHL)
  - Unspecified
- Ann Arbor classification of anatomic distribution of disease
  - **Stage I**: Single region, usually one LN, and surrounding area (I)
    - Or a single extranodal site in absence of LN involvement (IE)
    - Usually no "B" symptoms
  - **Stage II**: ≥ 2 separate regions on one side of diaphragm (II)
    - Or single extralymphatic site and associated regional LN involvement on one side of diaphragm (IIE)
  - **Stage III**: Spread to both sides of diaphragm (III)
    - May include extralymphatic extension with adjacent LN involvement (IIIE)
    - Splenic involvement (IIIS)
    - Both (IIIE,S)
  - **Stage IV**: Diffuse/disseminated involvement
    - ≥ 2 extralymphatic organs, (liver, marrow, or lung)
    - Location of stage IV disease indicated by modifier below
- Modifiers
  - A or B: Absence ("A") or presence ("B") of B-symptoms
  - E: Disease involves extralymphatic site(s) adjacent to site(s) of lymphatic involvement (± obvious direct extension)
  - X: Largest deposit is > 10 cm ("bulky disease") or mediastinum wider than 1/3 of the chest on a CXR
  - S: Splenic involvement; splenic nodule of any size, or histology proven

- Splenic enlargement alone insufficient to confirm involvement
  - H: Liver involvement = stage IV; liver nodules of any size or histology proven
    - Hepatomegaly alone insufficient to confirm involvement
  - M: Suspected bone marrow involvement by biopsy or imaging
  - L: Lung involvement; pulmonary nodule(s)
    - Or extension from adjacent mediastinal/hilar LN or extralymphatic extension (E lesion) = stage IV
  - Specific sites involved designated by letter subscripts
    - Includes "+" if biopsy-proven involvement; "-" if biopsy negative
    - Spleen (S), lung (L), marrow (M), hepatic (H), pericardium (Pcard), pleura (P), Waldeyer ring (W)
    - Osseous (bone) (O), gastrointestinal (GI), skin (D), soft tissue (Softis), thyroid (Thy)
- Limitations: Staging may not predict biological behavior
- International Prognostic Index (IPI) risk factors
  - Age > 60 years: Ann Arbor stage III or IV, elevated LDH, reduced performance status, extranodal disease
  - Patients assigned to 5 year survival risk categories
    - Low, low-intermediate, high-intermediate, high
    - Low (73%), high (26%)
  - Prognostic factors predict the success of conventional treatment in patients with locally extensive or advanced stage HD
    - Age ≥ 45 years; stage IV disease, Hb < 10.5 mg/dl, lymphocyte count < 600/µl or < 8%
    - Male, albumin < 4.0 mg/dl, WBC count ≥ 15,000/µl
  - Freedom from progression (FFP) at 5 years related to number of factors present
    - No factors (84%)
    - Each added factor lowers 5 year FFP by 7%
    - > 5 factors (42%)

CLINICAL ISSUES

Presentation
- Most common signs/symptoms
  - Most often asymptomatic and found incidentally
  - Painless LN enlargement (80% above diaphragm)
  - 40% present with systemic B-symptoms (weight loss, fever, night sweats)
  - 35% present with intermittent fever
- Other signs/symptoms
  - Enlarged LN painful for hours after alcohol consumption specific for HD, present in < 10%
  - Pel-Ebstein fever (rare): High fever 1-2 weeks alternates with afebrile period 1-2 weeks
  - Impingement on airway and vessels may produce corresponding symptoms

Demographics
- Age
  - Bimodal age incidence: 15-34 years and > 55 years
  - Young adults typically have NSHD
- Gender
  - M:F = 2.25:1

HODGKIN LYMPHOMA

○ Nodular sclerosis, M < F
○ Children: M:F = ~ 6:1

Natural History & Prognosis

• > 85% of HL is curable, but long-term toxicity from treatment is common
  ○ Significant rate of relapse
• Prognostic factors
  ○ Clinical stage (major factor)
  ○ Extent of involvement (number of regions, extranodal disease, disease bulk)
  ○ Presence of B-symptoms
  ○ Age
  ○ Blood counts, biochemical parameters
• HIV-associated HD markedly more aggressive than non-HIV type
  ○ Median survival 8-20 months
  ○ Extranodal and bone marrow involvement is common

Treatment

• 80% of patients with HL have event-free survival prolonged by treatment regimens
• Preferred approach to most cases involves combined modalities
  ○ Limits toxicity of individual agents and provides synergistic effect
• Radiotherapy vs. chemotherapy
  ○ Effective radiotherapy in patients with early stage HL depends on accurate delineation of tumor volume by PET/CT
  ○ Modern radiotherapy techniques include
    ▪ 3D-conformal radiotherapy, intensity-modulated radiotherapy, and respiratory gating
  ○ XRT used for initial disease as well as persistent disease following chemotherapy; also sites of original bulky disease
• Toxicity
  ○ Treatment may have serious long-term adverse effects
    ▪ Cardiopulmonary disease and secondary malignancies
  ○ PET is useful for minimizing toxicity
    ▪ Especially for patients with good response to treatment and for earlier adjustment in patients who are poor responders

DIAGNOSTIC CHECKLIST

Image Interpretation Pearls

• Always consider performing a PET/CT in patients newly diagnosed with HD
• Extensive literature to support using PET/CT for determining response to therapy
• Knowledge of staging systems critical to quality of imaging report

SELECTED REFERENCES

1. Ansquer C et al: 18-F FDG-PET in the staging of lymphocyte-predominant Hodgkin's disease. Haematologica. 93(1):128-31, 2008
2. Bartlett NL: Modern treatment of Hodgkin lymphoma. Curr Opin Hematol. 15(4):408-14, 2008
3. Friedmann AM et al: The evolving standard of care for hodgkin lymphoma. J Pediatr Hematol Oncol. 30(2):121-3, 2008
4. Hines-Thomas M et al: Comparison of gallium and PET scans at diagnosis and follow-up of pediatric patients with Hodgkin lymphoma. Pediatr Blood Cancer. 51(2):198-203, 2008
5. Juweid ME: 18F-FDG PET as a routine test for posttherapy assessment of Hodgkin's disease and aggressive non-Hodgkin's lymphoma: where is the evidence? J Nucl Med. 49(1):9-12, 2008
6. Kasamon YL et al: FDG PET and risk-adapted therapy in Hodgkin's and non-Hodgkin's lymphoma. Curr Opin Oncol. 20(2):206-19, 2008
7. Pelosi E et al: FDG-PET in the detection of bone marrow disease in Hodgkin's disease and aggressive non-Hodgkin's lymphoma and its impact on clinical management. Q J Nucl Med Mol Imaging. 52(1):9-16, 2008
8. Pelosi E et al: Role of whole-body [(18)F] fluorodeoxyglucose positron emission tomography/ computed tomography (FDG-PET/CT) and conventional techniques in the staging of patients with Hodgkin and aggressive non Hodgkin lymphoma. Radiol Med (Torino). 113(4):578-590, 2008
9. Terasawa T et al: 18F-FDG PET for posttherapy assessment of Hodgkin's disease and aggressive Non-Hodgkin's lymphoma: a systematic review. J Nucl Med. 49(1):13-21, 2008
10. Advani R et al: Impact of positive positron emission tomography on prediction of freedom from progression after Stanford V chemotherapy in Hodgkin's disease. J Clin Oncol. 25(25):3902-7, 2007
11. Brepoels L et al: Hodgkin lymphoma: Response assessment by revised International Workshop Criteria. Leuk Lymphoma. 48(8):1539-47, 2007
12. Girinsky T et al: Is FDG-PET scan in patients with early stage Hodgkin lymphoma of any value in the implementation of the involved-node radiotherapy concept and dose painting? Radiother Oncol. 85(2):178-86, 2007
13. Jabbour E et al: Pretransplant positive positron emission tomography/gallium scans predict poor outcome in patients with recurrent/refractory Hodgkin lymphoma. Cancer. 109(12):2481-9, 2007
14. Paolini R et al: The prognostic value of 18F-FDG PET-CT in the management of Hodgkin's lymphoma: preliminary results of a prospective study. Nucl Med Rev Cent East Eur. 10(2):87-90, 2007
15. Schaefer NG et al: Hodgkin disease: diagnostic value of FDG PET/CT after first-line therapy--is biopsy of FDG-avid lesions still needed? Radiology. 244(1):257-62, 2007
16. Specht L: FDG-PET scan and treatment planning for early stage Hodgkin lymphoma. Radiother Oncol. 85(2):176-7, 2007
17. Coleman M et al: Early 18F-labeled fluoro-2-deoxy-D-glucose positron emission tomography scanning in the lymphomas: changing the paradigms of treatments? Cancer. 107(7):1425-8, 2006
18. Hutchings M et al: FDG-PET after two cycles of chemotherapy predicts treatment failure and progression-free survival in Hodgkin lymphoma. Blood. 107(1):52-9, 2006

HODGKIN LYMPHOMA

CT Findings: Primary

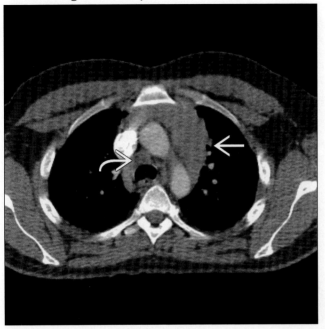
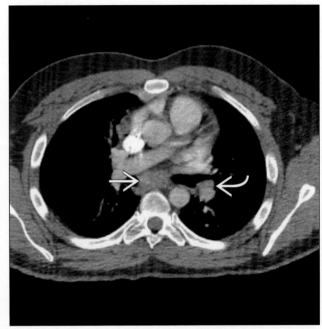

(Left) Axial CECT shows a soft tissue mass in the anterior mediastinum ➡ and a second focus of soft tissue in the pretracheal region ➡. (Right) Axial CECT shows subcarinal ➡ and left hilar adenopathy ➡.

CT Findings: Primary

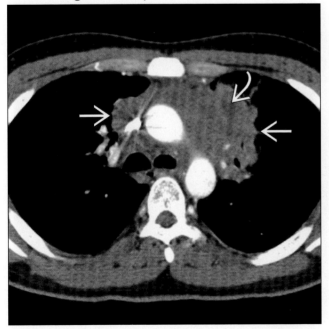
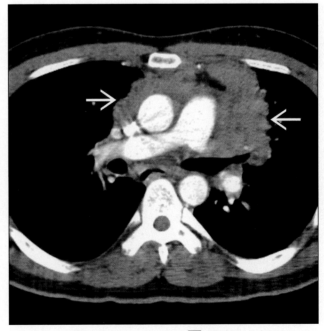

(Left) Axial CECT shows extensive mediastinal adenopathy ➡ with low attenuation, suggesting regions of necrosis ➡. (Right) Axial CECT shows extensive adenopathy presenting as a soft tissue mass ➡.

HODGKIN LYMPHOMA

PET/CT Findings: Staging

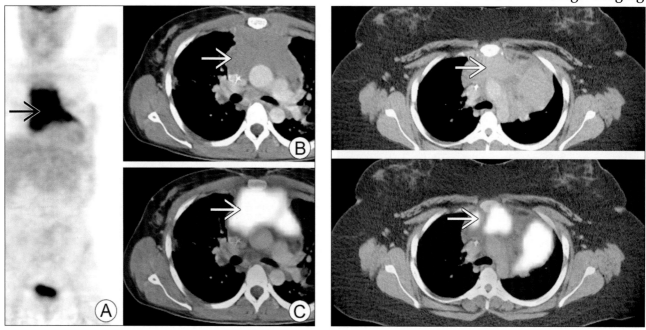

(Left) PET/CT study demonstrates intense FDG activity ➡ on the coronal PET (A) corresponding to a large anterior mediastinal mass ➡ on axial CT (B) and fused PET/CT (C). *(Right)* Axial CT (top) and fused PET/CT (bottom) demonstrate a large anterior mediastinal mass with intense FDG activity ➡, compatible with the patient's history of recently diagnosed Hodgkin lymphoma. The majority of Hodgkin lymphomas are FDG avid, and this is a typical representation.

PET/CT Findings: Staging

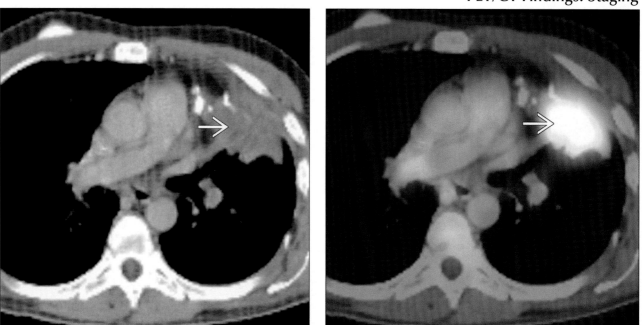

(Left) Axial CECT shows a mass in the superior lingula ➡ in this patient with recently diagnosed Hodgkin lymphoma. *(Right)* Axial fused PET/CT shows intense FDG activity in the superior segment lingular mass ➡, most compatible with Hodgkin lymphoma. Although this is atypical for Hodgkin lymphoma, approximately 10 to 20% of patients will have pulmonary involvement.

HODGKIN LYMPHOMA

PET/CT Findings: Staging

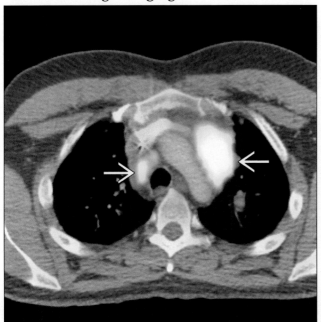 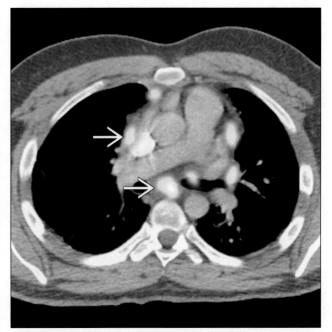

(Left) Axial fused PET/CT shows intense activity in the enlarged mediastinal nodes ➡ in this patient with documented Hodgkin lymphoma. *(Right)* Axial fused PET/CT of the same patient shows additional hypermetabolic mediastinal nodes ➡.

PET/CT Findings: Response to Therapy

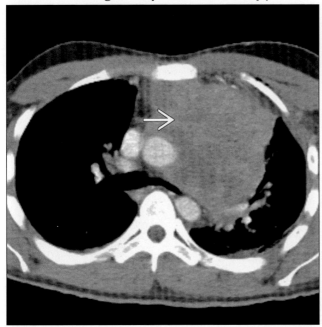 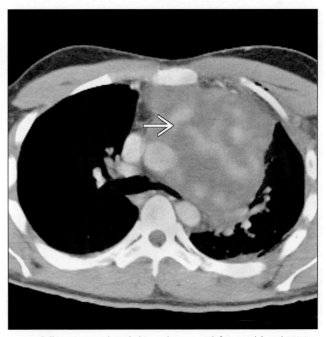

(Left) Axial CECT shows a large heterogeneous mediastinal mass ➡ that persists following 2 cycles of chemotherapy. *(Right)* Axial fused PET/CT of the same mediastinal lesion reveals mildly hypermetabolic activity within it ➡, compatible with persistent active disease.

HODGKIN LYMPHOMA

PET/CT Findings: Response to Therapy

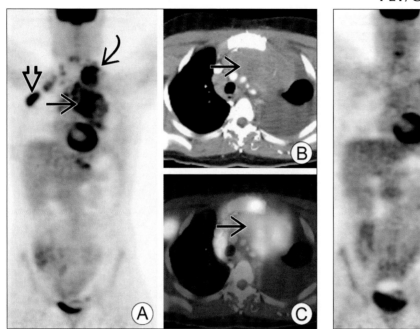

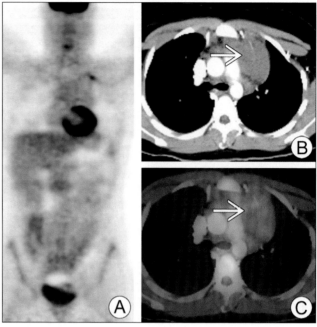

(Left) Multiple images (A, B, C) in a patient with Hodgkin lymphoma show FDG-avid masses in the anterior mediastinum ➡, left supraclavicular region ➡, and right axilla ➡. *(Right)* Multiple images (A, B, C) from a follow-up examination show complete response to therapy as evidenced by normalization of FDG activity in the anterior mediastinal mass ➡. Residual soft tissue in the early post-treatment period is common.

PET/CT Findings: Response to Therapy

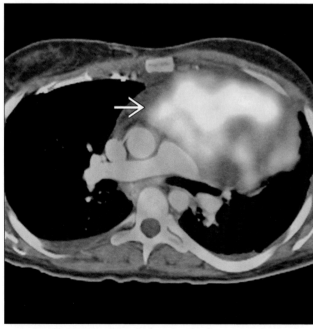

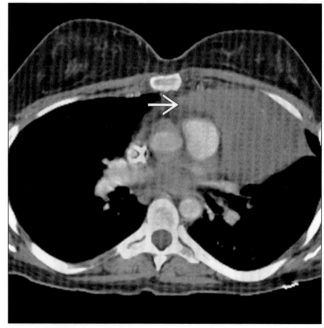

(Left) Axial fused PET/CT shows hypermetabolic activity within the mediastinal mass ➡ in this patient prior to the initiation of chemotherapy. *(Right)* Axial fused PET/CT shows almost no FDG activity within the residual mass ➡ in the same patient following treatment.

HODGKIN LYMPHOMA

PET/CT Findings: Response to Therapy

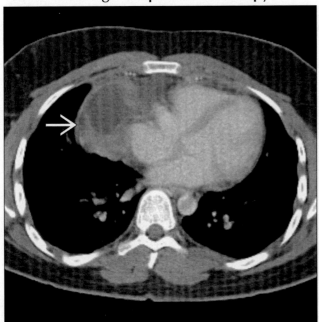 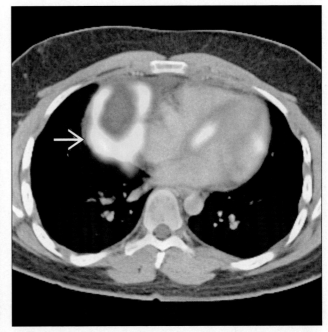

(Left) Axial CECT shows a necrotic mediastinal mass ➡. *(Right)* Axial fused PET/CT shows increased FDG activity within the nonnecrotic, peripheral aspect ➡ of the same mass.

PET/CT Findings: Response to Therapy

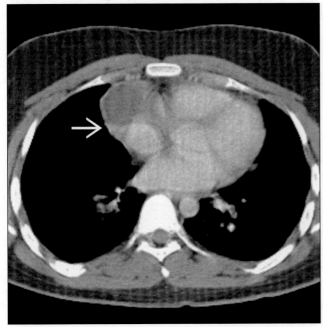 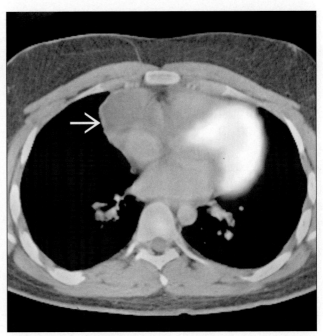

(Left) Axial CECT of the same patient shows some decrease in the size of the mediastinal mass ➡ after treatment. *(Right)* Axial fused PET/CT of the same lesion shows no increased FDG uptake ➡ following treatment.

HODGKIN LYMPHOMA

PET/CT Findings: Response to Therapy

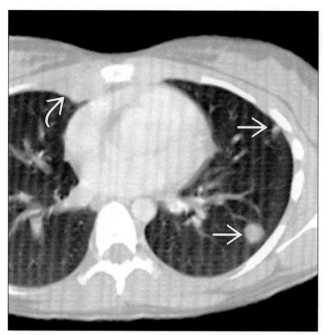
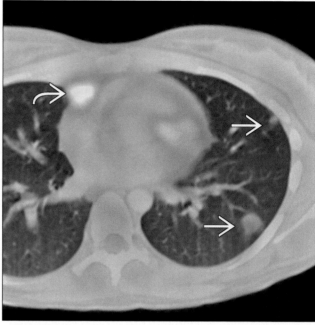

(Left) Axial NECT of a patient with Hodgkin lymphoma shows two pulmonary nodules in the left lower lobe and lingula, corresponding to pulmonary involvement ➡ and right internal mammary chain adenopathy ➡. *(Right)* Axial fused PET/CT of the same patient shows mildly increased FDG uptake in the nodules ➡ and marked FDG uptake in the internal mammary chain node ➡. Note that there is mild misregistration artifact.

PET/CT Findings: Response to Therapy

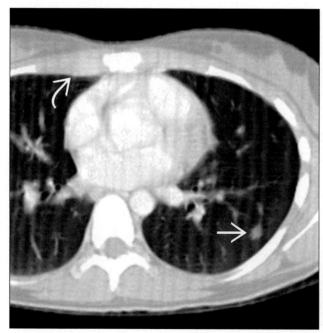
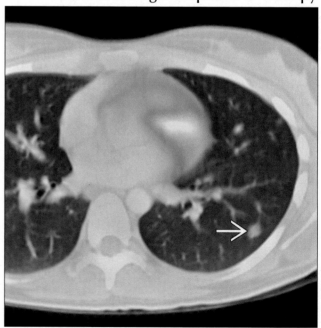

(Left) Axial NECT of the same patient shows the decreased size of the pulmonary nodules ➡ and adenopathy ➡ after treatment. *(Right)* Axial fused PET/CT shows no remaining increased FDG activity in the pulmonary lesion post therapy ➡, compatible with a complete response to therapy.

HODGKIN LYMPHOMA

PET/CT Findings: Response to Therapy

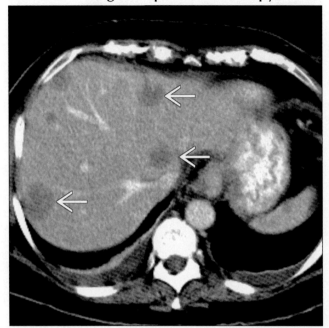 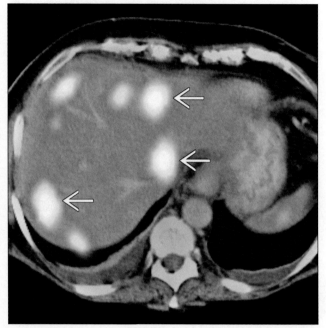

(Left) Axial CECT shows at least 5 hepatic lesions ➔ in a patient with known Hodgkin lymphoma. *(Right)* Axial fused PET/CT of the same patient shows increased FDG uptake ➔ in the hepatic lesions.

PET/CT Findings: Response to Therapy

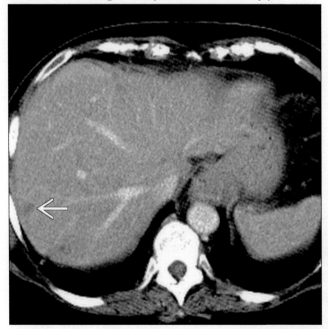 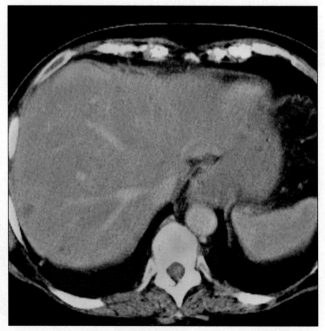

(Left) Axial CECT shows near complete resolution of the lymphomatous deposits in the liver ➔ following therapy. *(Right)* Axial fused PET/CT shows no residual increased focal FDG uptake above the background activity of the liver, compatible with a complete response to therapy.

NON-HODGKIN LYMPHOMA

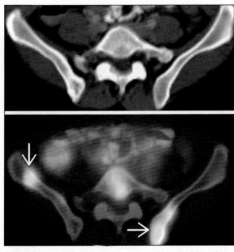

Although axial CT (top) shows no abnormalities, fused PET/CT (bottom) demonstrates multiple areas of osseous involvement ➡.

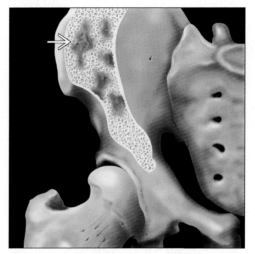

Graphic shows the infiltrative nature of lymphoma within the right iliac bone ➡.

TERMINOLOGY

Abbreviations and Synonyms
- Non-Hodgkin lymphoma (NHL)
- Large B-cell lymphoma
- Low grade follicular B-cell lymphoma (FL)
- Small lymphocytic lymphoma (SLL)
- Chronic lymphocytic leukemia (CLL)
- Marginal zone lymphoma (MZL)
- Mucosa-associated lymphoid tissue (MALT)
- Cutaneous T-cell lymphoma (CTCL)
- Post-transplant lymphoproliferative disease (PTLD)
- Hodgkin disease (HD)

Definitions
- **NHL**: Malignancy of B or T lymphocytes
- **Low grade lymphoma**
  - Slow growing, indolent non-Hodgkin lymphoma
  - Low grade diffuse B-cell lymphoma
    - SLL: Termed CLL when 1° in blood or marrow
    - Lymphoplasmacytic lymphoma (immunocytoma)
    - MZL: MALT; nodal marginal zone; splenic marginal zone
  - FL

- Small-cleaved cell type: < 20-25% large cells
- Mixed small-cleaved and large cell type: Survival inversely proportional to large cell percentage
- Large cell type: Intermediate grade but more aggressive in nature
  - CTCL: Mycosis fungoides (MF), Sézary syndrome (leukemic variant)
    - CTCL: Rarely transforms into more aggressive large cell lymphoma
    - Separate entity from aggressive peripheral T-cell lymphoma (PTL)
    - Also separate from adult T-cell lymphoma/ leukemia (ATLL)
- **Extranodal lymphomas**
  - Refer to lymphomas located in Waldeyer throat ring, thymus, and spleen

IMAGING FINDINGS

General Features
- Best diagnostic clue
  - Pre-therapy evaluation

DDx: FDG Avid Enlarged Nodes or Soft Tissue

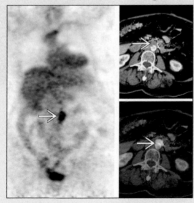

Retroperitoneal Fibrosis (Early)

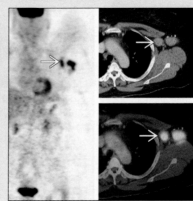

Reactive Lymph Nodes

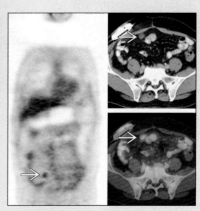

Metastatic Disease (Colon)

NON-HODGKIN LYMPHOMA

Key Facts

Terminology
- Non-Hodgkin lymphoma (NHL)
- NHL: Malignancy of B or T lymphocytes

Imaging Findings
- Spleen involved in 20% of patients with NHL
- Other extranodal lymphoma may arise in CNS, peripheral nervous system, lung and pleura, bone, skin, breast, testis, and GU tract
- PET/CT: Use with contrast-enhanced CT for staging
- Enlarged LN, extranodal mass with low to moderate FDG uptake
- Enlarged/normal-sized FDG-avid nodes in liver or spleen; "misty mesentery"
- PET excellent for predicting prognosis in aggressive NHL after therapy
- Post-therapy evaluation
  - Absence of metabolic activity on FDG PET following treatment (high predictive value for disease-free survival)
  - Persistent metabolic activity on FDG PET following treatment (moderate predictive value for recurrence)

Top Differential Diagnoses
- Normal Structures
- Reactive Lymph Node Hyperplasia
- Sarcoid
- Histoplasmosis
- Other Malignancy

Diagnostic Checklist
- Perform a baseline PET/CT in **all** patients with newly diagnosed NHL

- High grade NHL: Multiple enlarged lymph nodes or nodal groups with intense FDG activity ± splenic/other organ involvement
- Low grade NHL: Enlarged LN, extranodal mass with low to intense FDG uptake
- Marked FDG uptake may represent high grade transformation
- "Misty mesentery" also a common finding in NHL
- Occasionally normal-sized FDG-avid nodes
- PET/CT Post-therapy evaluation
  - Absence of metabolic activity on FDG PET following treatment (high predictive value for disease free survival)
  - Persistent metabolic activity on FDG PET following treatment (moderate predictive value for recurrence)
- Location
  - Superior mediastinal and paraaortic nodes common
  - NHL known for less predictable spread than HD
  - **Head and neck region**
    - Second most common site of NHL
    - Primary head and neck lymphoma accounts for 10-20% of all cases of NHL
    - Prone to be asymptomatic and unsuspected clinically
    - Usually presents on PET/CT as asymmetrical intense FDG activity in a lymphoid structure
    - Common locations: Palatine, lingual, sublingual tonsils, and adenoids
  - **Pulmonary**
    - Pulmonary involvement uncommon
    - Involvement without nodal disease seen more commonly in recurrent disease than at presentation
    - Also seen more commonly in PTLD
  - **Bone marrow**
    - PET/CT can help direct bone marrow biopsy to most metabolically active areas
    - Frequently have abnormal focal FDG activity without a correlative CT abnormality
    - Involvement found in 50-80% of low grade NHL and 25-40% of high grade NHL

- Tends to signify advanced stage disease
  - **Spleen**
    - Involved in 20% of patients with NHL
    - Defined as nodal in HD, extranodal in NHL
    - Organ size is poor predictor; spleen can be large but not involved or normal with infiltration
    - PET/CT significantly more accurate than CT alone for detecting splenic involvement
    - May appear as multiple lesions or diffuse involvement on FDG PET
  - **Other extranodal lymphoma**
    - CNS, peripheral nervous system, lung and pleura, bone, skin, breast, testis, and GU tract
    - GI lymphoma represents approximately 10-15% of all NHL
- Size
  - Most patients being evaluated for new onset lymphoma will have enlarged nodes
  - PET/CT will often detect additional normal-sized but malignant nodes
  - Lymph node size is a poor predictor of tumor involvement

Imaging Recommendations
- Best imaging tool
  - **PET/CT**
    - Preferred modality for staging NHL
    - Sensitivity/specificity for evaluating malignant nodes: PET/CT 91%, 90% vs. CT 88%, 86%
    - Sensitivity/specificity for extranodal involvement: PET/CT 88%, 100% vs. CT 50%, 90%
  - **Current and potential clinical applications of FDG PET/CT**
    - Initial diagnosis: Evaluate adenopathy ± systemic symptoms without current pathologic diagnosis of NHL
    - Determine staging
    - Guide biopsy
    - Assess conversion to higher grade
    - Evaluate early response to chemotherapy
    - Determine restaging
    - Monitor post-treatment progress

NON-HODGKIN LYMPHOMA

- o Conventional imaging staging technique
  - CECT of neck, chest, abdomen, pelvis; occasionally MR
  - Uni- or bilateral bone marrow biopsy
- Protocol advice
  - o Consider PET/CT with contrast-enhanced CT for staging
  - o Stage with PET/CT before any therapy is administered
    - One dose of chemotherapy may ↓ FDG uptake
  - o Consider low dose CT for restaging/surveillance after a negative PET/CT following therapy

CT Findings

- NECT
  - o Enlarged lymph nodes
  - o Can be large conglomerate masses with lobulated margins
  - o Calcification rarely seen prior to treatment; frequently seen after therapy in larger confluent nodal masses
  - o Size is not an independent predictive factor
- CECT
  - o Slight to moderate uniform enhancement following IV contrast
  - o Marked enhancement unusual (low attenuation in 20% of cases)
  - o Masses from lymphoma more likely to encase and displace the mediastinal structures
    - Unusual to constrict or invade them
  - o Lung/Mediastinum
    - Intrathoracic involvement in 50% of newly diagnosed cases (vs. 85% in HD)
    - 20% present with mediastinal adenopathy
    - Single or multiple discrete pulmonary nodules less well-defined and less dense than carcinoma
    - May cavitate (10-20%)
    - Consolidation with air bronchograms (solitary or multiple, includes pseudolymphoma)
    - Diffuse reticulonodular opacities (lymphocytic interstitial pneumonia)
    - Post-obstructive atelectasis due to nodal compression
  - o Pleura
    - Pleural effusions seen in 10% of patients at presentation, due to lymphatic or venous obstruction
    - Effusion, may resolve with irradiation of mediastinal lymph nodes
    - Pleural masses rare
  - o Pericardial
    - Pericardial effusion mostly coexists with adenopathy adjacent to pericardial margins
    - Associated with high grade peripheral T lymphoma, large B-cell lymphoma, and PTLD
  - o Chest wall
    - Invasion with rib destruction uncommon

Nuclear Medicine Findings

- Initial diagnosis
  - o PET/CT used to evaluate enlarged nodes in patients without a history of lymphoma

- Covered indication by CMS, but rarely used for initial diagnosis
- o Some NHL may not be FDG avid
  - MALT generally less FDG avid, but as a group MALTs have complex histology and may demonstrate uptake
- o PET for differentiation of indolent vs. aggressive lymphoma
  - Controversial topic
  - SUV ≥ 10 confers higher likelihood for aggressive disease (considerable overlap exists)
- Staging
  - o PET/CT more sensitive than CT for staging NHL
    - Consider baseline PET/CT for all patients with newly diagnosed NHL
    - Consider directed bone marrow biopsy to most metabolically active osseous structures detected on PET
  - o Splenic involvement much more accurately assessed with PET/CT than with CT alone
  - o Liver involvement may present as diffuse disease with patchy infiltrates originating in portal areas
    - Other patterns include miliary with multiple small lesions or, rarely, large focal lesions
  - o False negative bone marrow biopsy may result due to patchy nondisseminated marrow involvement
    - Bone marrow biopsy (BMB) alone can detect minimal bone marrow disease, which may escape detection by PET
  - o PET/CT shown to modify radiotherapy planning in 44% of patents with head/neck lymphoma
  - o CLL/SLL: PET of limited use in staging 2° ↓ FDG uptake (sensitivity 58%)
    - SUV > 3.5 suggests Richter transformation of CLL/SLL → diffuse large B-cell lymphoma (sensitivity 91%, specificity 80%, PPV 53%, NPV 97%)
  - o MZL: FDG PET staging sensitivity 71% (lower for extranodal)
    - MALT lymphoma: Typically no or low FDG uptake; SUV > 3.5 suggests plasmacytic differentiation
  - o CTCL: FDG PET useful in staging, especially in suspected single cutaneous site
    - CTCL: Intense nodal sites suspicious for large cell transformation
  - o FL: FDG PET useful in staging all grades (sensitivity 94%, specificity 100%)
    - Wide overlap between FDG uptake by lower (SUV 2.3-13) and higher grade (SUV 3.2-43) FL
    - Emergence of sites of ↑ FDG uptake (SUV > 10): Transformation to higher grade (specificity 81%)
  - o Upstaging of extranodal disease observed mostly in stage I and II disease
- Response to therapy
  - o FDG PET demonstrates poor sensitivity for predicting likelihood of response/progression in patients with indolent lymphoma
  - o PET excellent for predicting prognosis in aggressive NHL after therapy
    - Usefulness of follow-up scan hinges on existence of pre-therapy scan indicating FDG-avid disease

NON-HODGKIN LYMPHOMA

- Early identification of therapy response allows modification of ineffective treatment
- Nonresponders may avoid unnecessary side effects
- Tumor FDG uptake decreases dramatically as early as first week post-treatment in aggressive NHL
- Strong predictive value for 18 month outcome when imaged early in chemotherapy cycle, after only one cycle
- FDG PET in early response assessment (after 1-4 cycles): Sensitivity 79%, specificity 92%, PPV 90%, NPV 81%, accuracy 85%
- FDG PET in post-Rx assessment (mixed population HD, NHL): Sensitivity 79%, specificity 94%, PPV 82%, NPV 93%, accuracy 91%
- FDG PET in post-Rx assessment NHL: Sensitivity 67%, specificity 100%, PPV 100%, NPV 83%, accuracy 88%
- FDG PET in post reinduction chemo (before stem cell transplant): Sensitivity 84%, specificity 83%, PPV 84%, NPV 83%, accuracy 84%
  - 1999 European Organization for Research
    - Post-therapy SUV that increases 25% over baseline indicates progressive disease
    - SUV decrease of 15-25% after cycle 1 of chemotherapy and 25% after more than 1 cycle indicates partial metabolic response
  - Ga-67-citrate less sensitive and specific than FDG PET for aggressive lymphomas
  - Chemotherapy can cause marrow hyperplasia and also generalized FDG uptake
  - G-CSF and recombinant erythropoietin can result in diffusely increased FDG uptake bone marrow and spleen, limiting sensitivity
    - Uptake due to growth factors usually returns to baseline by one month post-therapy
- **Restaging**
  - Rationale for FDG PET imaging post-therapy
    - Allow for treatment of residual/progressive disease before it spreads further
  - PET can be positive months before histological confirmation of an asymptomatic relapse
    - Especially for diffuse large B-cell lymphoma patients
- **Benign FDG uptake patterns directly/indirectly associated with chemotherapy**
  - Low level, patchy uptake in residual fibrotic mass and scars
    - Decreases over months but may persist
    - Diffuse FDG uptake in all adipose tissue (brown + yellow fat), adrenal/periadrenal regions
  - Concurrent chemo + protease inhibitors (lymphoma + HIV)
    - Skeletal muscle uptake
    - Pattern similar to carbohydrate-insulin effect
  - Granulocyte colony stimulating factor (G-CSF) or other marrow stimulant drugs
    - Intense red bone marrow + splenic uptake/enlargement
    - May persist 2-3 months
  - Following cessation of chemotherapy

- Increased thymic uptake (thymic rebound); diffuse FDG activity in thymus usually 4-8 months following chemotherapy

DIFFERENTIAL DIAGNOSIS

Normal Structures
- Thymus, salivary glands, muscle, tonsils
- Look for symmetry
- Can be asymmetrical if contralateral normal structure paralyzed (vocal cord) or surgically removed (muscle, glands)
- Correlate with anatomical findings for confirmation of structure

Reactive Lymph Node Hyperplasia
- Typically ↑ FDG uptake
- Numerous sites, often symmetrical
- LN mildly to moderately enlarged
- May resolve over weeks to months
- When equivocal, short term follow-up exam is usually helpful

Granulomatous Disease
- FDG uptake moderate to marked
- Stable over time
- Often symmetrical hilar/mediastinal LN

Sarcoid
- Lung nodules: Sarcoid "galaxy" sign; multitude of tiny clustered lung nodules along bronchovascular bundle
- Garland triad (1-2-3 sign): Symmetrically enlarged bilateral hilar & right paratracheal LN
- Enlarged anterior mediastinal LN favors lymphoma

Viral Infections; Infectious Mononucleosis
- Minimally enlarged LN
- Sub-cm lung nodules that usually resolve completely

Histoplasmosis
- Sub-cm lung nodules that often calcify (granuloma)
- Calcified normal-sized mildly FDG-avid mediastinal & hilar LN, calcified splenic & hepatic granulomas

Tuberculosis (TB)
- Enlarged LN & ipsilateral consolidation in primary TB
- Lung nodules may calcify, apical scarring, positive PPD
- Cavitary lung lesion in the posterior segment right upper lobe or superior segment of the lower lobes

Cat-Scratch Fever
- Enlarged, painful LN
- Symptoms resolve over weeks

Whipple Disease
- Enlarged abdominal LN with low attenuation center

HIV, AIDS
- Enlarged LN in HIV
  - Reactive follicular hyperplasia (50%)
  - AIDS-related lymphoma (20%)
  - Mycobacterial infection (17%)
  - Kaposi sarcoma (10%)
  - Opportunistic infection (multiple pathogens)

2

NON-HODGKIN LYMPHOMA

o Metastases
o Drug reaction

Higher Grade Lymphomas on Therapy
- May show ↓ FDG uptake, mimicking low grade lymphoma

Other Malignancy
- FDG PET may identify best candidate site for biopsy

Thoracic, Extrathoracic Malignancy
- Enlarged FDG-avid LN accompanied by multiple FDG-avid lung nodules that increase in size and number over time

Small Cell Lung Carcinoma
- Markedly enlarged, prominently FDG-avid hilar and mediastinal LN

PATHOLOGY

General Features
- General path comments
  o Most common subtype in adults is diffuse large B-cell lymphoma
    - Most aggressive subtype with 60% of patients having disseminated disease at diagnosis
  o **More aggressive types**
    - Diffuse large B-cell
    - Mantle cell
    - Peripheral T-cell
  o **Fast-growing types**
    - Burkitt lymphoma
    - Lymphoblastic
  o **Slow-growing types**
    - Marginal zone
    - Small cell (= CLL when principally in lymph nodes)
    - Lymphoplasmacytic
    - Follicular
  o **Extranodal marginal zone lymphomas**
    - GI tract, lung, salivary gland, conjunctiva, and thyroid
    - Diagnosed as separate entity termed MALT
- Etiology
  o Unknown in most patients
  o MALT lymphoma (stomach) associated with H. pylori infection
  o Lymphoplasmacytic lymphoma: 1/3 associated with hepatitis C infection
  o Hashimoto thyroiditis associated with primary thyroid lymphoma
- Epidemiology
  o NHL incidence ↑ 75% in the past 20 years, with ↑ mortality
  o Primary NHL of thyroid unusual, only 3.4% of primary thyroid malignancies
  o Malignant lymphomas as a group compose 5th most frequently occurring type of cancer in the USA
  o **Most common NHL subtypes**
    - Diffuse large B-cell lymphoma, 31%
    - Follicular lymphoma, 22%
    - Small lymphocytic lymphoma, 16%
    - Mantle cell lymphoma, 6%
    - Peripheral T-cell lymphoma, 2%
    - Anaplastic large T-cell/null cell lymphoma, 2%
    - Burkitt-like lymphoma, 2%
    - Marginal zone nodal-type lymphoma, 1%
    - Lymphoplasmacytic lymphoma, 1%
    - Burkitt lymphoma, < 1%

Microscopic Features
- T- or B-cell clonality: No Reed-Sternberg cells
- Fine-needle aspiration is diagnostic in NHL
- FL: Aggressiveness proportionate to percentage of large cells

Staging, Grading, or Classification Criteria
- Histologic grading more important than staging of anatomic sites in NHL
- **Clinical staging**
  o Includes history & physical examination
  o Imaging of the chest, abdomen, & pelvis
  o Blood count, chemistry, and bone marrow biopsy
- **Pathologic staging**
  o Staging laparotomy & pathologic staging no longer routinely performed
- **REAL/WHO classification**
  o Revised European-American Classification of Lymphoid Neoplasms (REAL), adopted by World Health Organization (WHO)
  o Distinct disease entities defined by combination of morphology, immunophenotype & genetic features, and distinct clinical features
  o Relative importance of features varies by disease; no "gold standard"
  o Includes all lymphoid neoplasms: HD, NHL, lymphoid leukemias, & plasma cell neoplasms
  o Lymphomas & lymphoid leukemias included because solid + circulating phases are present in many lymphoid neoplasms
- **REAL/WHO classification of B-cell neoplasms**
  o Precursor B-cell neoplasm: Precursor B-lymphoblastic leukemia/lymphoma (precursor B-cell acute lymphoblastic leukemia)
  o Mature (peripheral) B-cell neoplasms
    - B-cell CLL/SLL; B-cell prolymphocytic leukemia
    - Lymphoplasmacytic lymphoma; splenic marginal zone B-cell lymphoma
    - Hairy cell leukemia; plasma cell myeloma/plasmacytoma
    - Marginal zone B-cell/MALT lymphoma
    - Nodal marginal zone B-cell lymphoma; follicular lymphoma; mantle cell lymphoma
    - Diffuse large B-cell lymphoma; Burkitt lymphoma/Burkitt cell leukemia
- **REAL/WHO classification of T-cell and natural killer (NK)-cell neoplasms**
  o Account for 10-15% of NHL
  o Precursor T-cell neoplasm: Precursor T-lymphoblastic lymphoma/leukemia (precursor T-cell ALL)
  o Mature (peripheral) T-/NK-cell neoplasms
    - T-cell prolymphocytic leukemia; T-cell granular lymphocytic leukemia; aggressive NK-cell leukemia

NON-HODGKIN LYMPHOMA

- Adult T-cell lymphoma/leukemia (HTLV1+); extranodal NK-/T-cell lymphoma, nasal type
- Enteropathy-type T-cell lymphoma; hepatosplenic T-cell lymphoma; subcutaneous panniculitis-like T-cell lymphoma
- Mycosis fungoides/Sézary syndrome; anaplastic large cell lymphoma, T/null cell, primary cutaneous type
- Peripheral T-cell lymphoma, not otherwise characterized; angioimmunoblastic T-cell lymphoma
- Anaplastic large cell lymphoma, T/null cell, primary systemic type
- **Ann Arbor classification**
  - Anatomic extent of disease in HD & NHL
  - **Stage I**
    - Single LN region (I)
    - Or localized involvement of a single extralymphatic site in the absence of LN involvement (IE) (rare in HD)
  - **Stage II**
    - ≥ 2 LN regions, same side of diaphragm (II); or single extralymphatic site with regional LN
    - ± Other LN stations, same side of diaphragm (IIE)
  - **Stage III**
    - LN regions, both sides of diaphragm (III)
    - May have extralymphatic extension with adjacent LNs (IIIE) or + spleen (IIIS) or both (IIIE, S)
  - **Stage IV**
    - Diffuse or disseminated disease in ≥ 1 extralymphatic organ
    - ± LN; or isolated extralymphatic organ with or without regional LN
    - Any liver, bone marrow, lung nodules
  - Presence or absence of systemic symptoms
    - A = asymptomatic, B = B-symptoms
- **International Prognostic Index (IPI)**
  - NHL prognostic factors of the International Prognostic Index used for Rx decisions along with histologic cell type
  - Additional factors reported to affect outcomes in preliminary studies include tumor β-2 microglobulin & S-phase fraction
  - Independent statistically significant pre-treatment risk factors
    - Age (60 vs. > 60 years)
    - Ann Arbor stage III or IV (advanced)
    - Serum LDH (normal vs. abnormal)
    - Reduced performance status (0 or 1 vs. > 2)
    - Extranodal sites of disease (1 vs. > 1)
  - Patients are assigned to 1 of 4 risk groups on the basis of presenting risk factors
    - Low (0 or 1); low intermediate (2); high intermediate (3); high (4, 5)
  - **Outcomes**
    - Low risk
    - 87% complete response
    - 73% 5 year survival in low risk patients
    - High risk
    - 44% complete response

CLINICAL ISSUES

Presentation
- Most common signs/symptoms
  - Asymptomatic
  - Loss of appetite
  - Fatigue
  - Enlarged LN
  - Flu-like symptoms
- Other signs/symptoms
  - Pruritus
  - Painful LN after drinking alcohol
  - Cough
  - **B-symptoms**
    - Unexplained persistent fever & chills, night sweats, fatigue, pruritus, weight loss
    - More common in aggressive (47%) than indolent lymphoma (25%)
    - Concern for progression to intermediate/high grade lymphoma with development of B-symptoms
  - Enlarged LN may be painful for hours after a person consumes large amounts of alcohol
  - Enlarging LN may narrow airways (cough, discomfort, stridor) or vessels (SVC syndrome)
  - Lymphoplasmacytic lymphoma: Hyperviscosity syndromes 2° IgM secretion (Waldenstrom macroglobulinemia)
  - **Cutaneous T-cell lymphoma spectrum**
    - Small raised red patches
    - Plaques, bumps, ulcers
    - Involvement of large areas of skin
    - Entire skin red, peeling (l'homme rouge)
    - LN, bone marrow (Sézary syndrome)

Demographics
- Age
  - Median age 55 years
  - Initial diagnosis usually > 50 years
  - > 90% NHL occurs in adults
  - Risk increases with age
- Gender: M:F = 1.4:1

Natural History & Prognosis
- Prognosis depends on histologic type, stage, and treatment
- Overall 5 year survival is ~ 50% to 60% with modern Rx
- 5 year survival with large B-cell lymphoma: 44%
- Vast majority of relapses occur in first 2 years after therapy
- **Two prognostic groups: Indolent and aggressive**
  - Indolent NHL: Relatively good prognosis, median survival up to 10 years, but usually not curable
  - Aggressive: 30% to 60% can be cured
  - Risk of late relapse > in patients with a divergent histology of both indolent and aggressive disease
- **Indolent lymphomas**
  - 20-45% of all lymphomas
  - Median survival ≥ 5 years
  - Treatment often deferred until morbidity occurs

NON-HODGKIN LYMPHOMA

○ Combination chemotherapy usually results in complete or partial response: Relapse rate 10-15%/year
- **Low grade lymphomas (Kiel/Lennert)**
  ○ Follicular small cleaved cell (22.5%): Median age 54 years, 70% 5 year survival
  ○ Follicular mixed (7.7%): Median age 56 years, 50% 5 year survival
  ○ Small lymphocytic (3.6%): Median age 61 years, 59% 5 year survival
- SLL/CLL
  ○ Median survival: 10 years
  ○ 30% progress to higher grade process, such as diffuse large cell lymphoma (Richter transformation) or prolymphocytic lymphoma
- MALT lymphoma: Plasmacytic differentiation to more aggressive diffuse large B-cell lymphoma
- Follicular lymphomas: Survival inversely proportionate to percentage of large cells

Treatment

- No standard approach to treatment of indolent lymphoma
- Can treat early indolent NHL (stage I, II) with deep X-ray therapy (XRT) alone
  ○ Extended (regional) radiation therapy to cover adjacent LN prophylactically may be curative in stage I or II
- Watchful waiting
  ○ Indolent lymphomas may be followed with no treatment until B-symptoms manifest
- Tailored therapy: Monoclonal autoantibodies ± radioligand (follicular lymphoma)
  ○ Monoclonal autoantibody therapy for FL ± chemotherapy; radioimmunotherapy (e.g., ibritumomab tiuxetan (Zevalin) or tositumomab and I-131 (Bexxar))
- Aggressive NHL has a shorter natural history
  ○ But significant number of patients can be cured with intensive combination chemotherapy
- Systemic chemotherapy
  ○ Stem cell transplant allows for higher dose chemotherapy
- Chemotherapy + XRT
- Investigational therapies
  ○ Combinations of antibodies ± radioimmunotherapy; vaccine therapy of FL; immune modulating therapy
- Cutaneous T-cell lymphomas
  ○ Topical chemotherapy, UV light for early (limited) stage
- Conventional chemotherapy regimens today give less than 50% prolonged disease-free survival rates for NHL

DIAGNOSTIC CHECKLIST

Consider

- Perform a baseline PET/CT in **all** patients with newly diagnosed NHL
- Good evidence to use FDG PET to evaluate response to therapy in aggressive NHL

Image Interpretation Pearls

- Staging FDG PET must be done prior to initiation of any therapy, as even one dose of chemotherapy may decrease sensitivity
- PET/CT: Intense uptake should suggest higher grade transformation and identify site to biopsy
- Proper localization of brown fat particularly important in areas like upper abdomen

SELECTED REFERENCES

1. Cheson BD: New staging and response criteria for non-hodgkin lymphoma and hodgkin lymphoma. Radiol Clin North Am. 46(2):213-23, 2008
2. Geus-Oei LF et al: Predictive and prognostic value of FDG-PET. Cancer Imaging. 8:70-80, 2008
3. Hampson FA et al: Response assessment in lymphoma. Clin Radiol. 63(2):125-35, 2008
4. Schöder H et al: PET Imaging for Response Assessment in Lymphoma: Potential and Limitations. Radiol Clin North Am. 46(2):225-41, 2008
5. Terasawa T et al: 18F-FDG PET for posttherapy assessment of Hodgkin's disease and aggressive Non-Hodgkin's lymphoma: a systematic review. J Nucl Med. 49(1):13-21, 2008
6. Ulaner GA et al: B-cell non-Hodgkin lymphoma: PET/CT evaluation after 90Y-ibritumomab tiuxetan radioimmunotherapy--initial experience. Radiology. 246(3):895-902, 2008
7. Wirth A et al: Impact of [18f] fluorodeoxyglucose positron emission tomography on staging and management of early-stage follicular non-hodgkin lymphoma. Int J Radiat Oncol Biol Phys. 71(1):213-9, 2008
8. Baudard M et al: Importance of [18F]fluorodeoxyglucose-positron emission tomography scanning for the monitoring of responses to immunotherapy in follicular lymphoma. Leuk Lymphoma. 48(2):381-8, 2007
9. Bishu S et al: F-18-fluoro-deoxy-glucose positron emission tomography in the assessment of peripheral T-cell lymphomas. Leuk Lymphoma. 48(8):1531-8, 2007
10. Bishu S et al: Predictive value and diagnostic accuracy of F-18-fluoro-deoxy-glucose positron emission tomography treated grade 1 and 2 follicular lymphoma. Leuk Lymphoma. 48(8):1548-55, 2007
11. Brepoels L et al: PET and PET/CT for response evaluation in lymphoma: current practice and developments. Leuk Lymphoma. 48(2):270-82, 2007
12. Cheson BD et al: Revised response criteria for malignant lymphoma. J Clin Oncol. 25(5):579-86, 2007
13. Lin C et al: Early 18F-FDG PET for prediction of prognosis in patients with diffuse large B-cell lymphoma: SUV-based assessment versus visual analysis. J Nucl Med. 48(10):1626-32, 2007
14. MacManus MP et al: Overview of early response assessment in lymphoma with FDG-PET. Cancer Imaging. 7:10-8, 2007
15. Weber WA: 18F-FDG PET in non-Hodgkin's lymphoma: qualitative or quantitative? J Nucl Med. 48(10):1580-2, 2007
16. Alinari L et al: 18F-FDG PET in mucosa-associated lymphoid tissue (MALT) lymphoma. Leuk Lymphoma. 47(10):2096-101, 2006
17. Kostakoglu L et al: FDG-PET after 1 cycle of therapy predicts outcome in diffuse large cell lymphoma and classic Hodgkin disease. Cancer. 107(11):2678-87, 2006

NON-HODGKIN LYMPHOMA

PET/CT: Staging

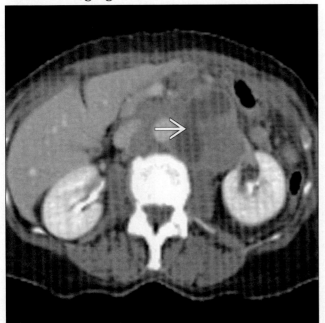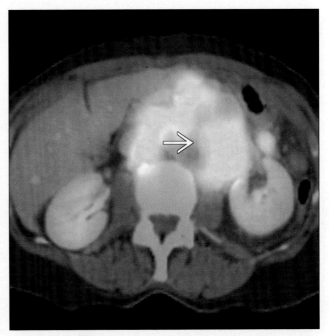

(Left) Axial CECT shows confluent mesenteric and retroperitoneal soft tissue involvement ➡ in this patient recently diagnosed with diffuse large B-cell lymphoma. *(Right)* Axial fused PET/CT shows intense increased FDG activity throughout the confluent adenopathy ➡. CT (not shown) revealed no definite evidence for disease above the diaphragm.

PET/CT: Staging

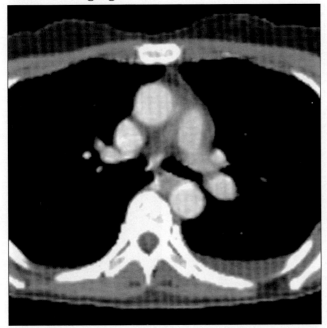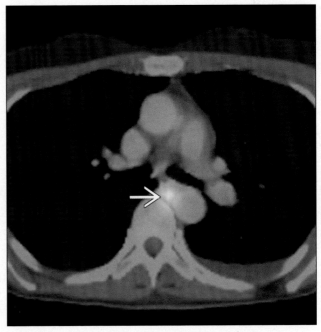

(Left) Axial CECT shows no definite abnormality. *(Right)* Axial fused PET/CT shows focal intense FDG activity in the paraspinal area corresponding to a small normal-sized lymph nodes ➡, compatible with active disease. The presence of a single lymph node above the diaphragm changes the stage of disease, although not the initial therapy of this patient.

NON-HODGKIN LYMPHOMA

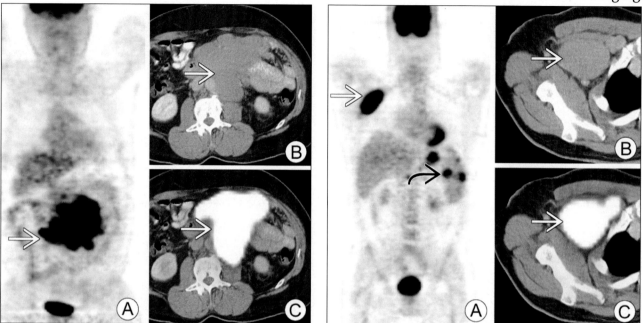

(Left) Coronal PET (A), axial CT (B) and fused PET/CT (C) from a restaging PET/CT examination show extensive mesenteric confluent adenopathy with intense FDG activity ➡, compatible with active lymphoma. *(Right)* Coronal PET (A), axial CT (B) and fused PET/CT (C) from a staging PET/CT examination show bulky right axillary lymph nodes with intense metabolic activity ➡ in addition to multifocal splenic involvement ➡.

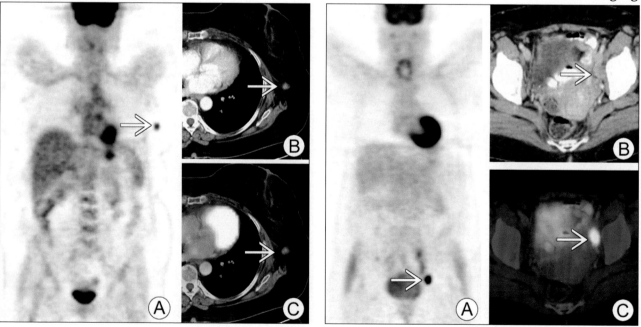

(Left) Coronal PET (A), axial CT (B)and fused PET/CT (C) from a staging PET/CT examination in a patient with primary disease below the diaphragm show a single normal-sized left axillary lymph node with intense FDG activity ➡, raising the initial stage of the patient's disease. *(Right)* Coronal PET (A), axial CT (B) and fused PET/CT (C) show a left external iliac hypermetabolic lymph node ➡ in this patient with newly diagnosed lymphoma with primary disease above the diaphragm.

NON-HODGKIN LYMPHOMA

PET/CT: Staging

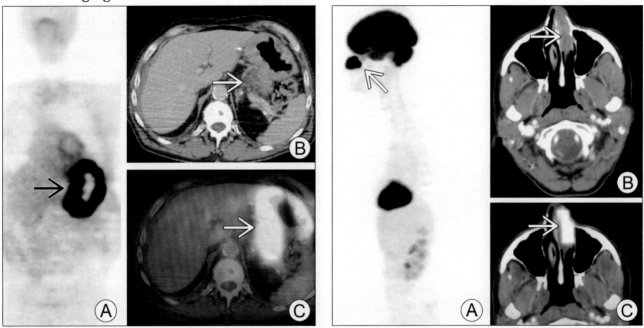

(Left) A staging PET/CT examination, in a patient with newly diagnosed gastric lymphoma, demonstrates circumferential intense gastric mucosal activity on coronal PET (A) ➡, which correlates with diffuse gastric wall thickening ➡ on axial CT (B) and fused PET/CT (C). *(Right)* Sagittal PET (A), axial CT (B) and fused PET/CT (C) from a PET/CT staging examination show an intranasal hypermetabolic mass ➡, compatible with the patient's history of recently diagnosed lymphoma.

PET/CT: Staging

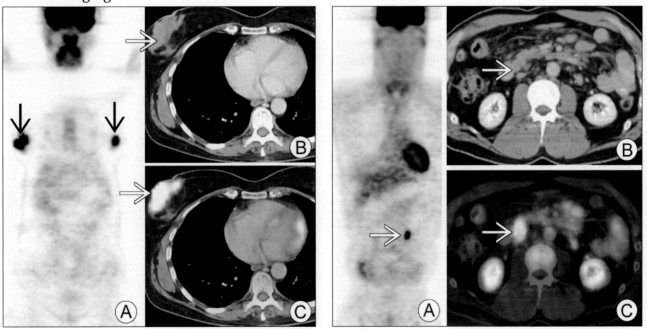

(Left) Coronal PET (A) demonstrates bilateral focal intense activity ➡ shown to be within the breast on axial CT (B) and fused PET/CT (C) ➡, compatible with bilateral breast carcinoma in this young patient who was BRCA positive. *(Right)* Coronal PET (A), axial CT (B) and fused PET/CT (C) show a focal area of intense activity corresponding to an approximately 1 cm retroperitoneal lymph node ➡.

NON-HODGKIN LYMPHOMA

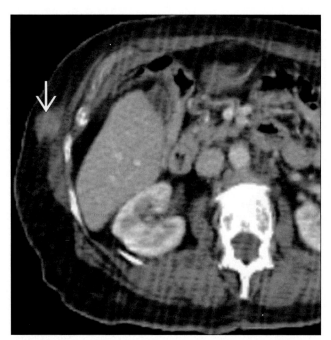 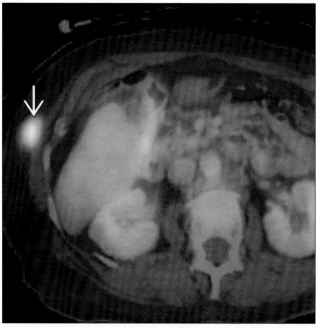

(Left) Axial CECT shows a subcutaneous soft tissue lesion in the adipose tissue of the right lateral abdominal wall ➡ in this patient with a history of non-Hodgkin lymphoma. *(Right)* Axial fused PET/CT shows focal intense FDG activity correlating with the subcutaneous lesion ➡, compatible with active lymphoma.

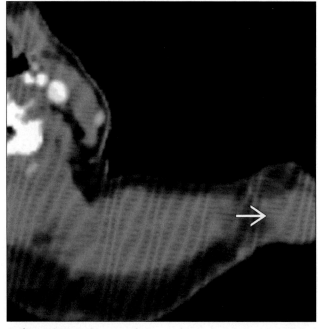 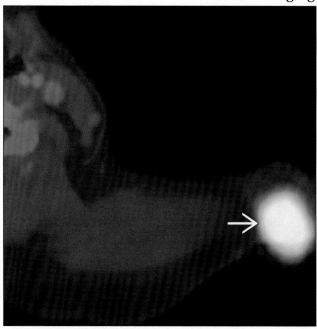

(Left) Axial CECT shows a soft tissue subcutaneous lesion around the left shoulder ➡ in this patient with a history of lymphoma. *(Right)* Axial fused PET/CT shows intense FDG activity ➡ correlating with the lesion in the left shoulder, compatible with active lymphoma.

NON-HODGKIN LYMPHOMA

PET/CT: Staging

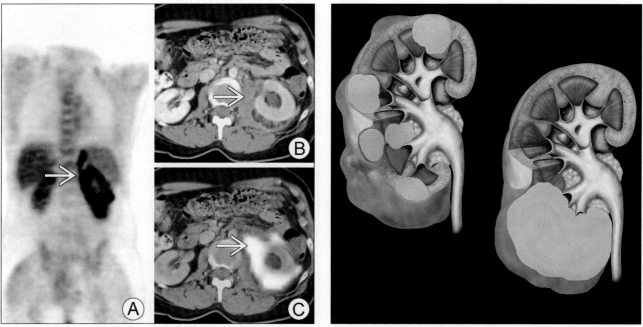

(Left) Coronal PET (A), axial CT (B) and fused PET/CT (C), in this patient recently diagnosed with renal lymphoma, demonstrate extensive perirenal nodular infiltration with intense FDG activity ➡, compatible with malignancy. *(Right)* Graphic shows examples of renal lymphoma as multiple masses (left) and one large mass (right).

PET/CT: Staging

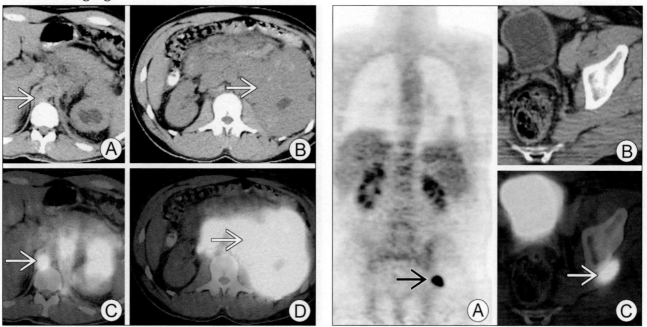

(Left) Axial CT (A, B) and fused PET/CT (C, D) of a patient newly diagnosed with primary renal lymphoma show extensive confluent soft tissue involvement in the perirenal space and extending into the retroperitoneal area ➡. *(Right)* Coronal PET image (A) demonstrates a focal abnormality in the left hemipelvis ➡ that is difficult to localize. Although no definite abnormality is seen on CECT (B), the axial fused PET/CT image (C) shows an intramuscular metastatic lesion ➡.

NON-HODGKIN LYMPHOMA

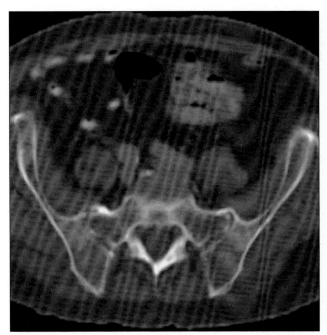 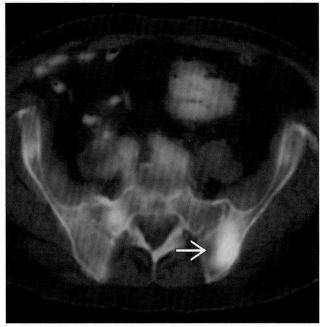

(Left) Axial CECT shows no definite abnormality on the staging PET/CT examination. *(Right)* Axial fused PET/CT shows asymmetrical focal intense activity in the left iliac bone ➡, compatible with lymphoma. The information from the fused PET/CT image can be used to direct a bone marrow biopsy.

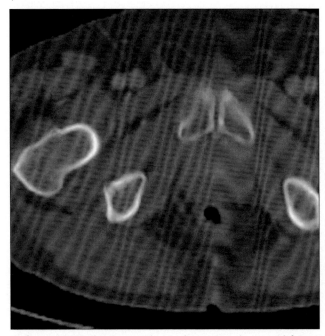 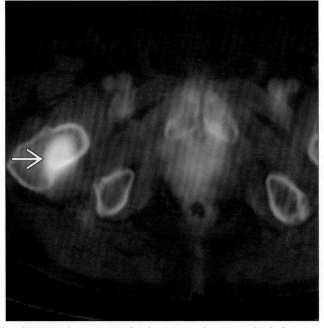

(Left) Axial CECT shows no evidence of metastatic disease. *(Right)* Axial fused PET/CT shows intense focal activity in the proximal right femur ➡, compatible with osseous involvement of non-Hodgkin lymphoma.

NON-HODGKIN LYMPHOMA

PET/CT: Staging

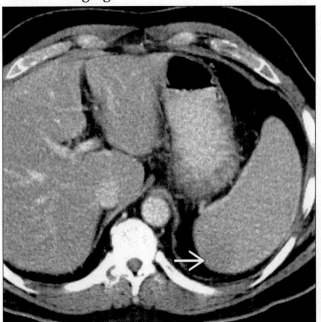 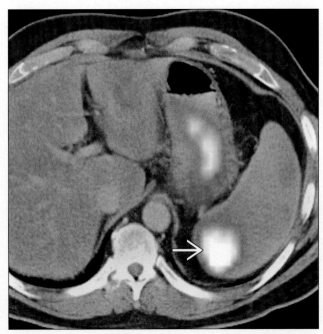

(Left) Axial CECT shows a questionable low attenuation lesion in the posterior aspect of the spleen ➡ in this patient with newly diagnosed lymphoma. *(Right)* Axial fused PET/CT image confirms the presence of a hypermetabolic lesion in the posterior aspect of the spleen ➡, compatible with active malignancy.

PET/CT: Staging

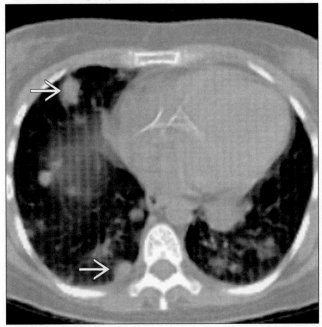 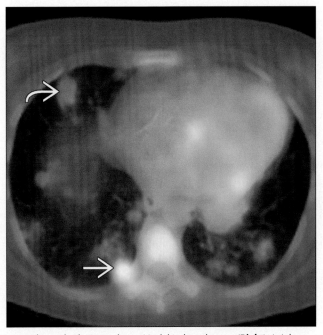

(Left) Axial CECT shows multifocal pulmonary involvement ➡ in this patient with newly diagnosed non-Hodgkin lymphoma. *(Right)* Axial fused PET/CT at the same level as the previous image shows one lesion in the right lower lobe with intense FDG activity ➡ as well as additional lesions with only mild to moderate FDG activity ➡. This type of variable FDG activity within metastatic lesions can occasionally be seen, particularly when the lesions are small.

NON-HODGKIN LYMPHOMA

PET/CT: Staging

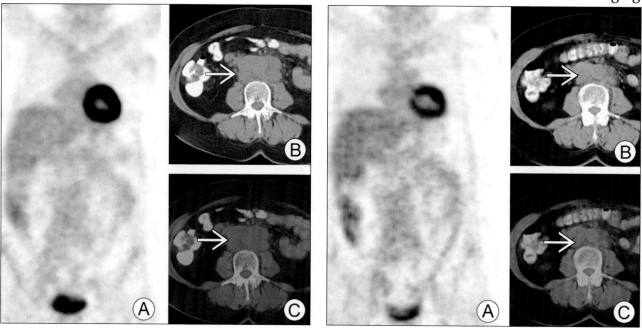

(Left) Coronal PET (A), axial CT (B) and fused PET/CT (C) show a large retroperitoneal nodal mass ➡ without increased metabolic activity, compatible with a low grade lymphoma. *(Right)* Follow-up coronal PET (A), axial CT (B) and fused PET/CT (C) show interval decrease in the size of the retroperitoneal mass ➡, although again no increased metabolic activity is identified, compatible with the patient's known history of low grade lymphoma.

PET/CT: Staging

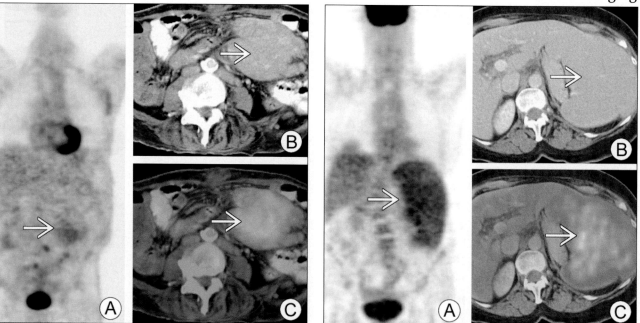

(Left) Coronal PET (A), axial CT (B) and fused PET/CT (C) demonstrate extensive mesenteric/retroperitoneal confluent adenopathy identified with mildly increased FDG activity ➡ in this patient with a newly diagnosed low grade lymphoma. *(Right)* Coronal PET (A), axial CT (B) and fused PET/CT (C) demonstrate mild to moderately increased FDG activity within an enlarged spleen ➡, compatible with splenic involvement with lymphoma.

NON-HODGKIN LYMPHOMA

PET/CT: Staging

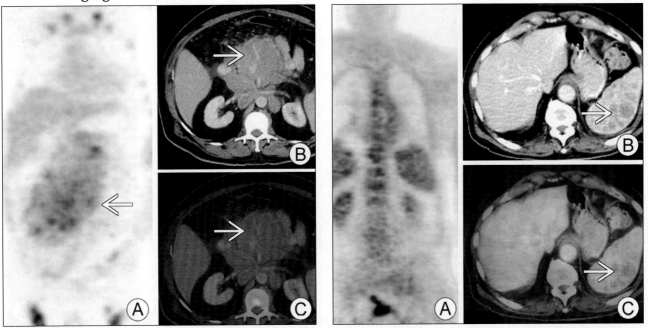

(Left) Coronal PET (A), axial CT (B) and fused PET/CT (C) demonstrate confluent masses ➡ in the mesentery and retroperitoneal area with only mild FDG uptake, compatible with a relatively low grade lymphoma. (Right) Coronal PET (A) shows no abnormal areas of FDG activity. However, axial CT (B) and fused PET/CT images (C) demonstrate multiple non-FDG splenic lesions ➡, compatible with non-FDG-avid lymphoma.

PET/CT: Restaging

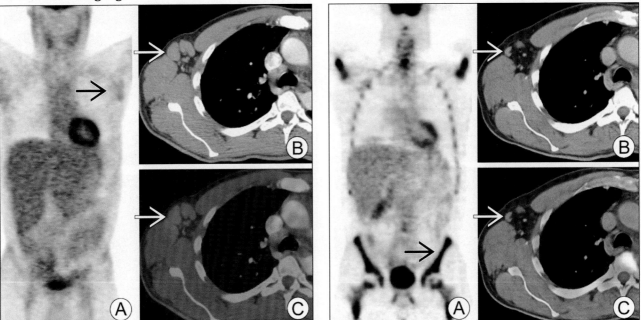

(Left) PET/CT in this patient with CLL shows only mildly increased FDG in the axillae ➡ on coronal PET (A), corresponding to markedly enlarged axillary nodes ➡ on the axial CT (B) and PET/CT (C). (Right) Post-treatment PET/CT shows diffusely increased metabolic activity throughout the osseous structures ➡ seen on coronal PET (A), compatible with marrow stimulation. Interval marked decrease in the enlarged axillary lymph nodes is apparent on axial CT (B) and fused PET/CT (C) ➡.

NON-HODGKIN LYMPHOMA

PET/CT: Restaging

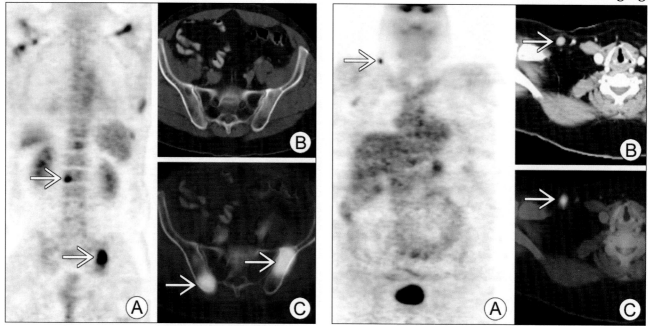

(Left) Coronal PET (A) and fused PET/CT (C) demonstrate multifocal osseous involvement ➡ without identifiable abnormalities on the CT (B) portion of the exam. *(Right)* This restaging PET/CT study was performed in a patient with a recent recurrence. Coronal PET (A), axial CT (B) and fused PET/CT (C) demonstrate an 8 mm, normal-sized right supraclavicular lymph node with intense FDG activity ➡, compatible with active lymphoma.

PET/CT: Restaging

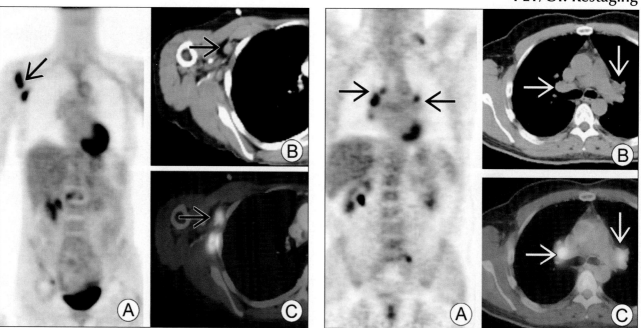

(Left) Coronal PET (A) and axial fused PET/CT (C) from a staging PET/CT examination show multiple right axillary hypermetabolic lymph nodes ➡ that were only borderline in size ➡ on the axial CT (B). *(Right)* Coronal PET (A), axial fused PET/CT (C) from a staging PET/CT examination show bilateral mediastinal and right paratracheal lymph node involvement ➡, correlating with the equivocal borderline enlarged lymph nodes ➡ on axial CT (B).

NON-HODGKIN LYMPHOMA

PET/CT: Restaging

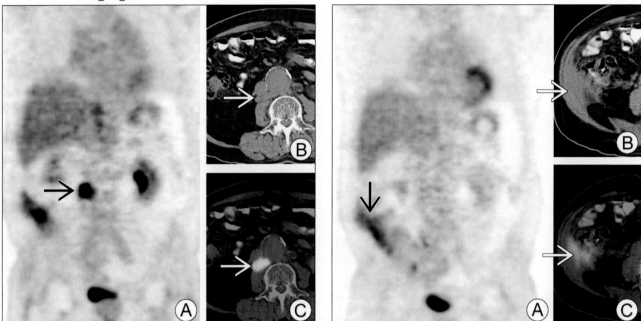

(Left) Coronal PET (A), axial CT (B) and fused PET/CT (C) from a restaging PET/CT in an asymptomatic patient show FDG activity ➡ within a retrocaval soft tissue lesion ➡, compatible with recurrent disease. *(Right)* Coronal PET (A) appears to show normal physiologic activity within the right colon ➡. However, the axial CT (B) and fused PET/CT (C) show abnormal soft tissue infiltration around the right hemicolon ➡, compatible with active lymphoma.

PET/CT: Restaging

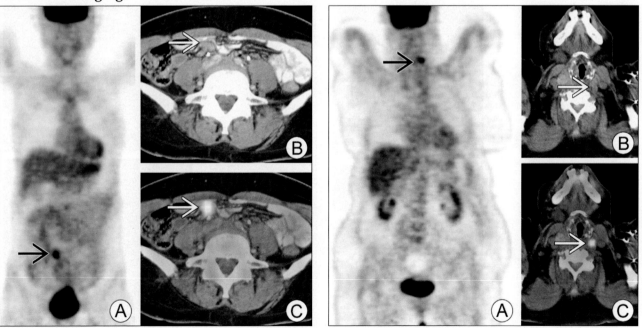

(Left) Coronal PET (A), axial CT (B) and fused PET/CT (C) from a restaging examination of an asymptomatic patient demonstrate a focal area of intense FDG activity ➡ that corresponds to a small mesenteric lymph node ➡, compatible with recurrent disease. *(Right)* Coronal PET (A), axial CT (B) and fused PET/CT (C) a show focal area of intense FDG activity ➡, correlating with a tiny lymph node in the lower left neck just anterior to a vertebral body ➡.

NON-HODGKIN LYMPHOMA

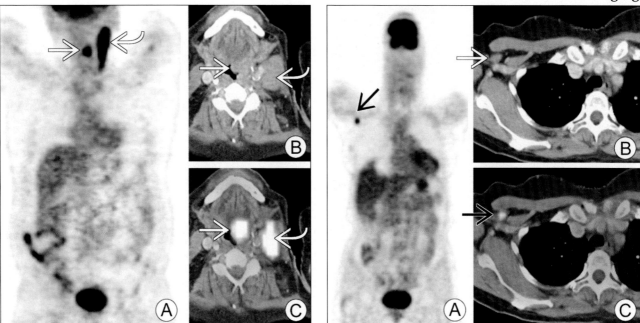

(Left) Coronal PET (A), axial CT (B) and fused PET/CT (C) from a restaging PET/CT show an area of intense FDG activity within the left lingual tonsil ➡ as well as extensive left-sided cervical hypermetabolic adenopathy ➡, compatible with malignancy. *(Right)* A staging CECT (B) shows a borderline enlarged right axillary lymph node ➡. A staging coronal PET (A) and axial PET/CT (C) show intense FDG uptake ➡, which raises the interpreting physician's confidence level in diagnosing malignancy.

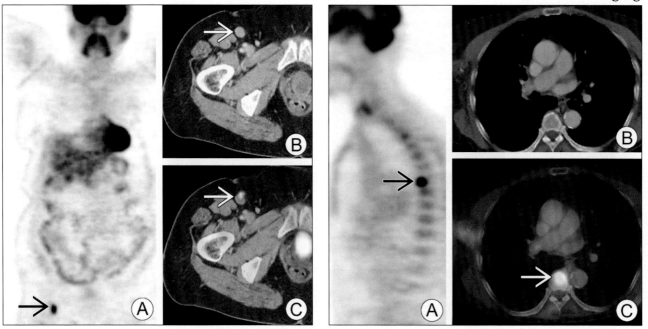

(Left) A restaging PET/CT in patient with a history of NHL shows a hypermetabolic node in the right inguinal area ➡ on coronal PET (A), correlating with a mildly enlarged lymph node ➡ on the axial CT (B) and PET/CT (C), compatible with recurrent disease. *(Right)* Sagittal PET (A) shows a focal abnormality in the mid-thoracic spine ➡ in this patient with a history of NHL. Although no definite abnormality is seen on axial CT (B), the axial fused PET/CT (C) localizes the lesion to a mid-thoracic vertebral body ➡.

NON-HODGKIN LYMPHOMA

PET/CT: Response to Therapy

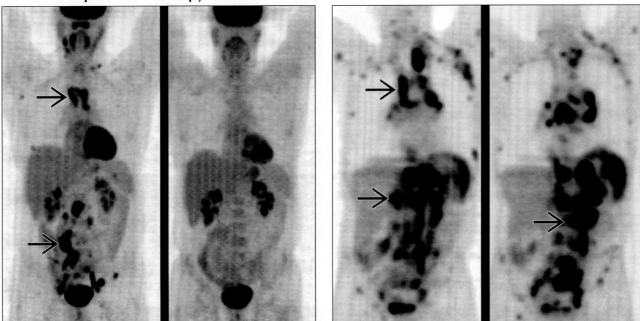

(Left) Coronal PET (left) shows a staging exam with multifocal disease above and below the diaphragm ➡. Coronal PET (right) shows a follow-up exam after approximately one to two cycles of chemotherapy, compatible with a complete response to therapy. (Right) Coronal PET shows extensive disease above and below the diaphragm ➡ with obvious splenic involvement. This staging PET/CT was performed on a patient recently diagnosed with diffuse large B-cell non-Hodgkin lymphoma.

PET/CT: Response to Therapy

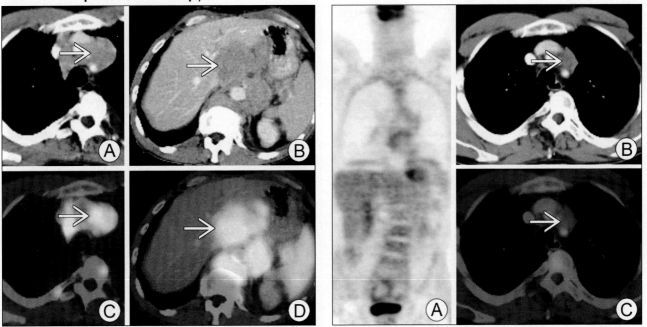

(Left) Axial CECT (A, B) and fused PET/CT (C, D) images of the same patient demonstrate multiple confluent masses ➡ in the mesentery retroperitoneal area and anterior mediastinum, compatible with active disease. (Right) Follow-up coronal PET (A), axial CT (B) and fused PET/CT (C) after one cycle of chemotherapy demonstrate complete resolution of the extensive disease, despite residual soft tissue in some areas ➡.

NON-HODGKIN LYMPHOMA

PET/CT: Response to Therapy

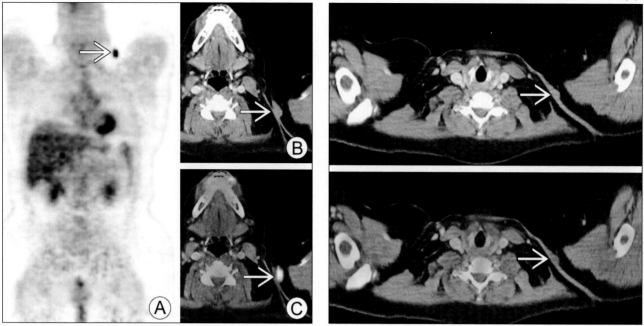

(Left) Coronal PET (A), axial CT (B) and fused PET/CT (C) images, from a staging examination of a patient with a newly diagnosed T-cell lymphoma, demonstrate a hypermetabolic subcutaneous soft tissue lesion near the left shoulder ➡, compatible with malignancy. **(Right)** Axial CT (top) and fused PET/CT (bottom) from a short-term follow-up examination approximately 2 cycles after chemotherapy initiation demonstrate interval decrease in size and metabolic activity ➡ of the subcutaneous lesion.

PET/CT: Response to Therapy

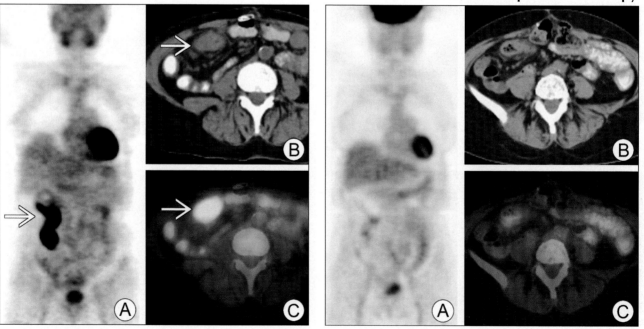

(Left) Coronal PET (A), axial CT (B) and fused PET/CT (C) of a patient recently diagnosed with PTLD of the bowel shows intense FDG activity in a loop of thickened bowel ➡, compatible with active PTLD. **(Right)** Coronal PET (A), axial CT (B) and fused PET/CT (C) of a follow-up PET/CT performed approximately 10 weeks after tapering immunosuppression shows almost complete resolution of the abnormal activity seen in the prior exam.

NON-HODGKIN LYMPHOMA

PET/CT: Response to Therapy

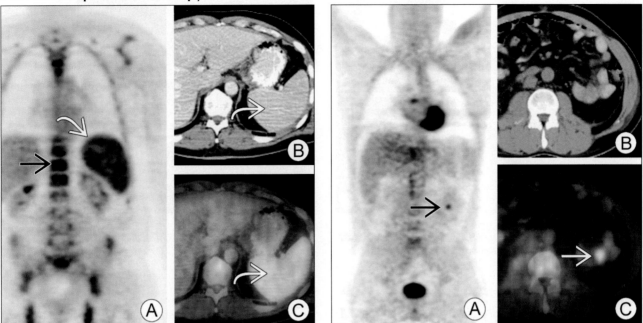

(Left) Coronal PET (A), axial CT (B) and PET/CT (C) show a typical post chemotherapy/G-CSF appearance on PET with diffusely increased FDG activity throughout the bone marrow ⇨ as well as diffusely increased activity in the spleen ⇨. *(Right)* Coronal PET (A) demonstrates a focal area of moderately increased FDG activity ⇨ without definite abnormality on CT (B). The fused PET/CT image (C) localizes the abnormality to a loop of jejunum ⇨ in this patient with a history of PTLD.

PET/CT: Response to Therapy

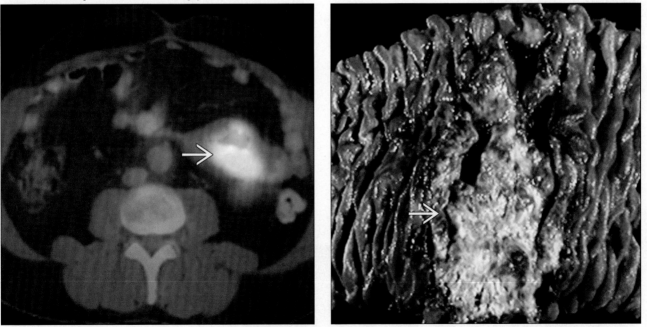

(Left) Axial image of a PET/CT in the same patient approximately two months later shows intense FDG activity, correlating with extensive circumferential thickening of the jejunal loop ⇨ that had the focal abnormality on the original PET/CT exam. *(Right)* Specimen from partial jejunal resection shows tumor infiltration ⇨, pathologically confirmed to be PTLD.

MELANOMA

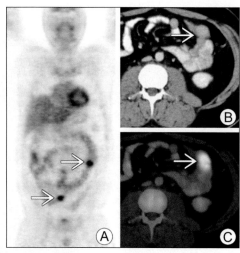

Coronal PET (A), axial CT (B) and fused PET/CT (C) show foci of increased FDG activity within the bowel ➡, corresponding to melanoma metastases.

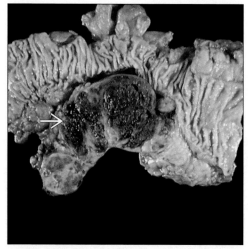

Gross pathology shows the partially hemorrhagic intraluminal bowel metastasis ➡ from the same patient as the previous image.

TERMINOLOGY

Abbreviations and Synonyms
- Malignant melanoma (MM)
- Skin cancer

Definitions
- Melanoma: Neoplasm of melanin-producing cells

IMAGING FINDINGS

General Features
- Best diagnostic clue: FDG-avid focal uptake on PET seen in primary, satellite lesions, lymph nodes (LN), visceral organs, and bone
- Location
  - **Primary melanoma**
    - Men: Torso most common
    - Women: Upper extremities most common
    - 4-5% of primary melanoma may arise in extracutaneous location
      - Locations include eye, meninges, mucous membranes of digestive, genitourinary, respiratory tracts
      - Multiple primaries occur in ~ 5% of patients
  - **Local spread**
    - At or near previous excision site
    - Recent biopsy or other inflammation may produce false positive on FDG PET
    - Sentinal node tumor may alter stage
  - **Metastatic disease**
    - In-transit nodal metastases: Between primary and regional lymph nodes
    - Regional lymph nodes
    - Common sites: Spine, brain, lung, liver, spleen, bowel
    - Clinically apparent brain metastases found in 18-46% of patients with stage IV disease
    - Conjunctival melanoma may present with systemic metastases in 26% of cases without regional lymph node involvement
- Size
  - Size considerations usually relative to depth of lesion
  - Stage is dependent on depth

DDx: Superficial FDG Activity or Skin Activity

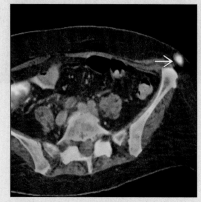

Metastasis

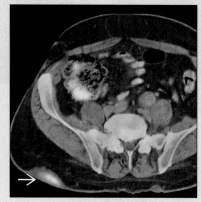

Neurofibroma

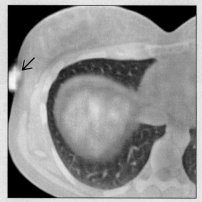

Contamination

MELANOMA

Key Facts

Terminology
- Malignant melanoma (MM)

Imaging Findings
- **CT**
  - CECT is better than FDG PET for detection of small pulmonary metastases
  - Less sensitive than FDG PET for bone, skin, lymph node, abdominal metastases
  - Combination of FDG PET and conventional imaging (CT/MR) more accurate than either one alone
  - CT generally performed for staging and restaging purposes
- **PET/CT**
  - Detects more lesions than CT, particularly intramuscular and other unsuspected metastases
  - More exact method of determining FDG uptake in a mass
  - Staging: Sensitivity 83%, specificity 91%
  - Restaging: 74% sensitivity 74%, specificity 86% for recurrence
- In one study, 16% of patients underwent further imaging &/or biopsies that ultimately had no effect on patient care

Top Differential Diagnoses
- Other Neoplasms
- Inflammation/Infection
- Brown Fat

Clinical Issues
- Tumor thickness = most important histologic prognostic indicator

---

- Morphology: Malignant lymph nodes are typically round with absence of fatty hilum

Imaging Recommendations
- Best imaging tool
  - **FDG PET**
    - May reveal focal increased uptake in lymph node bed, soft tissue, and organs
    - More sensitive than CT for skin, LN, bone, and abdominal metastases
  - **CECT**
    - Exclusion of benign structures with FDG uptake
    - Accurate delineation of primary and metastatic tumor in lymph node bed, soft tissue, and organs
    - Superior detection of small pulmonary metastases
    - Inclusion of lymph nodes by size or morphology (round without fatty hilum)
  - **MR**
    - For definition of brain metastases
- Protocol advice
  - FDG PET
    - Evaluate skin for lesions with non-attenuation corrected PET images
    - Attenuation correction can smooth data, obscuring lesions
    - PET scan often extended to true whole-body coverage due to metastatic behavior of melanoma
    - Clinical history crucial: False positives with recent surgery, biopsy, inflammation
  - Total lesion glycolysis (TLG) approach
    - More exact method of determining FDG uptake in a mass
    - Has failed to show superiority over simpler SUV measurement
  - Longer FDG uptake times may correlate to better overall sensitivity/specificity
    - In general, more uptake in malignant lesions and less uptake in benign lesions is seen at 2 or 3 hour time point

CT Findings
- CT generally performed for staging and restaging purposes
  - Not used to evaluate primary lesions
- **NECT**: Less sensitive for detecting metastatic lesions than CECT
- **CECT**: More sensitive for evaluation of organs and non-nodal soft tissue such as muscle
  - **General**
    - After typical search pattern, look again at muscle, gallbladder, and other subcutaneous soft tissues
  - **Brain**
    - Imaging performed for patients with known metastatic disease
    - Also performed for patients with neurological symptoms in the absence of known metastases
    - MR with contrast much more sensitive for detecting small brain metastases
  - **Chest**
    - May detect asymptomatic lesions
    - NECT and CECT approximately equal for detecting small pulmonary metastases
    - FDG PET less sensitive in general for detecting lung metastases ≤ 6 mm
  - **Abdomen**
    - Organ metastases may show hyperenhancement
    - Intramuscular metastases will generally show some abnormal enhancement, but may be otherwise undetectable
  - **Pelvis**
    - More likely positive in patients with primary disease below waist
  - **Bone**
    - Some may demonstrate enhancement, making them more conspicuous
    - Extensive bone metastasis may be missed altogether

Nuclear Medicine Findings
- **General**
  - Melanoma is almost always FDG avid

MELANOMA

- o True positives have significantly higher SUV than false positives in lesions > 1 cm on PET/CT
- o PET/CT has considerable but non-significant advantage over PET in characterization of lesions
  - Possibly due to high avidity of melanoma metastases
  - Certainty of lesion localization significantly improved with combined modality
  - Especially in detection of visceral metastases
- o Accuracy of PET/CT higher when equivocal lesions are considered negative
- o PET/CT recommended for stage III/IV patients
  - Thorough physical exam and US of draining nodes for lower stage patients
- o PET/CT may detect unheralded occult primary malignancy in patients with primary melanoma
- o Choroidal melanoma reported to have low FDG uptake
  - Correlated strongly to lesion size
- o Intra-operative FDG PET/CT
  - Handheld gamma probe used to find lesions during surgery
  - Used to verify intra-operative US findings
  - Used to verify excised tissue as being the FDG-avid lesion
  - Can evaluate residual sites of hypermetabolic activity immediately post-operatively
- • Staging
  - o PET established as useful modality for staging and restaging of cutaneous melanoma and for evaluating distant metastases
    - Large meta-analysis: Sensitivity 83% and specificity 91% for staging
    - Changes management in 26-50% of patients
    - In one study, 16% of patients underwent further imaging &/or biopsies that ultimately had no effect on patient care
  - o Local or early disease
    - PET/CT found to have high accuracy for evaluation of regional metastases
    - Sensitivity 23% if metastases ≤ 5 mm (e.g., small lung nodules)
    - One study concluded that PET reliably detects lymph node tumor deposits > 80 mm³
    - Loses sensitivity rapidly below that volume
    - Not reimbursable by Medicare for evaluation of regional lymph nodes in stage I/II disease
    - More sensitive in setting of clinical or radiographic evidence of disease
  - o Distant disease
    - Sensitivity ≥ 90% for lesions > 1 cm
    - Reimbursable by Medicare for evaluation of extranodal metastases during initial staging
    - Sensitivity of 60% with FDG PET for brain metastases due to high physiologic uptake in the brain
    - Organ-based accuracy in liver, lung, and brain variable
    - Accuracy of PET/CT for M-staging higher than that of PET or CT alone (98%, 93%, 84%, respectively)

- Superior sensitivity for lung metastases compared to MR
- o PET/CT of node positive melanoma at time of sentinal lymphadenectomy had management change in 31% of one patient cohort
  - CT/MR in this circumstance shown to yield less than 1%; not clinically indicated
  - Level of uptake in lymph node metastases correlates with recurrence risk
- • Restaging
  - o FDG PET detects recurrent disease with sensitivity/ specificity 74%/86%
  - o Elevated laboratory markers or clinical evidence of recurrence should prompt re-imaging
  - o Pre-surgical evaluation may detect more extensive disease and alter surgical planning
  - o FDG PET reimbursed by Medicare for pre-surgical evaluation of recurrence
- • Response to therapy
  - o PET/CT not routinely performed
    - Likely will play a more significant role in evaluating patients after various immunomodulating therapies
  - o One study showed complete agreement differentiating chemo-responders and nonresponders between CT and PET/CT
    - Baseline FDG PET very helpful for evaluating response to therapy
    - Melanoma differs from malignancies such as lymphoma, in which metabolic changes precede morphologic changes
    - PET/CT has benefit of relative ease of interpretation, but some controversy exists as to cost/benefit ratio
    - FDG PET pitfall: Cytokine therapy results in diffuse hypermetabolism in normal lymph nodes for months

MR Findings

- • More accurate in detection of mets to liver and bone
  - o Hepatic metastases ≤ 1 cm and containing melanin have bright signal on T1 weighted MR

DIFFERENTIAL DIAGNOSIS

Other Neoplasms

- • May appear similar to melanoma in FDG avidity
- • If suspicion of melanoma recurrence is low, consider
  - o Primary or metastatic disease from second primary
    - Unheralded second primary malignancies detected in 1.2% of patients (lung most common)
  - o Squamous or basal cell carcinoma
  - o Lymphoma in the presence of lymphadenopathy

Reactive Lymph Nodes

- • Look for CT evidence of other causes of reactive lymphadenopathy, e.g., colitis, pancreatitis, pneumonia

Inflammation/Infection

- • Pneumonia

- o May present with focal FDG uptake that mimics hypermetabolic nodule
- o CT correlation and follow-up studies are helpful to avoid unnecessary biopsy
- Granulomatous infection may manifest as enlarged, hypermetabolic lymph nodes
  - o Mycobacterium avium intracellulare
  - o Tuberculosis
  - o Sarcoidosis
  - o Histoplasmosis

Brown Fat

- Most prevalent in young males during cold-weather months
- Avoid cold temperatures prior to scan and employ warming maneuvers prior to FDG administration

Other

- Asymmetric muscle uptake
- Recent site of biopsy or other surgical procedure

PATHOLOGY

General Features

- Genetics
  - o 10-20% of melanoma patients have family history
    - Multiple dysplastic nevi and possible multiple primary melanoma
    - Tumors do not demonstrate increased aggressiveness
- Etiology
  - o UVA and UVB may work in concert as carcinogen
    - Damages melanocyte DNA
    - Suppresses dermal immune system
  - o Major risk factors
    - History of intermittent blistering sunburns
    - History of prior skin cancer, including non-melanoma
  - o Local recurrence due to 2 causes
    - Incomplete excision of original tumor
    - Microsatellite metastases with spread through surrounding lymphatics
- Epidemiology
  - o Accounts for 5% of skin cancer
  - o ~ 60,000 cases of invasive and ~ 50,000 cases of in-situ melanoma diagnosed per year in USA
  - o Incidence increasing at 5-7% per year
  - o 65% of all skin cancer deaths in the USA are due to cutaneous malignant melanoma
    - 3x the mortality of non-melanoma skin cancer
    - 5th most common cancer
- Associated abnormalities: Serum LDH (serum lactate dehydrogenase) may rise with recurrence

Gross Pathologic & Surgical Features

- Variable pigmentation
  - o Melanotic most common
  - o May present as non-pigmented lesion

Microscopic Features

- Large atypical intraepithelial melanocytes haphazardly arranged at dermoepidermal junction

- Vertical growth characteristics include evidence of proliferation (mitoses, MIB0-1 staining) and nuclear pleomorphism
- Tumor thickness defined by Breslow depth and is most important determinant of prognosis
  - o Measured vertically in millimeters from top of granular layer to deepest point of tumor involvement

Staging, Grading, or Classification Criteria

- Most significant prognostic factors include
  - o Sentinal node biopsy
  - o Breslow thickness and ulceration
  - o Tumor subtype
- American Joint Committee on Cancer staging system
  - o IA
    - < 1 mm thick, no ulceration/invasion
  - o IB
    - < 1 mm thick, + ulceration/invasion
    - 1-2 mm thick, no ulceration/invasion
  - o IIA
    - 1-2 mm thick, + ulceration/invasion
    - 2-4 mm thick, no ulceration
  - o IIB
    - 2-4 mm thick, + ulceration
    - > 4 mm, no ulceration
  - o IIC
    - > 4 mm, + ulceration
  - o IIIA
    - 1-3 mm + lymph nodes (microscopic), no ulceration
  - o IIIB
    - 1-3 mm + lymph nodes (microscopic), + ulceration
    - 1-3 mm + lymph nodes (macroscopic), no ulceration
  - o IIIC
    - 1-3 mm + lymph nodes (macroscopic), + ulceration
    - $\geq$ 4 mm + lymph nodes or matted node
  - o IV
    - Distant metastases
- Local staging by histologic analysis of tumor thickness and anatomic invasion
- Regional lymph node staging by surgical lymphadenectomy (sentinel lymph node)
- Distant staging by clinical exam, laboratory tests and imaging
  - o Whole-body: PET, CECT
  - o Brain: MR
- S-100B tumor marker used to indicate presence of distant metastases and tumor burden; also has prognostic implications
  - o Can be elevated in subarachnoid hemorrhage and stroke
  - o Clear drawback is false negative rate in 1/3 of patients with metastases

CLINICAL ISSUES

Presentation

- Most common signs/symptoms

MELANOMA

- o Clinical examination may reveal nevus with
  - Asymmetry
  - Irregular border
  - Color variation
  - Diameter ≥ 6 mm
  - Change over time
- o Signs and symptoms may be fairly nonspecific
  - ± Bleeding or itching of primary skin lesion
  - Palpable lymph nodes
  - Recurrent skin lesions following excision
  - Increased laboratory markers (LDH, liver function tests)
- Other signs/symptoms
  - o Signs/symptoms according to organ invasion
    - Bowel obstruction
    - Neurologic changes
    - Jaundice
    - Bone pain

Demographics

- Age
  - o Age is a risk factor for acquiring and dying from melanoma
  - o Average age at diagnosis is 55 years
  - o Second only to breast cancer in women aged 30-34 years
  - o Most common cancer in women aged 25-29 years
  - o In USA, 1-4% of all melanomas occur in patients ≤ 20 years old
- Gender: Slight female predominance below age 40; slight male predominance above age 40
- Ethnicity
  - o Fair skin is a risk factor
  - o Dark and easily tanned skin is protective

Natural History & Prognosis

- Prognosis depends heavily on tumor thickness and ulceration
  - o Thin primary without ulceration: 5 year survival 91-95%
  - o > 4 mm tumor with ulceration: 5 year survival 45%
  - o Regional lymph node metastasis: 5 year survival, 13-69% depending on extent
  - o Median survival time with distant metastases (stage IV) ~ 7.5 months
    - 5 year survival 7-19%
- Better prognosis
  - o Soft tissue, nodal, and isolated lung metastases
  - o Presence of nonvisceral (vs. visceral) metastases
- Worse prognosis
  - o Visceral metastases
  - o Higher number and palpability of metastatic lymph nodes
  - o Elevated LDH
- Recurrence
  - o 9% recurrence with negative sentinal lymph node
  - o 55% recurrence within 42 months with positive sentinal lymph node

Treatment

- No survival benefit demonstrated for adjuvant chemotherapy or radiotherapy

- Interferon alpha-2b currently the only adjuvant therapy approved by FDA for high risk melanoma
- For early stage melanoma, standard of care has become intra-operative lymphatic mapping
  - o Sentinal lymph node biopsy (SLNB) and selective complete lymph node dissection
  - o SLNB appears more sensitive than PET for lymphatic staging early in disease
  - o Current drugs have severe side effects and high cost, making early detection of success vs. failure of therapy important
- Lymph node dissection is the treatment of choice for localized disease but is an aggressive procedure
  - o Complication rates of 5-30% depending on technique, extent, and site
  - o Early disease detection can avoid unnecessary surgery

DIAGNOSTIC CHECKLIST

Consider

- Biopsy site may exhibit FDG uptake and obscure local recurrent tumor on PET
- Image entire body (including extremities) with FDG PET
- 50% of metastases are detected with skin examination by patient or doctor, or by lymph node sonography
- Small (< 1.5 cm) brain metastases may be missed on FDG PET

Image Interpretation Pearls

- Always examine non-attenuation corrected images for diagnosis and staging
- Cytokine therapy can result in symmetrical stimulation of lymphoid tissue (tonsils, nodes)

SELECTED REFERENCES

1. Akcali C et al: Detection of metastases in patients with cutaneous melanoma using FDG-PET/CT. J Int Med Res. 35(4):547-53, 2007
2. Choi EA et al: Imaging studies in patients with melanoma. Surg Oncol Clin N Am. 16(2):403-30, 2007
3. Gulec SA: A surgical perspective on positron emission tomography. J Surg Oncol. 95(6):443-6, 2007
4. Iagaru A et al: 2-Deoxy-2-[F-18]fluoro-D-glucose positron emission tomography/computed tomography in the management of melanoma. Mol Imaging Biol. 9(1):50-7, 2007
5. Koskivuo IO et al: Whole body positron emission tomography in follow-up of high risk melanoma. Acta Oncol. 46(5):685-90, 2007
6. Mottaghy FM et al: Direct comparison of [18F]FDG PET/CT with PET alone and with side-by-side PET and CT in patients with malignant melanoma. Eur J Nucl Med Mol Imaging. 34(9):1355-64, 2007
7. Nguyen NC et al: Prevalence and patterns of soft tissue metastasis: detection with true whole-body F-18 FDG PET/CT. BMC Med Imaging. 7:8, 2007
8. Strobel K et al: High-risk melanoma: accuracy of FDG PET/CT with added CT morphologic information for detection of metastases. Radiology. 244(2):566-74, 2007
9. Strobel K et al: S-100B and FDG-PET/CT in therapy response assessment of melanoma patients. Dermatology. 215(3):192-201, 2007

MELANOMA

CT Findings: Metastases

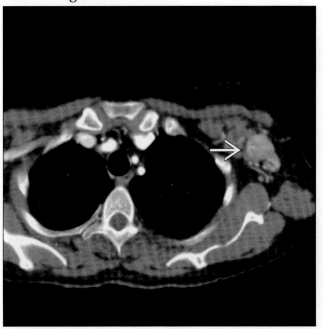 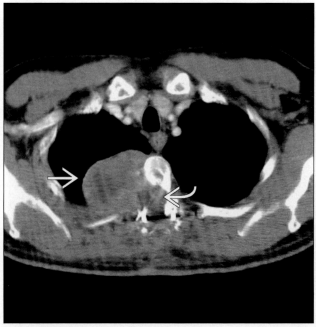

(Left) Axial CECT shows an axillary nodal metastasis in this patient with melanoma ➡. (Right) Axial CECT shows a large destructive melanotic metastasis ➡ that invades the adjacent pleura, rib, and vertebral body with encroachment on the thecal sac ➡.

CT Findings: Metastases

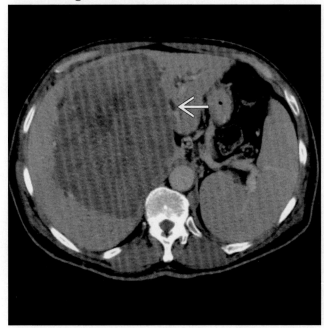 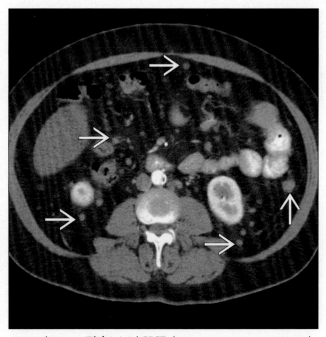

(Left) Axial CECT shows a large hepatic metastasis ➡ in a patient with known melanoma. (Right) Axial CECT shows numerous retroperitoneal and mesenteric soft tissue metastases in a patient with known melanoma ➡.

MELANOMA

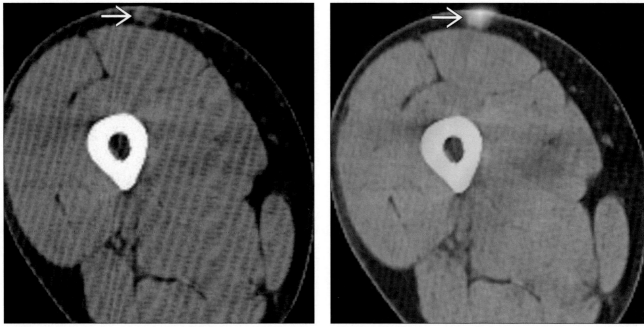

(Left) Axial NECT shows a superficial focus ➡ of soft tissue on the anterior thigh. *(Right)* Axial fused PET/CT shows increased FDG uptake ➡ in the soft tissue lesion, corresponding to primary melanoma lesion.

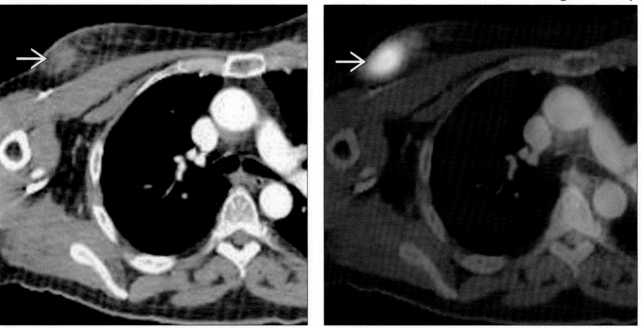

(Left) Axial CECT shows focal soft tissue infiltration ➡ anterior to the right pectoralis major. *(Right)* Axial fused PET/CT shows hypermetabolic activity in the same region of soft tissue infiltration ➡, corresponding to a primary melanotic lesion.

MELANOMA

PET/CT Findings: Regional Nodal Metastasis

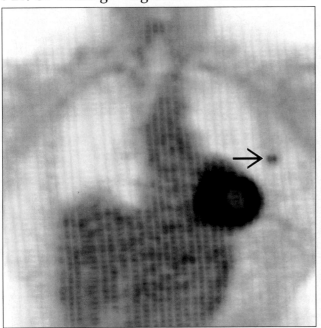 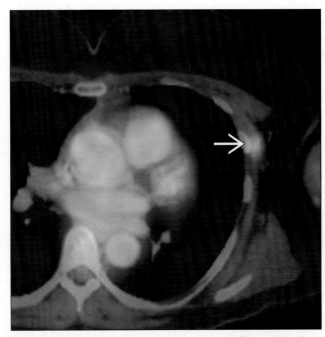

(Left) Coronal PET shows focal uptake in the rib ➡️*, corresponding to a metastasis in this patient with known melanoma. (Right) Axial fused PET/CT shows that the same lesion demonstrates increased FDG uptake* ➡️*.*

PET/CT Findings: Staging

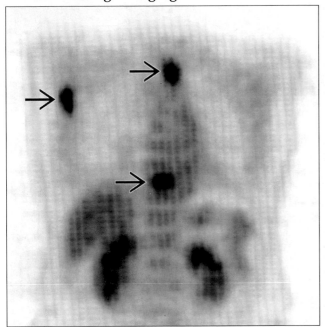 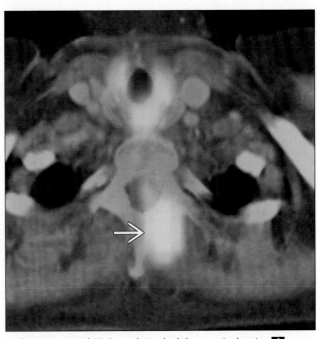

(Left) Coronal PET shows several metastases ➡️*. (Right) Axial fused PET/CT shows increased FDG uptake in the left paraspinal region* ➡️*, consistent with metastasis in this patient with melanoma.*

MELANOMA

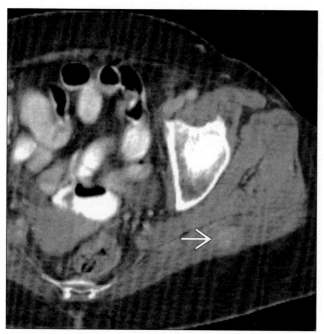
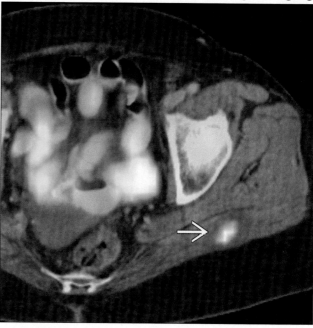

(Left) Axial CECT shows a focus of enhancement within the posterior musculature ➡, corresponding to a metastasis. *(Right)* Axial fused PET/CT shows the same lesion demonstrating increased FDG activity ➡.

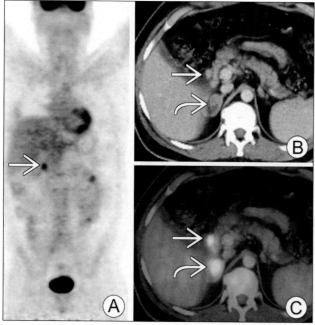
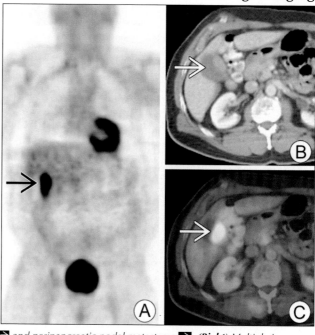

(Left) Coronal PET (A), axial CT (B) and fused PET/CT (C) show adrenal ➡ and peripancreatic nodal metastases ➡. *(Right)* Multiple images show a focus of increased activity on coronal PET (A) ➡ that was localized to a soft tissue focus ➡ in the gallbladder on axial CT (B) and fused PET/CT (C), confirmed to be a melanoma metastasis. Melanoma can metastasize anywhere including bowel, pancreas, gallbladder, soft tissue, heart, solid viscera, and even transplacentally in pregnant women! A high index of suspicion is always needed.

MELANOMA

PET/CT Findings: Restaging

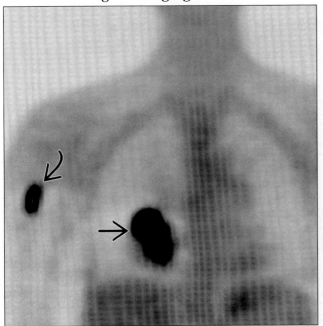
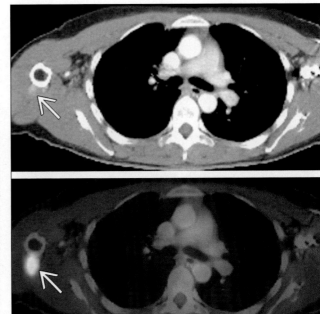

(Left) Coronal PET shows a large area of intense FDG activity ➡, compatible with metastatic disease. This patient with a history of stage IV melanoma had an abnormality on chest X-ray, prompting this scan. Although the patient was being considered for possible metastasectomy, she had unsuspected additional lesions ➡. *(Right)* Axial CECT (top) and fused PET/CT (bottom) show an enhancing soft tissue mass ➡ in the posterior musculature of the arm with increased FDG uptake, consistent with metastatic disease.

PET/CT Findings: Restaging

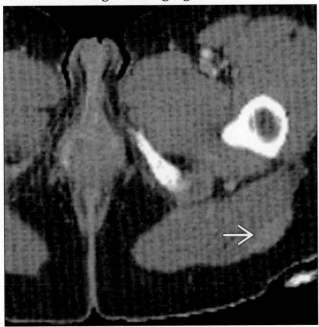
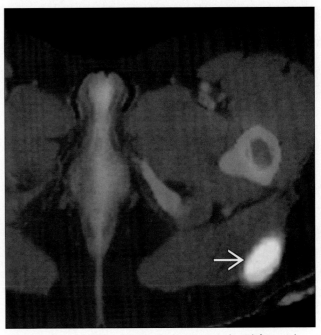

(Left) Axial CECT shows an enhancing lesion ➡ in the superficial aspect of the left gluteal muscle, not identified prospectively. *(Right)* Axial fused PET/CT in the same patient shows increased FDG activity ➡ in the left gluteal muscle, corresponding to melanoma metastasis.

MELANOMA

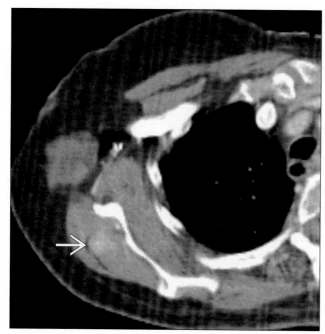 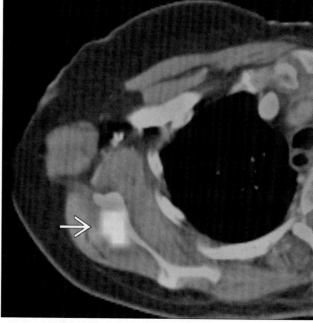

(Left) Axial CECT shows an enhancing lesion in the posterior musculature on the right ➡. *(Right)* Axial fused PET/CT shows increased FDG activity within a melanotic metastasis ➡.

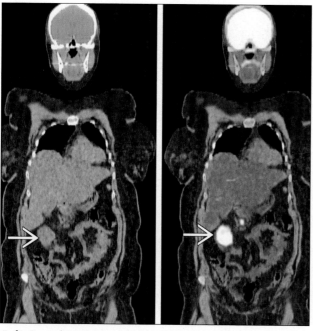 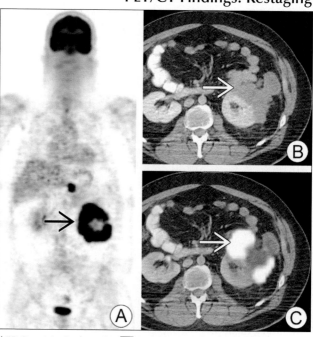

(Left) Coronal CT (left) and fused PET/CT (right) demonstrate intense focal FDG activity in the colon ➡ in this patient with a history of melanoma. A follow-up CT showed an intussusception caused by a metastatic focus in the bowel. *(Right)* Images show increased FDG uptake ➡ in the left upper abdomen on coronal PET (A), localized to the perinephric space as a soft tissue mass ➡ on axial CT (B) and fused PET/CT (C).

MELANOMA

PET/CT Findings: Restaging

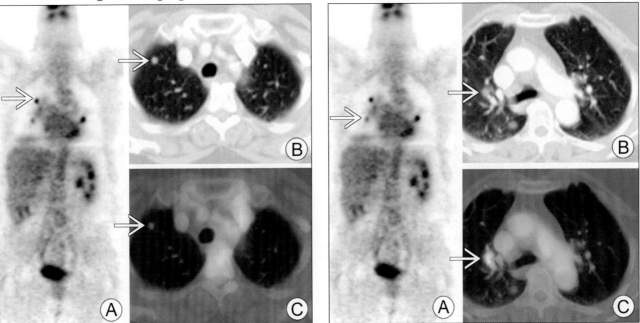

(Left) Coronal (A), axial CT (B) and fused PET/CT (C) show a tiny focus of increased FDG activity in the right upper lobe localized to a pulmonary nodule ➡, consistent with a metastasis. In cases such as this, biopsy may be required to differentiate between a metastasis and a primary lung neoplasm. *(Right)* Coronal (A), axial CT (B) and fused PET/CT (C) in the same patient show a second focus of increased FDG uptake in the right hilum ➡.

PET/CT Findings: Restaging

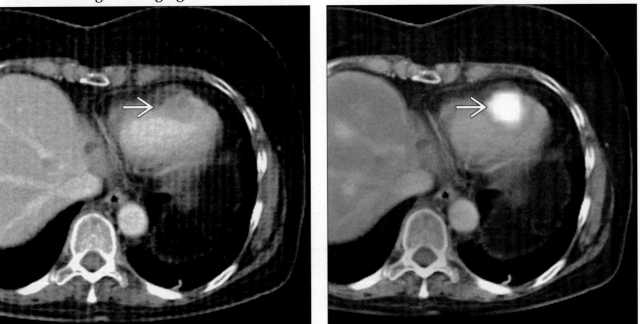

(Left) Axial CECT shows a questionable melanotic metastasis of the ventricular wall ➡. *(Right)* Axial fused PET/CT confirms the presence of the metastasis ➡ seen on the previous image.

CERVICAL CARCINOMA

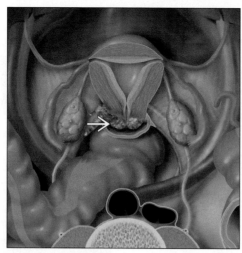

Graphic shows an irregular mass in the uterine cervix ➡, compatible with cervical carcinoma.

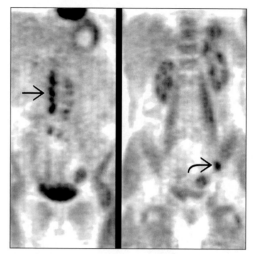

Coronal PET shows multiple periaortic lymph nodes ➡ and a left pelvic lymph node ↗, not previously identified. An additional IMRT plan was performed for the left pelvic lymph node.

TERMINOLOGY

Abbreviations and Synonyms

- Cervical cancer
- Cervical carcinoma
- Carcinoma of the cervix
- Squamous cell carcinoma of the uterine cervix
- Locally advanced cervical cancer (LACC)

Definitions

- Primary cancer that arises from intraepithelial neoplasia of cervical cells
  - Squamous cell carcinoma (SCCA): 80%
  - Adenocarcinoma: 15%
  - Adenosquamous: 3-5%
  - Rare: Lymphoma and sarcoma

IMAGING FINDINGS

General Features

- Best diagnostic clue
  - PET/CT

- Intense FDG activity in primary cervical mass, vagina, uterus, parametria
    - ± Lymphadenopathy, visceral metastases
  - CT/MR
    - Enhancing mass in expected location of cervix
    - ± Extension into vagina, uterus, parametria
    - ± Lymphadenopathy, visceral metastases
- Location
  - Primary
    - Cervix
  - Local
    - Vaginal mucosa
    - Extension into endometrium or myometrium
    - Direct extension into parametrium or adjacent structures
  - Regional LN
    - Para-aortic
    - Common iliac
    - External iliac
  - Metastatic
    - Distant nodes
    - Organs
- Size
  - Varies, from microscopic to several centimeters

DDx: Benign Mimics of Cervical Carcinoma

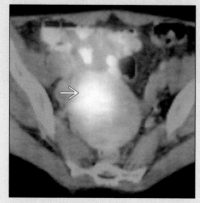

Leiomyoma

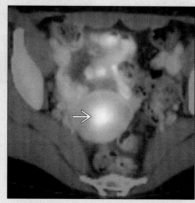

Endometrial Cavity, Menstruation

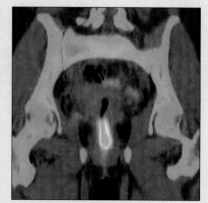

Vaginal Canal, Menstruation

CERVICAL CARCINOMA

Key Facts

Imaging Findings
- PET/CT: Intense FDG activity in primary cervical mass, vagina, uterus, parametria; ± lymphadenopathy, visceral metastases
- Primary tumor: CEMR
- Most cervical SCCA is avid on FDG → high sensitivity for sizable lesions
- Evaluation of pelvic and para-aortic LN
- LN detection on PET: Sensitivity 75-91%, specificity 93-100%
- When PET/CT is performed with diagnostic quality CT, including IV and oral contrast, quality of the overall procedure is improved
- Sensitivity and specificity for post-therapy of patients with cervical cancer: 90-93%, 91-100%

Top Differential Diagnoses
- Other Female Reproductive Tract Malignancy
- Ovarian Cancer
- Leiomyoma
- Physiologic FDG Activity in Female Reproductive Organs
- Urine Contamination

Clinical Issues
- Often asymptomatic
- Clinical staging accurate in ~ 60% of patients

Diagnostic Checklist
- PET/CT for optimal staging
- Physical exam, MR for evaluation of primary tumor

- o Many small cervical masses will not be apparent on CT

Imaging Recommendations
- Best imaging tool
  - o **Primary tumor**
    - CEMR probably best modality for evaluating the primary lesion
  - o **Local and distant metastases**
    - PET/CT (consider with contrast-enhanced CT)
    - CT reveals ~ 1/3 para-aortic mets
    - MR and CT: Moderate sensitivity and specificity for detecting pelvic, para-aortic lymphadenopathy; may fail to identify small metastases
    - MR for detecting cervical cancer lymphadenopathy: Sensitivity 36-71%, specificity 76-100%
  - o Combination of tumor markers and PET/CT may be highly efficient for detecting recurrence
- Protocol advice
  - o FDG excretion through urinary tract and bladder can cause false positive
    - Bladder voiding prior to imaging important to minimize FDG accumulation within the bladder (may cause artifact in pelvis)
    - However, primary tumor likely well characterized on anatomic imaging modality (MR)
    - Image from thighs toward head to minimize excretory FDG within the bladder
    - Can repeat a bed position after voiding if unclear on initial PET scan
    - Lasix may be useful, although not routinely used

CT Findings
- **Local tumor**
  - o Primary tumor arises in cervical canal
    - Extension into peripheral parenchyma can be evaluated with CT
  - o Compared to normal cervical stroma, primary tumor may be hypo- or isoattenuating

- Stage IB tumors frequently are isoattenuating to normal cervical tissue (50%)
  - May not be apparent on CT
- o Larger lesions will show variable diffuse enhancement pattern seen in delayed images of normal cervix
- o Tumor extension outside cervix is less likely when cervical margins are smooth and well defined
- o Enlargement of endometrial cavity with blood, serous fluid, or pus can follow obstruction of endocervical canal status post radiotherapy
- o Necrosis or prior biopsy of lesion may produce intratumoral gas
- o Poorer outcome associated with cervical enlargement > 3.5 cm and an AP size > 6 cm
- **Extension/metastasis**
  - o CT useful for the depiction of
    - Adenopathy
    - Pelvic side wall extension
    - Advanced bladder and rectal invasion
    - Ureteral obstruction
    - Extrapelvic spread of disease
  - o Tumor extension within 3 mm of pelvic side wall fulfills criterion for invasion
  - o Tumor extension into uterine body careful evaluation for metastic spread
  - o Ureteral encasement may result secondary to tumor extension into parametrium
    - Ureteral encasement is specific for parametrial invasion
    - Stage IIIB disease indicated by presence of hydronephrosis
    - Parametrial invasion may also result in perivascular invasion and uterosacral ligament thickening
  - o Muscular enlargement and enhancing soft tissue mass may be seen with frank invasion of piriformis and obturator internus
  - o Direct extension to pelvic bones results in bony destruction
  - o Tumor may encase and narrow iliac vessels
  - o Signs of bladder or rectal involvement

CERVICAL CARCINOMA

- Intraluminal mass
- Loss of perivesical or perirectal fat plane
- Asymmetric nodular thickening of bladder or rectal wall
- Fistula formation with intravesical air
  - Cystic appearance of recurrent pelvic disease can be confused with post-surgical fluid collection
    - Recurrence has minimal soft tissue and generally occurs more than 6 months after surgery
  - Distant metastases
    - 30% of patients have liver metastases
    - Appear as solid masses with variable enhancement
    - 15% of patients have adrenal metastases
    - 35-40% of patients with thoracic metastatic disease have this presentation
    - Multiple pulmonary nodules may represent thoracic metastasis
    - Minority of cases demonstrate cavitation
- **Lymph nodes**
  - Cutoff for suspicion of malignancy is size > 1 cm in short axis
    - 90% of metastatic retroperitoneal LNs are normal-sized
    - Sensitivity for retroperitoneal metastases: 44%
    - Sensitivity for para-aortic metastases: 34%
  - Enhancement pattern rarely helps differentiate benign from malignant disease
    - Central necrosis has ~ 100% PPV
  - Parametrial station is usually the first to be infiltrated by disease
  - Tumor spreads through 3 lymphatic pathways most commonly
    - Laterally along external iliacs
    - Hypogastric route along internal iliacs
    - Presacrally along uterosacral ligament
    - Each pathway leads to common iliac lymph nodes, then leads to para-aortic nodes

Nuclear Medicine Findings

- PET/CT performed with diagnostic CT
  - Quality of the overall procedure is improved
  - Much easier to identify focal abdominopelvic lesions from opacified bowel if oral contrast is used
- **Initial diagnosis**
  - Evaluation of primary cervical tumor
    - Generally not performed to look at primary tumor
    - However, most cervical SCCA is FDG-avid → high sensitivity for sizable lesions
    - PET/CT reliable in advanced disease
    - May help avoid unnecessary operations
    - May help with radiation therapy planning
    - Primary tumor SUV ≥ 10 associated with significantly lower 5 year disease-free survival than tumors with lower SUV (52% vs. 71%)
    - Overall survival comparable whether SUV < or > 10
- **Staging**
  - Evaluation of pelvic and para-aortic LN
    - LN detection on PET: Sensitivity 75-91%, specificity 93-100%
    - PET sensitivity for advanced disease 87%, specificity 100%

- Low sensitivity in LN < 1 cm
- Pelvic LN: Sensitivity 46%, specificity 91%
- Para-aortic LN: Sensitivity 40%, specificity 99%
- Presence or absence of para-aortic LN on PET correlates most significantly with disease-free survival
- Knowledge of para-aortic lymph node status is crucial for treatment planning
- Invasive surgery, with laparotomy or laparoscopy, has traditionally been used
  - Evaluation of distant metastases
    - In one study, ~ 8% of patients had distant supraclavicular lymphadenopathy detected only by PET
- **PET/CT**
  - Useful supplement to clinical staging procedures
    - Sensitivity of 75% and specificity of 87-96% for detection of nodal metastases in the pelvis
  - High sensitivity/specificity for newly diagnosed cervical cancer with FIGO stage IB or higher
  - Useful for planning treatment strategy
  - Histologic confirmation of results should be obtained prior to change of treatment plan
  - Can be used for biopsy guidance
- **PET/CT vs. conventional imaging for detecting metastatic lymph nodes**
  - Sensitivity 97% vs. 40%
  - Specificity 94% vs. 65%
  - PPV 97% vs. 70%
  - NPV 94% vs. 34%
- **False positives**
  - Inflammatory/infectious lesions
    - Pulmonary tuberculosis
    - Acute cholangitis
  - Physiologic uptake
    - Physiologic uptake in bowel, vessels, ureter
    - Ovarian uptake, depending on phase of cycle: Around ovulation and early luteal phase
    - Functional ovarian cysts, such as hemorrhagic corpus luteum cyst, may mimic lymph node metastases
  - Other
    - Post-operative changes
    - Benign thyroid tumor
- **False negatives**
  - Low tumor volumes
- **Restaging**
  - Sensitivity and specificity for post-therapy of patients with cervical cancer: 90-93%, 91-100%

DIFFERENTIAL DIAGNOSIS

Other Female Reproductive Tract Malignancy
- Endometrial cancer
- Ovarian cancer

Leiomyoma
- Variable FDG avidity, ranging from very minimal to intense
- Often distinguishable from cervical mass on CT portion of PET/CT

CERVICAL CARCINOMA

Physiologic FDG Activity in Female Reproductive Organs

- Menstruation: FDG activity in endometrial cavity, less frequently in vagina, associated with normal menstruation
  - Clinical history of current menstruation important
  - May need ultrasound, clinical correlation if patient not currently menstruating
- Ovaries: Benign and malignant etiologies
  - May need ultrasound to distinguish

Urine Contamination

- May need ultrasound to distinguish
- Incontinence can cause contamination of external genitalia

Endometrial Carcinoma

- Usually spares cervix, though may spread to cervix if diagnosed late
- Generally older patient population

PATHOLOGY

General Features

- General path comments
  - Glut-1: Overexpressed in cervical carcinoma, may be correlated with tumor grade
    - Absence of glut-1 correlated with improved metastasis-free survival
  - In women with LN positive cervical carcinoma, 80% of involved LN are < 1.0 cm in greatest dimension
- Etiology
  - Likely multifactorial
  - Associated with human papillomavirus (HPV) infection (strains 16, 18, 31, 33, 45)
  - Other risk factors
    - Multiple sexual partners
    - Sex before age 18
    - Tobacco use
    - Diethylstilbestrol
- Epidemiology
  - In USA: ~ 10,000 cases per year
    - ~ 1/3 die of disease
  - HPV vaccination programs widely instituted with goal of eradicating cervical cancer
  - However, cervical cancer remains an important public health problem
  - Worldwide:
    - > 300,000 cases diagnosed per year
    - 2nd most frequently diagnosed gynecologic malignancy in women
    - 50% mortality rate
  - 5 year recurrence: 28%
  - 5 year overall mortality: 27.8%

Staging, Grading, or Classification Criteria

- In contrast to other gynecologic malignancies, cervical cancer is staged clinically
- FIGO staging
  - Allows only the following diagnostic tests to be used in determining the stage

- Palpation, inspection, colposcopy, endocervical curettage, hysteroscopy, cystoscopy, proctoscopy, and intravenous urography
- X-ray examination of the lungs and skeleton, and cervical conization
  - Most important limitation: Does not provide any information about retroperitoneal lymph node status
    - Especially para-aortic nodal metastases
  - Discrepancies between FIGO staging and surgical/histopathologic findings
    - Occurs in about 30% of patients with locally advanced cervical cancer
- Clinical staging accurate in ~ 60% of patients
  - Undiagnosed lymphadenopathy is a major problem
- American Joint Committee on Cancer (AJCC) staging
  - Stage 0
    - Carcinoma in situ
  - Stage I
    - Confined to uterus
  - Stage II
    - Beyond uterus, but not to pelvic side wall, lower third of vagina
  - Stage IIIA
    - Extends to pelvic wall, lower third of vagina
    - Causes hydronephrosis/nonfunctioning kidney
    - Negative lymph nodes (LN)
  - Stage IIIB
    - Extends to pelvic wall, lower third of vagina
    - Causes hydronephrosis/nonfunctioning kidney
    - Positive LN
  - Stage IVA
    - Beyond true pelvis, bladder mucosa, rectal mucosa
    - Positive LN
  - Stage IVB
    - Distant metastases
- Pre-treatment surgical staging issues
  - Risks of laparotomy for nodal staging include
    - Bowel obstruction
    - Infection
    - Vascular damage
    - Ureteral injury
    - Fistula formation
    - Lymphocyst/lymphedema
    - Thrombophlebitis
  - Surgical staging results in treatment modification in 18-44% of patients
  - Negative sentinal lymph node biopsy accurately predicts negative status of retroperitoneal lymph nodes in early cervical cancer
    - NPV: 92-97%
  - Sentinal node biopsy has limited value in locally advanced disease due to high false negative rate
  - Many centers defer surgical staging due to high morbidity

CLINICAL ISSUES

Presentation

- Most common signs/symptoms
  - Often asymptomatic

CERVICAL CARCINOMA

- ▪ Abnormal cells typically found during a cervical screening test (Pap smear)
  - ○ Later symptoms
    - ▪ Abnormal vaginal bleeding/discharge
    - ▪ Discomfort during/after sexual intercourse
- • Other signs/symptoms: Smaller lesions often asymptomatic

Demographics

- • Age: Primarily affects younger women, although can be seen at any age

Natural History & Prognosis

- • 5 year survival
  - ○ No lymphadenopathy: 57%
  - ○ Positive pelvic lymphadenopathy: 34%
  - ○ Positive para-aortic lymphadenopathy: 12%
- • Despite advances in screening and treatment programs, mortality from cervical cancer has not decreased in the past 3 decades
- • Para-aortic lymph node metastasis is the most important prognostic factor for progression-free survival & recurrence
  - ○ Observed in about 1/3 of locally advanced cervical cancer patients
  - ○ Knowledge of para-aortic nodal status crucial for choice of ideal treatment method
  - ○ 24% of patients with FIGO stage IIB-IVA have para-aortic spreading after surgical staging at time of diagnosis

Treatment

- • Surgery or radiotherapy in early stages
  - ○ Single treatment modality preferred
- • Chemotherapy + radiotherapy in advanced stages
- • Evaluation of disseminated recurrence essential to selecting optimal therapy and avoiding unnecessary surgical intervention

DIAGNOSTIC CHECKLIST

Consider

- • PET/CT for optimal staging
- • Physical exam, MR for evaluation of primary tumor

SELECTED REFERENCES

1. Boughanim M et al: Histologic results of para-aortic lymphadenectomy in patients treated for stage IB2/II cervical cancer with negative [18F]fluorodeoxyglucose positron emission tomography scans in the para-aortic area. J Clin Oncol. 26(15):2558-61, 2008
2. Gold MA et al: Surgical versus radiographic determination of para-aortic lymph node metastases before chemoradiation for locally advanced cervical carcinoma: a Gynecologic Oncology Group Study. Cancer. 112(9):1954-63, 2008
3. Macdonald DM et al: Combined intensity-modulated radiation therapy and brachytherapy in the treatment of cervical cancer. Int J Radiat Oncol Biol Phys. 71(2):618-24, 2008
4. Selman TJ et al: Diagnostic accuracy of tests for lymph node status in primary cervical cancer: a systematic review and meta-analysis. CMAJ. 178(7):855-62, 2008
5. Beriwal S et al: Early clinical outcome with concurrent chemotherapy and extended-field, intensity-modulated radiotherapy for cervical cancer. Int J Radiat Oncol Biol Phys. 68(1):166-71, 2007
6. Chung HH et al: Clinical impact of integrated PET/CT on the management of suspected cervical cancer recurrence. Gynecol Oncol. 104(3):529-34, 2007
7. Grigsby PW: The contribution of new imaging techniques in staging cervical cancer. Gynecol Oncol. 107(1 Suppl 1):S10-2, 2007
8. Grigsby PW: The role of FDG-PET/CT imaging after radiation therapy. Gynecol Oncol. 107(1 Suppl 1):S27-9, 2007
9. Jewell EL et al: Primary surgery versus chemoradiation in the treatment of IB2 cervical carcinoma: a cost effectiveness analysis. Gynecol Oncol. 107(3):532-40, 2007
10. Kidd EA et al: The standardized uptake value for F-18 fluorodeoxyglucose is a sensitive predictive biomarker for cervical cancer treatment response and survival. Cancer. 110(8):1738-44, 2007
11. Kumar R et al: 18F-fluoro-2-deoxy-D-glucose-positron emission tomography (PET)/PET-computed tomography in carcinoma of the cervix. Cancer. 110(8):1650-3, 2007
12. Lin LL et al: Adaptive brachytherapy treatment planning for cervical cancer using FDG-PET. Int J Radiat Oncol Biol Phys. 67(1):91-6, 2007
13. Loft A et al: The diagnostic value of PET/CT scanning in patients with cervical cancer: a prospective study. Gynecol Oncol. 106(1):29-34, 2007
14. Schwarz JK et al: Association of posttherapy positron emission tomography with tumor response and survival in cervical carcinoma. JAMA. 298(19):2289-95, 2007
15. Unger JB et al: The prognostic value of pretreatment 2-[18F]-fluoro-2-deoxy-D-glucose positron emission tomography scan in women with cervical cancer. Int J Gynecol Cancer. 17(5):1062-7, 2007
16. Choi HJ et al: Comparison of the accuracy of magnetic resonance imaging and positron emission tomography/computed tomography in the presurgical detection of lymph node metastases in patients with uterine cervical carcinoma: a prospective study. Cancer. 106(4):914-22, 2006
17. Chou HH et al: Low value of [18F]-fluoro-2-deoxy-D-glucose positron emission tomography in primary staging of early-stage cervical cancer before radical hysterectomy. J Clin Oncol. 24(1):123-8, 2006
18. Grigsby PW et al: Gene expression patterns in advanced human cervical cancer. Int J Gynecol Cancer. 16(2):562-7, 2006
19. Hope AJ et al: FDG-PET in carcinoma of the uterine cervix with endometrial extension. Cancer. 106(1):196-200, 2006
20. Kumar R et al: Positron emission tomography in gynecological malignancies. Expert Rev Anticancer Ther. 6(7):1033-44, 2006
21. Sironi S et al: Lymph node metastasis in patients with clinical early-stage cervical cancer: detection with integrated FDG PET/CT. Radiology. 238(1):272-9, 2006
22. Grigsby PW et al: Lack of benefit of concurrent chemotherapy in patients with cervical cancer and negative lymph nodes by FDG-PET. Int J Radiat Oncol Biol Phys. 61(2):444-9, 2005
23. Grigsby PW: 4th International Cervical Cancer Conference: update on PET and cervical cancer. Gynecol Oncol. 99(3 Suppl 1):S173-5, 2005

CERVICAL CARCINOMA

CT Findings: Primary

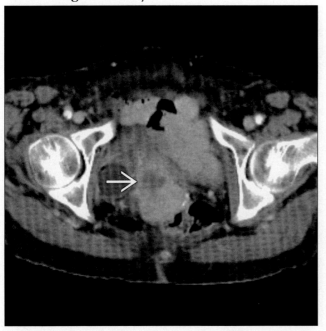
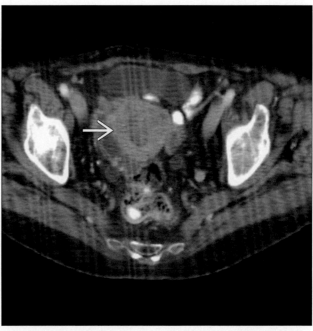

(Left) Axial CECT shows a mixed attenuation mass ⮕ that corresponds to the patient's recently diagnosed cervical carcinoma. *(Right)* Axial CECT shows a heterogeneously enhancing mass in the inferior aspect of the uterus ⮕, corresponding to the patient's recently diagnosed squamous cell carcinoma of the uterine cervix.

CT Findings: Primary with Metastases

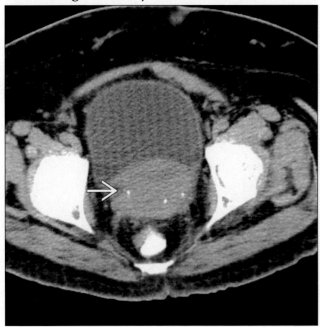
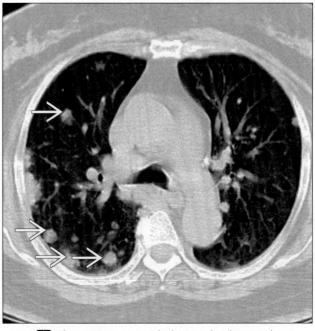

(Left) Axial CECT shows nonspecific questionable thickening of the uterine cervix ⮕. The patient was recently diagnosed with cervical carcinoma. Often the CT findings are nonspecific and may not show a definite cervical mass. *(Right)* Axial NECT shows innumerable bilateral pulmonary metastases ⮕ in a patient with stage IV cervical carcinoma.

CERVICAL CARCINOMA

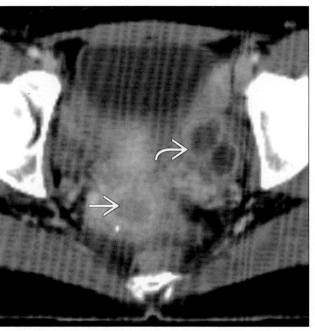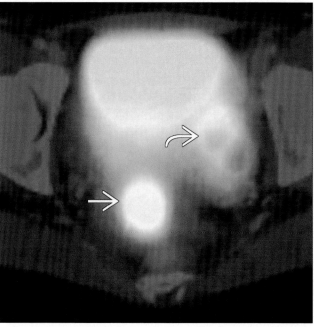

(Left) Axial CECT shows a heterogeneously enhancing cervical mass ➡, compatible with the patient's primary cervical carcinoma. In addition, there are cystic metastases involving the left adnexa ➡. *(Right)* Axial fused PET/CT shows intense FDG activity within both the primary cervical mass ➡ and the left adnexa ➡. In general, cervical carcinoma tends to be FDG avid, as are most squamous cell carcinomas throughout the body.

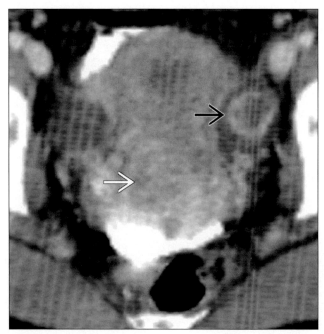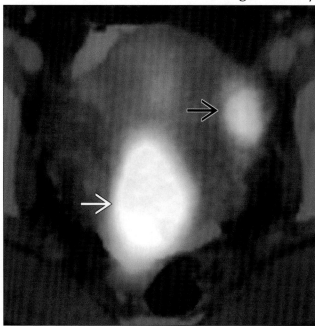

(Left) Axial CECT shows a primary cervical mass ➡ in addition to a rim-enhancing left ovarian mass ➡ in an otherwise normal-appearing ovary, suggestive of a corpus luteal cyst. *(Right)* Axial fused PET/CT shows intense FDG activity that corresponds to the primary cervical mass ➡ and moderate FDG activity that correlates with the left ovarian mass ➡. Although the differential diagnosis includes ovarian metastasis, the appearance is most compatible with a normal corpus luteum cyst, which was proven by laparoscopic excision and pathologic evaluation.

CERVICAL CARCINOMA

PET/CT Findings: Staging

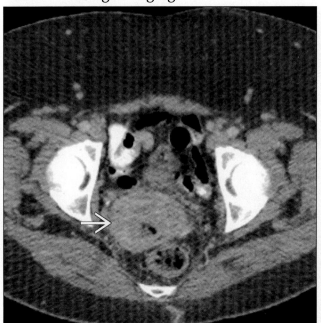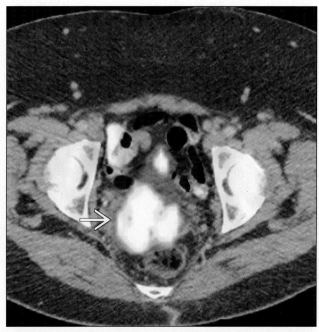

(Left) Axial NECT shows prominent cervical soft tissue ➔ in this patient with diagnosed cervical carcinoma. *(Right)* Axial fused PET/CT shows intense FDG activity within the patient's primary cervical mass ➔, compatible with cervical carcinoma.

PET/CT Findings: Staging

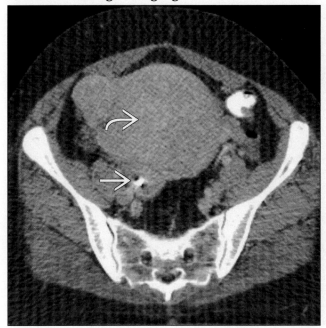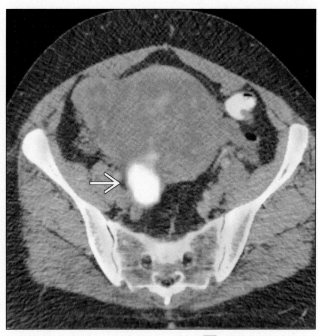

(Left) Axial CECT shows an enlarged fibroid uterus ➔ in addition to a cervical mass with a stent within the cervical os ➔. *(Right)* Axial fused PET/CT shows intense FDG activity in the area of the cervical mass ➔, compatible with primary cervical carcinoma.

CERVICAL CARCINOMA

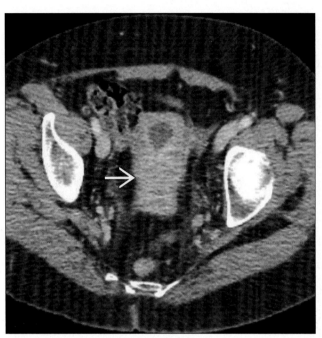 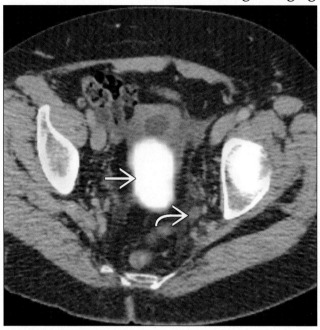

(Left) Axial CECT shows irregular thickening in the area of the cervix ➡, compatible with patient's history of recently diagnosed cervical cancer. *(Right)* Axial fused PET/CT shows focal intense activity within the cervix ➡, corresponding to the patient's cervical carcinoma. In addition, there is a small 5 to 6 mm left pelvic lymph node with mild FDG activity ➡, compatible with malignancy. The FDG activity within the lymph node is underestimated due to partial volume averaging.

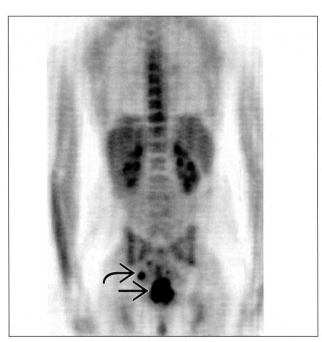 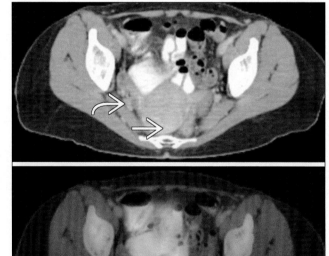

(Left) Coronal PET shows a large area of intense FDG activity in the pelvis ➡, which correlates with the patient's primary cervical carcinoma. An unsuspected right pelvic lymph node was also identified ➡. *(Right)* Axial CT (top) and fused PET/CT (bottom) images demonstrate focal intense activity within the patient's primary cervical carcinoma ➡, in addition to focal activity within a suspected pelvic lymph node immediately adjacent to the cervix ➡.

CERVICAL CARCINOMA

PET/CT Findings: Staging

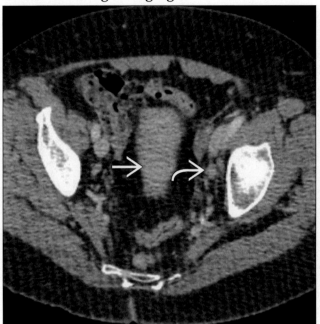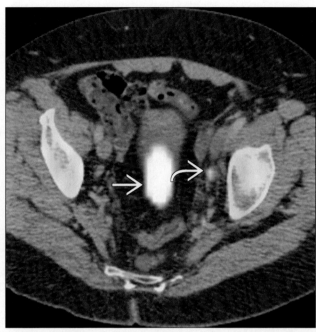

(Left) Axial CECT shows no definite cervical thickening or mass in the area of the cervix ➡. However, a borderline enlarged left external iliac lymph node is noted ➡. *(Right)* Axial fused PET/CT shows intense FDG activity in the area of the cervix ➡, corresponding to the patient's primary cervical carcinoma. In addition, intense activity within the questionable left-sided pelvic lymph node ➡ confirms metastatic disease.

PET/CT Findings: Staging

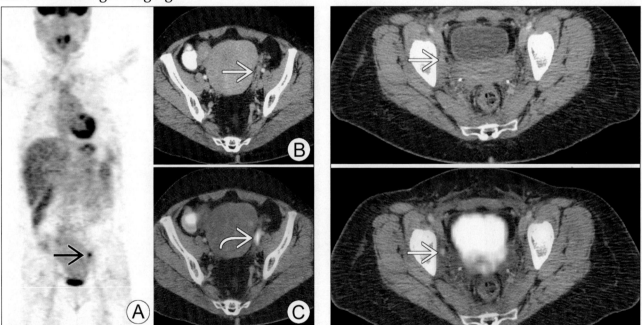

(Left) PET/CT (A) performed for restaging demonstrated a focal area of intense FDG activity ➡, which raised the suspicion for metastatic disease to the pelvic lymph nodes. While the CT portion of the exam (B) demonstrates normal-sized pelvic lymph nodes ➡, the fused PET/ CT (C) shows hypermetabolism ➡, suggesting metastases. *(Right)* Axial CT (top) and fused PET/CT (bottom) images show a tiny lymph node measuring approximately 4 to 5 mm ➡ in this patient with newly diagnosed cervical carcinoma. The lymph nodes were found to be malignant during surgery.

CERVICAL CARCINOMA

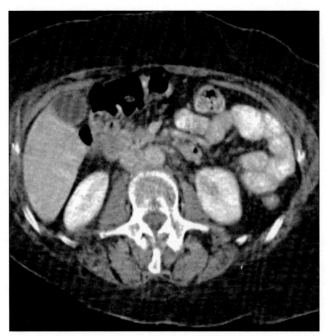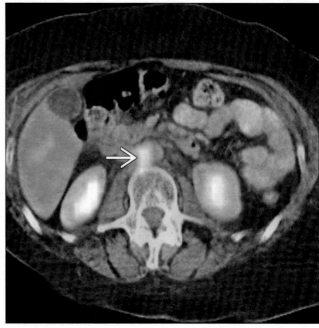

(Left) Axial CECT shows no definite evidence for metastatic disease. *(Right)* Axial fused PET/CT shows intense FDG activity in the aortocaval region, corresponding to a small lymph node ➡ not identified on the CT portion of the exam.

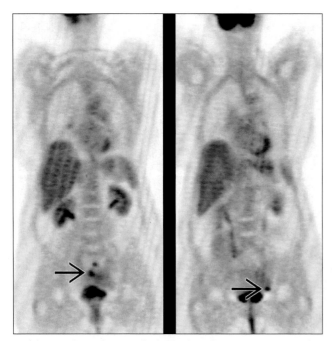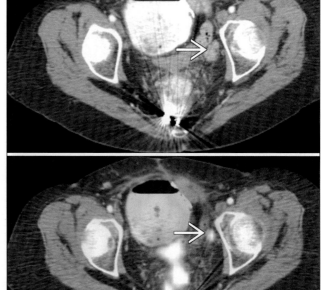

(Left) Coronal PET shows multiple tiny foci of intense activity correlating with unsuspected pelvic lymph nodes ➡ in this patient with newly diagnosed cervical carcinoma. *(Right)* Axial CT (top) and fused PET/CT (bottom) images show a borderline enlarged left external iliac lymph node with intense FDG activity ➡, compatible with malignancy.

CERVICAL CARCINOMA

PET/CT Findings: Staging

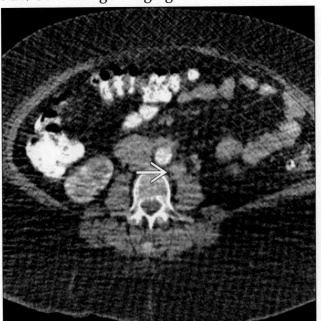 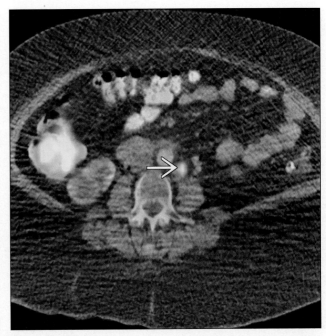

(Left) Axial CECT shows borderline enlarged left periaortic lymph nodes ➡ in this patient with newly diagnosed cervical carcinoma. *(Right)* Axial fused PET/CT shows intense focal activity correlating with the questionable lymph node in the left periaortic area ➡, confirming malignancy.

PET/CT Findings: Staging

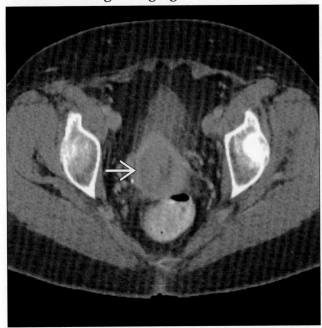 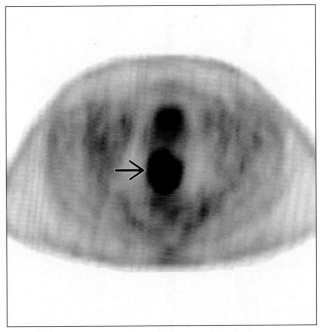

(Left) Axial CECT shows a partially cystic mass in the region of the uterine cervix ➡ in this patient with newly diagnosed cervical carcinoma. *(Right)* Axial PET shows focal intense FDG activity correlating with the cervical mass ➡. Most squamous cell carcinomas of the uterine cervix tend to be FDG avid.

CERVICAL CARCINOMA

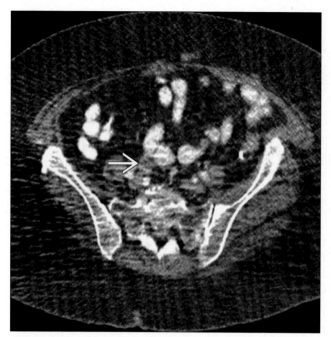 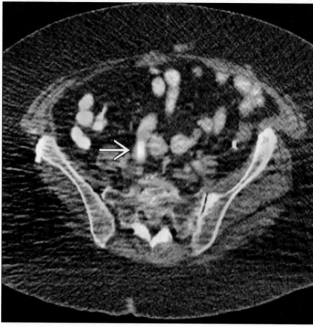

(Left) Axial CECT shows the opacification of small bowel with a soft tissue lesion of uncertain etiology adjacent to a loop of small bowel ➡. *(Right)* Axial fused PET/CT shows focal intense FDG activity corresponding to the soft tissue lesion ➡, which confirms metastatic disease in this patient with newly diagnosed cervical carcinoma.

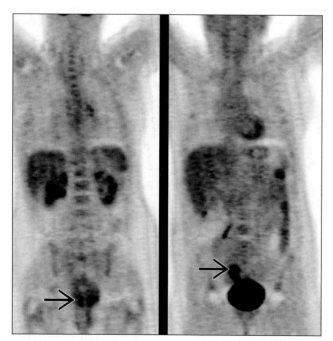 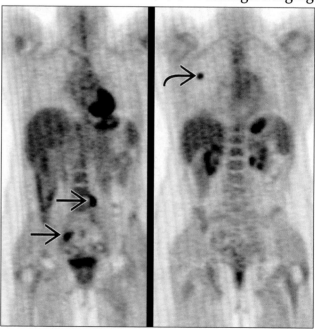

(Left) Coronal PET shows intense activity superior to the urinary bladder ➡ that corresponds to the patient's recently diagnosed cervical carcinoma. *(Right)* Coronal PET shows 3 metastatic lesions, 2 in the retroperitoneal area ➡ and 1 in the right lung ➡ in this patient with stage IV cervical carcinoma.

CERVICAL CARCINOMA

PET/CT Findings: Staging

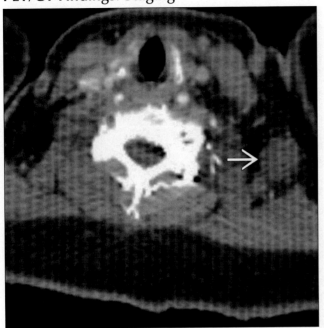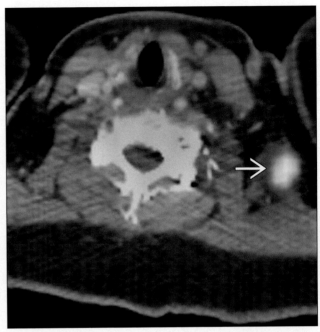

(Left) Axial NECT shows an enlarged left supraclavicular lymph node ➡ in this patient with newly diagnosed cervical cancer. *(Right)* Axial fused PET/CT shows intense activity within the enlarged left supraclavicular lymph node ➡, compatible with malignancy.

PET/CT Findings: Staging

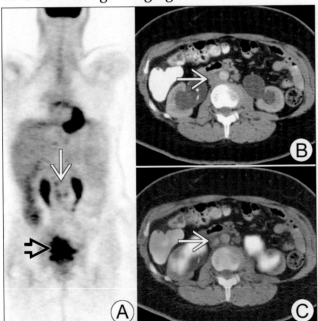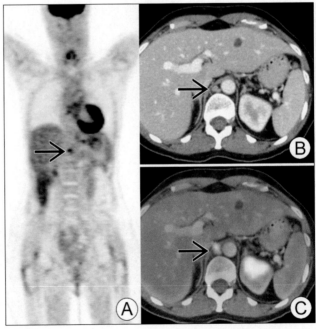

(Left) Coronal PET (A), axial CT (B) and fused PET/CT (C) images demonstrate a large area of intense activity within the pelvis ➡, compatible with the patient's primary cervical carcinoma. In addition, multiple small aortocaval and left periaortic lymph nodes showing moderate FDG avidity ➡ were identified on this patient's staging PET/CT examination. *(Right)* Coronal PET (A), axial CT (B) and fused PET/CT (C) demonstrate subtle focal intense activity in the right retrocrural area ➡, corresponding to a small malignant lymph node on this staging PET/CT examination.

CERVICAL CARCINOMA

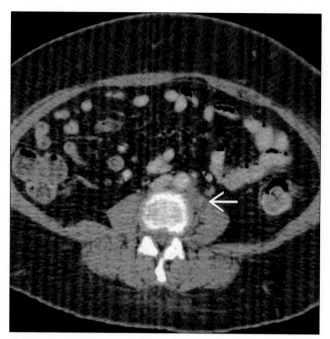 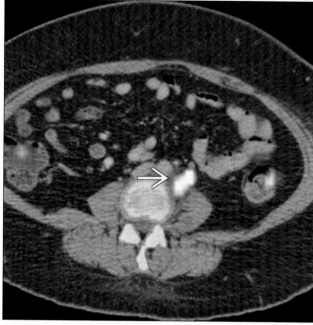

(Left) Axial CECT prospectively interpreted as negative for malignancy shows some subtle soft tissue in the left para-aortic area ➡. *(Right)* Axial fused PET/CT shows intense FDG uptake within the para-aortic soft tissue ➡, confirming malignancy.

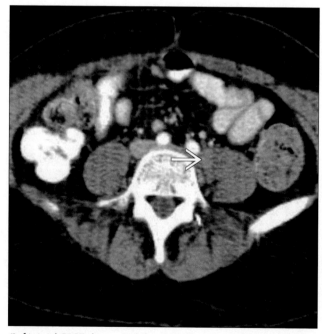 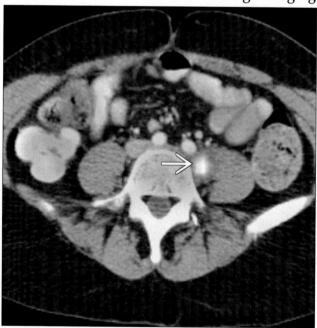

(Left) Axial CECT shows a subtle minimally enhancing lesion adjacent to the left psoas muscle ➡ not identified prospectively. *(Right)* Axial fused PET/CT shows intense activity ➡ correlating with the questionable area on CT, confirming metastatic disease in this patient with a history of cervical cancer.

CERVICAL CARCINOMA

PET/CT Findings: Staging

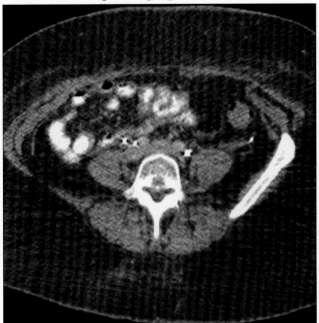 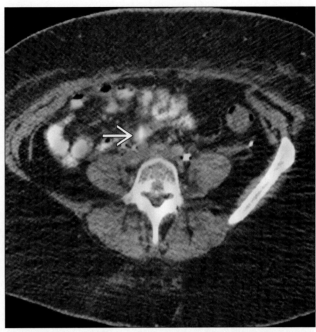

(Left) Axial NECT shows no definite evidence for malignancy within the abdomen or pelvis. *(Right)* Axial fused PET/CT shows focal intense activity within a small retroperitoneal lymph node ➡, not identified on the CT portion of the exam but compatible with malignancy.

PET/CT Findings: Staging

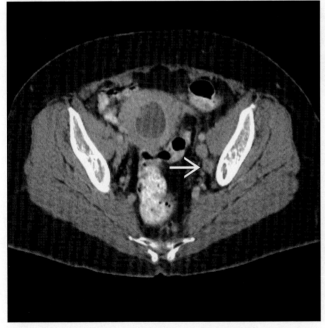 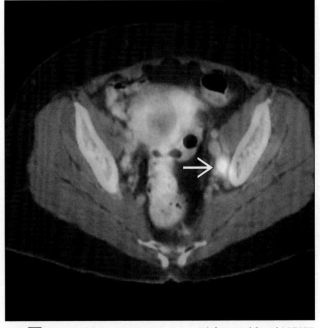

(Left) Axial CECT shows a borderline enlarged left pelvic side wall lymph node ➡ equivocal for regional metastases. *(Right)* Axial fused PET/CT shows focal intense FDG activity correlating with the equivocal left pelvic side wall lymph node ➡, compatible with metastatic disease.

CERVICAL CARCINOMA

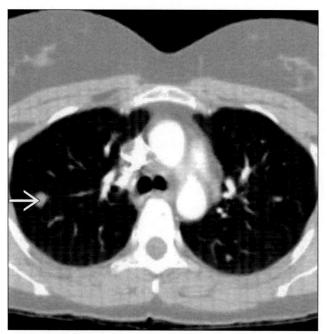 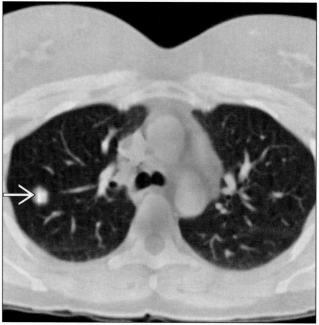

(Left) Axial CECT shows an unsuspected right upper lobe well-rounded pulmonary nodule ➡ in this patient without a history of a pulmonary nodule but with recently diagnosed cervical cancer. *(Right)* Axial fused PET/CT shows intense activity correlating with the right upper lobe pulmonary nodule ➡, compatible with lung metastases from cervical cancer.

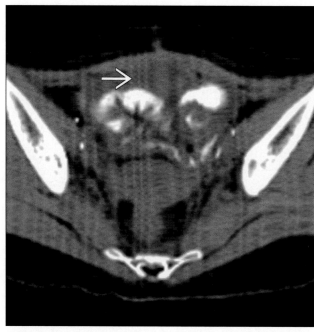 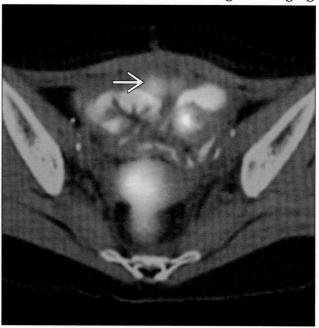

(Left) Axial NECT with good opacification of the small bowel shows a thick rind of tissue ➡ anterior to the bowel, representing metastatic disease in this patient with cervical carcinoma. *(Right)* Axial fused PET/CT shows moderate FDG activity corresponding to the soft tissue ➡, compatible with metastatic disease.

CERVICAL CARCINOMA

PET/CT Findings: Restaging

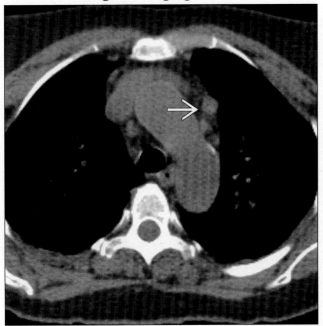 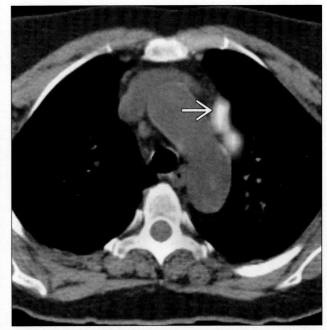

(Left) Axial NECT shows prominent prevascular lymph nodes of uncertain clinical significance ➡ in this patient with newly diagnosed cervical cancer. (Right) Axial fused PET/CT shows intense activity within the prevascular lymphadenopathy ➡, compatible with metastatic disease.

PET/CT Findings: Restaging

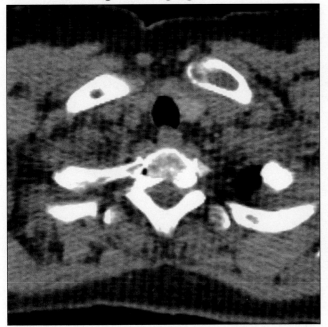 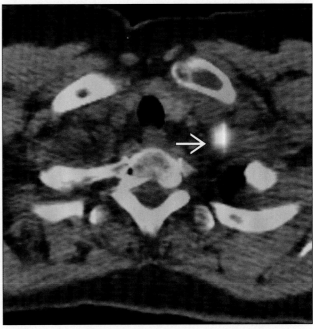

(Left) Axial NECT was originally interpreted as negative for metastatic disease in the neck or chest. (Right) Axial fused PET/CT in the same patient shows focal intense activity correlating with a small left supraclavicular lymph node ➡, compatible with metastatic disease.

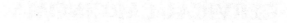

SECTION 3
Emerging Clinical Applications of PET/CT

NEUROENDOCRINE TUMORS

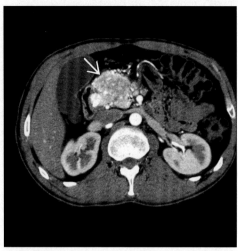

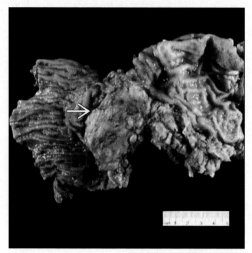

Axial CECT shows a hypervascular mass on arterial phase in the pancreatic head →. The location and hypervascularity are characteristic of a neuroendocrine tumor.

Gross pathology specimen shows the mass ➡ following surgical resection.

TERMINOLOGY

Abbreviations and Synonyms

- Neuroendocrine tumor (NET)
- Small cell undifferentiated carcinoma
- Neoplasm of the endocrine pancreas (NEP)
- Pancreatic islet cell tumor
  - Also known as amine precursor uptake and decarboxylation (APUD) cells

Definitions

- Heterogeneous group of tumors of neuroendocrine origin
- Islet cell tumors include
  - Insulinoma
  - Glucagonoma
  - Gastrinoma
  - VIPoma
  - Somatostatinoma

IMAGING FINDINGS

General Features

- Best diagnostic clue
  - Aggressive neuroendocrine tumors generally demonstrate hypervascularity
    - Look for hypervascular lesions in pancreas, liver, &/or bowel
- Location
  - Many gastrinomas and somatostatinomas are found close to, but not within, the pancreatic parenchyma
    - Suggests possible extrapancreatic development
  - **Extrapancreatic locations**
    - Duodenum
    - Stomach
    - Lymph nodes
    - Ovaries
- Size
  - Large tumors, independent of functional status, are generally highly malignant
    - Look for calcification and local invasion
    - Liver metastases often arise secondary to early portal vein invasion

---

DDx: Malignant Liver Lesion on PET/CT

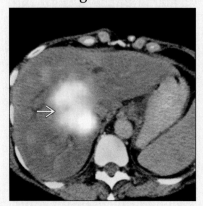

Cholangiocarcinoma

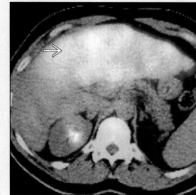

Hepatocellular Carcinoma

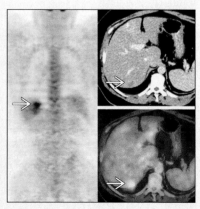

Metastasis

NEUROENDOCRINE TUMORS

Key Facts

Terminology
- Neuroendocrine tumor (NET), small cell undifferentiated carcinoma
- Pancreatic islet cell tumor; neoplasm of the endocrine pancreas (NEP)
- Heterogeneous group of tumors of neuroendocrine origin

Imaging Findings
- High-resolution image through pancreas to localize and stage most NEPs
  - May still fail to identify as many as 70% of these lesions
- CT scan with contrast or PET/CT with contrast
- FDG PET tends to have variable degrees of success with NET due to variability in FDG uptake

- CECT: Variable enhancement in arterial and portal venous phases
  - Typically intense arterial phase enhancement is observed
  - Useful to identify tumors characterized by rapid growth or aggressive behavior
- FDG PET mainly useful with poorly differentiated neuroendocrine tumors

Top Differential Diagnoses
- Metastatic Disease
- Lymphoma
- Sarcoma
- Pancreatic Adenocarcinoma

Diagnostic Checklist
- Contrast-enhanced CT or FDG PET/CT

- Range in size from a few millimeters to several centimeters
  - Average size ≤ 2 cm
  - Patients generally symptomatic with small primary lesions
- Lymphadenopathy ranges in size from 1-11 cm, average 4 cm
- Morphology
  - Generally start as well-rounded areas of hyperenhancement
    - Seen best on hepatic arterial phase of imaging
    - May not be identifiable on portal venous and noncontrast phases

Imaging Recommendations
- Best imaging tool
  - CT with contrast or PET/CT with contrast
    - More helpful if a hepatic arterial phase is included
  - FDG PET tends to have variable degrees of success with NET
    - Due to variability in FDG uptake
- Protocol advice: IV contrast for CT; arms down for PET or PET/CT
- Additional nuclear medicine imaging options
  - Octreotide probably best test
    - In conjunction with CT or PET/CT for non-head and non-neck neuroendocrine tumors

CT Findings
- 70% of NEP lesions may go undetected, even with high-resolution CT through pancreas
- NECT
  - Masses have mixed hyper- and isodensity (compared to normal pancreas)
  - Cystic and necrotic areas seen in larger non-insulin and nonfunctioning tumors
  - Smaller lesions often undetectable
  - Variable calcification
  - Marked edema of the stromal tissue may be appreciated separating nests of endocrine cells
  - Nonfunctioning tumors usually
    - Larger

- More complex internal architecture
- More calcification
- CECT
  - 90% are hypervascular and hyperintense on arterial phase
  - Cystic and necrotic areas hypodense
  - Liver and nodal metastases enhance on arterial phase
  - Insulinoma shows solid or ring enhancement on delayed scan
  - Nonfunctioning liver metastases may be extensive in asymptomatic patient

Nuclear Medicine Findings
- FDG may show variability
  - Some NET may show very little FDG activity (falsely negative)
    - Metastatic lesions may show photopenia compared to background normal activity
  - F-DOPA PET also shows some variability in uptake
- FDG PET mainly useful with poorly differentiated neuroendocrine tumors
  - Useful to identify tumors characterized by rapid growth or aggressive behavior
  - FDG uptake may be related to worse prognosis
  - Contributes to improved staging of advanced disease
  - FDG PET should be reserved for patients with negative results on somatostatin-receptor scintigraphy
- Somatostatin-receptor scintigraphy
  - NEP expresses many active somatostatin receptors on lipid membrane
    - With exception of somatostatinomas
  - Radiolabeled somatostatin-analog octreotide is used as radiotracer
  - Low resolution for exact localization of primary
  - Useful for identification of metastases

DIFFERENTIAL DIAGNOSIS

Pancreatic Adenocarcinoma
- Usually associated with jaundice

3

NEUROENDOCRINE TUMORS

- CT findings helpful
  - Obstructive ductal enlargement in pancreatic carcinoma demonstrated on imaging
  - Pancreatic adenocarcinomas are often poorly marginated infiltrative tumor vs. well-demarcated margins with NEP
  - Retropancreatic fat is obliterated
  - NEP hypervascular vs. hypovascular pancreatic adenocarcinoma

Mucinous Cystic Tumor of Pancreas
- Multiloculated hypodense mass with enhancement of thin internal septa and wall
- Difficult to distinguish from cystic/necrotic islet cell tumor
- Most common in tail of pancreas

Serous Cystadenoma
- Benign cystadenoma of pancreas
- Most common in head of pancreas
- Glycogen-rich tumor with honeycomb or sponge appearance
- Enhancing septations delineate small cysts

Metastatic Disease
- Hypervascular metastases to pancreas are rare but can occur
  - Caused by renal cell carcinoma, leiomyosarcoma, melanoma, carcinoid, thyroid carcinoma, and angiosarcoma
- Round, well-defined hypervascular lesions indistinguishable from islet cell tumor metastases

Lymphoma
- Primary or secondary lymphoma may occur in pancreas
- Large homogeneous hypovascular mass, infrequently with cystic areas
- Secondary lymphoma demonstrates peripancreatic lymphadenopathy with displacement of vessels

Sarcoma
- Rare in pancreas
- Primary sarcomas are occasionally hypervascular

PATHOLOGY

General Features
- General path comments: Neoplasms of the endocrine pancreas are classified as functional and nonfunctional subtypes
- Genetics
  - Clonal chromosomal abnormalities have been identified in pancreatic endocrine tumors
  - Related to MEN1 and von Hippel-Lindau syndromes
- Etiology
  - No clear etiologic environmental factors
  - Idiopathic or iatrogenic immunosuppression has been implicated
- Epidemiology
  - Solitary NEP, without personal or family history, is rare
  - NEP associated with MEN1syndrome more common

- Autosomal dominant inheritance
- 80% have one or more pancreatic neoplasms in lifetime
- Gastrinoma and insulinoma most common
  - Overall annual incidence of NEP: 3-10 cases per 1,000,000
    - Prevalence in nonselected autopsy specimens: 0.5-1.5%
    - Indicates indolent nature of tumors
  - Insulinoma and gastrinoma occur with roughly equal annual incidence
  - Nonfunctional tumors account for 14-48% of all recognized neoplasms of endocrine pancreas
  - VIPoma are 1/8 as common and glucagonoma 1/17 as common as insulinoma
  - Somatostatinoma more rare
  - 15-25% of patients with APUDomas have MEN1
  - Patients with NEP account for less than 2% of cases of pancreatic cancer in USA
- Associated abnormalities
  - Variety of syndromes
    - Zollinger-Ellison syndrome with gastrinoma
    - Insulinoma syndrome
    - Verner-Morrison syndrome (VIPoma)
    - Glucagonoma syndrome
    - Somatostatinoma syndrome

Gross Pathologic & Surgical Features
- Firm, encapsulated tumor
- May develop calcifications and cystic or necrotic areas when large

Microscopic Features
- APUD cells contain enzyme neuron-specific enolase
  - Universal marker for hyperplasia and neoplasia of such cells
- All neuroendocrine tumor cells appear similar under light microscopy
- Benign and malignant cells are generally indistinguishable
  - Histologic staging depends on invasion

Staging, Grading, or Classification Criteria
- Three major divisions for staging involve number and location of tumor
  - Solitary intraparenchymal lesions
  - Multiple intraparenchymal lesions
  - Spread beyond pancreas to lymph nodes or distant sites

CLINICAL ISSUES

Presentation
- Most common signs/symptoms
  - **Insulinoma**
    - Symptoms related to hypoglycemia and compensatory catecholamine excess
  - **ZE syndrome**
    - Hypersecretion of gastric acid leading to peptic ulcers refractory to medical/surgical therapy
  - **VIPoma**
    - Watery diarrhea, weakness related to hypokalemia
  - **Glucagonoma**

NEUROENDOCRINE TUMORS

- ▪ Dermatitis, stomatitis, weight loss, anemia
  - **Somatostatinoma**
    - ▪ Gallstones, steatorrhea, diabetes mellitus-like symptoms
  - Patients with nonfunctioning tumors present later with mass effect
- Other signs/symptoms: Pain may be secondary symptom

Demographics
- Age
  - Sporadic NEP age 30-50 years
  - MEN1-related NEP age 10-30 years
- Gender: Slightly higher incidence of NEP in women (except gastrinoma)
- Ethnicity: No racial differences in NEP

Natural History & Prognosis
- **Prognosis**
  - Insulinoma > gastrinoma
  - Major factor is presence of liver metastases
  - Invasion of regional lymph nodes does not ↑ stage
  - Usually poor for patients with MEN1, as islet cell tumors in this group are often multiple and malignant
  - Patients with nonfunctional tumors present later, with correspondingly poorer survival
- In many patients with NEP, metastases progress slowly
  - Watchful waiting is often advocated for nonsecreting liver metastases
  - Many of these patients may die of causes unrelated to tumor

Treatment
- Initial treatment aimed at stabilizing patients with endocrine syndrome for pre-operative evaluation
  - Long-acting octreotide works for all but somatostatinoma
- Surgery involves local excision for small tumors distant from the duct
  - Pancreatectomy for more advanced disease
  - Excision of primary tumor and hepatic metastases may provide long-term cure
  - More often curative for insulinoma than gastrinoma

DIAGNOSTIC CHECKLIST

Consider
- Correlate with clinical/biochemical profile
- Contrast-enhanced CT or FDG PET/CT in conjunction with octreotide study are likely best diagnostic tests
  - Small tumors may not be visualized unless an arterial phase CECT is performed
- Baseline PET/CT will also establish inherent FDG activity of the lesions
  - If non-FDG-avid, likely no future benefit in using PET/CT

SELECTED REFERENCES

1. Alexakis N et al: Pancreatic neuroendocrine tumours. Best Pract Res Clin Gastroenterol. 22(1):183-205, 2008
2. Baum RP et al: Receptor PET/CT imaging of neuroendocrine tumors. Recent Results Cancer Res. 170:225-42, 2008
3. Gustafsson BI et al: Neuroendocrine tumors of the diffuse neuroendocrine system. Curr Opin Oncol. 20(1):1-12, 2008
4. Kayani I et al: Functional imaging of neuroendocrine tumors with combined PET/CT using (68)Ga-DOTATATE (DOTA-DPhe(1),Tyr(3)-octreotate) and (18)F-FDG. Cancer. 112(11):2447-55, 2008
5. Song YS et al: Correlation between FDG uptake and glucose transporter type 1 expression in neuroendocrine tumors of the lung. Lung Cancer. 61(1):54-60, 2008
6. Chong S et al: Integrated PET/CT of pulmonary neuroendocrine tumors: diagnostic and prognostic implications. AJR Am J Roentgenol. 188(5):1223-31, 2007
7. Chong S et al: Spectrum of findings and usefulness of integrated PET/CT in patients with known or suspected neuroendocrine tumors of the lung. Cancer Imaging. 7:195-201, 2007
8. Cwikla JB et al: Diagnostic imaging approach to gastro-entero-pancreatic carcinomas of neuroendocrine origin - single NET center experience in Poland. Neuro Endocrinol Lett. 28(6):789-800, 2007
9. Howman-Giles R et al: Neuroblastoma and other neuroendocrine tumors. Semin Nucl Med. 37(4):286-302, 2007
10. Pfannenberg AC et al: Value of contrast-enhanced multiphase CT in combined PET/CT protocols for oncological imaging. Br J Radiol. 80(954):437-45, 2007
11. Seemann MD: Detection of metastases from gastrointestinal neuroendocrine tumors: prospective comparison of 18F-TOCA PET, triple-phase CT, and PET/CT. Technol Cancer Res Treat. 6(3):213-20, 2007
12. Sundin A et al: Nuclear imaging of neuroendocrine tumours. Best Pract Res Clin Endocrinol Metab. 21(1):69-85, 2007
13. Tamm EP et al: Imaging of neuroendocrine tumors. Hematol Oncol Clin North Am. 21(3):409-32; vii, 2007
14. von Falck C et al: Neuroendocrine tumour of the mediastinum: fusion of 18F-FDG and 68Ga-DOTATOC PET/CT datasets demonstrates different degrees of differentiation. Eur J Nucl Med Mol Imaging. 34(5):812, 2007
15. Junik R et al: The role of positron emission tomography (PET) in diagnostics of gastroenteropancreatic neuroendocrine tumours (GEP NET). Adv Med Sci. 51:66-8, 2006
16. Melen-Mucha G et al: The place of somatostatin analogs in the diagnosis and treatment of the neuoroendocrine glands tumors. Recent Patents Anticancer Drug Discov. 1(2):237-54, 2006
17. Mottaghy FM et al: Functional imaging of neuroendocrine tumours with PET. Pituitary. 9(3):237-42, 2006
18. Niederhuber JE et al: Treatment of metastatic disease in patients with neuroendocrine tumors. Surg Oncol Clin N Am. 15(3):511-33, viii, 2006
19. Oberg K: Molecular imaging in diagnosis of neuroendocrine tumours. Lancet Oncol. 7(10):790-2, 2006
20. Rufini V et al: Imaging of neuroendocrine tumors. Semin Nucl Med. 36(3):228-47, 2006

3

NEUROENDOCRINE TUMORS

CT Findings: Neuroendocrine Tumor

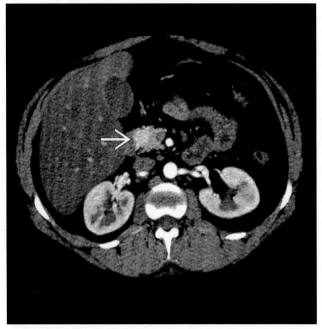 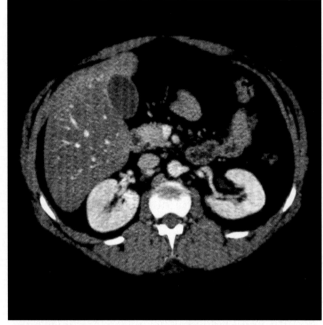

(Left) Axial CECT shows a small hypervascular mass in the pancreatic head ➡, consistent with an insulinoma. *(Right)* Axial CECT of the same patient as previous image, during the portal venous phase of imaging, reveals that the hypervascular tumor is no longer evident.

CT Findings: Neuroendocrine Tumor

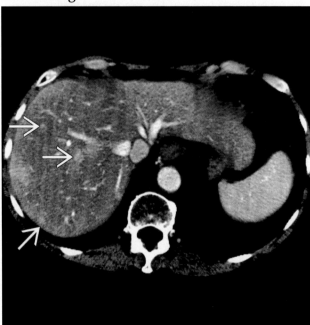 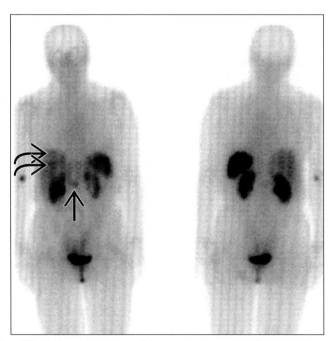

(Left) Axial CECT shows several scattered hypervascular foci within the liver ➡ in this same patient with known insulinoma. *(Right)* Coronal octreotide scan shows a focal area of moderate activity, correlating with the primary pancreatic lesion ➡, in addition to several foci of activity correlating with the hepatic metastases ➡.

NEUROENDOCRINE TUMORS

CT Findings: Neuroendocrine Tumor

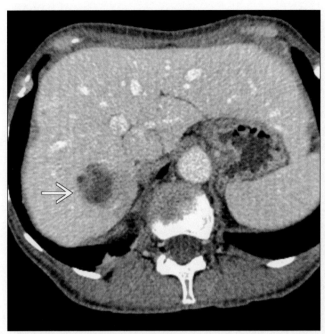

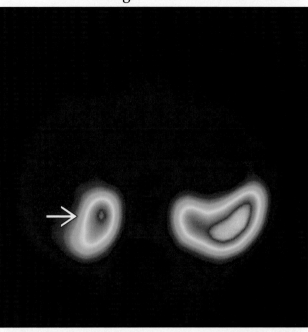

(Left) Axial CECT during the portal venous phase of imaging shows a hepatic metastasis with variable contrast enhancement and questionable peripheral nodular enhancement ➡ in this patient with known neuroendocrine neoplasm. *(Right)* Axial octreotide scan shows intense activity in the hepatic lesion ➡, confirming this to be a neuroendocrine metastasis rather than a hemangioma.

CT Findings: Neuroendocrine Tumor

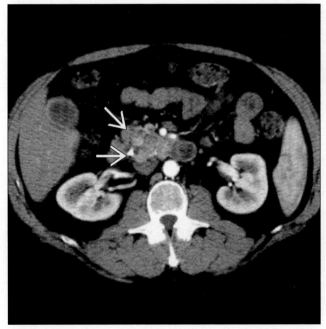

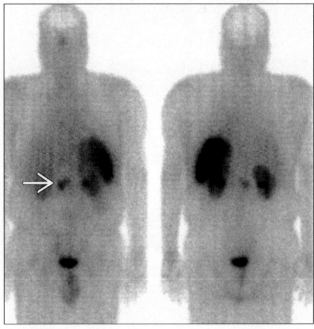

(Left) Axial CECT shows at least two hypervascular lesions in the pancreatic head ➡, consistent with multifocal insulinoma. *(Right)* Coronal octreotide scan shows foci of increased radiotracer activity correlating to the pancreatic lesions ➡.

NEUROENDOCRINE TUMORS

CT Findings: Neuroendocrine Tumor

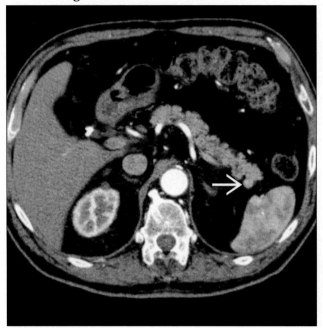 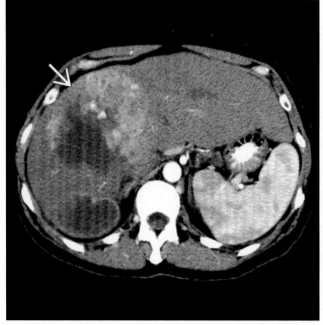

(Left) Axial CECT shows a tiny hypervascular lesion ➡ in the tail of the pancreas, subsequently confirmed to be a VIPoma. *(Right)* Axial CECT shows a heterogeneously enhancing mass with necrosis and areas of hypervascularity ➡, consistent with a metastatic lesion from a neuroendocrine primary.

CT Findings: Neuroendocrine Tumor

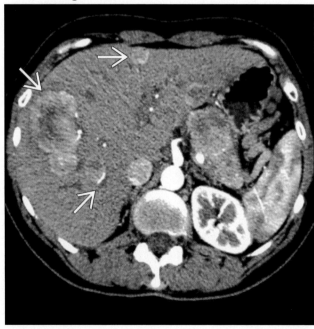 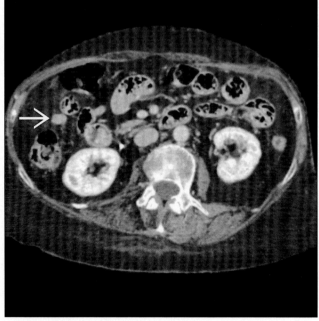

(Left) Axial CECT shows several hypervascular hepatic metastases ➡ in a patient with a known insulinoma. *(Right)* Axial CECT shows a small mesenteric hypervascular lesion ➡, consistent with a metastatic lesion from a glucagonoma.

NEUROENDOCRINE TUMORS

CT Findings: Neuroendocrine Tumor

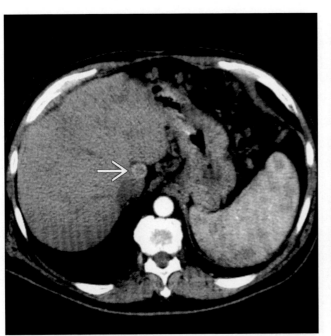 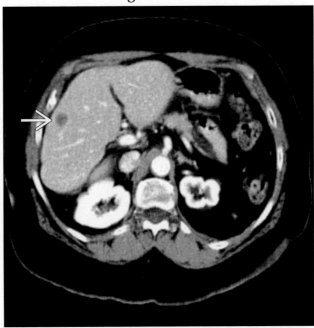

(Left) Axial CECT shows a small caudate lesion with continuous rim enhancement ➡, consistent with a neuroendocrine metastasis. Liver lesions with continuous rim enhancement have a limited differential, including metastasis or abscess. Pyogenic abscesses tend to have a multiloculated appearance. *(Right)* Axial CECT shows a hepatic metastasis in the right lobe of the liver ➡.

PET/CT Findings: Neuroendocrine Tumor

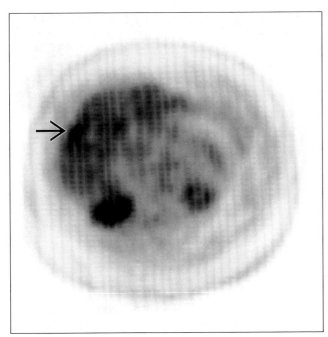 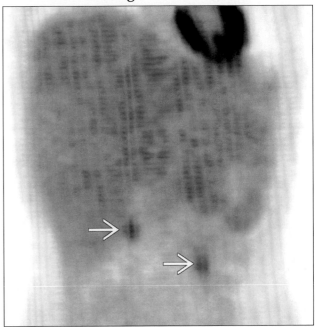

(Left) Axial PET shows the same metastasis with moderate to intense FDG activity ➡. *(Right)* Coronal PET shows no areas of focal FDG activity in this patient with a history of a neuroendocrine tumor. Note the foci of FDG activity within the ureters bilaterally ➡.

NEUROENDOCRINE TUMORS

PET/CT Findings: Neuroendocrine Tumor

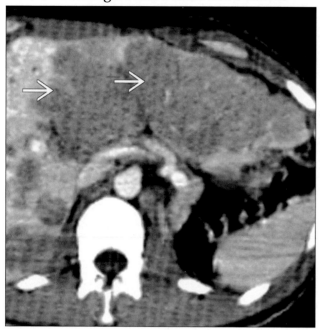
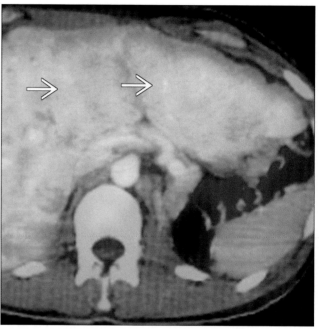

(Left) Axial CECT shows diffuse, infiltrative tumor throughout the left hepatic lobe and smaller lesions in the right hepatic lobe ➡ in this patient with a history of neuroendocrine tumor. Neuroendocrine tumors commonly invade the portal vein and often metastasize to the liver. *(Right)* Axial fused PET/CT shows mild increased FDG activity relative to the background liver ➡, a common finding with neuroendocrine tumors.

PET/CT Findings: Neuroendocrine Tumor

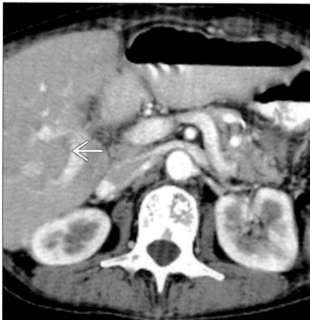
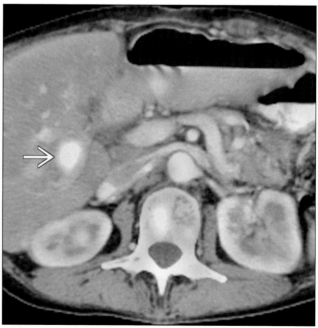

(Left) Axial CECT shows no definite lesion, or perhaps a very subtle lesion ➡, displacing portal venous branches. *(Right)* Axial fused PET/CT in the same patient as the previous image confirms the presence of a hypermetabolic metastasis ➡.

NEUROENDOCRINE TUMORS

PET/CT Findings: Neuroendocrine Tumor

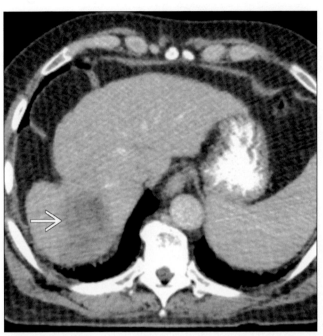 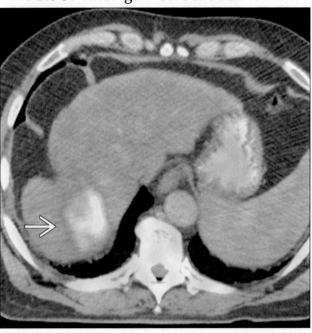

(Left) Axial CECT shows a large posterior right hepatic lobe metastasis ➜ in this patient with a history of neuroendocrine tumor. *(Right)* Axial fused PET/CT shows moderately increased metabolic activity in this lesion ➜.

PET/CT Findings: Neuroendocrine Tumor

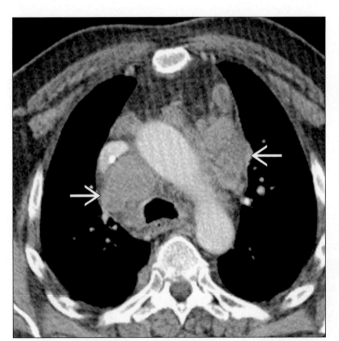 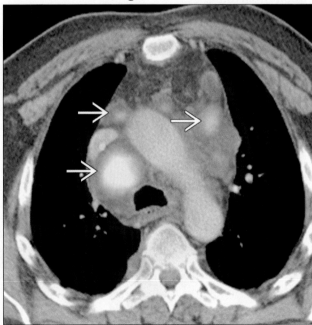

(Left) Axial CECT shows bulky mediastinal adenopathy ➜ with areas of necrosis. *(Right)* Axial fused PET/CT in the same patient as the previous image shows the metastatic nodes to be variably hypermetabolic ➜.

PRIMARY BONE NEOPLASMS

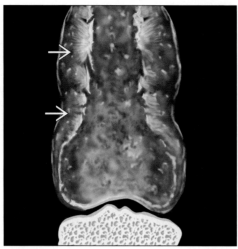

Graphic shows the typical appearance of a primary sarcoma of the femur ➡.

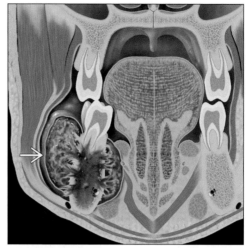

Coronal graphic shows the typical appearance of a mandibular osteosarcoma ➡.

TERMINOLOGY

Abbreviations and Synonyms
- Chondrosarcoma
- Ewing sarcoma
- Osteogenic sarcoma, osteosarcoma, primary bone sarcoma

Definitions
- **Chondrosarcoma**
  - Primary malignant tumor of bone
  - Produces hyaline cartilage leading to abnormal cartilage &/or bone
- **Ewing sarcoma**
  - Primary malignant tumor of bone
- **Osteosarcoma**
  - Primary malignant tumor of bone
  - Contains osteoid with osteoblastic differentiation

IMAGING FINDINGS

General Features
- Best diagnostic clue

- o **Chondrosarcoma**
  - Mass with variable chondroid matrix
  - May have cortical disruption &/or soft tissue extension
  - FDG uptake tends to correlate with tumor grade
- o **Ewing sarcoma**
  - Permeative appearance ± extraosseous large soft tissue component adjacent to bone
- o **Osteosarcoma**
  - Heterogeneous metaphyseal mass
  - Increased FDG uptake with high grade osteosarcoma
  - May have characteristic starburst appearance
- Location
  - o **Chondrosarcoma**
    - Most common areas: Pelvis, femur, and humerus
    - Mostly in proximal aspect of long bones
    - Peripheral, periosteal, or central intraosseous locations
  - o **Ewing sarcoma**
    - Most common in metaphysis or diaphysis of long bones
    - May arise in any bone
  - o **Osteosarcoma**

DDx: FDG Avid Bone Lesion Mimicking Primary Bone Lesion

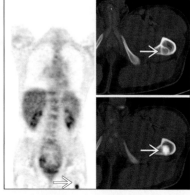

Non-Ossifying Fibroma

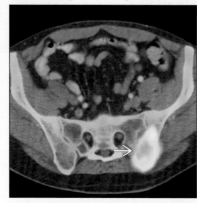

Metastasis

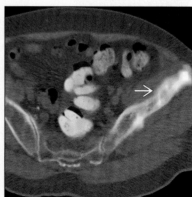

Paget Disease

PRIMARY BONE NEOPLASMS

Key Facts

Terminology
- Chondrosarcoma
- Ewing sarcoma
- Osteogenic sarcoma

Imaging Findings
- PET/CT improves accuracy of identification and localization of invasive disease
- Crucial for determining therapeutic strategy
- FDG PET superior for detection of osseous lesions; CT for lung lesions
- Low FDG uptake and metabolic activity in cartilaginous tissue
- FDG uptake increases with more aggressive histologic tumor types
- High pre-treatment SUV sensitive for higher grade tumor

- PET/CT superior to CT alone for detection of minimal malignant residue

Top Differential Diagnoses
- Bone Metastases
- Other Bone Tumors
- Acute Leukemia
- Benign Bone Lesions
- Fracture
- Abscess/Osteomyelitis
- Bone Infarction
- Paget Disease

Diagnostic Checklist
- Best time to perform FDG PET or PET/CT is prior to therapy to establish inherent FDG activity
- Many sarcomas, including primary osseous sarcomas, may not be FDG avid

---

- Metaphyseal long bone
- Distal femur
- Size: Variable
- Morphology
  - **Ewing sarcoma**
    - Obscured margins
    - Aggressive periosteal invasion
  - **Osteosarcoma**
    - Bone mass with destruction of bone elements
    - Cortical expansion
    - Large zone of transition
  - **Chondrosarcoma**
    - Endosteal scalloping
    - May have cortical destruction
    - Typically associated with a large soft tissue mass

Imaging Recommendations
- Best imaging tool
  - FDG PET and PET/CT may be useful for staging, restaging, and response to therapy
    - Both have current insurance coverage limitations

CT Findings
- **Chondrosarcoma**
  - Lytic mass with medullary cavity expansion
  - Variable amounts of calcification and chondroid matrix
  - Often have cortical thickening
  - ± Soft tissue mass
  - ± Endosteal scalloping
- **Ewing sarcoma**
  - Commonly involves long bones (metaphysis or diaphysis)
  - Intramedullary mass ± involvement of the cortex
    - Permeative/"moth-eaten" appearance
    - Heterogeneous contrast enhancement
  - Periosteal reaction often described as "sunburst"
    - Large zone of transition
  - Soft tissue mass frequently present
  - Frequently metastasizes to lung, bone, and marrow
- **Osteosarcoma**
  - Intramedullary mass

- "Moth-eaten" appearance of osseous destruction
- Indistinct borders
- Wide zone of transition
- Cortical break through
- Most common in distal femur
- Sunburst pattern of periosteal reaction
- May have contrast enhancement

Nuclear Medicine Findings
- **Initial diagnosis**
  - High grade tumors typically have intense FDG activity
  - FDG PET is sensitive for osteosarcoma and Ewing sarcoma
  - Chondrosarcoma shown to have low FDG uptake (average SUV of 4.5)
  - Histologic grade correlates well with SUV between high and low grade bone sarcomas
- **Staging**
  - PET/CT improves accuracy of identification and localization of invasive disease
    - Crucial for determining approach to therapy
    - Invasion of adjacent structures can be determined
    - FDG PET superior for detection of osseous lesions
    - Useful for estimating percentage of tumor necrosis
    - PET/CT may offer additional biopsy localization information
    - CT more sensitive for lung lesions
  - **Ewing sarcoma**
    - Tend to be FDG avid
    - Small study reported overall sensitivity 96% and specificity 78%
    - PET/CT more sensitive than bone scan for osseous metastases
    - Degree of FDG uptake indicates disease stage and may have prognostic value
  - **Chondrosarcoma**
    - Low FDG uptake and metabolic activity in cartilaginous tissue
    - FDG uptake increases with more aggressive histologic tumor types

PRIMARY BONE NEOPLASMS

- Cannot differentiate grade I chondrosarcoma from benign cartilage tumors
  - High pre-treatment SUV sensitive for higher grade tumor
  - High sensitivity for high grade mets
  - SUV may be as accurate as tumor grade for prognosis of overall survival
- **Restaging**
  - PET/CT superior to CT alone for
    - Detection of minimal malignant residue
    - Distinction between vital and necrotic tumor regions
    - Improved detection and localization of recurrence in patients with implanted orthopedic devices
- **Response to therapy**
  - Treated lesions may not change size after treatment, making metabolic imaging useful for evaluating response to therapy
  - Change in post-treatment maximum SUV correlates well with tumor response
    - Average SUV measurement prone to inconsistency based on tumor area chosen
  - Useful in Ewing sarcoma to assess response to induction chemotherapy
  - Less than 90% tumor necrosis response following pre-surgical treatment
    - Denotes poor response and is associated with less favorable outcome in Ewing and osteosarcoma

DIFFERENTIAL DIAGNOSIS

Bone Metastases
- Hypermetabolic foci in typical distribution for given primary

Other Bone Tumors
- Primary bone lymphoma

Benign Bone Lesions
- Some benign lesions associated with increased FDG activity
  - Aneurysmal bone cyst
  - Eosinophilic granuloma
  - Osteoid osteoma
  - Giant cell tumor
  - Enchondroma
  - Osteochondroma
  - Fibrous dysplasia
  - Hereditary multiple exostoses
  - Chronic osteomyelitis

Fracture
- Correlate with clinical history
- Intense FDG uptake during subacute phase with callous formation
- FDG uptake in acute phase may prompt evaluation for pathologic fracture

Abscess/Osteomyelitis
- FDG uptake especially with abscess and extensive erosive osteomyelitis
- Purulent aspiration material with negative culture: Suspect tumor

- Correlate with fever &/or other clinical symptoms of infection

Bone Infarction
- FDG uptake depends on phase of healing
- Decreased in early and increased in reparative phase

Paget Disease
- Bone scan strongly positive
- FDG PET shows mild to moderate activity

PATHOLOGY

General Features
- Genetics
  - **Osteosarcoma**
    - Hereditary risk factors: Paget disease, fibrous dysplasia, enchondromatosis, hereditary multiple exostoses
  - **Chondrosarcoma**
    - Maffucci syndrome, Ollier disease, and multiple hereditary exostosis raise risk
  - **Ewing sarcoma**
    - Family members have increased risk of neuroectodermal and stomach malignancies
- Etiology
  - **Chondrosarcoma**
    - Unclear in most cases
    - Higher risk in patients with Paget disease, prior radiation treatments, chemotherapy
  - **Ewing sarcoma**
    - Cause is unknown
    - Increased incidence in children whose parents work on farms
  - **Osteosarcoma**
    - Exact cause unknown
    - Risk factors include rapid bone growth, radiation exposure, and genetic predisposition
- Epidemiology
  - **Osteosarcoma**
    - Second to multiple myeloma in overall frequency among primary bone tumors
    - Radiation-induced osteosarcoma peak occurrence ~ 12-16 years
    - Accounts for 5% of childhood tumors
    - USA incidence of 4.8 cases per 1,000,000 per year in patients under age 20
  - **Chondrosarcoma**
    - Follow osteosarcoma and multiple myeloma as most common primary bone tumor
    - Accounts for 1/4 of primary bone tumors
  - **Ewing sarcoma**
    - Rare (2 per 1,000,000 children worldwide)
    - Incidence in Caucasians > > > African-Americans
- Associated abnormalities: Benign bone disorders such as Paget disease, enchondroma, osteochondroma (chondro-/osteosarcoma)

Staging, Grading, or Classification Criteria
- **Chondrosarcoma**
  - Musculoskeletal Tumor Society stages
    - IA: Low grade, within bone, no metastasis
    - IB: Low grade, outside bone, no metastasis

PRIMARY BONE NEOPLASMS

- IIA: High grade, within bone, no metastasis
- IIB: High grade, outside bone, no metastasis
- IIIA: Any grade, inside bone, with metastasis
- IIIB: Any grade, outside bone, with metastasis
- Grade
  - I: Low grade, closely resembling normal cartilage, but may surround lamellar bone and contain atypical cells
  - II: Intermediate grade, with more cells, nuclear atypia, hyperchromatic nuclei, larger nuclear size than grade I
  - III: High grade, with marked pleomorphism, large cells, marked hyperchromatic nuclei, occasional giant cells, frequent mitosis, necrosis
- Osteosarcoma
  - Enneking system staging
    - IA: Low grade tumor, intracompartmental
    - IB: Low grade tumor, extracompartmental
    - IIA: High grade tumor, intracompartmental
    - IIB: High grade tumor, extracompartmental
    - III: Any grade tumor with metastasis
  - Staging system for spinal tumors: Complex, based on anatomic location of a spinal segment about a clock face and location
- Ewing sarcoma
  - No formal staging method

CLINICAL ISSUES

Presentation
- Most common signs/symptoms: Most patient present with some combination of pain, swelling, fever, weight loss, or fracture

Demographics
- Age
  - Chondrosarcoma: Low incidence in children
  - Ewing: Typically 5-20 years
  - Osteosarcoma: Bimodal distribution
    - 75% < 20 years; 15-20% > 65 years
- Gender: Slightly higher incidence in males

Natural History & Prognosis
- Chondrosarcoma
  - Most cases represent low grade disease
  - Metastatic potential, 5 year survival, and recurrence rate depend on grade
    - Grade I: 0%, 90%, low
    - Grade II: 10-15%, 81%, fair
    - Grade III: > 50%, 29%, high
    - Dedifferentiated: > 95%, < 10% (1 year), high
- Ewing sarcoma
  - Negative prognostic factors
    - Metastatic vs. localized disease: 30% vs. 75% overall survival
    - Adolescence vs. childhood: 30% vs. 62% 5 year survival
    - Large tumor size
    - Primary located in pelvis
- Osteosarcoma
  - Prognosis depends heavily on successful resection and good response to neoadjuvant therapy

- Overall survival 60-70%
- High grade tumors metastasize rapidly, often to lung and bone

Treatment
- Chondrosarcoma
  - Complete resection, with limb-salvage when possible, may be curative
  - Resection of high grade tumor accompanied by adjuvant chemoradiation (often poor response)
- Ewing sarcoma
  - Fairly radiosensitive tumor
  - Surgery alone often ineffective due to high rate of subclinical metastasis
  - Combination therapy is standard of care
- Osteosarcoma
  - Highest likelihood of cure is achieved with combination chemotherapy and surgery, with follow-up chemotherapy
  - 10-20% 5 year survival with surgery alone
  - Pelvic tumors may prompt radiotherapy adjuvant to surgical resection

DIAGNOSTIC CHECKLIST

Image Interpretation Pearls
- General
  - FDG PET not currently covered by insurance for evaluating primary bone neoplasms
  - Best time to perform FDG PET or PET/CT is prior to therapy to establish inherent FDG activity
  - Many sarcomas, including primary osseous sarcomas, may not have increased levels of FDG activity

SELECTED REFERENCES

1. Arush MW et al: Positron emission tomography/computed tomography with 18fluoro-deoxyglucose in the detection of local recurrence and distant metastases of pediatric sarcoma. Pediatr Blood Cancer. 49(7):901-5, 2007
2. Tateishi U et al: Bone and soft-tissue sarcoma: preoperative staging with fluorine 18 fluorodeoxyglucose PET/CT and conventional imaging. Radiology. 245(3):839-47, 2007
3. Tateishi U et al: Staging performance of carbon-11 choline positron emission tomography/computed tomography in patients with bone and soft tissue sarcoma: comparison with conventional imaging. Cancer Sci. 97(10):1125-8, 2006
4. McCarville MB et al: PET/CT in the evaluation of childhood sarcomas. AJR Am J Roentgenol. 184(4):1293-304, 2005

PRIMARY BONE NEOPLASMS

Typical

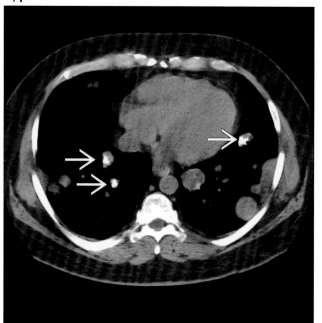 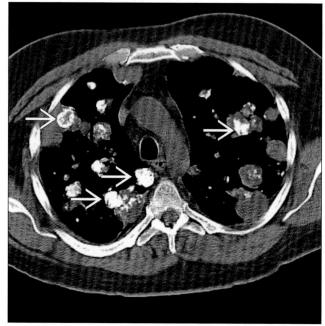

(Left) Axial NECT shows several pulmonary metastases ➡, some of which contain calcifications, in a patient with known osteosarcoma. *(Right)* Axial NECT of the same patient a few months later shows marked progression of the partly calcified metastases ➡. Calcified metastases are characteristic of metastatic osteosarcoma.

Typical

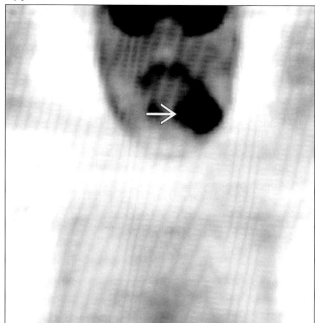 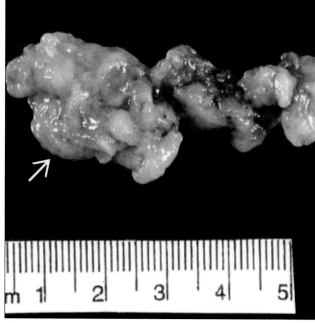

(Left) Coronal PET shows an intense region of uptake in the left jaw ➡ of this patient with osteosarcoma. *(Right)* Gross pathology shows the resected jaw osteosarcoma ➡ from the patient in the previous image.

PRIMARY BONE NEOPLASMS

Typical

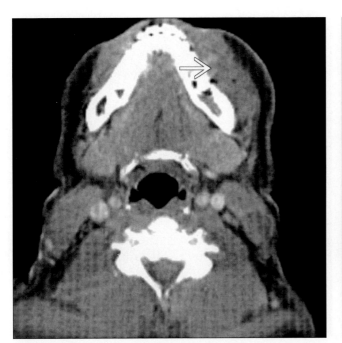
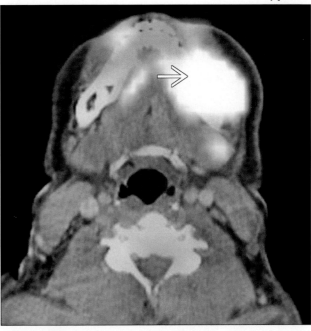

(Left) Axial CECT shows a small, almost imperceptible region of increased soft tissue ➡ superficial to the body of the left mandible. *(Right)* Axial fused PET/CT of the same patient as the previous image reveals intense FDG uptake in the same region ➡, compatible with malignancy.

Typical

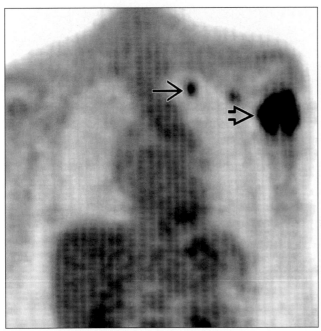
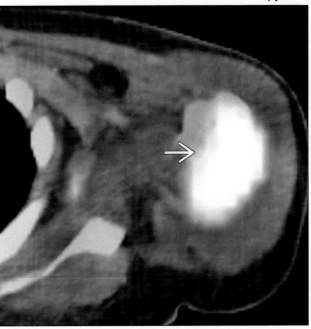

(Left) Coronal PET shows intense FDG activity in the proximal diaphysis and metaphysis of the left humerus ➡ and a focal region of uptake in the left upper lobe apical segment ➡, suspicious for metastasis. *(Right)* Axial fused PET/CT of the same patient localizes the intense FDG uptake to the left humerus ➡.

3

PRIMARY BONE NEOPLASMS

Typical

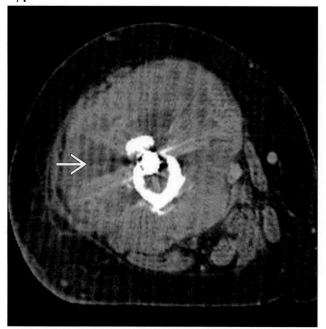 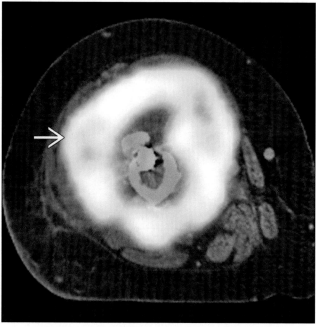

(Left) Axial NECT shows obliteration of the deep fascial planes by soft tissue enlargement/infiltration ➡ that surrounds the femur and the fixation device. (Right) Axial fused PET/CT shows intense diffuse FDG uptake in the region of deep soft tissue infiltration ➡, compatible with malignancy.

Typical

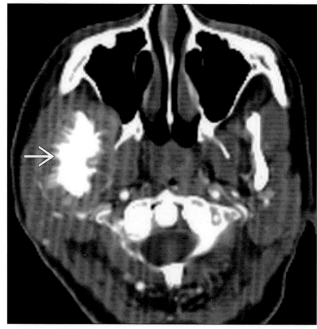 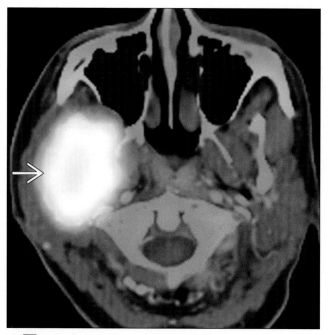

(Left) Axial CECT shows a classic "sunburst" appearance of an osteosarcoma ➡ of the right mandible. (Right) Axial fused PET/CT of the same patient shows intense metabolic activity ➡ in the same region, typical of an osteosarcoma.

3

PRIMARY BONE NEOPLASMS

Typical

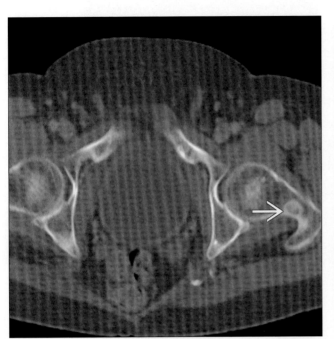 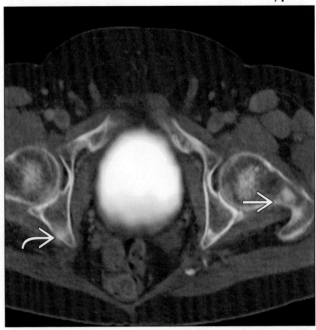

(Left) Axial CECT on bone windows shows a sclerotic lesion ➡ in the left femoral neck in this patient with a history of chondrosarcoma. *(Right)* Axial fused PET/CT of the same patient shows this lesion ➡ to be hypermetabolic. A second lesion ➡ is noted in the posterior right acetabulum.

Typical

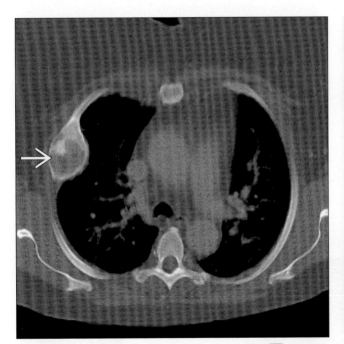 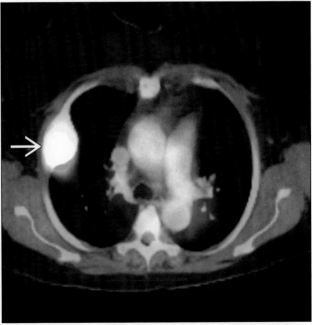

(Left) Axial CECT shows an expansile lesion of a right rib ➡. *(Right)* Axial fused PET/CT of the same patient as the previous image shows the lesion ➡ to be hypermetabolic, with subsequent pathology proving a Ewing sarcoma.

METASTATIC LESIONS OF THE BONES

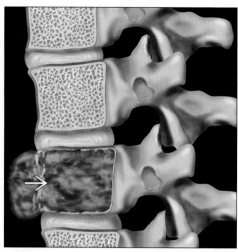

Graphic shows a vertebral body ➡ that has been completely replaced with metastatic disease.

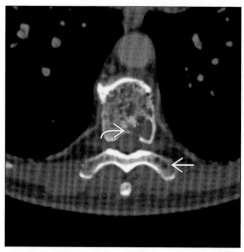

Axial CECT shows lytic foci within a vertebral body ➡ in a patient with multiple myeloma; one lesion erodes the posterior vertebral body cortex ➡.

TERMINOLOGY

Abbreviations and Synonyms
- Bone metastases, metastatic lesions to bone, secondary bone tumors
  - Sclerotic/osteosclerotic metastases
  - Osteolytic metastases

Definitions
- Malignant extension to bone, often by carcinoma, due to direct extension, retrograde venous flow, or hematogenous metastasis

IMAGING FINDINGS

General Features
- Best diagnostic clue: Typical presentation includes scattered lesions in areas of osteoblastic or osteolytic activity
- Location
  - Seeding occurs mostly in red marrow where blood flow is high
    - (80%) axial skeleton
    - Spine, pelvis, ribs, sternum, calvaria, proximal limb bones
    - Random distribution typical
    - More common proximally in long bones
  - Cortical involvement can occur secondary to direct invasion
- Size: Ranges from small, solitary lesion to replacement of the entire marrow space
- Morphology
  - Often infiltrating, elongated, or expansile
  - Focal or regional pattern more characteristic of fracture or arthropathy
  - May not be identifiable on CT

Imaging Recommendations
- Best imaging tool
  - PET/CT very sensitive for detection of bone metastases
    - FDG PET sensitive for osteolytic lesions and CT sensitive for osteoblastic lesions
    - PET/CT more sensitive and specific than bone scan for delineation of disease and for surgical planning

DDx: FDG Activity in Bones, Other than Malignancy

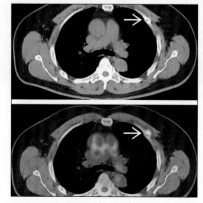

Fracture

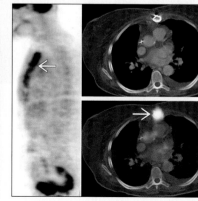

Post-Operative: Recent CABG

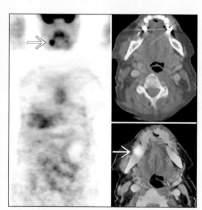

Infection: Dental Abscess

METASTATIC LESIONS OF THE BONES

Key Facts

Terminology
- Bone metastases, metastatic lesions to bone, secondary bone tumors

Imaging Findings
- More than 80% of metastases to bone are located in axial skeleton where red marrow blood flow is high
  ○ Vertebrae, ribs, and hips
- FDG PET generally ineffective for tumors that are not FDG avid
  ○ Prostate cancer, highly mucinous tumors, occasionally renal cell carcinoma
  ○ Also limited in some sclerotic metastases
  ○ Reveals marrow lesions in FDG-avid disease prior to cortical effects (often before bone scan becomes positive)
- CT may miss many early infiltrative or osteolytic lesions
- CT has higher sensitivity for osteoblastic/sclerotic bone metastases
- F-18 NaF PET: Excellent PET bone agent, currently not reimbursed by Medicare and most third party payers

Top Differential Diagnoses
- Degenerative Processes, Arthropathies
- Healing Fracture or Bone Injury
- Iatrogenic: Vertebroplasty, Kyphoplasty
- Physiologic Activity
- Primary Bone Tumors

Pathology
- Most common childhood primaries: Neuroblastoma, Ewing sarcoma, rhabdosarcoma

---

  ○ Tc-99m whole body bone scan often used as initial screening due to low cost
    ■ Sensitivity 80-90%, better than plain radiograph or CT but nonspecific
    ■ More sensitive than FDG PET for osteoblastic lesions
    ■ Plain film correlation for further characterization/ambiguity; additional evaluation with CT or MR as necessary
- Protocol advice
  ○ FDG PET/CT
    ■ Position arms above head for whole body scan

CT Findings
- More sensitive for osteoblastic/sclerotic lesions
- Insensitive for early infiltrative or osteolytic lesions
- Early bone infiltration (before destruction) appears as increased attenuation of the normally fatty bone marrow
- Increased attenuation of lesions generally correlates with lowered FDG uptake
- Overall sensitivity for bone-seeking cancers: 71-100%
- Spine
  ○ Posterior vertebral body almost always involved
  ○ 80% also in anterior body
  ○ Enhancement often not detectable

Nuclear Medicine Findings
- **General applications**
  ○ FDG PET/CT more sensitive and specific than bone scan
    ■ Earlier detection of FDG-avid osteolytic marrow lesions (before cortical changes become evident)
    ■ Reveals 75% more metastases from breast cancer and to long bones
    ■ Exceptions include primaries with low FDG avidity, which are typically osteoblastic
    ■ Osteoblastic metastases include prostate, highly mucinous tumors, and occasionally renal cell carcinoma
    ■ Sclerotic metastases may not be FDG avid

  ○ Prediction of bone metastasis in the absence of associated CT findings is hindered by false positives
    ■ Especially with solitary foci
    ■ PPV of lesions with negative CT and positive FDG PET: 61%
    ■ PPV of lesions positive on CT but negative on PET: 17%
  ○ PET/CT may be cost-effective following screening bone scan for more detailed evaluation of bone metastases
- **Restaging**
  ○ Overall rate of detection of recurrence for FDG PET and CT separately were 47% and 96%
  ○ Following therapy, "flare" phenomenon may present
    ■ Treated lesions may have increased FDG uptake during healing and osteoblastic remodeling
    ■ Bone pain may increase as well
    ■ Typically arises 4-6 weeks post-therapy and resolves within 3-6 months
    ■ May show "mixed" response, with a variety of resolved, stable, and new lesions
- **Response to therapy**
  ○ Reduction in SUV of metastatic bone lesions following therapy is highly predictive of response
  ○ Total lesion glycolysis (TLG) changes were a poor indicator of response duration
    ■ Possibly due to lack of volume change in treated lesions
- **Findings/anatomy**
  ○ Most common finding: Scattered osseous lesions focused in regions of red marrow, i.e., axial and proximal appendicular skeleton
    ■ Solitary lesions more likely inflammatory or degenerative than metastatic
    ■ Linear uptake along ribs (single focus of activity in ribs more likely fracture)
    ■ Vertebral mets often asymmetric and not confined to endplate
    ■ Proximal long bone involvement more common; distal long bone mets seen in lung, thyroid, and renal cell carcinoma
  ○ PET can detect tumors confined to marrow space

METASTATIC LESIONS OF THE BONES

- May have no detectable cortical remodeling and thus not be seen on bone scan
  - Multiple myeloma, lymphoma, leukemia
  - Aggressive tumors with overwhelming osteolytic/osteoblastic activity may be photopenic
    - Renal cell carcinoma, thyroid carcinoma, poorly differentiated anaplastic tumors
    - Occasionally lung, breast, neuroblastoma, myeloma
    - Lytic lesions may become photopenic following radiotherapy, often surrounded by reactive rim of activity
  - "Superscan" MDP bone scan
    - Diffusely increased activity due to disseminated bone lesions
    - May show relative absence of normal renal and soft tissue activity
    - Breast and prostate cancer most common causes
- Findings by primary
  - Breast
    - FDG PET is sensitive for detection of predominantly osteolytic metastatic breast cancer
    - Decreased FDG uptake may be seen in sclerotic metastases
    - Treated, previously lytic metastases may have post-therapy sclerotic changes and lose FDG avidity
    - Loss of FDG avidity post-treatment may reflect diminished malignant potential
  - Prostate
    - Variable sensitivity
    - Sensitivity as low as 18% for treated bone metastases from prostate cancer
    - Sensitivity as high as 65% in selected untreated patients; usually more aggressive pathology
  - Lymphoma
    - FDG PET much more sensitive than CT for early infiltrative lesions
    - Higher sensitivity than routine scintigraphy
  - Thyroid
    - Useful in patients with a history of well-differentiated cancer with high thyroglobulin levels and negative I-131
    - Positive PET has strong NPV and is associated with an 8-fold increased risk of death
    - Among patients with differentiated thyroid carcinoma, 25% of metastases were to bone
- False positives
  - Benign fractures or other trauma
    - Acute fracture may show no FDG uptake
    - Uptake is often focal and solitary
    - FDG PET may return to baseline 8 weeks after injury (longer in elderly)
  - Hyperparathyroidism may result in diffusely increased uptake in whole skeleton
    - Especially calvaria, pelvis, and lower extremities
  - Polymethylmethacrylate vertebroplasty may be FDG avid and mimic spinal metastases

Other Modality Findings
- F-18 NaF PET: Excellent PET bone agent, currently investigational

- Tc-99m-methylene diphosphonate bone scintigraphy identifies osteoblastic response
  - Most metastases demonstrate cortical remodeling as increased focal tracer accumulation on bone scan

DIFFERENTIAL DIAGNOSIS

Physiologic Activity
- Baseline mild FDG uptake is common in vascular regions of red marrow of axial skeleton
- Growth plates in prepubescent individuals
- Muscle parallel to ribs and long bones

Metabolic Disease, Infection, or Inflammation
- Hypercortisol states, e.g., Cushing, steroid usage
- Periodontal disease
- Paget disease
- Brown tumor of hyperparathyroidism

Degenerative Processes, Arthropathies
- Seen in common sites of degenerative or rheumatic joint disease
  - Disc spaces and facet joints
  - Knees, hands
  - Acromioclavicular/sternoclavicular joints

Orthopedic Intervention
- Orthopedic devices
  - Loosening, infection
- Vertebroplasty, kyphoplasty
- Focal sclerotic areas in bone
- Uptake often artifactual; examine non-AC-corrected PET image

Healing Fracture or Bone Injury
- Usually focal rather than infiltrative or elongated
- Correlate with patient history
- Exclude pathologic fracture

Sacral Insufficiency Fracture
- Fractures with fractures lines, sclerotic lines, or both
- Areas of sclerosis within the sacral alae parallel to sacroiliac joints

Primary Bone Tumors
- Lymphoma, myeloma, enchondroma, osteoma, fibrous dysplasia
  - Stable activity in enchondroma may be benign

Osseous Infarction, Avascular Necrosis, Osteonecrosis
- Common in knees and heads of femur and humerus
- Etiologies include steroids, radiation, alcohol, trauma, sickle cell, etc.

PATHOLOGY

General Features
- Etiology
  - Common adult primaries

METASTATIC LESIONS OF THE BONES

- ■ Breast, prostate, bronchogenic, colon, renal cell, and carcinoid
  - o Common childhood primaries
    - ■ Neuroblastoma, Ewing sarcoma, rhabdosarcoma, retinoblastoma, medulloblastoma
  - o Arterial and venous vascular spread to red marrow
  - o Direct invasion to cortical bone
  - o Lymphangitic spread
- • Epidemiology
  - o Incidence of bone metastases is not fully known
  - o Diagnosed in up to 85% of advanced breast and prostate cancer patients
    - ■ Also in 15-30% of patients with carcinoma of lung, colon, stomach, bladder, uterus, rectum, thyroid, or kidney
- • Associated abnormalities: Pathologic fractures

Gross Pathologic & Surgical Features
- • Lesions from breast cancer are predominantly osteolytic (15-20% are osteoblastic)

CLINICAL ISSUES

Presentation
- • Most common signs/symptoms
  - o Most common manifestations are pain, fractures, and spinal cord compression
  - o Note: Development of bone pain in patient with known primary is highly suspicious for metastasis
    - ■ However, 36% of patients with spinal metastases in one study did not complain of bone pain
    - ■ 66% of patients with back pain and a history of previous malignancy had no bone metastasis
  - o Lesions are often detected incidentally
- • Other signs/symptoms: Elevated alkaline phosphatase in 50% of patients

Demographics
- • Age
  - o Varies according to age of incidence of primary
  - o Overall incidence of bone metastases increases with age and a history of malignancy

Natural History & Prognosis
- • Bone metastasis indicates advanced disease and poor prognosis
  - o 20% 5 year survival in breast cancer patients
  - o Prognosis better with decreased SUV and increased attenuation of lesion post-therapy
- • Complications
  - o Pathologic fracture due to demineralization and disorganized repair
  - o Pain decreasing quality of life
  - o Hypercalcemia
  - o Spinal cord compression

Treatment
- • Bone-seeking radiopharmaceutical agents
  - o Increasing palliative use for unremitting bone pain from metastases
  - o Agents include strontium-89 (80% rate of relief) and rhenium-186 stannum-ethylhydroxydiphosphonate
  - o Does not improve survival

- • Vertebroplasty
  - o Often used to treat osteoporotic fractures
  - o 70% rate of pain relief when used for spinal metastases
  - o Involves percutaneous injection of polymethylmethacrylate
  - o May result in neurologic damage
- • Systemic chemotherapy and targeted external beam radiotherapy are also used

DIAGNOSTIC CHECKLIST

Image Interpretation Pearls
- • Suspicious findings include
  - o FDG uptake not attributable to physiologic activity or nonmalignant pathology (infection, trauma, degenerative joint disease)
- • Single lesions may be difficult to categorize, necessitating additional imaging
  - o Solitary skull lesions are often benign (can be seen in about 10% of patients without metastatic disease)

SELECTED REFERENCES

1. Kumar J et al: Whole-body MR imaging with the use of parallel imaging for detection of skeletal metastases in pediatric patients with small-cell neoplasms: comparison with skeletal scintigraphy and FDG PET/CT. Pediatr Radiol. 38(9):953-62, 2008
2. Palmedo H et al: PET and PET/CT with F-18 fluoride in bone metastases. Recent Results Cancer Res. 170:213-24, 2008
3. Shie P et al: Meta-analysis: comparison of F-18 Fluorodeoxyglucose-positron emission tomography and bone scintigraphy in the detection of bone metastases in patients with breast cancer. Clin Nucl Med. 33(2):97-101, 2008
4. Tateishi U et al: Bone metastases in patients with metastatic breast cancer: morphologic and metabolic monitoring of response to systemic therapy with integrated PET/CT. Radiology. 247(1):189-96, 2008
5. Chen YW et al: Discordant findings of skeletal metastasis between tc 99M MDP bone scans and F18 FDG PET/CT imaging for advanced breast and lung cancers--two case reports and literature review. Kaohsiung J Med Sci. 23(12):639-46, 2007
6. Du Y et al: Fusion of metabolic function and morphology: sequential [18F]fluorodeoxyglucose positron-emission tomography/computed tomography studies yield new insights into the natural history of bone metastases in breast cancer. J Clin Oncol. 25(23):3440-7, 2007
7. Hur J et al: Accuracy of fluorodeoxyglucose-positron emission tomography for diagnosis of single bone metastasis: comparison with bone scintigraphy. J Comput Assist Tomogr. 31(5):812-9, 2007
8. Ito S et al: Comparison of 18F-FDG PET and bone scintigraphy in detection of bone metastases of thyroid cancer. J Nucl Med. 48(6):889-95, 2007
9. Schirrmeister H: Detection of bone metastases in breast cancer by positron emission tomography. Radiol Clin North Am. 45(4):669-76, vi, 2007
10. Taira AV et al: Detection of bone metastases: assessment of integrated FDG PET/CT imaging. Radiology. 243(1):204-11, 2007

METASTATIC LESIONS OF THE BONES

Typical

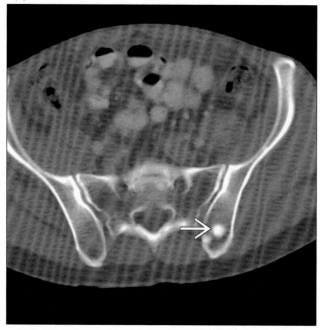 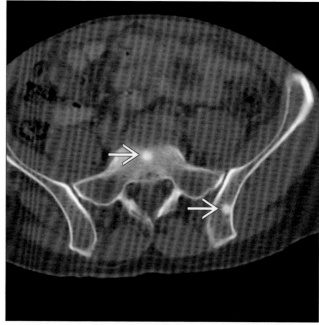

(Left) Axial CECT reveals a sclerotic metastasis ➡ in the left iliac bone in a patient with prostate cancer. *(Right)* Axial CECT shows sclerotic metastases ➡ in the sacrum and left iliac bone in another patient with prostate cancer. Bone scanning is more sensitive for osteoblastic lesions than FDG PET.

Typical

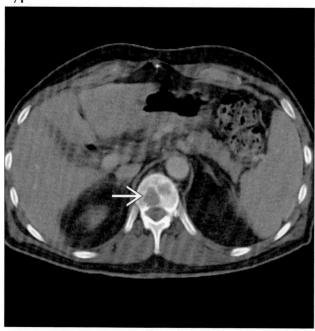 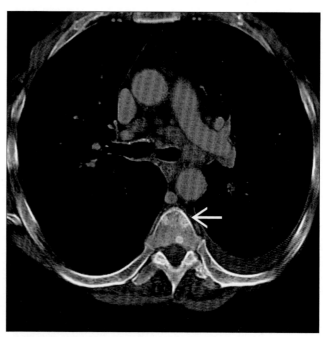

(Left) Axial CECT shows typical lytic foci in a thoracic vertebral body ➡ in a patient with myeloma. *(Right)* Axial CECT reveals sclerotic metastases ➡ in a thoracic vertebral body of a patient with transitional cell carcinoma of the bladder.

METASTATIC LESIONS OF THE BONES

Typical

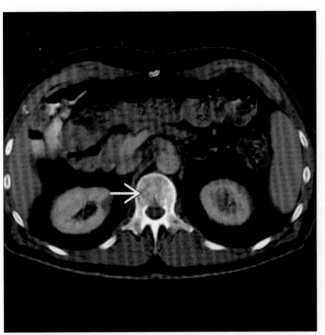

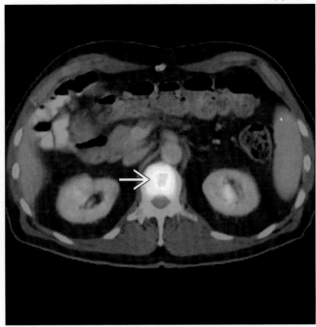

(Left) Axial CECT shows subtle mixed lytic metastases ➡ throughout this vertebral body in a patient with breast cancer. *(Right)* Axial fused PET/CT of the same patient shows diffuse FDG activity ➡ from the numerous small lytic metastases.

Typical

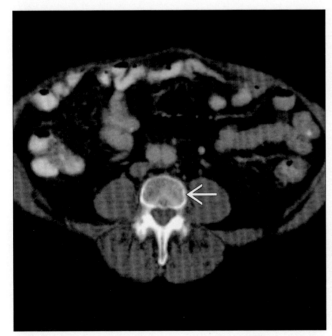

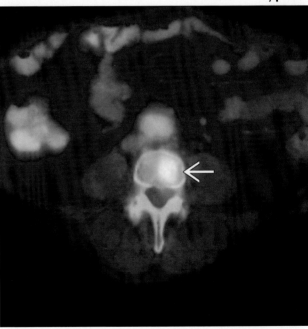

(Left) Axial CECT shows a subtle sclerotic metastasis ➡ in the left aspect of the vertebral body in a patient with lung cancer. *(Right)* Axial fused PET/CT of the same patient easily documents intense increased FDG uptake in the metastasis ➡, making this patient's disease stage IV.

3

METASTATIC LESIONS OF THE BONES

Typical

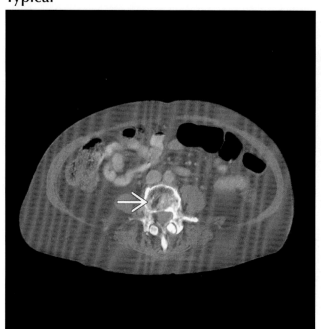 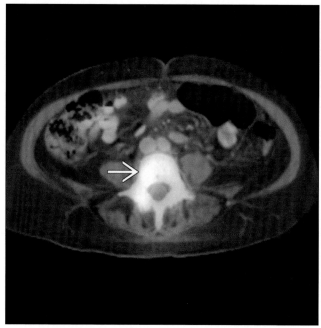

(Left) Axial CECT shows a small lytic lesion ➡ in a vertebral body in a patient with breast cancer. *(Right)* Axial fused PET/CT of the same patient shows the increased FDG uptake in the lesion ➡.

Typical

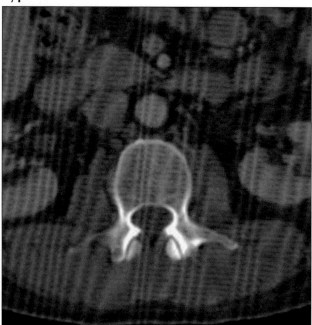 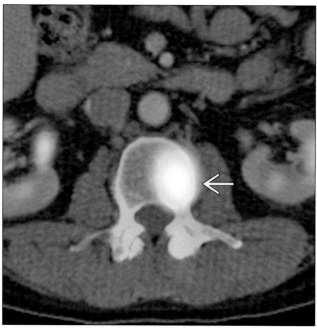

(Left) Axial CECT shows no definite abnormality within this lumbar vertebral body in a patient with breast cancer. *(Right)* Axial fused PET/CT of the same patient shows a markedly FDG-avid metastasis ➡ at this level.

METASTATIC LESIONS OF THE BONES

Typical

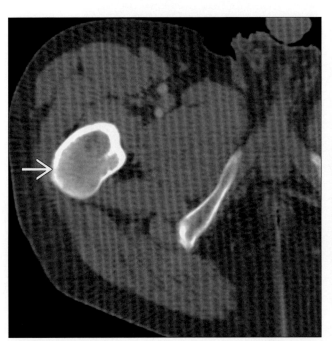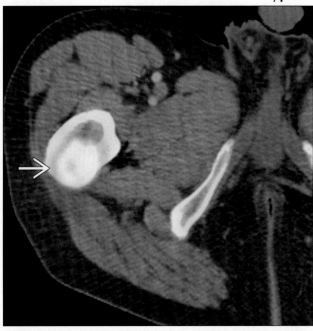

(Left) Axial CECT shows a very subtle sclerotic metastasis ➡ in the right femur in a patient with known breast cancer. *(Right)* Axial fused PET/CT of the same patient shows marked FDG uptake in the metastatic lesion ➡.

Typical

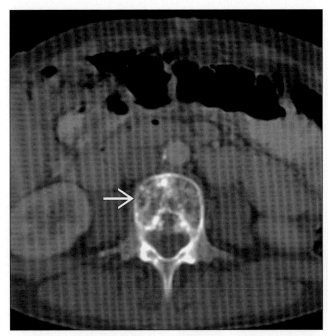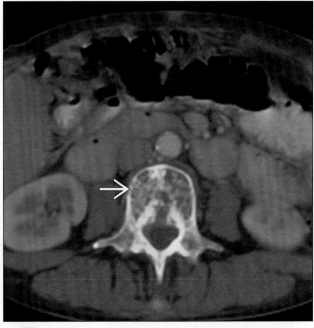

(Left) Axial CECT shows numerous lytic lesions throughout the vertebral body ➡ in a patient with known myeloma. *(Right)* Axial fused PET/CT of the same patient does not show any increased activity in the lytic lesions ➡. Lytic lesions of multiple myeloma may not be hypermetabolic.

MULTIPLE MYELOMA

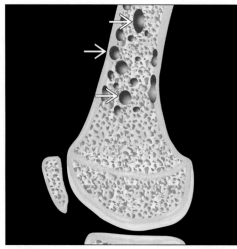

Graphic shows the typical punched out appearance of bone with multiple lytic lesions ➡, representing the changes of multiple myeloma.

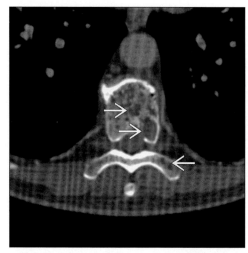

Axial CECT shows several lytic lesions ➡ within a vertebral body and with the typical appearance of myeloma.

TERMINOLOGY

Abbreviations and Synonyms
- Multiple myeloma (MM), monoclonal gammopathy of undetermined significance (MGUS)

Definitions
- Malignancy of antibody-forming plasma cells in bone marrow
  - Overproduction of monoclonal immunoglobulins
  - Causes a wide variety of manifestations

IMAGING FINDINGS

General Features
- Best diagnostic clue
  - Multiple lytic or punched out lesions are diagnostic of MM
    - Present in 75-90% of patients at diagnosis
  - PET: Increased activity in lytic lesion or extramedullary site
    - Not all lesions are hypermetabolic
- Location
  - 97% of cases present in bone and bone marrow
    - Spine is the most common site of involvement of myeloma
    - Due to presence of red marrow in axial skeleton throughout life
  - Common extramedullary sites of occurrence: Paranasal sinuses, nasopharynx, tonsils
    - Less common: Lung, spleen, liver
  - Osteonecrosis of humeral and femoral heads reported in up to 10% of MM patients
    - Area of involvement is often asymptomatic
    - Risk factors include treatment with dexamethasone, male gender, younger age
- Morphology
  - Increased complement of plasma cells in marrow and lytic bone lesions
    - Plasma cells > 10-15% of marrow cells
  - May present as solid mass (plasmacytoma) in bone or soft tissue

Imaging Recommendations
- Best imaging tool
  - Prior to imaging, confirm disease via lab work and analysis of bone marrow aspiration

DDx: Mimics of Multiple Myeloma

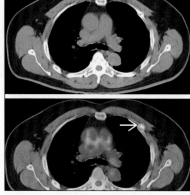

Benign Fracture

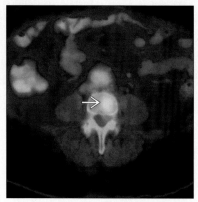

Metastatic Disease

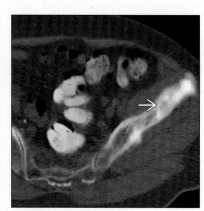

Paget Disease

MULTIPLE MYELOMA

Key Facts

Terminology
- Multiple myeloma (MM), monoclonal gammopathy of undetermined significance (MGUS)
- Myeloma: Proliferation of clonal plasma cells and overproduction of monoclonal immunoglobulins

Imaging Findings
- Increased activity in lytic lesion or extramedullary site on PET/CT
- Multiple lytic or punched-out lesions are diagnostic of MM and are present in 75-90% of patients at diagnosis
- Bone marrow and bone (97%)
- PET/CT performs better than MR in the detection of focal lesions
- Most studies have shown PET/CT reliable for bone lesions ≥ 1 cm using standard SUV cutoff of 2.5

- PET provides accurate staging of untreated MM (solitary, multifocal)
- Diffuse marrow uptake on PET usually indicates elevated plasma cell population
- PET exceptionally useful in monitoring disease activity in patients with nonsecretory myeloma

Top Differential Diagnoses
- Lytic Skeletal Metastases
- Osteopenia, Osteoporosis
- Other Bone + Soft Tissue Malignancy
- Other Plasma Cell Neoplasms

Diagnostic Checklist
- FDG PET/CT to stage and establish baseline for monitoring therapy (especially in nonsecretory myeloma)

- FDG PET useful for
  - Evaluation of disease activity
  - Detection of extraosseous disease involvement
  - Direction of local therapy (e.g., radiation)
  - Assessment of patients with nonsecretory myeloma
  - Evaluation of response to therapy
- FDG PET/CT with contrast
  - Superior to MR in the detection of focal lesions
- MR better for diagnosis of diffuse disease pattern
  - Limited window (spine and pelvis) reduces sensitivity
  - Generally reserved for evaluation of bone marrow in spine and pelvis
  - Improved ability to detect both focal and diffuse disease
- Protocol advice
  - For detection of diffuse disease, obtain PET/CT from top of head to toes
  - For patients not affected by renal failure (which is common in MM), use oral and IV contrast-enhanced CT
  - Marrow stimulant drugs may mask underlying MM lesions

CT Findings
- Plasma cell tumors in bone → ↑ osteoclasts and ↓ osteoblasts → "punched out" lesions in flat and long bones
- NECT is indicated for evaluation of cortical destruction and intra-/extraosseous extent of tumor
- Up to 30% demineralization required before lytic lesion may be detected
- CT useful to guide percutaneous biopsies
- Findings
  - Multiple well-defined, rounded, lytic, punched out lesions
    - Usual sites: Skull, spine, pelvis
  - Cortical and cancellous bone erosion
  - Endosteal scalloping (may be subtle)
  - Diffuse osteopenia, osteoporosis, osteolysis, with accentuated trabecular pattern

- Minimal periosteal new bone formation
- Lesions often become sclerotic after therapy
- Spine
  - Vertebral collapse
    - Large endplate depressions
    - Sparing of posterior elements
  - Paraspinal/epidural soft tissue mass adjacent to bone destruction
- Plasmacytoma
  - Solitary expansile lesions present in 10% of cases
  - May appear as bubbly expansion of single bone
  - Occasionally associated with soft tissue mass
  - Represents early stage of melanoma (progresses to multiple lesions)
  - Presents most commonly in ribs, pelvis, long bones
  - Discovery of second myeloma lesion upstages patient's disease from I to III
- Benign fracture suggested by
  - Retropulsed posterior fragment
  - Cortical fragments without destruction
  - Identifiable fragment lines within cancellous bone
  - Intravertebral vacuum phenomenon
  - Thin diffuse paraspinal soft tissue mass

Nuclear Medicine Findings
- General
  - False positives seen with infection, inflammation, post-surgical changes, and hemangioma
- Initial diagnosis
  - Most studies have shown PET/CT reliable for bone lesions of at least 1 cm using standard SUV cutoff of 2.5
    - Any lesions smaller than 5 mm with uptake should be considered positive, regardless of SUV
  - Stable MGUS may be diagnosed based on negative whole body PET in patients with monoclonal gammopathy
  - PET/CT can be useful for diagnosing infection, even with severe neutropenia/lymphopenia
    - Nearly 10% of newly diagnosed patients die within 60 days of complications due to infection or renal failure

MULTIPLE MYELOMA

- Silent infections are also detected and should be considered in the differential diagnosis of FDG-avid foci
- **Staging**
  o FDG PET highly accurate for staging of untreated MM (solitary and multifocal)
    - Accurate staging is critical for treatment decisions and prognosis
  o FDG PET helps accurately delineate target volumes for radiotherapy planning
  o PET/CT leads to change in management in up to 70% of cases and upstaging of disease in up to 37.5%
  o Extramedullary plasmacytoma: FDG PET leads to management changes in more than 25% of patients
    - Due to presence of additional sites of disease in 33% of cases
  o Prognosis dismal for patients with extramedullary FDG-avid disease
- **Restaging**
  o Sites of disease relapse often represent new lesions
  o PET highly sensitive for monitoring disease activity in patients with nonsecretory myeloma
    - Transplanted patients no longer secrete abnormal immunoglobulin
    - Recurrent foci of disease are still avid for FDG
    - Any sizable new foci will be readily evident
  o Diffuse marrow uptake on PET usually indicates elevated plasma cell population
    - Meaning of diffuse bone marrow uptake in MM patients must be further investigated
    - Mild and diffuse FDG uptake in the spine is also found in young or mildly anemic patients
- **Response to therapy**
  o Early relapse is predicted by persistent FDG activity following induction therapy
  o Prognosis is excellent for patients with no FDG-avid disease following stem cell transplant

DIFFERENTIAL DIAGNOSIS

Lytic Skeletal Metastases
- Most common primaries include breast, prostate, thyroid, and renal cell carcinoma

Osteopenia, Osteoporosis
- Numerous etiologies lead to decreased bone mineral density
- Appears as increased radiolucency of bone

Other Bone and Soft Tissue Malignancy
- Lymphoma
- Chondrosarcoma
- Osteosarcoma

Other Plasma Cell Neoplasms
- Plasma cell leukemia
- MGUS

PATHOLOGY

General Features
- General path comments
  o **MM spectrum encompasses**
    - Premalignant stage of MGUS (progresses to malignant MM at rate of 1% per year)
    - Progresses to malignant MM at rate of 1% per year
    - Amyloidosis with soft tissue deposit of fibrils related to monoclonal immunoglobulin light chains
    - Intramedullary MM with symptomatic osteolytic lesions
    - Smoldering myeloma with intramedullary tumor and without complications of intramedullary MM
    - More aggressive extramedullary MM mostly involving blood, pleura, and skin
  o Unchecked proliferation of plasma cells results in both local mass effect and systemic effect
    - Due to overproduction of monoclonal protein
- Genetics: Possible HLA type-related pathogenesis of MM
- Etiology
  o Unclear link to radiation exposure
  o Exposure to variety of environmental factors
    - DDT, wood dust, hair dye, and unknown toxins in agriculture and petrochemical industries
  o MGUS: 20% develop MM within 20 years
- Epidemiology
  o Most common primary bone cancer and plasma cell neoplasm
  o 16,000 new cases and 11,000 deaths yearly in USA
  o Accounts for
    - 2% of all cancer deaths
    - 10% of all hematologic malignancies
    - 20% of fatalities from hematologic malignancies

Gross Pathologic & Surgical Features
- Pathologic bone fractures
- Amyloidosis (joint thickening, subcutaneous nodules)

Microscopic Features
- Histologic variables that play a role in prognosis
  o Proportion of plasma cells in bone marrow (< 30%)
  o IgG and IgA peaks > 3.5 g/dL and 2 g/dL
  o Low residual normal immunoglobulin
- Proliferation of plasma cells may interfere with the normal production of blood cells
  o Results in leukopenia, anemia, and thrombocytopenia

Staging, Grading, or Classification Criteria
- Newer International Staging System does not include imaging criteria
- International Staging System
  o Based solely on serum beta-2 microglobulin and albumin levels
- Durie-Salmon staging system
  o Stage I
    - Small number of myeloma cells
    - Slightly ↓ hemoglobin
    - Plain films with ≤ 1 lesion or area of bone involvement

- Normal calcium
- Small amount of monoclonal immunoglobulin in blood/urine
  - Stage II
    - Moderate number of myeloma cells
    - Labs and plain films intermediate between stage I and III
  - Stage III
    - Large number of myeloma cells
    - Severely ↓ hemoglobin
    - Hypercalcemia
    - ≥ 3 sites of bone involvement on plain films
    - Large amount of monoclonal immunoglobulin in blood/urine

CLINICAL ISSUES

Presentation
- Most common signs/symptoms
  - Bone damage is present in more than 80% of patients at diagnosis
    - Focal disease causes bone pain and pathologic fractures
    - Pain usually worse supine and at night; not relieved by rest or NSAIDs
    - May also present with diffuse osteoporotic pattern
  - Weakness, fever, weight loss
  - Anemia, pneumococcal infection, hypercalcemia, renal failure
- Other signs/symptoms
  - Spinal cord compression
    - Emergency as it may progress rapidly
- Clinical Profile
  - Patient with > 10% plasma cells in marrow
    - With lytic lesions on X-ray and monoclonal immunoglobulins in blood/urine (diagnostic of MM)

Demographics
- Age: Incidence increases with age and reaches a peak during 7th decade of life
- Gender: M:F = 3:2
- Ethnicity: African-American:Caucasian ≈ 2:1

Natural History & Prognosis
- MM is a relatively slowly proliferative malignant plasma cell tumor
  - Until advanced stages of disease
- Five year survival
  - Stage I: > 60 months
  - Stage II: 40-45 months
  - Stage III: 23-29 months
- Overall median survival in all patients: 3 years
- Indicators of poor prognosis include
  - Renal impairment
  - Extraosseous disease (median survival 7 months)

Treatment
- Therapy is initiated as soon as end-organ damage is seen
  - Including bone disease, renal impairment, anemia, &/or hypercalcemia

- Survival improving from usual 30-36 months with introduction of novel therapeutics including
  - Thalidomide, lenalidomide, bortezomib and potential success of stem cell transplant
- In patients with bone involvement the incidence of vertebral fractures can be reduced
  - Use a potent IV bisphosphonates
- External beam radiation only for solitary plasmacytoma of bone; no proven benefit of chemotherapy
  - Bone patients' survival of solitary plasmacytoma > 50% if disease does not progress to MM

DIAGNOSTIC CHECKLIST

Consider
- Follow-up imaging not routinely indicated, as lytic bone lesions rarely show radiographic evidence of healing
  - Even in patients with complete remission
  - However, any myeloma patient with new pain or neurologic symptoms should have repeat studies
- Insufficiency fractures when new site of abnormality is discovered in one or both pubic rami or in sacrum
  - Especially within one or both sacral alae
- Patient with negative PET/CT in setting of monoclonal gammopathy has an excellent prognosis

SELECTED REFERENCES

1. Fonti R et al: 18F-FDG PET/CT, 99mTc-MIBI, and MRI in evaluation of patients with multiple myeloma. J Nucl Med. 49(2):195-200, 2008
2. D'Sa S et al: Guidelines for the use of imaging in the management of myeloma. Br J Haematol. 137(1):49-63, 2007
3. Even-Sapir E: PET/CT in malignant bone disease. Semin Musculoskelet Radiol. 11(4):312-21, 2007
4. Ghesani M et al: Multiple myeloma presenting with [18F]fluorodeoxyglucose avid liver lesions diagnosed on positron emission tomography scan. J Clin Oncol. 25(33):5319-20, 2007
5. Nanni C et al: 11C-choline vs. 18F-FDG PET/CT in assessing bone involvement in patients with multiple myeloma. World J Surg Oncol. 5:68, 2007
6. Zamagni E et al: A prospective comparison of 18F-fluorodeoxyglucose positron emission tomography-computed tomography, magnetic resonance imaging and whole-body planar radiographs in the assessment of bone disease in newly diagnosed multiple myeloma. Haematologica. 92(1):50-5, 2007
7. Breyer RJ 3rd et al: Comparison of imaging with FDG PET/CT with other imaging modalities in myeloma. Skeletal Radiol. 35(9):632-40, 2006
8. Nanni C et al: Role of 18F-FDG PET/CT in the assessment of bone involvement in newly diagnosed multiple myeloma: preliminary results. Eur J Nucl Med Mol Imaging. 33(5):525-31, 2006
9. Bredella MA et al: Value of FDG PET in the assessment of patients with multiple myeloma. AJR Am J Roentgenol. 184(4):1199-204, 2005
10. Wang K et al: Bone scintigraphy in common tumors with osteolytic components. Clin Nucl Med. 30(10):655-71, 2005

3

MULTIPLE MYELOMA

CT Findings: Multiple Myeloma

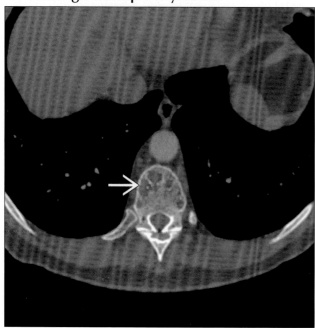 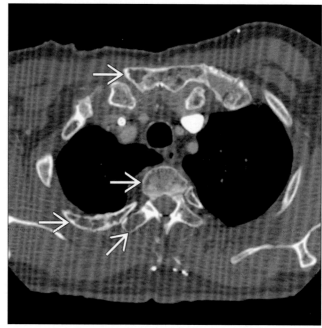

(Left) Axial CECT shows several lytic lesions ➡ within a thoracic vertebral body in a patient with myeloma. *(Right)* Axial CECT shows numerous lytic lesions ➡ in ribs, vertebral body, transverse process, and sternum in a patient with multiple myeloma.

PET/CT Findings: Multiple Myeloma

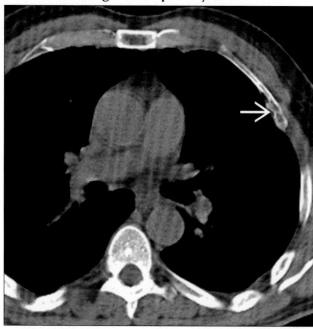 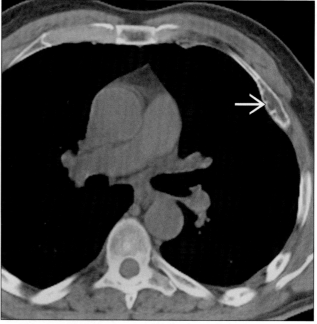

(Left) Axial NECT shows a slightly expansile left anterior rib lesion ➡ in a patient with multiple myeloma. *(Right)* Axial fused PET/CT shows only minimal FDG activity correlating with the rib lesion ➡. Myeloma lesions may have variable activity ranging from almost no increased FDG uptake to fairly intense activity.

MULTIPLE MYELOMA

PET/CT Findings: Multiple Myeloma

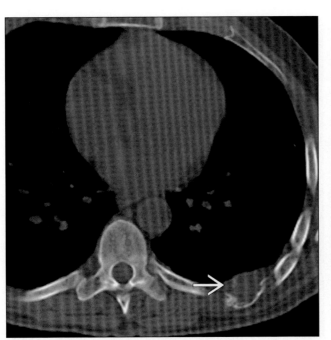
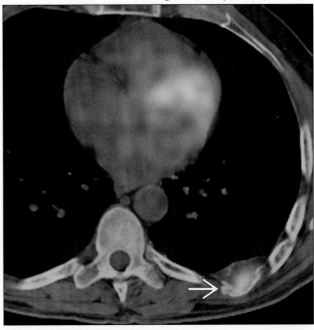

(Left) Axial CECT shows an expansile, lytic lesion ➡ in a rib with cortical disruption. *(Right)* Axial fused PET/CT of the same patient shows moderately increased FDG activity ➡ within the lesion.

PET/CT Findings: Multiple Myeloma

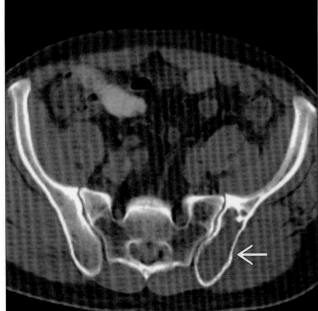
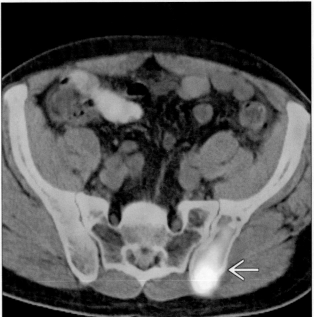

(Left) Axial NECT shows an expansile lytic lesion in the left iliac bone ➡. *(Right)* Axial fused PET/CT of the same patient shows intense FDG uptake in the expansile lesion ➡, compatible with multiple myeloma.

3

MULTIPLE MYELOMA

PET/CT Findings: Multiple Myeloma

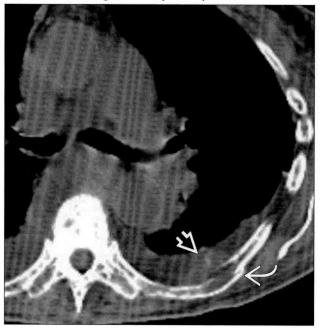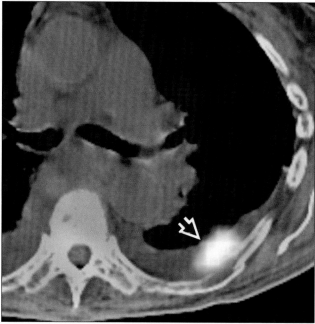

(Left) Axial NECT shows a soft tissue, pleural-based mass (plasmacytoma) ⬂ atop a pathologic rib fracture ➡ in a patient with multiple myeloma. *(Right)* Axial fused PET/CT in the same patient shows the pleural-based lesion to be hypermetabolic ➡.

PET/CT Findings: Multiple Myeloma

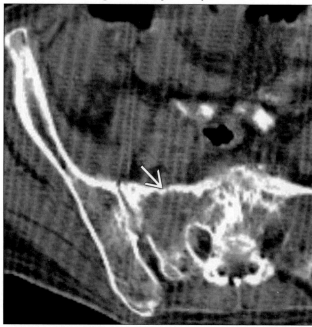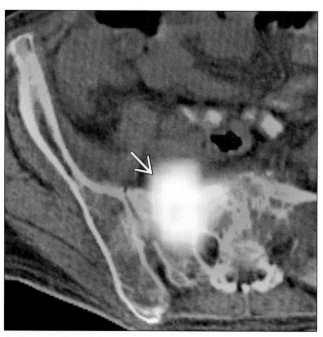

(Left) Axial NECT shows a lytic, expansile right sacral lesion ➡. *(Right)* Axial fused PET/CT of the same patient shows the right sacral lesion to be hypermetabolic ➡.

MULTIPLE MYELOMA

PET/CT Findings: Multiple Myeloma

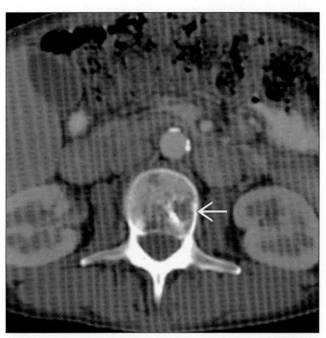

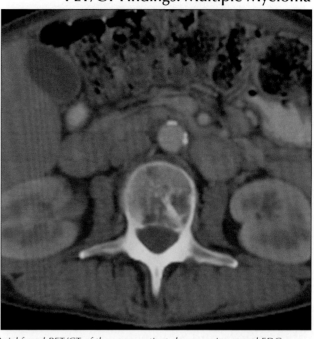

(Left) Axial CECT shows lytic foci in a lumbar vertebral body ➡. *(Right)* Axial fused PET/CT of the same patient shows no increased FDG uptake in the lytic lesions.

PET/CT Findings: Multiple Myeloma

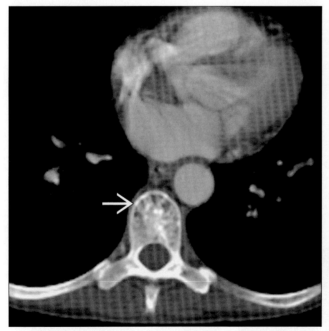

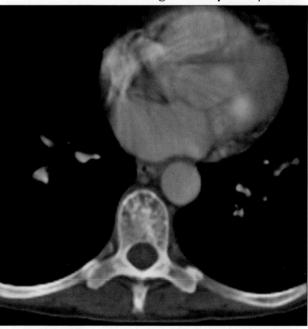

(Left) Axial CECT shows tiny lytic lesions in the anterior aspect of the vertebral body ➡. *(Right)* Axial fused PET/CT of the same patient shows no hypermetabolic activity in the lytic lesions.

SOFT TISSUE SARCOMAS

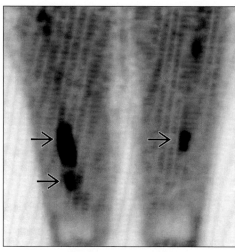

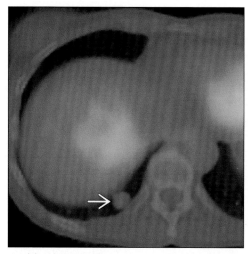

Coronal PET shows lesions with intense FDG activity in both legs ⇨ in this patient with a newly diagnosed sarcoma.

Axial fused PET/CT shows a non-FDG avid pulmonary metastasis ⇨ in the same patient as the previous image.

TERMINOLOGY

Abbreviations and Synonyms
- Liposarcoma
- Leiomyosarcoma
- Rhabdomyosarcoma
- Synovial sarcoma
- Fibrosarcoma
- Malignant fibrous histiocytoma (MFH)
- Angiosarcoma

Definitions
- Heterogeneous group of malignancies arising from mesenchymal tissues

IMAGING FINDINGS

General Features
- Best diagnostic clue
  - Large mixed-attenuation mass
  - Variable FDG activity within larger masses
    - Usually with peripheral ring-like FDG activity and central photopenia
- Small lesions will demonstrate a wide range of FDG activity
  - Central necrosis
  - Peripheral contrast enhancement
- Location
  - Location of primary lesion depends on primary mesenchymal tissue affected
  - Sarcomas tend to have very unpredictable patterns of metastatic disease
- Size
  - Variable from subcentimeter to very large
    - Often present as large tumors 10-15 cm
- Morphology
  - Variable, but larger metastatic lesions tend to outgrow blood supply
  - Often contain large areas of central necrosis
  - Usually well-circumscribed lesions
  - Following therapy, minimal change may be seen in tumor morphology in spite of significant changes in viability

Imaging Recommendations
- Best imaging tool

DDx: FDG Avid Soft Tissue Mass

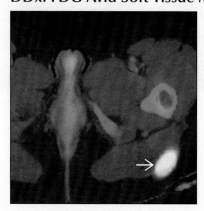

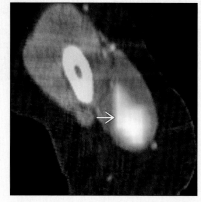

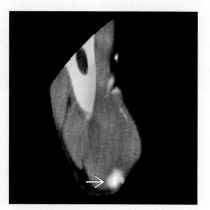

Metastasis: Melanoma

Physiologic Muscular FDG Activity

Injection Site

SOFT TISSUE SARCOMAS

Key Facts

Terminology
- Heterogeneous group of malignancies arising from mesenchymal tissues

Imaging Findings
- Overall accuracy of combined PET/CT and conventional imaging in preoperative TNM staging for soft tissue sarcoma was 87%
- PET/CT useful mainly for more accurate M-staging
- FDG-avid primary does not imply equally intense FDG uptake in pulmonary metastases
- FDG PET has been shown to have low sensitivity for detection of nodal metastases during chemotherapy with rhabdomyosarcoma
- Useful for therapeutic monitoring and distinguishing chronic scar from sarcoma
- Large mixed attenuation mass
- Variable FDG activity within larger masses
- Central necrosis
- Peripheral contrast enhancement

Top Differential Diagnoses
- Fibrosarcoma
- Malignant Fibrous Histiocytoma
- Synovial Sarcoma
- Leiomyosarcoma
- Liposarcoma
- Melanoma
- Metastases

Diagnostic Checklist
- PET/CT may be helpful
  - Remember that some sarcomas may not be FDG-avid, and some metastases will show variable FDG activity

---

- Combination of imaging modalities, including CT, MR, and PET/CT
- Overall accuracy of combined PET/CT and conventional imaging
  - Pre-operative TNM staging for soft tissue sarcoma 87% accurate
  - Used to grade sarcomas and assess response to therapy in advanced disease
  - Good for clinical applications of detecting & grading sarcomas and treatment evaluation of locally advanced disease
- Protocol advice
  - Consider performing PET/CT with a dedicated contrast-enhanced CT for staging
  - If tumor is not FDG avid, follow-up with CT or MR

CT Findings
- **Malignant fibrous histiocytoma (MFH)**
  - Typically a nonspecific, large, lobulated soft tissue mass
    - Predominantly muscle density, with nodular and peripheral enhancement of solid portions
  - Central areas of low attenuation may be present
    - Correspond to myxoid regions, old hemorrhage, or necrosis
  - Fat attenuation is not observed in the tumors
    - Can be useful in distinguishing MFH from some well-differentiated liposarcomas
  - CT may be used to evaluate potential internal matrix &/or cortical erosion
  - Retroperitoneal tumors manifest as heterogeneous masses
    - May have areas of hemorrhage &/or necrosis
    - Occasionally focal or diffuse coarse calcifications (approximately 10%)
    - May invade the abdominal musculature
    - Do not invade the renal veins or inferior vena cava
- **Liposarcoma**
  - CT scans demonstrate 3 distinct patterns
    - Enhancing, solid, inhomogeneous, poorly defined, infiltrating mass
    - Mixed-pattern tumor with foci of fat interspersed in high-attenuating tissue
    - Pseudocystic water-density tumor
  - Liposarcomas of the myxoid, mixed myxoid and round cell, round cell, and pleomorphic types are usually poorly defined
    - Attenuation values of 12-38 HU
    - Varying degrees of contrast enhancement
    - Calcification is detectable in as many as 12% of the tumors
  - Occasionally, the mass may appear inhomogeneous
    - Low-attenuation, fatty components
    - Soft tissue elements
- **Synovial sarcoma**
  - Findings are nonspecific and usually demonstrate a single round or lobulated mass with a soft tissue density
  - Lesions measure approximately 3-12 cm in their largest dimension
  - Usually found near a joint
  - Mass is typically well-defined
    - Occasionally appear infiltrative and can be homogeneous and show homogeneous enhancement
    - Particularly in smaller lesions
    - Alternatively, if hemorrhage or necrosis has occurred, the lesion may be multiloculated and show heterogeneous enhancement
  - Calcifications are demonstrated in 30% of patients
    - Typically diffuse and punctate; more often concentrated at periphery than at center
  - Extensive calcifications can be similar in appearance to osteosarcoma or a calcified chondroid lesion
  - Densely calcified lesions, when found near a joint, may simulate tumoral calcinosis
  - Involvement of the adjacent bone can cause changes
    - Including cortical invasion with a wide zone of transition
    - Bone remodeling from pressure erosion
    - Adjacent periosteal reaction
- **Rhabdomyosarcoma**
  - Isodense to muscle

3

SOFT TISSUE SARCOMAS

- o Heterogeneous enhancement
- o Younger patient population
- o Orbit: Large soft tissue mass with ill-defined margins
  - Destruction of orbital wall
  - Extension into preseptal space, sinuses, intracranial cavity
  - Associated sclerosis and periosteal reaction

Nuclear Medicine Findings

- **Initial diagnosis**
  - o Substantial differences have been seen in FDG uptake between low and high grade soft tissue sarcomas
    - Uptake values correlate with histologic grade in heterogeneous series of soft tissue sarcomas
  - o Studies show that FDG PET may discriminate between sarcomas and benign tumors as well as between low and high grade sarcomas
    - Small study found cutoff SUV value of 1.6 for stratifying low and high grade tumors
    - Correlation has not been seen in all studies
  - o FDG PET useful for identifying the most metabolically active portion of tumor mass to increase accuracy in biopsy
  - o Sarcomas with significant amount of acellular matrix material can have dilution of FDG signal and underestimation of biological aggressiveness
    - Examples include myxoid liposarcomas and chondrosarcomas
  - o Some sarcomas may have variable FDG uptake
  - o Metastatic lesions also may have variable FDG activity
    - Staging study with an FDG-avid primary and a non-FDG-avid lesion suspicious for metastatic disease will usually represent metastis
- **Staging**
  - o PET/CT useful mainly for more accurate M-staging
  - o FDG-avid primary does not imply equally intense FDG uptake in pulmonary metastases
    - CT superior for detection of pulmonary mets
    - However, also a higher false positive rate
  - o Using tumor-to-background SUV ratio cutoff of 3.0
    - Sensitivity for detection of malignancy was 93%, specificity 67%, and accuracy 82%
- **Restaging**
  - o PET/CT may be helpful for restaging patients with a variety of soft tissue sarcomas
  - o Major limitation is that many sarcomas show variability in their FDG uptake
    - May lead to false negatives
    - PET/CT more helpful when positive, as a negative study may indicate a non-FDG-avid tumor
- **Response to therapy**
  - o Evaluation of response to chemotherapy is crucial
    - May impact surgical planning for amputation or limb saving procedures
  - o FDG PET useful for prediction of outcomes in patients with high grade extremity soft tissue sarcomas treated with chemotherapy
  - o Patients with high grade localized sarcomas showing SUV max > 6.0 and having less than 40% decreased in SUV after chemotherapy

- 90% risk of systemic recurrence 4 years from time of initial diagnosis
- Another study used SUV cutoff of 4.0 and tumor grade of III to provide prediction of relapse (PPV = 90%, NPV = 95%)
- Max SUV recorded in a variety of tumors treated with neoadjuvant chemotherapy or resection
- Shown to be a statistically significant predictor of survival after adjusting for standard clinical prognostic factors, including grade
  - o Used for treatment monitoring
    - FDG PET may help clinicians decide to prolong chemotherapy or proceed with surgery
  - o Persistent accumulation of FDG has been reported within benign therapy-related fibrous tissue
    - Fibrous pseudocapsule with inflammatory tissue that can form around tumor after treatment
    - Inflammatory response on post-chemotherapy scans appears as a rim of increased FDG activity around tumor
    - Using SUV max as tool for assessment of response to therapy may prove difficult
  - o Useful for therapeutic monitoring and distinguishing chronic scar from sarcoma

DIFFERENTIAL DIAGNOSIS

Fibrosarcoma
- Nonspecific findings
- Overlap with many other sarcomas

Malignant Fibrous Histiocytoma
- Nonspecific findings
- Overlap with many other sarcomas

Synovial Sarcoma
- Proximity to joint
- Overlap with many other sarcomas

Leiomyosarcoma
- Nonspecific findings
- Overlap with many other sarcomas

Liposarcoma
- Typically contain variable amounts of fat
- Presence of any enhancement or any complexity of the lesion should discourage a diagnosis of lipoma
- Often appear in the retroperitoneal space

Melanoma
- History is essential
- May be indistinguishable from sarcoma metastases

Metastases
- Will have variable appearance depending on the primary tumor type
- History is crucial
- Often indistinguishable from sarcoma metastases

SOFT TISSUE SARCOMAS

PATHOLOGY

General Features
- General path comments: Mixed cellularity of mesenchymal tissues
- Epidemiology
  - Soft tissue sarcomas are rare tumors, approximately 0.7% of adult malignancies
    - In children younger than 15 years, soft tissue sarcomas represent 6.5% of all cancers
    - Rhabdomyosarcoma most common pediatric sarcoma

Microscopic Features
- In surgically treated patients, the most important prognostic factor has been shown by some groups to be chemotherapy-induced necrosis
- Histopathologic examination of surgical specimens post-therapy is difficult because of abundance of fibroblasts
  - Identification of tumor necrosis vs. chemo-induced inflammatory response is therefore also difficult

CLINICAL ISSUES

Presentation
- Most common signs/symptoms: Variable, depending on the primary tumor type

Natural History & Prognosis
- Patients with high grade soft tissue sarcoma are at high risk for developing distant pulmonary metastases

Treatment
- Anthracyclines and ifosfamide
  - Established as the most active drugs for treatment of patients with advanced soft tissue sarcoma
  - Few treatment options remain in the case of failure of these drugs
  - Effective for most histologic subtypes (except GIST)
- Ifosfamide thought to induce inflammatory response in tumor bed
  - Can make interpretation of post-therapy FDG PET scan difficult
- FDG PET results for treatment monitoring may determine type of surgical intervention
  - Limb salvage cannot be recommended to patients in whom wide margins cannot safely be achieved
- Curative treatment approach typically includes surgery
  - Often combined with chemoradiation therapy

DIAGNOSTIC CHECKLIST

Consider
- PET/CT may be helpful for staging, restaging, and response to therapy
  - However, some sarcomas may not be FDG avid, and some metastases will show variable FDG activity
- If lesions are not FDG avid on PET, follow-up with CT or MR

SELECTED REFERENCES

1. Buck AK et al: Imaging bone and soft tissue tumors with the proliferation marker [18F]fluorodeoxythymidine. Clin Cancer Res. 14(10):2970-7, 2008
2. Conill C et al: Diagnostic efficacy of bone scintigraphy, magnetic resonance imaging, and positron emission tomography in bone metastases of myxoid liposarcoma. J Magn Reson Imaging. 27(3):625-8, 2008
3. Evilevitch V et al: Reduction of glucose metabolic activity is more accurate than change in size at predicting histopathologic response to neoadjuvant therapy in high-grade soft-tissue sarcomas. Clin Cancer Res. 14(3):715-20, 2008
4. Fadul D et al: Advanced modalities for the imaging of sarcoma. Surg Clin North Am. 88(3):521-37, vi, 2008
5. James SL et al: Post-operative imaging of soft tissue sarcomas. Cancer Imaging. 8:8-18, 2008
6. Kasper B et al: Early prediction of therapy outcome in patients with high-risk soft tissue sarcoma using positron emission tomography. Onkologie. 31(3):107-12, 2008
7. Nakamura-Horigome M et al: Successful treatment of primary cardiac angiosarcoma with docetaxel and radiotherapy. Angiology. 59(3):368-71, 2008
8. Park K et al: The role of radiology in paediatric soft tissue sarcomas. Cancer Imaging. 8:102-15, 2008
9. Schuetze SM et al: Selection of response criteria for clinical trials of sarcoma treatment. Oncologist. 13 Suppl 2:32-40, 2008
10. Sheah K et al: Metastatic myxoid liposarcomas: imaging and histopathologic findings. Skeletal Radiol. 37(3):251-8, 2008
11. Sung PL et al: Whole-body positron emission tomography with 18F-fluorodeoxyglucose is an effective method to detect extra-pelvic recurrence in uterine sarcomas. Eur J Gynaecol Oncol. 29(3):246-51, 2008
12. Tewfik JN et al: Fluorine-18-deoxyglucose-positron emission tomography imaging with magnetic resonance and computed tomographic correlation in the evaluation of bone and soft-tissue sarcomas: a pictorial essay. Curr Probl Diagn Radiol. 37(4):178-88, 2008
13. Toner GC et al: PET for sarcomas other than gastrointestinal stromal tumors. Oncologist. 13 Suppl 2:22-6, 2008
14. Reddy MP et al: Accurate grading of 3 synchronous liposarcomas assessed by PET-CT in a single patient. Clin Nucl Med. 32(12):937-9, 2007
15. Brenner W et al: Risk assessment in liposarcoma patients based on FDG PET imaging. Eur J Nucl Med Mol Imaging. 33(11):1290-5, 2006
16. Suzuki R et al: PET evaluation of fatty tumors in the extremity: possibility of using the standardized uptake value (SUV) to differentiate benign tumors from liposarcoma. Ann Nucl Med. 19(8):661-70, 2005
17. Schwarzbach MH et al: Assessment of soft tissue lesions suspicious for liposarcoma by F18-deoxyglucose (FDG) positron emission tomography (PET). Anticancer Res. 21(5):3609-14, 2001
18. Jadvar H et al: Evaluation of Rare Tumors with [F-18]Fluorodeoxyglucose Positron Emission Tomography. Clin Positron Imaging. 2(3):153-158, 1999
19. Adler LP et al: Grading liposarcomas with PET using [18F]FDG. J Comput Assist Tomogr. 14(6):960-2, 1990
20. Kern KA et al: Metabolic imaging of human extremity musculoskeletal tumors by PET. J Nucl Med. 29(2):181-6, 1988
21. Kalender ME et al: Detection of complete response to imatinib mesylate (Glivec((R))/Gleevec ((R))) with 18F-FDG PET/CT for low-grade endometrial stromal sarcoma. Cancer Chemother Pharmacol. (In Press)

SOFT TISSUE SARCOMAS

CT Findings: Primary

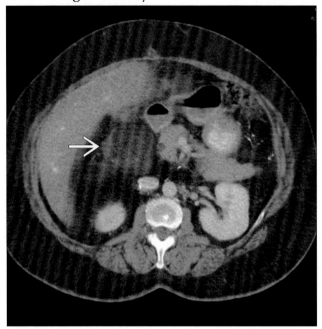
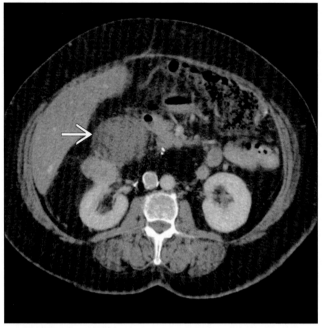

(Left) Axial CECT shows a "hazy" fat-containing lesion ➡ that was subsequently proven to be a liposarcoma. *(Right)* Axial CECT shows the same lesion ➡ more inferiorly, where it displays a more solid enhancing component.

CT Findings: Primary

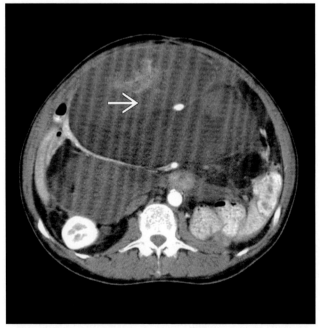
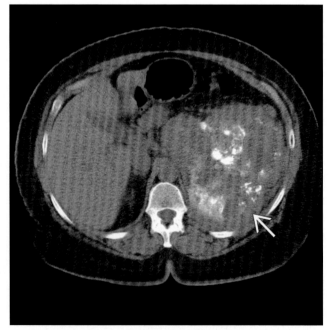

(Left) Axial CECT shows a very large lesion ➡ in the abdomen containing fat, hemorrhage, and central enhancement, consistent with a large soft tissue sarcoma. *(Right)* Axial NECT shows a large soft tissue mass containing calcifications ➡, subsequently proven to be a sarcoma.

SOFT TISSUE SARCOMAS

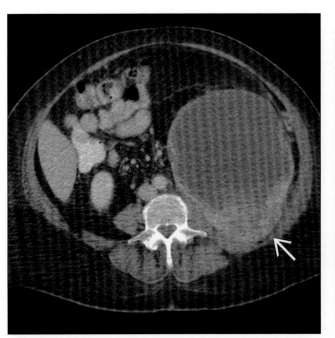
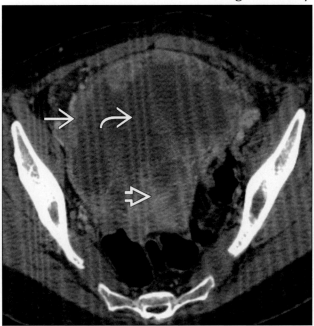

(Left) Axial CECT shows a mass with regions of necrosis enhancing centrally and peripherally ➡ in the left retroperitoneal space. *(Right)* Axial CECT shows the same lesion ➡ extending into the pelvis with central necrosis ➡ and peripheral enhancement ➡, consistent with leiomyosarcoma.

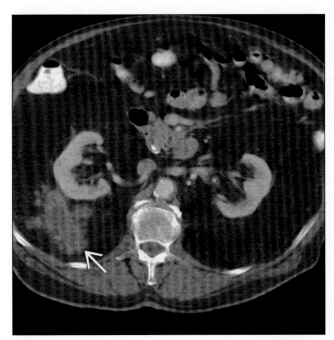
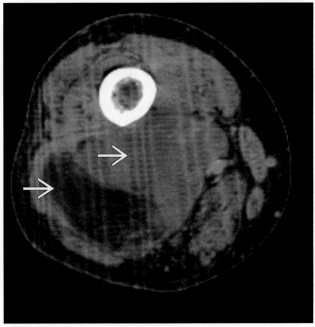

(Left) Axial CECT shows a heterogeneously enhancing mass ➡ in the left posterior pararenal space, consistent with a high grade liposarcoma. *(Right)* Axial CECT shows a large, mixed fat/soft tissue attenuation mass in the right thigh ➡. Biopsy proved this to be a high grade sarcoma.

SOFT TISSUE SARCOMAS

CT Findings: Primary

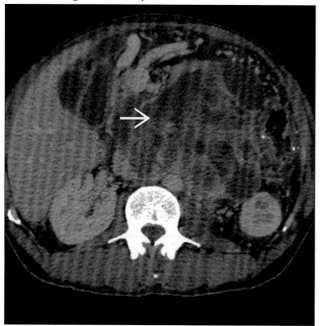 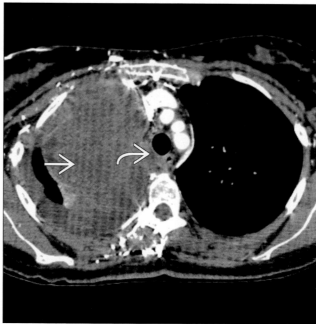

(Left) Axial CECT shows a very large mixed attenuation mass centered in the retroperitoneal area ➡, proven at biopsy to be a poorly differentiated liposarcoma. (Right) Axial CECT shows a large heterogeneously enhancing mass at the right apex ➡ with probable pleural invasion ➡.

CT Findings: Primary

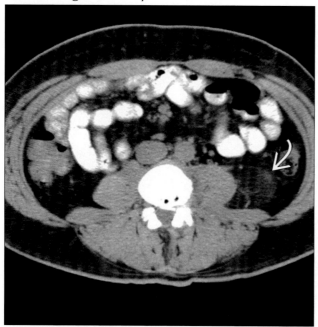 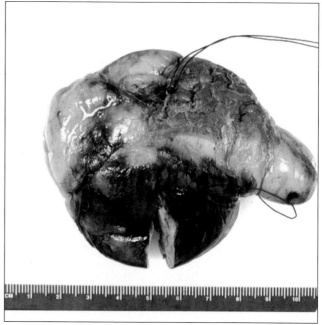

(Left) Axial CECT shows a mostly fat attenuation mass, later found to be a liposarcoma. Note the focal region of enhancement peripherally ➡. Soft tissue component or enhancement should raise the suspicion for a liposarcoma, rather than a lipoma. (Right) Gross pathology shows the specimen of the left retroperitoneal lesion following resection.

SOFT TISSUE SARCOMAS

CT Findings: Staging

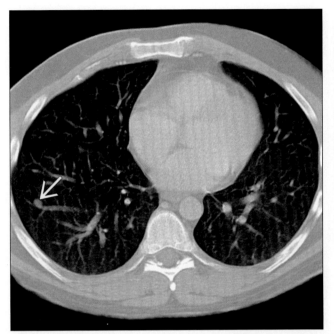

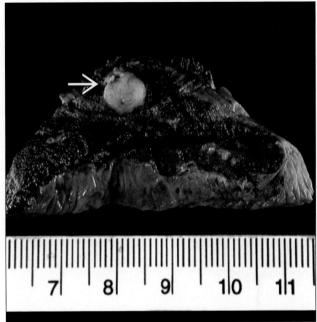

(Left) Axial NECT shows a new pulmonary nodule ➡ in this patient with a history of sarcoma, compatible with a small pulmonary metastasis. *(Right)* Surgical pathology specimen of the same lesion following resection shows a well-rounded tan nodular mass ➡. If the lesion is close to the pleural surface, the patient may present with a pneumothorax.

CT Findings: Restaging

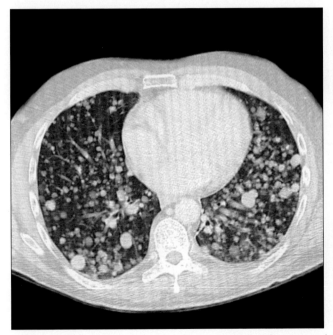

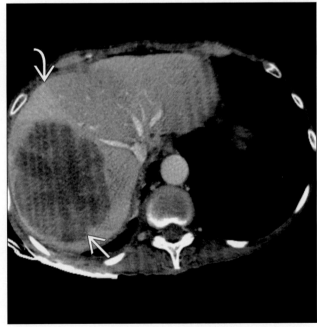

(Left) Axial NECT in the same patient shows numerous pulmonary nodules in both lower lobes, consistent with pulmonary metastases from a sarcoma. *(Right)* Axial CECT shows a large necrotic heterogeneously enhancing mass in the posterior right hepatic lobe ➡ in this patient with a history of a sarcoma. Note the sharp demarcation of enhancement ➡, greater in the right hepatic lobe, created by impaired portal venous inflow from pressure exerted by the tumor, creating a transient hepatic attenuation difference or THAD.

SOFT TISSUE SARCOMAS

CT Findings: Restaging

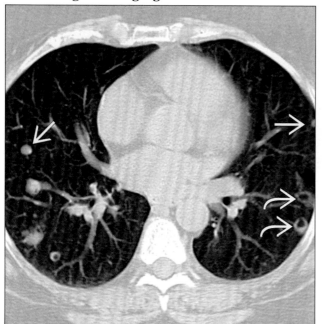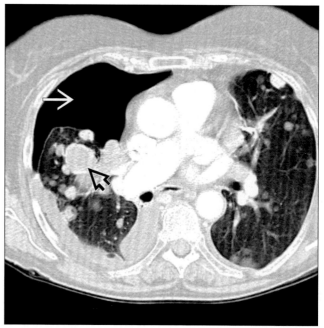

(Left) Axial CECT shows several pulmonary metastases ➡ bilaterally. Note that several have slight cavitation ➡, a nonspecific finding that may be seen with sarcomatous metastases. *(Right)* Axial CECT of the same patient performed several months later shows progression of the metastases ➡; one of them has caused a pneumothorax ➡.

Typical

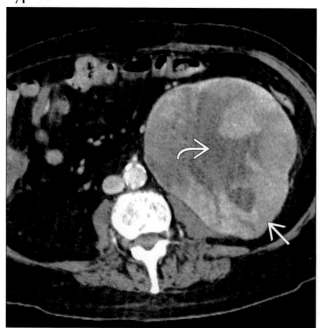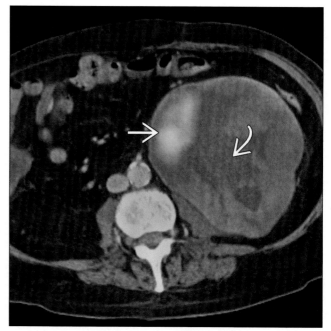

(Left) Axial CECT shows a large retroperitoneal mass ➡ that is heterogeneously enhancing and centrally necrotic ➡. *(Right)* Axial fused PET/CT of the same patient shows the more solid appearing components ➡ to be FDG avid, although the central necrotic portion does not have any FDG uptake ➡. These findings are characteristic of sarcoma metastases.

SOFT TISSUE SARCOMAS

Typical

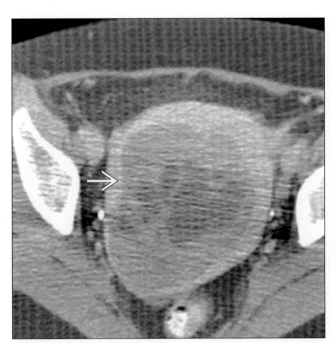 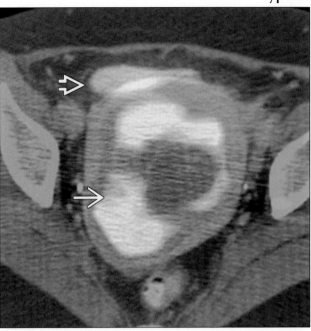

(Left) Axial CECT shows a large heterogeneously enhancing mass in the pelvis ➡ immediately superior to the bladder, proven at biopsy to be uterine leiomyosarcoma. *(Right)* Axial fused PET/CT of the same patient shows intense FDG uptake in the more solid components of the tumor ➡. Note the misregistration artifact ➡ from the bladder, which is immediately below the tumor.

PET/CT Findings: Staging

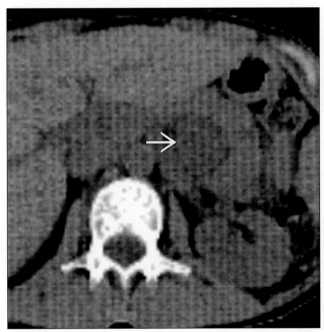 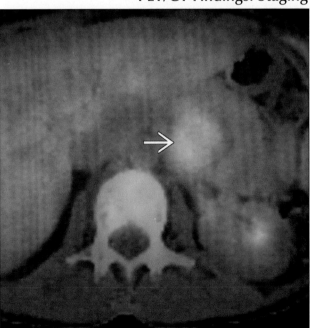

(Left) Axial NECT shows metastatic upper abdominal adenopathy ➡ in a patient with a history of sarcoma. *(Right)* Axial fused PET/CT shows mildly to moderately increased FDG activity within the upper abdominal metastases ➡. In general, sarcomas may have variably FDG-avid metastases compared to the primary lesion.

SOFT TISSUE SARCOMAS

PET/CT Findings: Staging

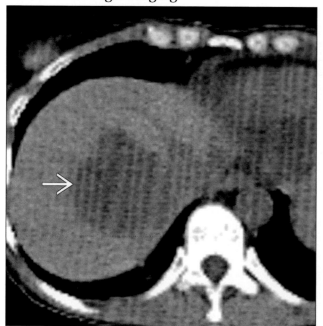 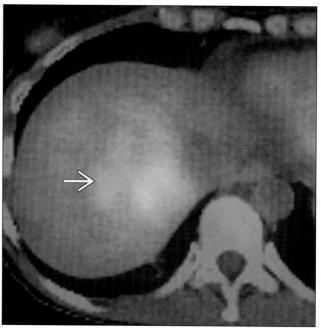

(Left) Axial NECT shows a large low attenuation lesion in the dome of the liver ➡ in this patient with a large primary sarcoma. *(Right)* Axial fused PET/CT shows areas of mildly and moderately increased FDG activity that correspond to the large low attenuation hepatic lesion ➡, compatible with metastatic disease from the patient's known sarcoma.

PET/CT Findings: Staging

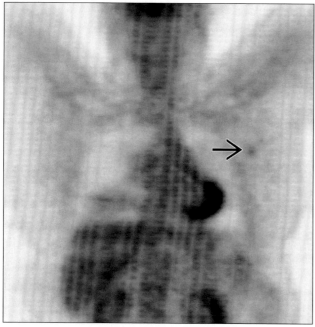 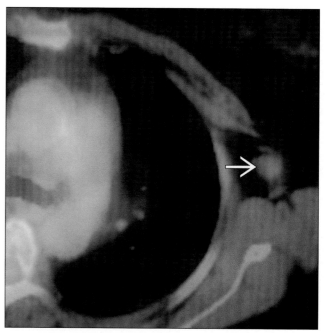

(Left) Coronal PET shows a mildly hypermetabolic left axillary lymph node ➡ in a patient with a history of soft tissue sarcoma of the chest wall. *(Right)* Axial fused PET/CT shows mildly increased FDG activity in a left axillary lymph node ➡, which was biopsy-proven to be metastasis from the patient's primary sarcoma of the chest wall.

SOFT TISSUE SARCOMAS

PET/CT Findings: Staging

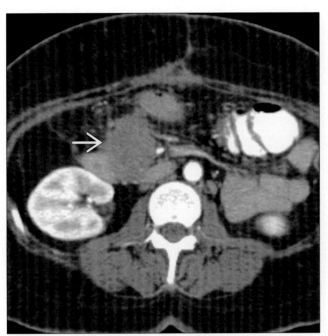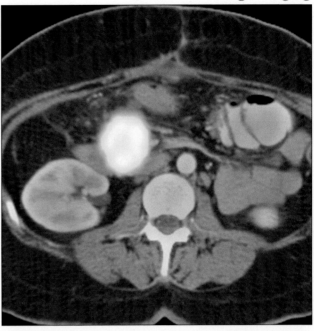

(Left) Axial CECT shows a soft tissue mass ➡ in the retroperitoneal area in this patient with a history of metastatic sarcoma. *(Right)* Axial fused PET/CT shows intense FDG uptake in the same lesion, compatible with metastatic disease.

PET/CT Findings: Restaging

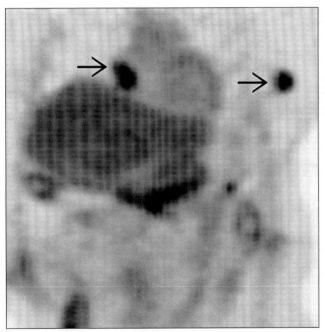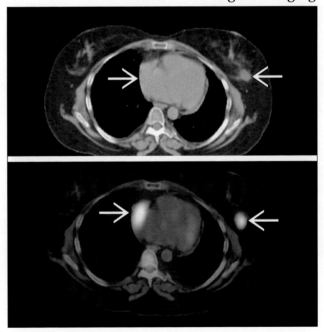

(Left) Coronal PET shows foci of increased activity at the right heart border and in the left breast ➡ in this patient with a history of sarcoma. *(Right)* Axial NECT (top) and fused PET/CT (bottom) show soft tissue lesions ➡ in the right pericardial region and left breast, both with increased FDG activity, consistent with metastases.

SOFT TISSUE SARCOMAS

PET/CT Findings: Restaging

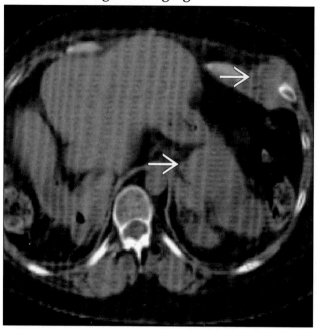 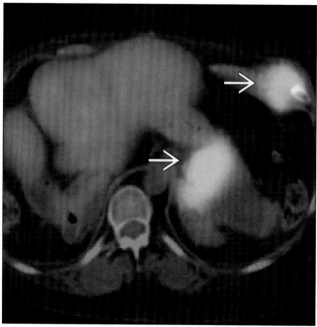

(Left) Axial NECT shows soft tissue masses ➡ anterior to the left adrenal and in the anterior intercostal space on the left. *(Right)* Axial fused PET/CT shows FDG activity in the region of the soft tissue lesions ➡ shown on the previous image.

PET/CT Findings: Restaging

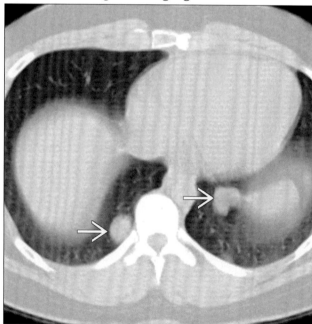 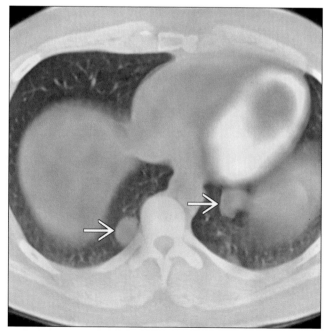

(Left) Axial NECT shows two lower lobe, well-demarcated lesions ➡ in this patient with a history of a sarcoma, compatible with metastatic disease. *(Right)* Axial fused PET/CT shows only mildly increased metabolic activity within the lower lobe metastases ➡. Sarcomas may show variability in FDG activity in metastatic lesions.

SOFT TISSUE SARCOMAS

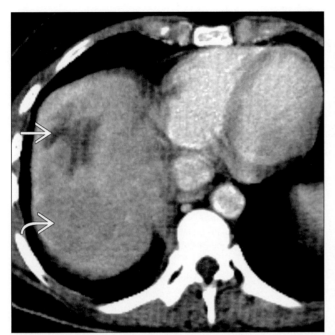 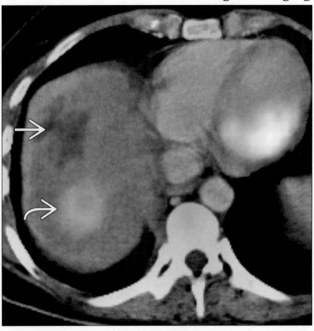

(Left) Axial CECT shows a mostly low attenuation sarcoma metastasis ➡, in addition to a subtle but large lesion ➡ more posteriorly. *(Right)* Axial fused PET/CT shows no increased activity correlating to the more anterior lesion ➡ and mild to moderately increased activity in the more posterior lesion ➡. Variability in FDG activity within multiple metastases is characteristic of sarcomas on FDG PET.

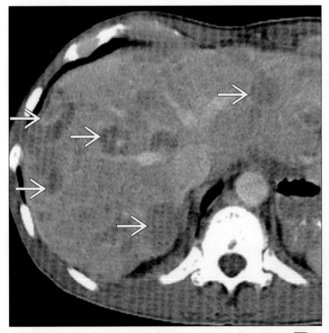 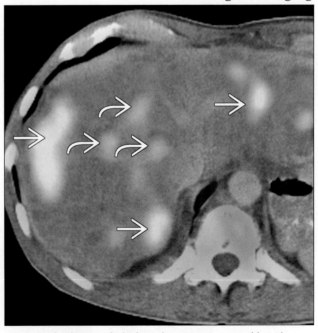

(Left) Axial CECT shows bilobar low attenuation hepatic lesions ➡ in this patient with a history of a high grade sarcoma, compatible with metastatic disease. *(Right)* Axial fused PET/CT shows corresponding metabolic activity in the bilobar hepatic metastases. Note that the larger lesions have moderate to intense FDG activity ➡, while the smaller lesions have milder FDG activity ➡.

MESOTHELIOMA

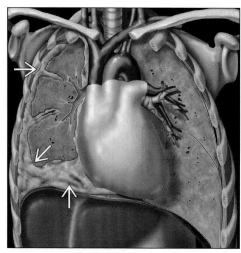

Graphic shows nodular thickening of the right pleura ➡, representing mesothelioma.

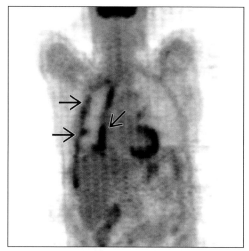

Coronal PET shows increased FDG activity ➡ in the right pleura in a patient with mesothelioma.

TERMINOLOGY

Abbreviations and Synonyms
- Malignant mesothelioma (MM)
- Peritoneal mesothelioma (PM)
- Benign variant: Asbestos-related benign pleural disease

Definitions
- Primary neoplasm arising from mesothelial cells that line body cavities

IMAGING FINDINGS

General Features
- Best diagnostic clue
  - Chest: Pleural effusion, thickening, calcification
  - Abdomen: Omental caking or peritoneal masses
- Location
  - 60-80% of cases have primary arising from mesothelial surfaces of pleura
    - Also seen in peritoneum, pericardium, and tunica vaginalis
  - Compared with other intrathoracic malignancies, lymphatic pattern of spread of mesothelioma is unpredictable
  - Distant metastases historically uncommon due to poor prognosis and rapid demise of patients
    - Recent reports more common
    - Reported in brain, lung, bone, adrenals, peritoneum, abdominal lymph nodes, and abdominal wall
- Size: Focal masses may grow to several centimeters
- Morphology
  - 75% of pleural mesotheliomas are diffuse desmoplastic type (usually malignant)
    - Diffuse disease may envelop abdominal viscera
  - Remainder are focal, producing large mass with scattered pleural/peritoneal nodules

Imaging Recommendations
- Best imaging tool
  - Although not routinely used, PET/CECT may offer best information for diagnosis, staging, and response to therapy
  - CT sensitive but not specific for invasion
- Protocol advice

DDx: FDG Activity in Pleura or Pleural Space

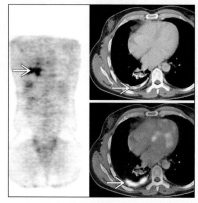

Inflammation: Talc Pleurodesis

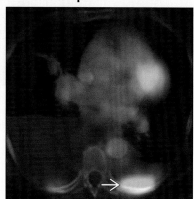

Malignant Pleural Effusion

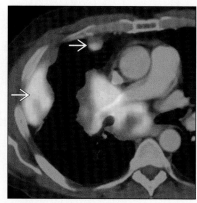

Pleura Metastases

MESOTHELIOMA

Key Facts

Imaging Findings

- Pleural effusion &/or pleural thickening
- 80% of cases have primary arising from mesothelial surfaces of pleura
  - Also seen in peritoneum, pericardium, and tunica vaginalis
- Distant metastases historically uncommon due to poor prognosis and rapid demise of patients
- 75% of pleural mesotheliomas are diffuse (usually malignant)
- Nodular, irregular, unilateral pleural thickening
- CT findings in mesothelioma by frequency
  - Pleural thickening
  - Thickening of interlobular fissures
  - Pleural effusion
  - Pleural calcification

- Features helpful in distinguishing malignant from benign pleural disease include
  - Circumferential pleural thickening
  - Nodular pleural thickening
  - Mesothelioma generally FDG avid
- FDG PET accurate for prediction of response with serial changes in tumor tracer uptake following one cycle of chemotherapy

Top Differential Diagnoses

- Chronic Organized Empyema
- Metastatic Tumor to Pleura, Especially Adenocarcinoma
- Infection Processes (e.g., Actinomycosis, Tuberculosis, Nocardiosis)
- Asbestos-related Pleural Disease

- Modified breathing algorithms to reduce misregistration along diaphragm
  - Coronal reformation of CECT may aid in detection of mesothelioma
- Water or oral contrast to distend bowel loops

CT Findings

- Pleural disease best imaged with contrast enhancement at 45-60 second delayed scan time
- Extent of pleural and extrapleural involvement is well-evaluated on CT
- **Most common findings**
  - Irregular, unilateral thickening of the pleura in a nodular, concentric, or plaque-like configuration
  - Pleural effusion
    - Pleural effusion commonly fills 1/3 to 2/3 of hemithorax
- **Pleural thickening may present with**
  - Greater thickness at bases
  - Thickening of interlobular fissures
  - Calcification
  - Contraction of hemithorax in 40%
  - Chest wall invasion (difficult to detect based on irregularity alone)
  - Bilaterality in 20%
- **Findings of local invasion**
  - Irregular contour along inferior aspect of diaphragm
  - Invasion of endothoracic fat
  - Loss of normal adjacent fat planes
  - Infiltration along biopsy tract or surgical incision seen in 20%
  - Greater than 50% circumferential encasement of mediastinal structure
- **Findings of extrathoracic spread**
  - Soft tissue mass encasing hemidiaphragm
  - Absence of fat plane between diaphragm and abdominal organs
  - Liver metastases may rarely present with diffuse calcification
- **Findings typical of malignant vs. benign disease**
  - Involvement of mediastinal pleura
  - Nodular pleural thickening

- Greater than 1 cm thickening of parietal pleura
  - Circumferential pleural thickening
- **Response to therapy**
  - Modified RECIST criteria evaluating thickness of involved pleura
    - Must decrease by 30% to indicate partial response to therapy
  - In one study, 47% of partial responders imaged with CT were detected after one cycle of chemotherapy

Nuclear Medicine Findings

- **Initial Diagnosis**
  - Mesothelioma generally FDG avid
    - Mild or absent FDG uptake has been reported in some patients with mesothelioma of epithelial subtype
  - SUV of 2.0 used as cutoff for suspicion of malignancy in pleural lesions
  - FDG PET pattern and intensity do not allow differentiation of
    - Subtypes of malignant pleural mesothelioma
    - Mesothelioma from adenocarcinoma or sarcoma
- **Staging**
  - PET/CT suited for
    - Detection of unsuspected nodal and occult distant metastases
    - Particularly useful for staging mediastinal nodal involvement
    - Sensitivity, specificity for T4 disease: 67% and 93%
    - PET alone sensitivity 19%
  - Limited for evaluation of nodal mets
    - 38% sensitivity in one study
    - Insensitive for microscopic disease
    - False positives from inflammatory/infectious etiologies
    - e.g., talc pleurodesis, benign inflammatory pleuritis, parapneumonic effusion, tuberculous pleuritis
  - Limited for determining presence/extent of local tumor invasion
- **Response to therapy**

3

MESOTHELIOMA

- o FDG PET accurate for prediction of response following one cycle of chemotherapy
- o Defining tumor volume is laborious and error-prone due to "rind-like" morphology of mesothelioma
  - Tumor glycolysis volume (TGV) has been used effectively for accurate prognostic information
  - TGV superior to max SUV or CT response after one cycle of chemotherapy for predicting survival
- • Morphology
  - o Tumors at earlier stage tend to have focal or linear patterns
  - o Mixed and encasing patterns are indicative of more advanced disease
- • PET/CT and CT alone differ in TNM classification in up to 50% of patients
  - o 50% of discordances clinically relevant
  - o PET/CT upstaged 12% of patients with noncurable disease and downstaged 12% of patients to curable disease
- • Prognosis
  - o Best: Low SUV and epithelial histology; median survival 24 months
  - o Worst: High SUV and sarcomatoid histology; median survival 14 months
  - o High SUV tumors associated with 3.3x higher risk of death than low SUV tumors
  - o Intensity of FDG uptake by primary shown to have poor correlation with histologic grade, good correlation with surgical stage

DIFFERENTIAL DIAGNOSIS

Asbestos Related Pleural Disease
- • Typically less FDG avid
- • Often indistinguishable from mesothelioma on CT
- • Look for absence of malignant findings
  - o Continuous pleural "rind"
  - o Pleural nodularity
  - o Thickening > 1 cm
  - o Involvement of mediastinal pleura
- • Benign disease may also demonstrate nodular pleural thickening
- • Biopsy recommended for equivocal cases
- • Calcified plaques are sign of asbestos exposure, not precursor to mesothelioma

Congestive Heart Failure
- • Interstitial and perivascular edema may develop, most prominent at lung bases
- • Large pleural effusions and alveolar edema in perihilar and lower lobe distribution
- • Correlate clinically with follow-up imaging

Chronic Organized Empyema
- • Gas bubbles in pleural fluid collection virtually diagnostic of empyema
- • Pleural thickening and enhancement very common
- • Rarely involves entire pleural space
- • Pleural tap is indicated

Malignant Fibrosing Histiocytoma
- • Typical findings include large lobulated soft tissue mass of muscle density

- • Central areas of low attenuation represent myxoid region, old hemorrhage, or necrosis
- • No fat attenuation
- • Tumors do not invade renal veins or inferior vena cava

Localized Fibrosing Tumor of the Pleura
- • Not associated with metastasis or lymphadenopathy

Metastatic Tumor to Pleura, Especially Adenocarcinoma
- • Noncalcified lesions
- • Spherical or ovoid lesions (vs. linear or irregular)
- • Close proximity to adjacent vessels
- • Pleural effusion in 50%

Other Causes of Pleural Effusion
- • CHF, PE
- • Para-pneumonic effusion
- • Acute pancreatitis
- • Systemic lupus erythematosus
- • Traumatic chylothorax
- • Uremia
- • Generally resolve spontaneously within 2 months

Infection Processes (e.g., Actinomycosis, Tuberculosis, Nocardiosis)
- • May invade chest wall but usually at single focus rather than multiple sites

PATHOLOGY

General Features
- • General path comments
  - o Three histologic categories
    - Epithelial: 55-65%
    - Sarcomatoid: 10-15%
    - Mixed: 20-35%
- • Etiology
  - o 77% of patients with pleural mesothelioma have history of asbestos exposure
    - e.g., mining, milling, manufacturing, shipyard work, building construction
    - Family members may be exposed to asbestos fibers in workers' clothing
    - Lifetime risk for asbestos workers of 8%
  - o Smoking is a significant risk factor in those with history of asbestos exposure
    - NO association between smoking and mesothelioma independent of asbestos
- • Epidemiology: ~ 3,000 cases per year in USA

Gross Pathologic & Surgical Features
- • Pleural surfaces become seeded with malignant cells, leading to grouped nodularity
- • Entire pleural space becomes covered; invasion into chest wall, mediastinum, and diaphragm is seen

Microscopic Features
- • Pleural fluid and tissue reveal malignant cells of epithelial, sarcomatous, or mixed subtype
- • Hemorrhagic exudate common in pleural fluid

MESOTHELIOMA

CLINICAL ISSUES

Presentation
- Most common signs/symptoms
  - Progressive dyspnea and non-pleuritic chest pain
  - Also fatigue, night sweats, weight loss, clubbing
  - Metastatic disease uncommon at presentation
    - Contralateral findings usually due to benign asbestos-related pleural disease

Demographics
- Age
  - Mean age of onset is 40-60 years
    - Incidence peaks 25-40 years after asbestos exposure
- Gender: M:F = 3:1

Natural History & Prognosis
- Marked by rapid spread along pleural surfaces and involvement of pericardium, mediastinum, and contralateral pleura
- Distant metastasis eventually may occur to abdominal lymph nodes and organs
- Complications due to local invasion, include SVC syndrome, hoarseness, Horner syndrome, and dysphagia
- Paraneoplastic syndromes include DIC, hemolytic anemia, thrombocytosis, migratory thrombophlebitis
- Prognosis
  - Dismal for local or advanced disease
  - Localized: 5 months
  - Extensive: 16 months
  - 1 year survival: 25%
  - Best survival with limited primary, no nodal involvement, and epithelial subtype

Treatment
- On the whole, chemoradiation ineffective as primary treatment
  - Most chemo regimens are cisplatin-based and have failed to show survival benefit
  - Cisplatin and pemetrexed (antifolate agent) may improve survival by 3 months
- Extrapleural pneumonectomy or pleurectomy with decortication are indicated for patients with limited disease
  - Local control with surgery often plagued by presence of undetected distant metastasis
  - Pleurectomy with decortication is more limited procedure
    - Used for patients with inadequate cardiopulmonary reserve
  - EPP involves en-bloc resection of lung, pleura, and pericardium followed by reconstruction
  - Survival may be improved to 74% at 2 years and 39% at 5 years
- Palliative therapy
  - Resection may offer symptomatic benefits
  - Pleurodesis, drainage of effusions, and radiotherapy

DIAGNOSTIC CHECKLIST

Consider
- Adequate histologic specimen may require open pleural biopsy
- PET/CT superior to mediastinoscopy in sensitivity for depiction of local involvement

SELECTED REFERENCES

1. Fennell DA et al: Advances in the systemic therapy of malignant pleural mesothelioma. Nat Clin Pract Oncol. 5(3):136-47, 2008
2. Ceresoli GL et al: Assessment of tumor response in malignant pleural mesothelioma. Cancer Treat Rev. 33(6):533-41, 2007
3. Francis RJ et al: Early prediction of response to chemotherapy and survival in malignant pleural mesothelioma using a novel semiautomated 3-dimensional volume-based analysis of serial 18F-FDG PET scans. J Nucl Med. 48(9):1449-58, 2007
4. Spitilli MG et al: Malignant pleural mesothelioma: utility of 18 F-FDG PET. Ann Ital Chir. 78(5):393-6, 2007
5. Yamamuro M et al: Morphologic and functional imaging of malignant pleural mesothelioma. Eur J Radiol. 64(3):356-66, 2007
6. Ceresoli GL et al: Early response evaluation in malignant pleural mesothelioma by positron emission tomography with [18F]fluorodeoxyglucose. J Clin Oncol. 24(28):4587-93, 2006
7. Fiore D et al: Imaging before and after multimodal treatment for malignant pleural mesothelioma. Radiol Med (Torino). 111(3):355-64, 2006
8. Flores RM et al: Positron emission tomography predicts survival in malignant pleural mesothelioma. J Thorac Cardiovasc Surg. 132(4):763-8, 2006
9. Quint LE: PET: other thoracic malignancies. Cancer Imaging. 6:S82-8, 2006
10. Truong MT et al: Preoperative evaluation of patients with malignant pleural mesothelioma: role of integrated CT-PET imaging. J Thorac Imaging. 21(2):146-53, 2006
11. West SD et al: Management of malignant pleural mesothelioma. Clin Chest Med. 27(2):335-54, 2006
12. Ambrosini V et al: Additional value of hybrid PET/CT fusion imaging vs. conventional CT scan alone in the staging and management of patients with malignant pleural mesothelioma. Nucl Med Rev Cent East Eur. 8(2):111-5, 2005
13. Benamore RE et al: Use of imaging in the management of malignant pleural mesothelioma. Clin Radiol. 60(12):1237-47, 2005
14. Erasmus JJ et al: Integrated computed tomography-positron emission tomography in patients with potentially resectable malignant pleural mesothelioma: Staging implications. J Thorac Cardiovasc Surg. 129(6):1364-70, 2005
15. Flores RM: The role of PET in the surgical management of malignant pleural mesothelioma. Lung Cancer. 49 Suppl 1:S27-32, 2005
16. Rice DC et al: Extended surgical staging for potentially resectable malignant pleural mesothelioma. Ann Thorac Surg. 80(6):1988-92; discussion 1992-3, 2005
17. Salgado RA et al: Malignant pleural mesothelioma with heterologous osteoblastic elements: computed tomography, magnetic resonance, and positron emission tomography imaging characteristics of a rare tumor. J Comput Assist Tomogr. 29(5):653-6, 2005

MESOTHELIOMA

Typical

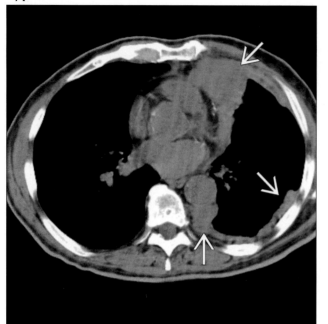 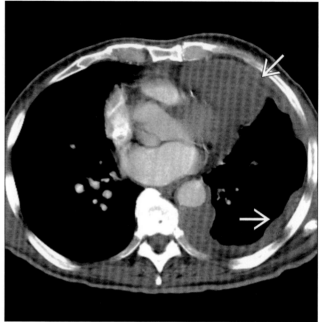

(Left) Axial NECT shows soft tissue nodular thickening involving the pleura ➡. Note anteriorly the soft tissue along the pleura that does not invade the mediastinum. The differential diagnostic considerations include metastasis, mesothelioma, fibrothorax, or prior pleurodesis. The marked soft tissue thickening anteriorly should raise concern for neoplasm. *(Right)* Axial CECT of the same patient as previous image shows interval progression ➡.

Typical

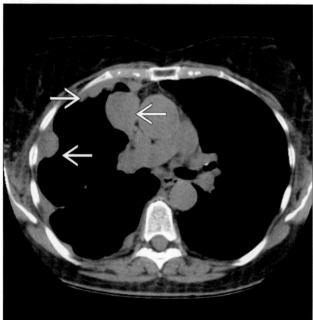 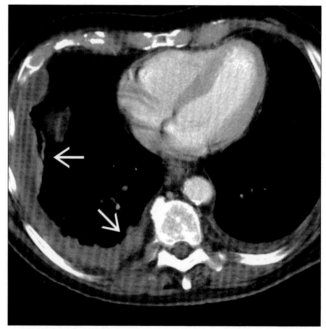

(Left) Axial NECT shows nodular soft tissue thickening of the pleura ➡, subsequently biopsy-proven to be mesothelioma. *(Right)* Axial CECT shows continuous but nodular soft tissue thickening of the pleura ➡ in this patient with mesothelioma.

MESOTHELIOMA

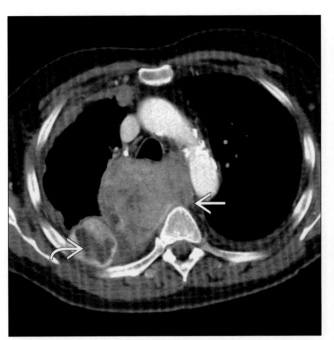
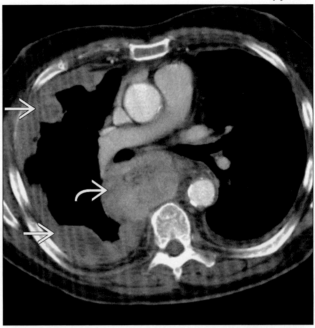

(Left) Axial CECT shows circumferential, heterogeneously enhancing soft tissue in the pleura with invasion into the mediastinum ➡ and regions of necrosis ➡. *(Right)* Axial CECT of the same patient more inferiorly shows continuous pleural involvement ➡ and mediastinal invasion by tumor ➡.

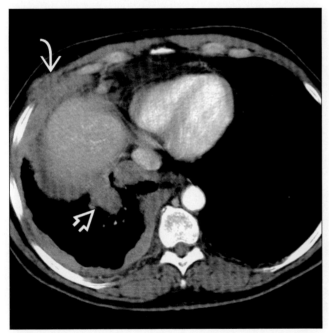
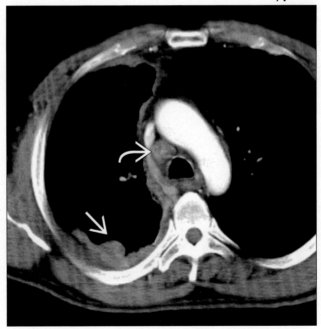

(Left) Axial CECT of the same patient at the level of the diaphragm shows that the tumor now invades the chest wall ➡ and the diaphragm ➡, in addition to the extensive pleural involvement and mediastinal invasion seen more superiorly. *(Right)* Axial CECT of a patient with mesothelioma shows nodular, enhancing soft tissue involving pleura ➡ and a mediastinal nodal metastasis ➡.

MESOTHELIOMA

Typical

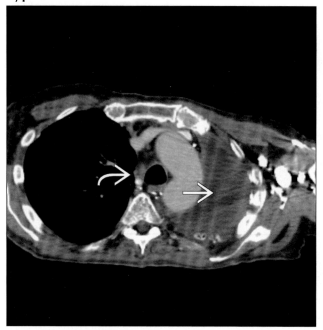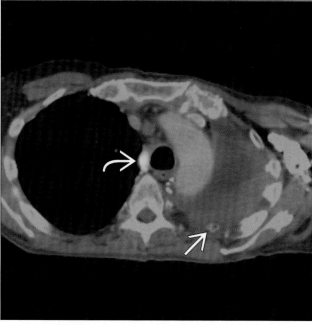

(Left) Axial CECT shows complete pleural involvement at the apex with necrosis and fluid ➡ in the pleural cavity. Note the small paratracheal lymph node ➡. *(Right)* Axial fused PET/CT shows a hypermetabolic paratracheal node that is not enlarged ➡. Very little metabolic activity is appreciated in the pleural-based tumor ➡.

Typical

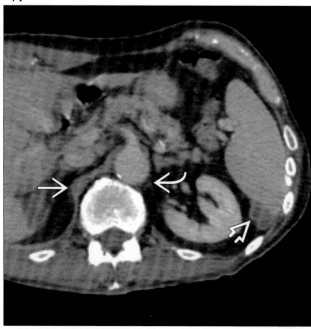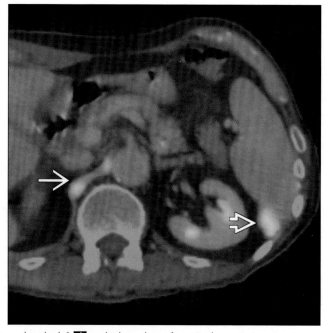

(Left) Axial CECT shows asymmetric thickening of the right crus ➡ compared to the left ➡ and a hypodense focus in the posterior aspect of the spleen ➡. *(Right)* Axial fused PET/CT of the same patient demonstrates that the right crus ➡ and posterior splenic lesion ➡ are hypermetabolic metastases.

MESOTHELIOMA

Typical

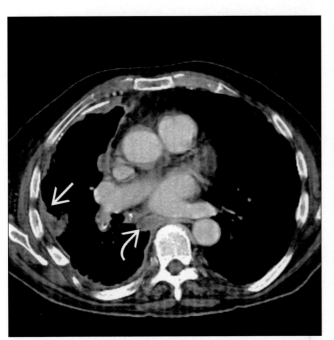 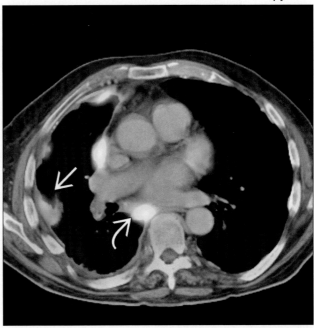

(Left) Axial CECT shows nodular circumferential pleural thickening ➜ and an enlarged subcarinal lymph node ➜. *(Right)* Axial fused PET/CT of the same patient shows the pleural thickening ➜ and node ➜ to be hypermetabolic, demonstrating the extent of tumor involvement.

Typical

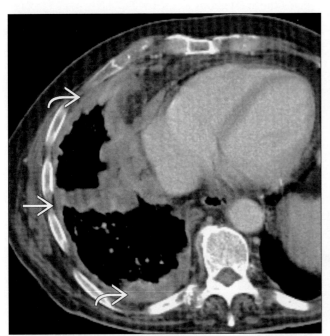 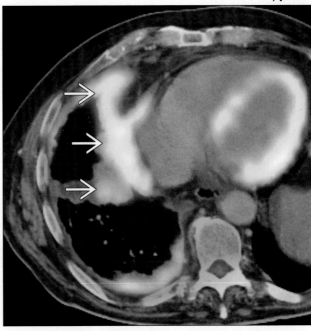

(Left) Axial CECT shows circumferential pleural thickening ➜ that also involves the major fissure ➜. *(Right)* Axial fused PET/CT shows intense uptake to the pleural thickening, including the major fissure ➜, demonstrating the extent of the mesothelioma.

THYMIC PROCESSES

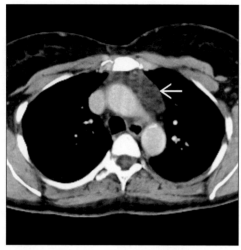

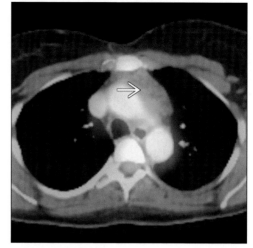

Axial CECT shows normal thymic tissue ➡ with a mix of fatty and soft tissue.

Axial fused PET/CT shows minimal or no FDG activity within a normal thymus ➡.

TERMINOLOGY

Abbreviations and Synonyms
- Thymic hyperplasia
- Thymic rebound
- Thymic cysts
- Thymic carcinoma
- Thymoma
- Thymic teratoma
- Thymolipoma

Definitions
- Variety of etiologies leading to thymic enlargement or architectural change on morphologic imaging

IMAGING FINDINGS

General Features
- Best diagnostic clue: Mass in the anterior mediastinum
- Location
  ○ Thymus resides in anterior mediastinum
    ■ Posterior to sternum and sternohyoid/thyroid muscles
    ■ Anterior to surface of pericardium, arch of aorta, brachiocephalic vein, and trachea
  ○ Efferent lymphatics drain to parasternal, tracheobronchial, and brachiocephalic veins
  ○ Prevalence of ectopic thymic tissue up to 40% in patients with myasthenia gravis
- Size
  ○ Size, weight, and consistency vary greatly with patient's age
    ■ Infant: 20 grams
    ■ Puberty: 30 grams
    ■ 40 years: Dominated by fatty tissue
    ■ 60 years: Entirely replaced by fat
- Morphology
  ○ Thymus divided into right and left lobe
    ■ Left slightly larger than right and comprises main caudal aspect of organ
  ○ Usually prominent in children
    ■ Spans from lower pole of thyroid to 4th costal cartilage
  ○ Predominantly composed of epithelial cells and lymphocytes

DDx: Thymic FDG Activity

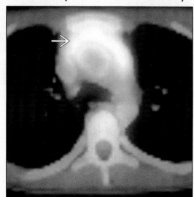

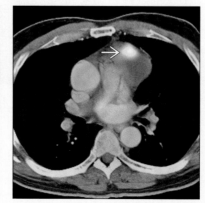

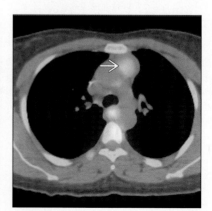

Normal Thymus in Young Patient

Cystic Thymic Carcinoid

Thymoma

THYMIC PROCESSES

Key Facts

Terminology
- Thymic hyperplasia, thymic rebound, thymic cysts, thymic carcinoma
- Variety of etiologies leading to thymic enlargement or architectural change on morphologic imaging

Imaging Findings
- Indicators of malignancy
  - Bilateral extension of mass
  - Invasion of adjacent structures
- Gross asymmetry (to one side of mediastinum) or lobulation of thymus strongly suggests diagnosis of thymoma
  - Thymoma cannot be distinguished from other thymic masses unless fat is visible

- Thymus may not be enlarged in cases of lymphoid follicular hyperplasia and may be easily overlooked on CT
- Thymic FDG uptake may be normal in patients up to age 30
- Thymus resides in anterior mediastinum

Top Differential Diagnoses
- Thymic Hyperplasia
- Thymic Neuroendocrine Tumor (Thymic Carcinoid)
- Thymic Carcinoma
  - May also show infiltration of adjacent structures in mediastinum
- Thymic Rebound
- Lymphoma
- Thymic Cyst

Imaging Recommendations
- Best imaging tool: CECT probably best modality for differentiating between various anterior mediastinal masses
- Protocol advice: Consider noncontrast and contrast-enhanced CT to evaluated thymic masses

CT Findings
- Contrast enhancement often helpful for differentiating mass from surrounding vascular structures
- Indicators of malignancy
  - Bilateral extension of mass
  - Absence of fat planes
  - Invasion of adjacent structures
- Gross asymmetry (to one side of mediastinum) or lobulation of thymus strongly suggests diagnosis of thymoma
  - Thymoma cannot be distinguished from other thymic masses unless fat is visible
  - Thymoma is usually homogeneous and shows mild contrast enhancement
- Well-defined and homogeneously enhancing capsule strongly suggests benign lesion
- Normal thymic findings by age group
  - Birth through puberty
    - CT attenuation similar to chest wall musculature
    - Outer contours may be convex laterally
    - Lobes may be triangular and slightly rotated to the left
    - Junction of lobes is 2 cm to the left of midline
  - Puberty through age 30
    - Attenuation less than skeletal muscle
    - Seen as discrete triangular or bilobed structures
    - Outer border may appear straight or slightly concave laterally
    - Normal thickness approximately 1.8 cm
  - Age > 30
    - Thymic remnants appear as small islands of soft tissue attenuation

    - Linear, oval, or small/round configurations of background of more abundant fat
    - Normal thickness less than 1 cm
  - Elderly
    - Thymus entirely replaced by fat
    - Thin fibrous skeleton of thymic tissue may remain
- Thymus may not be enlarged in cases of lymphoid follicular hyperplasia and may be easily overlooked on CT
- Carcinoma
  - Usually lacks well-defined capsule
  - Commonly contains areas of necrosis and hemorrhage
  - Carcinoma arising from thymic cyst may have prominent cystic changes
- Thymic carcinoid
  - Usually encapsulated
  - Large size, average 11 cm

Nuclear Medicine Findings
- FDG accumulation in thymus is suggestive of malignancy when
  - Activity is intense compared to normal surrounding structures
  - Typical triangular shape of thyroid is abolished
- Thymic FDG uptake may be normal in patients up to age 30
- Correlation may be seen between FDG uptake and attenuation on CT
- SUV of 4.0 has been used as cutoff for suspicion of malignancy
  - In one study, mean SUV for thymic hyperplasia vs. thymoma: 1.89 vs. 4.75
- Mean SUV for thymic carcinoma in one study was 7.2 ± 2.9
- Treatment with therapeutic dose of I-131 has been shown to contribute to increased thymic uptake
  - Time course not known
- No significant difference in SUV has been shown to distinguish invasive from non-invasive thymoma
- Small nodules < 7 mm may be falsely negative on FDG PET

THYMIC PROCESSES

- FDG PET important for detection and localization of early recurrence for planning further therapeutic modalities
  - CT alone cannot reliably detect or localize early tumor recurrence

DIFFERENTIAL DIAGNOSIS

Thymic Hyperplasia
- Associated with myasthenia gravis (MG)
  - 2/3 of MG patients demonstrate thymic hyperplasia
  - 25-50% of these patients have normal thymus by CT
- Defined histologically as the presence of numerous lymphoid follicles with active germinal centers
- May also accompany acromegaly, Addison disease, and Graves disease

Thymic Neuroendocrine Tumor (Thymic Carcinoid)
- Carcinoid is most common tumor
- Invasive, spreading to lungs, lymph nodes, liver, and bone
- 33% produce ACTH and cause Cushing syndrome
- CT findings are nonspecific and cannot differentiate this entity from other thymic masses

Thymic Carcinoma
- Aggressive tumor that commonly produces hematogenous and lymphatic spread locally and distally
- May demonstrate central necrosis in large tumor masses
- May also show infiltration of adjacent structures in mediastinum

Thymic Rebound
- True thymic hyperplasia, including increased size and weight of organ
- Cortex and medulla involved in hypertrophic process
- May occur several months after recovery from chronic illness, chemotherapy, Cushing syndrome, or other stressor
- More common in younger age groups
- Increase in volume of 50% or more from baseline is criterion for rebound

Thymic Teratoma
- Sharply defined, low attenuation cystic components predominate
- Fatty tissue present in 50% of cases, with occasional fat-fluid level
- Foci of calcification and ossification are common
- Soft tissue attenuation may be seen

Seminoma
- Large homogeneous mass with soft tissue attenuation
- Low attenuation areas may be seen secondary to necrosis and hemorrhage

Non-Seminomatous Tumor
- Large heterogeneous tumor with large areas of low attenuation
- Occasional areas of calcification

Lymphoma
- Enlarged thymus, symmetrically or asymmetrically
- Difficult to differentiate from enlarged surrounding lymph nodes

Thymolipoma
- Fatty mass interspersed with varying amounts of thymic tissue
- Typically demonstrates thin rim of thymic tissue
- Mimics pure lipoma of mediastinum

Thymic Cyst
- Homogeneous with water attenuation
- Attenuation can vary if proteinaceous fluid or blood is present
- Neoplasm with cystic degeneration can mimic cyst

PATHOLOGY

General Features
- General path comments
  - Three divisions of epithelial thymic tumors
    - Benign thymoma
    - Type 1 malignant (invasive)
    - Type 2 malignant (carcinoma)
- Etiology
  - Common causes of cancer identified in the thymus
    - Leukemia
    - Non-Hodgkin Lymphoma (NHL)
    - Hodgkin disease
    - Histiocytosis X
    - Metastases from lung, GU tract, GI tract, breast
- Epidemiology
  - 50% of thymic tumors are malignant in patients between 20 and 40 years old
    - 33% are malignant in those outside this age range
  - Thymic mass incidence varies with age
  - Thymic masses in adults by decreasing frequency
    - Thymoma
    - Neurogenic tumor
    - Lymphoma
    - Germ cell tumor
  - Thymic masses in children by decreasing frequency
    - Neurogenic tumors
    - Foregut cysts
    - Germ cell tumors
    - Lymphoma (1/3 to 1/2 of cases are lymphoblastic lymphoma)
  - Thymic Ca accounts for 0.06% of thymic neoplasms
  - Hodgkin and NHL account for 20% of all anterior mediastinal tumors

Gross Pathologic & Surgical Features
- Biopsy specimens are difficult to obtain, often are crushed and inadequate

Microscopic Features
- Type 1 thymoma is often indistinguishable cytoarchitecturally from benign thymoma
- Thymoma and thymic carcinoid are similar under microscope

THYMIC PROCESSES

CLINICAL ISSUES

Presentation
- Most common signs/symptoms
  - 55% of benign thymic masses are asymptomatic at presentation
    - 15% of malignant masses are asymptomatic
- Other signs/symptoms
  - Incidental widening of the mediastinum on a chest radiograph
  - Chest pain
  - Shortness of breath

Demographics
- Age
  - Thymoma most common over age 30
    - 70% of cases seen in 5th and 6th decades
    - Rare in children
  - Thymic carcinoma has wide age range, with mean incidence in the 40s
- Gender
  - Slight female predominance of thyroid neoplasm
    - Greater among thymic carcinoids: M:F = 1:3

Natural History & Prognosis
- Thymic carcinoid histologically similar to thymoma but more aggressive
- Thymoma: Typically indolent and more likely to relapse locally post-therapy than to metastasize
- Thymic carcinoma: Invasive tumor with high risk of relapse and death

Treatment
- Depends on pathology, but most are amenable to surgical intervention

SELECTED REFERENCES

1. Lee JW et al: Clinical influence of 18F-fluorodeoxyglucose positron emission tomography on the management of primary tumours of the thymus. J Med Imaging Radiat Oncol. 52(3):254-61, 2008
2. Maeda R et al: Thymic carcinoma with combined resection of the hemisternum. Gen Thorac Cardiovasc Surg. 56(7):361-4, 2008
3. Osaki T et al: Multilocular mediastinal cyst with rim calcification: report of a case. Surg Today. 38(1):52-5, 2008
4. Rosado-de-Christenson ML et al: Imaging of thymic epithelial neoplasms. Hematol Oncol Clin North Am. 22(3):409-31, 2008
5. Srirajaskanthan R et al: A review of thymic tumours. Lung Cancer. 60(1):4-13, 2008
6. El-Bawab H et al: Role of flourine-18 fluorodeoxyglucose positron emission tomography in thymic pathology. Eur J Cardiothorac Surg. 31(4):731-6, 2007
7. Fujishita T et al: Detection of primary and metastatic lesions by [18F]fluoro-2-deoxy-D-glucose PET in a patient with thymic carcinoid. Respirology. 12(6):928-30, 2007
8. Palmieri G et al: Cetuximab is an active treatment of metastatic and chemorefractory thymoma. Front Biosci. 12:757-61, 2007
9. Priola SM et al: The anterior mediastinum: anatomy and imaging procedures. Radiol Med (Torino). 111(3):295-311, 2006
10. Quint LE: PET: other thoracic malignancies. Cancer Imaging. 6:S82-8, 2006
11. Sung YM et al: 18F-FDG PET/CT of thymic epithelial tumors: usefulness for distinguishing and staging tumor subgroups. J Nucl Med. 47(10):1628-34, 2006
12. Castellucci P et al: Potential pitfalls of 18F-FDG PET in a large series of patients treated for malignant lymphoma: prevalence and scan interpretation. Nucl Med Commun. 26(8):689-94, 2005
13. Ferolla P et al: Thymic neuroendocrine carcinoma (carcinoid) in multiple endocrine neoplasia type 1 syndrome: the Italian series. J Clin Endocrinol Metab. 90(5):2603-9, 2005
14. Godart V et al: Intense 18-fluorodeoxyglucose uptake by the thymus on PET scan does not necessarily herald recurrence of thyroid carcinoma. J Endocrinol Invest. 28(11):1024-8, 2005
15. Markou A et al: [18F]fluoro-2-deoxy-D-glucose ([18F]FDG) positron emission tomography imaging of thymic carcinoid tumor presenting with recurrent Cushing's syndrome. Eur J Endocrinol. 152(4):521-5, 2005
16. Ferdinand B et al: Spectrum of thymic uptake at 18F-FDG PET. Radiographics. 24(6):1611-6, 2004
17. Groves AM et al: Positron emission tomography with FDG to show thymic carcinoid. AJR Am J Roentgenol. 182(2):511-3, 2004
18. Kawano T et al: The clinical relevance of thymic fluorodeoxyglucose uptake in pediatric patients after chemotherapy. Eur J Nucl Med Mol Imaging. 31(6):831-6, 2004
19. Karapetis CS et al: Use of fluorodeoxyglucose positron emission tomography scans in patients with advanced germ cell tumour following chemotherapy: single-centre experience with long-term follow up. Intern Med J. 33(9-10):427-35, 2003
20. Pagliai F et al: PET scan evaluation of thymic mass after autologous peripheral blood stem-cell transplantation in an adult with non-Hodgkin's lymphoma. Leuk Lymphoma. 44(11):2015-8, 2003
21. Wittram C et al: Thymic enlargement and FDG uptake in three patients: CT and FDG positron emission tomography correlated with pathology. AJR Am J Roentgenol. 180(2):519-22, 2003
22. Brink I et al: Increased metabolic activity in the thymus gland studied with 18F-FDG PET: age dependency and frequency after chemotherapy. J Nucl Med. 42(4):591-5, 2001
23. Rini JN et al: 18F-FDG Uptake in the Anterior Mediastinum. Physiologic Thymic Uptake or Disease? Clin Positron Imaging. 3(3):115-125, 2000
24. Alibazoglu H et al: Normal thymic uptake of 2-deoxy-2[F-18]fluoro-D-glucose. Clin Nucl Med. 24(8):597-600, 1999
25. Kubota K et al: PET imaging of primary mediastinal tumours. Br J Cancer. 73(7):882-6, 1996
26. Patel PM et al: Normal thymic uptake of FDG on PET imaging. Clin Nucl Med. 21(10):772-5, 1996
27. Smith SM et al: Adenocarcinoma of a foregut cyst: detection with positron emission tomography. AJR Am J Roentgenol. 167(5):1153-4, 1996

THYMIC PROCESSES

CT: Normal Thymus

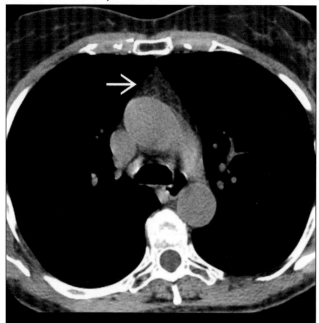
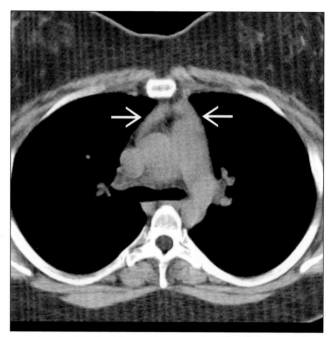

(Left) Axial NECT shows minimal residual normal thymic tissue ➔. (Right) Axial NECT shows both lobes of a normal thymus ➔.

CT: Normal Thymus

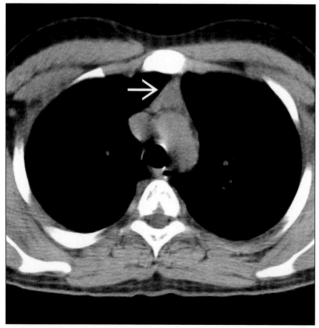
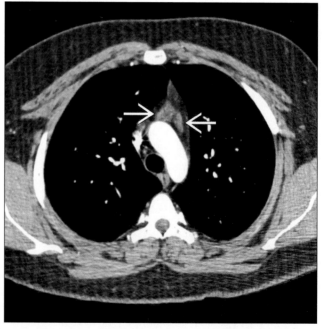

(Left) Axial NECT shows a normal thymus. Note that the margins of the thymus as it interfaces with the pleura are concave ➔. (Right) Axial CECT shows a normal thymus ➔. Both lobes are well seen.

THYMIC PROCESSES

CT: Normal Thymus and Hyperplasia

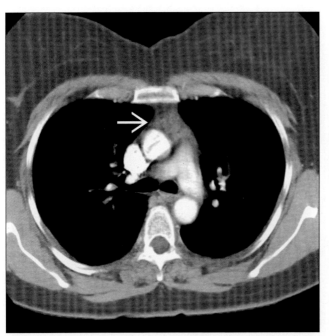 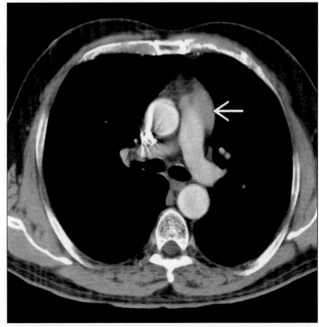

(Left) *Axial CECT shows a normal thymus* ➜. *(Right)* *Axial CECT shows prominent asymmetric soft tissue in the anterior mediastinum, corresponding to thymic hyperplasia* ➜. *The patient received chemotherapy approximately 6 months prior to this imaging.*

CT: Thymic Cyst

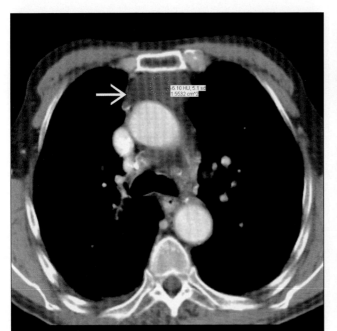 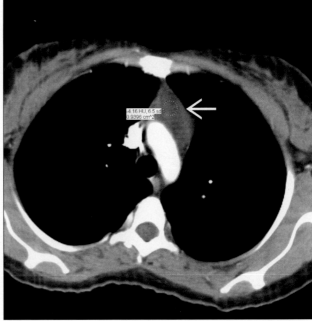

(Left) *Axial CECT shows a near water density lesion* ➜ *in the anterior mediastinum, corresponding to a thymic cyst.* *(Right)* *Axial CECT shows a cystic focus in the anterior mediastinum* ➜, *corresponding to a thymic cyst.*

THYMIC PROCESSES

CT: Thymic Cyst and Thymoma

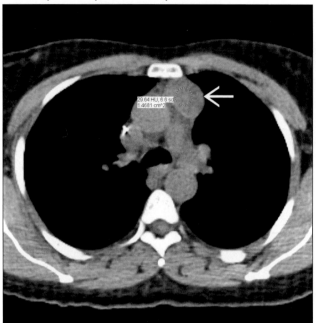 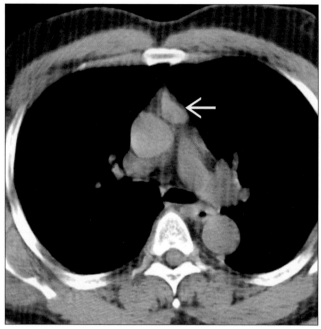

(Left) Axial NECT shows a near water density lesion in the anterior mediastinum ➡, consistent with thymic cyst. (Right) Axial CECT shows a soft tissue mass ➡ within the left aspect of the anterior mediastinum in a patient with myasthenic symptoms. The mass was found to be a thymoma. Differentiation between invasive and non-invasive thymoma is often difficult with imaging alone and is determined at surgical pathology.

CT: Thymoma

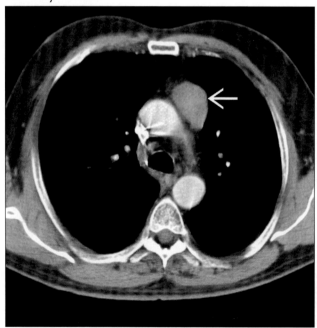 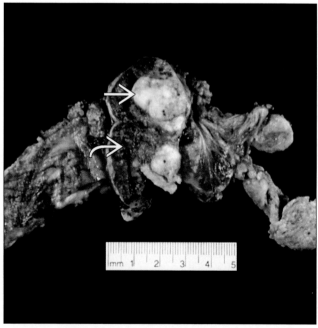

(Left) Axial CECT shows a soft tissue mass in the left aspect of the anterior mediastinum ➡, confirmed to be a thymoma at surgical excision. Notice the convex margin at the pleural interface. These tumors have associations with autoimmune disorders such as myasthenia gravis, hypogammaglobulinemia, and pure red cell aplasia. (Right) Gross pathology of the thymoma seen on the previous image after surgical excision shows the tan nodular thymoma ➡ with a background of normal thymic tissue ➡.

THYMIC PROCESSES

CT: Thymoma and Cystic Teratoma

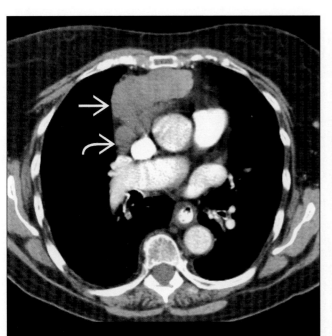
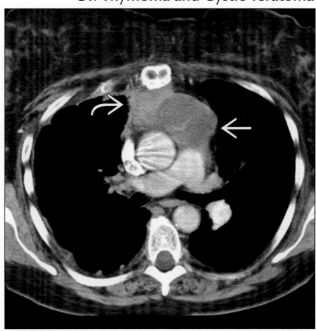

(Left) Axial CECT shows a soft tissue mass ➡ that is not localized to the right or left aspect of the mediastinum and crosses midline, a finding that suggests invasion. Note the satellite lesion ➡ corresponding to metastatic disease. *(Right)* Axial CECT shows a mixed cystic ➡ and solid ➡ lesion that was confirmed to be a cystic teratoma after surgical excision.

CT: Cystic Teratoma and Thymolipoma

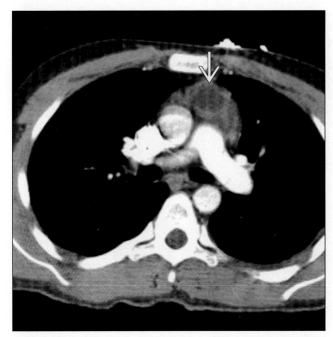
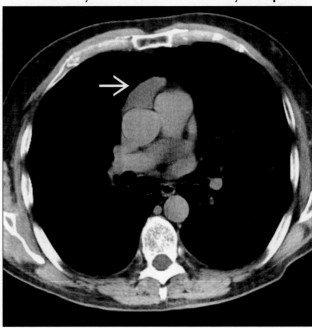

(Left) Axial CECT shows a low attenuation solid anterior mediastinal mass with heterogeneous peripheral enhancement ➡. *(Right)* Axial NECT demonstrates a fat attenuation anterior mediastinal mass ➡, consistent with thymolipoma.

THYMIC PROCESSES

CT: Thymoma

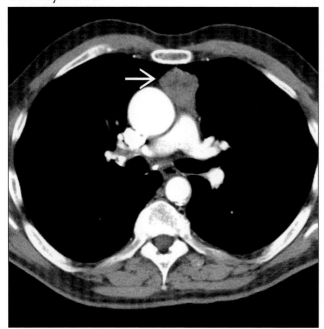
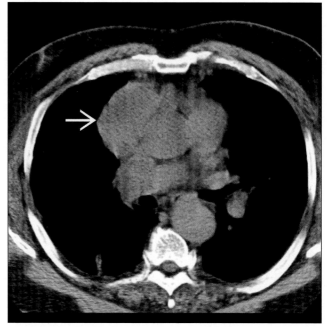

(Left) Axial CECT shows an enhancing lesion crossing midline ➡, pathologically proven to be invasive thymoma. In addition to parenchymal metastases, thymomas can metastasize along pleural surfaces, so pleural nodularity should raise suspicion for metastases. *(Right)* Axial CECT shows a soft tissue mass with convex borders ➡. In the absence of associated autoimmune disorders or metastases, a diagnosis of thymoma is difficult to render since other mediastinal lesions may have a similar appearance.

CT: Thymoma

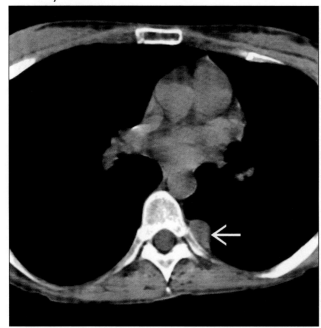
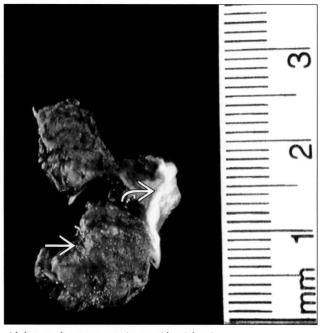

(Left) Axial NECT shows a soft tissue pleural-based lesion ➡ in a patient with known thymoma, consistent with a "drop" metastasis. *(Right)* Gross pathology surgical specimen of the "drop" metastasis shows a partially hemorrhagic lesion ➡ with normal adjacent rib ➡.

THYMIC PROCESSES

PET/CT: Thymic Hyperplasia

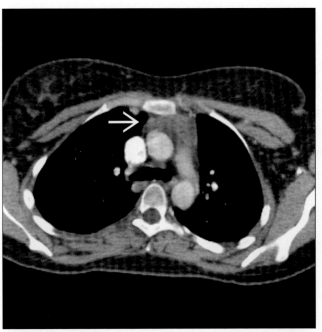

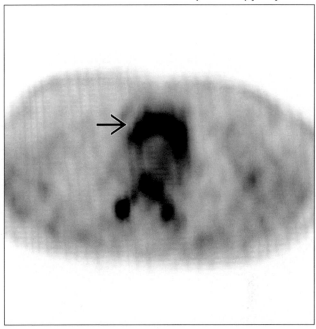

(Left) Axial CECT shows soft tissue in the anterior mediastinum ➡ in a patient following chemotherapy. *(Right)* Axial PET shows increased FDG activity in the region of anterior mediastinal soft tissue ➡. A subsequent 3 month follow-up PET/CT showed resolution of the activity, indicating likely thymic rebound.

PET/CT: Thymic Hyperplasia

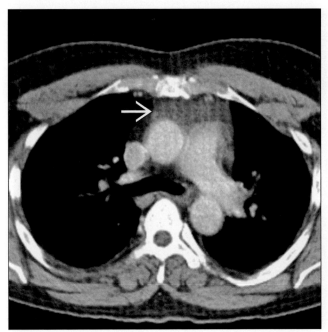

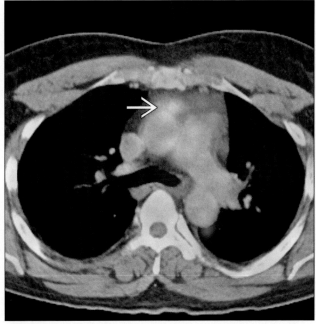

(Left) Axial CECT shows infiltrative soft tissue in the anterior mediastinum ➡, which was diagnosed as thymic hyperplasia. *(Right)* Axial fused PET/CT shows a small focus of increased FDG activity ➡ in the anterior mediastinum within the same soft tissue region. The finding is consistent with thymic hyperplasia.

3

THYMIC PROCESSES

PET/CT: Thymic Cyst

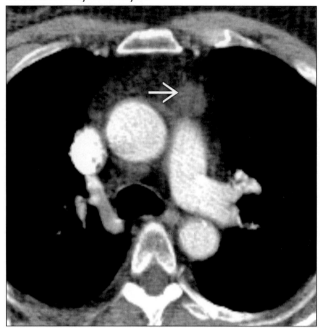 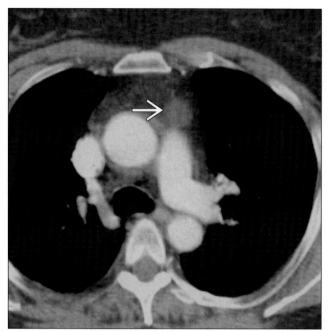

(Left) Axial CECT shows a well-defined, near water density mass in the anterior mediastinum ➡, consistent with thymic cyst. *(Right)* Axial fused PET/CT shows no FDG activity in the region of the cystic focus ➡ seen on the previous image.

PET/CT: Thymic Cyst

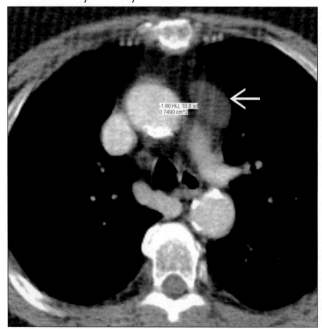 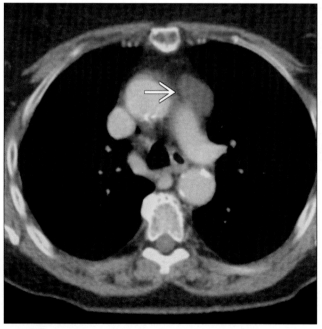

(Left) Axial CECT demonstrates another thymic cyst in the anterior mediastinum ➡. *(Right)* Axial fused PET/CT in the same patient shows no FDG activity within the cyst ➡.

THYMIC PROCESSES

PET/CT: Thymoma

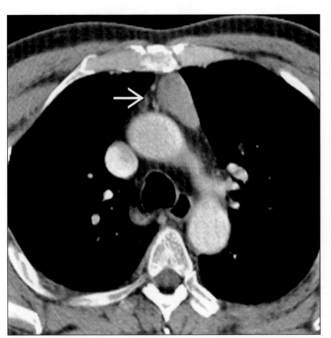
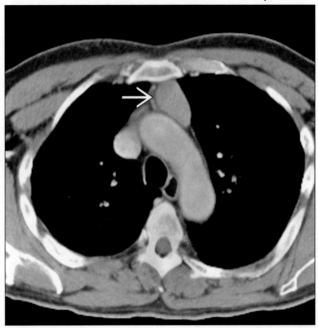

(Left) Axial CECT shows a homogeneously enhancing soft tissue lesion ➡ in a patient with no autoimmune disorder. This was surgically proven to be a non-invasive thymoma. *(Right)* Axial fused PET/CT shows no FDG activity within the thymoma ➡.

PET/CT: Thymoma

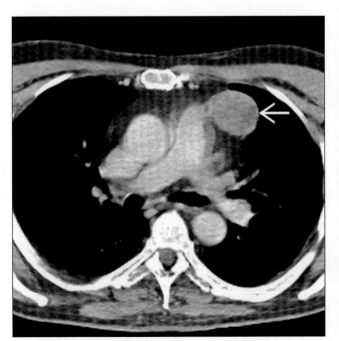
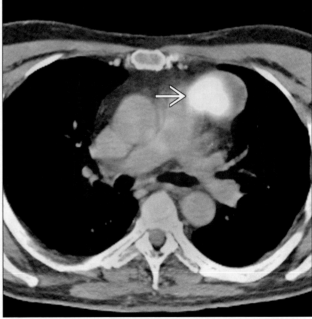

(Left) Axial CECT shows a heterogeneously enhancing soft tissue lesion that has convex margins ➡ with the left mediastinal surface and may invade the pleura. This was pathologically proven to be invasive thymoma. *(Right)* Axial fused PET/CT shows asymmetric increased FDG activity in the right aspect ➡ of the invasive thymoma, which corresponds to the more solid-appearing component of the lesion.

CHOLANGIOCARCINOMA

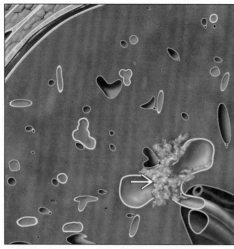

Graphic shows a typical Klatskin tumor ➜, which is cholangiocarcinoma near the bifurcation of the main right and left intrahepatic bile ducts.

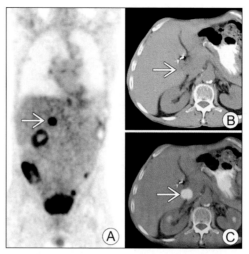

Coronal PET (A), axial CT (B) and fused PET/CT (C) show focal intense activity in the portacaval region ➜ of this patient with a history of cholangiocarcinoma.

TERMINOLOGY

Abbreviations and Synonyms
- Cholangiocarcinoma (CC), Klatskin tumor, malignant bile duct tumor

Definitions
- Malignancy that arises from ductular epithelium of intrahepatic biliary tree and extrahepatic bile ducts
  - Note: Gallbladder cancer 9x more common than CC
- Klatskin tumor: Perihilar cholangiocarcinoma involving bifurcation of hepatic duct; accounts for more than 70% of all bile duct cancers

IMAGING FINDINGS

General Features
- Best diagnostic clue
  - **PET**: Hypermetabolic activity corresponding to primary tumor in liver, extrahepatic metastatic disease
  - **Ultrasound, CT, MR**: Bile duct obstruction w/small central mass suggests hilar lesion (Klatskin tumor)

- Location
  - Extrahepatic tumors (87-92% of CC): Proximal, middle, distal ductal tumors
  - Extrahepatic tumor at bifurcation of proximal common hepatic duct = Klatskin tumor
  - Intrahepatic tumors (8-13% of CC) arise from small ducts
  - Nodular or papillary type is most common in distal duct and periampullary region
  - Intrahepatic tumors have tendency for perineural spread, but spread to liver, peritoneum, lung is extremely rare
  - Extrahepatic tumors spread to celiac nodes in ~ 16% of cases
- Size
  - Peripheral lesions are usually larger, measuring 5-20 cm at presentation
  - More central lesions (Klatskin) smaller at diagnosis
- Morphology
  - Variable
  - Most intrahepatic CC present as mass, whereas 90% of extrahepatic CC reveal diffusely infiltrating growth pattern

DDx: FDG Activity in the Liver Mimicking Cholangiocarcinoma

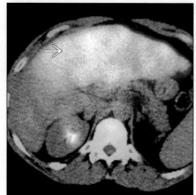
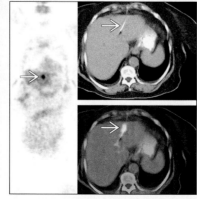
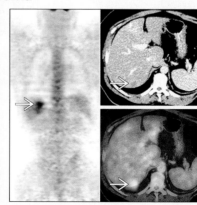

Hepatocellular Carcinoma　　　*Inflammation around PTC*　　　*Metastatic Disease*

CHOLANGIOCARCINOMA

Key Facts

Terminology
- Malignancy that arises from ductular epithelium of intrahepatic biliary tree, extrahepatic bile ducts

Imaging Findings
- PET: Hypermetabolic activity corresponding to primary tumor in liver, extrahepatic metastatic disease
- Ultrasound (US), CT, MR: For hilar lesions (Klatskin tumor), bile duct obstruction with small central mass
- Extrahepatic tumors (87-92% of CC): Proximal, middle, distal ductal tumors
- PET for staging distant metastases; characterizing peripheral CC
- Delayed enhancement with increasing attenuation seen in up to 74% of lesions, usually ↑ CT sensitivity/specificity

- Hilar CC: Low FDG activity with focal nodular or linear branching pattern

Top Differential Diagnoses
- Hepatocellular Carcinoma (HCC)
- Primary Sclerosing Cholangitis (PSC)
- Focal Nodular Hyperplasia (FNH)
- Cavernous Hemangioma
- Pancreatic Carcinoma

Clinical Issues
- Obstructive jaundice (90%)

Diagnostic Checklist
- Ability of PET to detect distant metastases alters surgical management (reportedly up to 30% of cases)
- PET sensitivity for distant mets 65-70%
- PET sensitivity for regional or hepatoduodenal mets is approximately 13%

Imaging Recommendations
- Best imaging tool
  - CT: Staging regional/distant metastases; similar to US for demonstrating ductal dilation, large mass lesions
  - MRCP/ERCP: Sensitivity of 71-81% for detecting tumor in malignant stenoses, particularly central lesions
  - PET for staging distant metastases and characterizing peripheral CC
  - ERCP with brush cytology, DNA analysis, and serum analysis of CA 19-9 and CEA for initial workup
    - Have been shown to increase sensitivity significantly
    - Diagnosis of CC, especially in primary sclerosing cholangitis (PSC), may remain uncertain until invasive and aggressive approaches such as exploratory laparotomy provide biopsy
- Protocol advice
  - Delayed PET imaging at ~ 120 minute time point shown to better discriminate tumor from inflammation
  - Delayed imaging helps differentiate tumor from background liver activity

CT Findings
- NECT
  - Mass predominantly hypoattenuating with irregular margins
  - Intrahepatic biliary duct (IHBD) dilation common with obstruction
  - Larger peripheral lesions may be isodense with central low attenuation and scarring
    - Central and satellite lesions
  - Hilar masses often not visible on NECT
    - IHBD dilation = clue
  - Capsular retraction may reveal intrahepatic tumor
  - Large common duct (extrahepatic) masses may be identified on NECT
- CECT

  - Solitary, small, well-demarcated tumors are difficult to differentiate from primary hepatocellular carcinoma (HCC)
  - Arterial phase: Peripheral CC seen as intrahepatic mass showing early peripheral rim enhancement and progressive patchy central enhancement
  - Portal phase: Portal vein invasion, ductal wall thickening with minimal enhancement, and portal lymphadenopathy
  - Delayed phase
    - Enhancement with increasing attenuation seen in up to 74% of lesions, usually ↑ CT sensitivity/specificity
    - Persistent tumor enhancement due to fibrous stroma
  - Low reported sensitivity for small hilar lesions (approximately 50%)
  - Regional lymph node spread rarely detected (24-40% of cases)

Nuclear Medicine Findings
- FDG PET
  - Primary uses
    - Identification of new lesions
    - Evaluation of metabolic activity and associated malignancy
    - Characterization of response to neoadjuvant therapy
    - Detection of lesions in liver that are not suspected on US or MR in up to 50% of patients
  - Peripheral CC: Intensely hypermetabolic activity, may be ring-shaped
  - Hilar CC: Low activity with focal nodular or linear branching pattern
    - Lower FDG uptake may be related to tumor size or arrangement of fibrous stroma and mucin pool in tumor
    - Can be difficult to discriminate between extrahepatic tumor itself and FDG-accumulating lymph nodes in perihilar region

CHOLANGIOCARCINOMA

- Extrahepatic CC may have low uptake due to loosely connected cell nests and poor detection with PET due to infrequency of evident mass formation
  - PET sensitivity
    - 61-90% for primary CC
    - 85% for nodular CC
    - 18% for infiltrating CC
    - 65-70% for distant metastases
    - Only 13% for regional or hepatoduodenal mets
  - False negatives are seen with mucinous adenocarcinomas (rare)
  - False positives are seen due to foci of inflammation (e.g., intrahepatic stone)
    - Uptake likely to be seen along tract of biliary stents
  - Primary sclerosing cholangitis (PSC)
    - PET can be used to discriminate between PSC with and without CC
    - Not reliable for early diagnosis of CC in patients with PSC
    - Liver in patients with PSC may have ↑ background signal than those of healthy control patients
- PET/CT
  - Allows better identification of non-FDG avid tumors & carcinomatosis and helps distinguish stent-related uptake from malignant disease
  - Shown to change oncological management in up to 17% of patients
  - No diagnostic advantage over CECT in detection of intrahepatic CC or primary tumor site of extrahepatic CC
  - Generally cost-effective method, avoids unnecessary surgery
- **Hepatobiliary scintigraphy**: Focal photopenic lesion
- **Tc-99m sulfur colloid**: Focal photopenic lesion
- **Ga-67 scintigraphy**: Variable Ga-67 uptake

DIFFERENTIAL DIAGNOSIS

Hepatocellular Carcinoma (HCC)
- NECT typically shows an iso- or hypodense mass
- Shows early enhancement on CECT (vs. late enhancement in CC)
- Variable FDG uptake with ~ 50% having little/no FDG uptake due to ↑ glucose-6-phosphatase

Primary Sclerosing Cholangitis (PSC)
- Isolated dilation of intrahepatic bile ducts, known as skip dilations, strongly suggestive of PSC

Focal Nodular Hyperplasia (FNH)
- On NECT scans, FNH may appear as isoattenuating or slightly hypoattenuating mass
- After contrast administration, FNH becomes hyperattenuating relative to surrounding liver in arterial phase
- Larger lesions may have characteristic central scar

Cavernous Hemangioma
- NECT: Hemangiomas appear hypo-attenuating relative to adjacent liver

- Arterial phase CECT: Small hemangiomas show intense, uniform enhancement and retain enhancement during portal venous phase
- Portal venous phase CECT: Characteristic peripheral nodular enhancement with continued centripetal filling in most larger lesions

Pancreatic Carcinoma
- Abrupt obstruction of pancreatic &/or distal common bile duct
- Look for dilated pancreatic duct distal to mass lesion

PATHOLOGY

General Features
- General path comments
  - Extent of duct involvement by perihilar tumors assigned according to Bismuth classification
  - > 95% are cancers of biliary tree, and 90% of CC are adenocarcinomas
  - Hilar type
    - Develops from large bile ducts of hepatic hilum, symptomatic early due to central bile duct obstruction and jaundice
  - Peripheral type
    - Originates from interlobular bile ducts, tends to form mass, attains large size before becoming clinically apparent (no central biliary obstruction)
    - 60-70% of CC are Klatskin tumors
    - 20-30% arise in distal common bile duct
    - 5-10% are peripheral
    - Increased glucose transporter and hexokinase activity relative to surrounding tissue
- Etiology
  - Risk factors
    - PSC: 10% average risk of developing cholangiocarcinoma among PSC patients
    - Parasitic infection
    - Fibropolycystic liver disease
    - Intrahepatic biliary stones
    - Carcinogen exposure
    - Viral hepatitis
  - Known risk factors account for only a few cases of CC
  - Thorotrast (intravascular contrast agent used until 1950s) strongly associated; ↑ risk 300x many years after exposure
- Epidemiology
  - 2nd most common primary hepatic malignancy after HCC
  - Incidence of intrahepatic CC increasing worldwide, cause unclear
  - Incidence of extrahepatic CC declining
  - 10% prevalence of CC among PSC patients

Microscopic Features
- More than 95% of all cancers of the biliary tree are adenocarcinomas

CHOLANGIOCARCINOMA

CLINICAL ISSUES

Presentation
- Most common signs/symptoms
  - Obstructive jaundice (90%)
  - Abdominal pain (47%)
  - Palpable mass (18%)

Demographics
- Age: Peak incidence in 7th decade
- Gender: Slight male predominance

Natural History & Prognosis
- Overall 5 year survival < 5%
- Unresected cholangiocarcinoma has no five year survival
- With aggressive surgical treatment, 5 year survival rate 22-32%, complication rates ≤ 36-59%, 60 day mortality 8-10%
- Biliary neoplasm with distant metastases associated with survival of only a few months, regardless of therapy

Treatment
- Surgical resection = only curative treatment
- Intrahepatic and Klatskin tumors require liver resection
- Liver transplantation combined with chemoradiotherapy may improve survival
- Chemotherapy and radiotherapy generally ineffective for inoperable tumors
- Biliary drainage: Mainstay of palliation
- Photodynamic therapy: New palliative technique that may improve quality of life
- No patient with suspected CC should be excluded from surgery on basis of positive PET/CT finding, due to likelihood of false positives
  - But detection and confirmation of distant mets paramount to offer surgery only to those who may benefit from it
- Regional lymph node involvement does not demonstrate contraindications for surgery in most centers and does not alter surgical approach

DIAGNOSTIC CHECKLIST

Consider
- Ability of PET to detect distant metastases alters surgical management (reportedly up to 30% of cases)
- PET sensitivity for distant mets 65-70%
- PET sensitivity for regional or hepatoduodenal mets approximately 13%
- Diaphragmatic respiratory motion can create challenges in detection of liver lesions

Image Interpretation Pearls
- In general, FDG activity in primary tumor is variable: Larger, more peripheral lesions are detected more often
- In patients with biliary stents: 58% of cases have hypermetabolic activity along stent tract
- False positive on PET due to inflammation, e.g., intrahepatic stone, biliary stent
- False negative on PET with mucinous adenocarcinomas

SELECTED REFERENCES

1. Corvera CU et al: 18F-fluorodeoxyglucose positron emission tomography influences management decisions in patients with biliary cancer. J Am Coll Surg. 206(1):57-65, 2008
2. Kim JY et al: Clinical role of 18F-FDG PET-CT in suspected and potentially operable cholangiocarcinoma: a prospective study compared with conventional imaging. Am J Gastroenterol. 103(5):1145-51, 2008
3. Moon CM et al: Usefulness of 18F-fluorodeoxyglucose positron emission tomography in differential diagnosis and staging of cholangiocarcinomas. J Gastroenterol Hepatol. 23(5):759-65, 2008
4. Paudyal B et al: Clinicopathological presentation of varying 18F-FDG uptake and expression of glucose transporter 1 and hexokinase II in cases of hepatocellular carcinoma and cholangiocellular carcinoma. Ann Nucl Med. 22(1):83-6, 2008
5. Seo S et al: Fluorine-18 fluorodeoxyglucose positron emission tomography predicts lymph node metastasis, P-glycoprotein expression, and recurrence after resection in mass-forming intrahepatic cholangiocarcinoma. Surgery. 143(6):769-77, 2008
6. Fevery J et al: Incidence, diagnosis, and therapy of cholangiocarcinoma in patients with primary sclerosing cholangitis. Dig Dis Sci. 52(11):3123-35, 2007
7. Jadvar H et al: [F-18]fluorodeoxyglucose positron emission tomography and positron emission tomography: computed tomography in recurrent and metastatic cholangiocarcinoma. J Comput Assist Tomogr. 31(2):223-8, 2007
8. Kuker RA et al: Optimization of FDG-PET/CT imaging protocol for evaluation of patients with primary and metastatic liver disease. Int Semin Surg Oncol. 4:17, 2007
9. Laverman P et al: [(18)F]FDG accumulation in an experimental model of multistage progression of cholangiocarcinoma. Hepatol Res. 37(2):127-32, 2007
10. Miller G et al: The use of imaging in the diagnosis and staging of hepatobiliary malignancies. Surg Oncol Clin N Am. 16(2):343-68, 2007
11. Nishiyama Y et al: Comparison of early and delayed FDG PET for evaluation of biliary stricture. Nucl Med Commun. 28(12):914-9, 2007
12. Patel T et al: Cholangiocarcinoma: emerging approaches to a challenging cancer. Curr Opin Gastroenterol. 23(3):317-23, 2007
13. Sun L et al: Positron emission tomography/computer tomography: challenge to conventional imaging modalities in evaluating primary and metastatic liver malignancies. World J Gastroenterol. 13(20):2775-83, 2007
14. Grobmyer SR et al: Perihepatic lymph node assessment in patients undergoing partial hepatectomy for malignancy. Ann Surg. 244(2):260-4, 2006
15. Nagaoka S et al: Value of fusing PET plus CT images in hepatocellular carcinoma and combined hepatocellular and cholangiocarcinoma patients with extrahepatic metastases: preliminary findings. Liver Int. 26(7):781-8, 2006
16. Sotiropoulos GC et al: Liver transplantation for double primary hepatic cancer-hepatocellular carcinoma and intrahepatic cholangiocarcinoma. Transplantation. 82(5):718-9, 2006

3

CHOLANGIOCARCINOMA

CT Findings

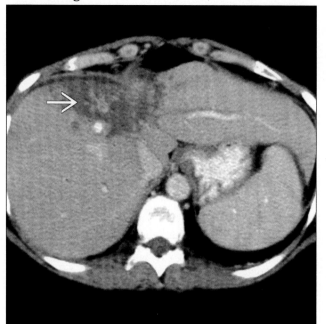 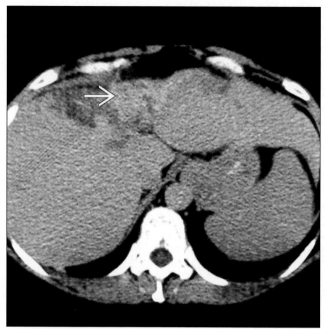

(Left) Axial CECT shows a large low attenuation mass with heterogeneous enhancement on portal venous phase involving the anterior and medial segments of the liver, which is compatible with this patient's history of cholangiocarcinoma. *(Right)* Axial CECT with a 10 minute delay shows subtle increased enhancement along the anterior portions of the mass ➡. Delayed contrast enhancement is a characteristic of cholangiocarcinoma.

CT Findings

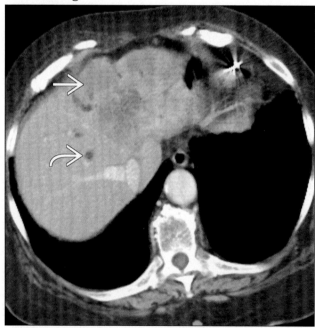 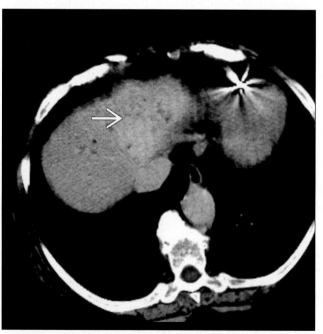

(Left) Axial CECT shows a large heterogeneous mass with variable enhancement ➡ in the left hepatic lobe, compatible with cholangiocarcinoma. Also note intrahepatic biliary duct dilatation in the right hepatic lobe ➡. *(Right)* Axial CECT with a 10 minute delay shows subtly increased contrast enhancement within the entire left hepatic lobe mass ➡.

CHOLANGIOCARCINOMA

CT Findings

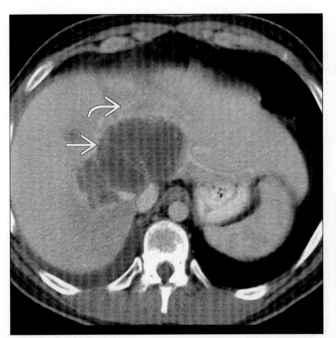
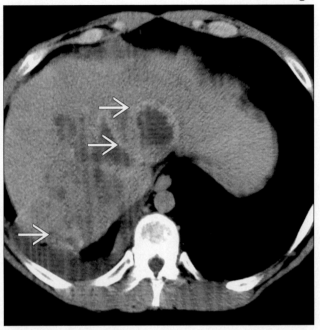

(Left) Axial CECT during the portal venous phase imaging shows a primarily low attenuation mass ➡ surrounding the confluence of the hepatic veins. Minimal peripheral enhancement is also present ➡. *(Right)* Axial CECT with a 10 minute delay shows increased areas of delayed contrast enhancement ➡, a characteristic finding of cholangiocarcinoma.

CT Findings

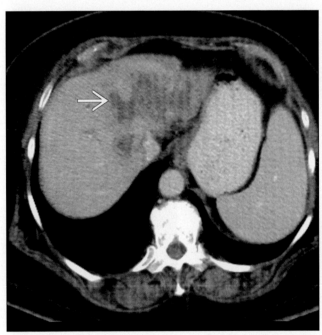
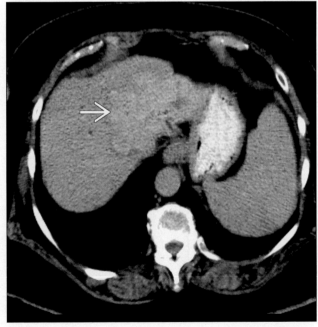

(Left) Axial CECT during the portal venous phase imaging shows a heterogeneous mass rarely involving the left hepatic lobe superiorly ➡ with areas of central low attenuation, compatible with cholangiocarcinoma. *(Right)* Axial CECT with a 10 minute delay shows fairly marked diffuse delayed contrast enhancement within the hepatic lesion ➡. With a history of cholangiocarcinoma, consider performing a 10 minute delayed CT acquisition along with a contrast-enhanced CT as part of a PET/CT.

CHOLANGIOCARCINOMA

CT Findings

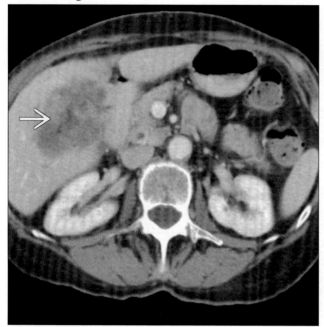 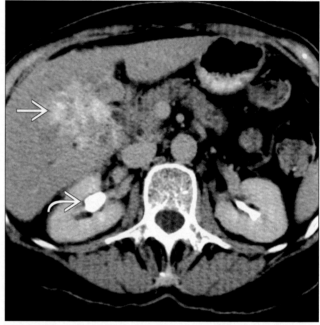

(Left) Axial CECT during the portal venous phase of enhancement shows a low attenuation mass in the right hepatic lobe ➡ with heterogeneous areas of mild enhancement. *(Right)* Axial CECT after a 10 minute delay shows a focal area of increased enhancement ➡, characteristic of cholangiocarcinoma. Very concentrated contrast material is present within the urinary collecting system ➡, compatible with the pyelographic or delayed phase of imaging.

PET/CT Findings

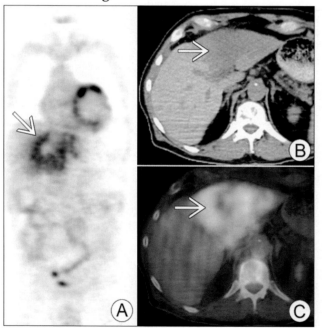 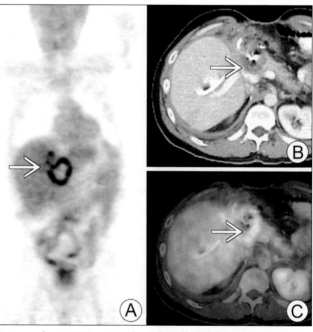

(Left) Coronal PET (A), axial CT (B) and fused PET/CT (C) images demonstrate moderate FDG activity throughout the left lobe of the liver ➡ in this patient with newly diagnosed cholangiocarcinoma. *(Right)* This patient underwent a left hepatectomy after being diagnosed with cholangiocarcinoma. This examination was performed for restaging; coronal PET (A), axial CT (B) and fused PET/CT (C) demonstrate ring-like activity in the resection bed ➡, compatible with recurrent disease.

CHOLANGIOCARCINOMA

PET/CT Findings

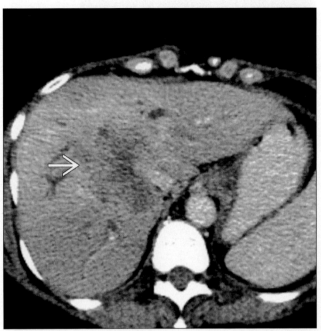 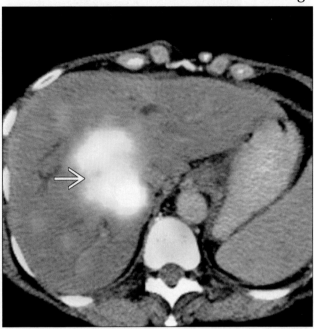

(Left) Axial CECT shows an infiltrative mass in the liver ➡ with heterogeneous enhancement in this patient with a recent biopsy showing cholangiocarcinoma. *(Right)* Axial fused PET/CT shows intense FDG activity corresponding to the infiltrative hepatic mass ➡. In general, smaller, more central primary tumors may be missed on FDG PET, whereas the larger or peripherally based tumors will usually be easily identified on PET.

PET/CT Findings

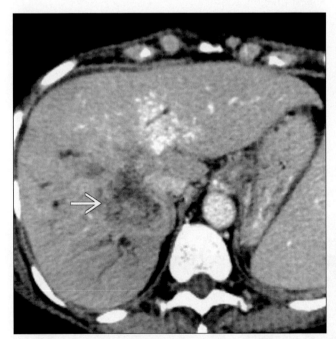 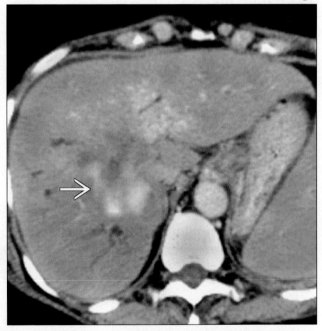

(Left) Axial CECT shows an infiltrative mass in the liver ➡ with heterogeneous enhancement in a patient with a recent biopsy showing cholangiocarcinoma. *(Right)* Axial fused PET/CT shows more moderate FDG activity than in the previous patient, corresponding to the known cholangiocarcinoma ➡.

GALLBLADDER CARCINOMA

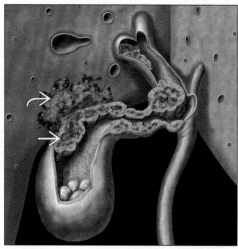

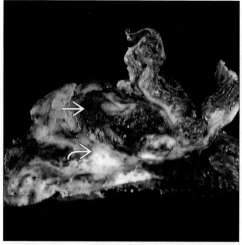

Graphic shows typical appearance for gallbladder carcinoma ➡ with hepatic invasion ➡.

Specimen shows a tannish red mass in the gallbladder ➡ with extension outside the walls of the gallbladder ➡, compatible with carcinoma of the gallbladder.

TERMINOLOGY

Abbreviations and Synonyms
- Gallbladder (GB), gallbladder cancer (GBC)

Definitions
- Malignant neoplasm arising from epithelial layer of the gallbladder mucosa

IMAGING FINDINGS

General Features
- Best diagnostic clue: FDG-avid mass of the gallbladder with invasion of liver
- Location
  o Most common site of recurrence is laparoscopic port incision
  o Most frequent sites of lymph node invasion are pericholedocal and cystic
- Size
  o Variable, but usually large at diagnosis
  o Can be polypoid lesion if detected incidentally on CT

- Morphology
  o Early disease presents as diffuse wall thickening or polyp
    ■ Rarely seen, as disease frequently presents in advanced stages
  o Advanced disease usually appears as large mass with signs of infiltration

Imaging Recommendations
- Best imaging tool
  o **Ultrasound**
    ■ Mass within the gallbladder or focal thickening of the gallbladder wall
  o **Endoscopic retrograde cholangiopancreatography (ERCP)**
    ■ Obtain tissue sample for histologic diagnosis
    ■ Localize obstruction in jaundiced patients
    ■ Stent placement in the case of obstruction
  o **CT/MR**
    ■ Delineation of local invasion and metastatic disease, particularly in relation to vascular structures
  o **FDG PET**
    ■ Initial diagnosis when clinically indicated (rare)

DDx: FDG Uptake in or near the Gallbladder

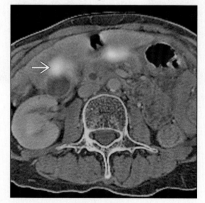

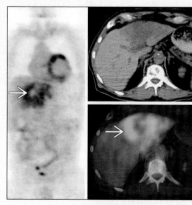

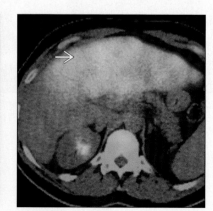

Metastasis

Cholangiocarcinoma

Hepatocellular Carcinoma

GALLBLADDER CARCINOMA

Key Facts

Imaging Findings
- GB mass with intense uptake often invading into liver
- FDG PET for evaluation of localized or metastatic GBC
- Also for staging and restaging malignant tumors leading to detection of unsuspected mets in 25-30% and leading to major changes in therapy in 15-20% of cases
- CECT can demonstrate tumor extension outside GB and identify metastatic disease in the abdomen and pelvis
- Intense FDG uptake in the primary GB mass often directly extends into liver
- Abnormal uptake along bile ducts with subserosal and regional lymph node invasion

- PET often reveals disease in nonenlarged lymph nodes
- Distant hematogenous metastasis and peritoneal seeding may occur

Top Differential Diagnoses
- Cholecystitis
- Cholangiocarcinoma
- Metastases
- Gallbladder Polyp
  - Benign polyps in 4-6% of the general population; most show no radiotracer uptake

Diagnostic Checklist
- Pitfall: Misregistered normal bowel activity onto liver or GB can be misleading without CT correlation for presence of mass lesions

---

        - Staging and restaging (25-30% rate of detection of unsuspected metastatic disease, 15-20% rate of major change in therapeutic planning)
- Protocol advice
  - Use contrast-enhanced CT when possible for patients with suspected or known GB malignancy
  - FDG PET protocol
    - ≥ 6 hour fast prior to scan
    - Patient with serum glucose ≥ 200 mg/dl should be rescheduled
    - Avoid exercise or cold temperatures prior to scan
    - Administer 370-555 MB (10-15 mCi) F-18 FDG IV 1-2 hours before scan
    - Scan with arms above head
    - Post-operative patients should be given 4-6 weeks to resolve inflammation prior to scan

CT Findings
- **Mass and thickening**
  - Mass form is more common due to late diagnosis of most cases
    - Heterogeneous
    - Hyperdense areas due to necrosis
    - Hypovascular, poorly enhancing mass infiltrating GB fossa
    - Often direct extension to liver along main lobar fissure
    - Common duct invasion and periportal adenopathy present as hazy density around duct
  - Early disease presents as wall thickening
    - Focal and irregular
    - Disease may originate at site of chronic cholecystitis
    - Sometimes indistinguishable from inflammatory conditions
    - Evidence for neoplasm includes hyperemia of thick inner layer that is iso- or hyperattenuating to liver in portal phase
- **Gallstones**
  - Association with porcelain gallbladder unclear, but its presence is frequently reported

  - Calcific gallstones present in 65-75% of patients with GBC
    - Less than 1% of patients with gallstones develop GBC
- **Staging**
  - CT limited in staging the following entities
    - Nonenlarged malignant lymph nodes
    - Distant lymph nodes
    - Small liver metastases
    - Peritoneal seeding
    - Early vs. benign lesions
  - Invasion of liver and porta hepatis common
  - Whole body scanning important for detection of distant lung and bone metastases
  - Intraperitoneal metastasis and carcinomatosis indicate advanced disease
- **Lymph nodes**
  - CECT may reveal lymphadenopathy in the porta hepatis
  - Involved lymph nodes appear ring-shaped with heterogeneous contrast enhancement
  - Metastasis to peripancreatic lymph nodes easily confused for pancreatic carcinoma

Nuclear Medicine Findings
- **FDG PET and PET/CT**
  - **Initial diagnosis**
    - FDG PET has limited role in initial diagnosis because most GBC is diagnosed incidentally within the gallbladder after cholecystectomy
    - Tumor masses show peripheral uptake with areas of low uptake when there is necrosis
    - Uptake in primary mass may be seen to extend into liver in the presence of hepatic invasion
    - Mucinous tumors often demonstrate low FDG avidity
  - **Staging**
    - According to one study, typical SUV of metastatic disease ranges from 2.7-7.5
    - FDG PET often detects distant disease unsuspected on CT alone, particularly in nonenlarged lymph nodes

3

GALLBLADDER CARCINOMA

- Major weakness of FDG PET alone is poor sensitivity for carcinomatosis
- Metastasis tends to show increased radiotracer uptake
- Combined-modality PET/CT superior to CECT for detection of metastasis
- Low sensitivity for regional lymph node detection (vs. 24-40% sensitivity with CECT)
- Regional and subserosal lymph node invasion may appear as abnormal uptake along bile ducts
  - Restaging
    - Most important contribution of FDG PET and PET/CT is identification of recurrent and metastatic disease
    - Interpretation of residual tumor in gallbladder fossa following cholecystectomy can be obscured by post-surgical inflammation
    - Sensitivity and specificity for recurrent disease approximately 80% and 80%
  - **Response to therapy**
    - FDG PET has been used for determination of therapy response, although there is a paucity of studies in the current literature

DIFFERENTIAL DIAGNOSIS

Cholecystitis

- Acute cholecystitis
  - Intense FDG uptake
    - Must be differentiated clinically from malignancy
  - Ring-like appearance
- Chronic cholecystitis
  - May predispose to GBC, which often originates at site of inflammatory change
  - Difficult to distinguish from carcinoma clinically and on morphologic imaging
  - Findings common to GBC and chronic cholecystitis
    - Wall thickening
    - Gallstones
    - Porcelain gallbladder
- Xanthomatous cholangitis
  - FDG uptake has been reported
  - Benign process characterized by inflammation
  - Difficult to distinguish from carcinoma by morphologic imaging

Cholangiocarcinoma

- Similar appearance to GBC on PET/CT
- Distribution usually different

Metastases

- Other primary tumors may metastasize to gallbladder, periportal lymph nodes, and liver

Gallbladder Polyp

- May mimic early GBC, but rarely FDG avid
- Present in 4-6% of population

Adenomyomatosis

- Benign finding with no FDG avidity
- Rokitansky-Aschoff sinuses may be identified on morphologic imaging as outpouching of mucosa into or through thickened muscular layer

- Usually localized to fundus; present in ~ 5% of population

PATHOLOGY

General Features

- Genetics
  - Associated with Gardner syndrome, neurofibromatosis type 1, and hereditary non-polyposis colon cancer
  - Oncogenic mutations are actively being researched
- Etiology
  - Arises in the setting of chronic inflammation
    - Highest risk in patients with years of biliary pain from chronic cholecystitis
  - Gallstones
    - > 75% of patients have cholesterol gallstones
    - Incidence of 0.3-3% among gallstone carriers
    - Incidence rises to 10-25% with porcelain gallbladder
  - Other inflammatory causes
    - Salmonella
    - Pancreatic reflux to biliary tree
- Epidemiology
  - Most common malignant tumor of the biliary tract
    - Occurs in about 2% of all people operated on for biliary tract disease
    - Fifth most common tumor of digestive system
  - 9,000 new cases of GBC per year in USA
- Associated abnormalities: Cholelithiasis, porcelain gallbladder

Gross Pathologic & Surgical Features

- Proximity of GBC tumors to major vessels frequently results in unresectability because of direct invasion of these critical structures
- Patients with limited nodal disease within the hepatoduodenal ligament may benefit from resection
  - Those with involvement of more distant nodal basins such as retropancreatic, celiac, and para-aortic do not usually benefit from resection

Microscopic Features

- Cellular classifications include
  - Adenocarcinoma (intestinal type, papillary, mucinous, clear cell)
  - Signet ring cell
  - Adenosquamous
  - Squamous cell
  - Small cell
  - Undifferentiated
  - Carcinoma sarcoma
  - Carcinoma NOS
- F-18 FDG PET may show less uptake in mucinous tumors causing false negatives

Staging, Grading, or Classification Criteria

- Stage I: Tumor limited to gallbladder
  - IA: T1N0M0 invades GB lamina propria
  - IB: T2N0M0 invades perimuscular connective tissue layer
- Stage II: Tumor invades serosa or has spread to regional lymph nodes

GALLBLADDER CARCINOMA

- o IIA: T3N0M0 tumor invades serosa/visceral peritoneum
- o IIB: T1-3N1M0
- Stage III: Involves main portal vein or hepatic artery, directly invades liver and/or adjacent organ: T4N0-1M0
- Stage IV: Tumor invades multiple organs, &/or distant metastases (any T, any N, M1)

CLINICAL ISSUES

Presentation
- Most common signs/symptoms
  - o Biliary colic: RUQ pain, vomiting, weight loss, jaundice
  - o Symptoms are identical to those of gallstone disease
  - o 34% of patients present with jaundice
  - o No specific biochemical alterations of utility for early diagnosis
- Other signs/symptoms: Elevated bilirubin and alkaline phosphatase when biliary obstruction present
- Clinical profile
  - o GBC usually manifests in one of the three following situations
    - ▪ Incidental finding after cholecystectomy for benign disease
    - ▪ Lesion detected in vesicular wall and resectable after extension study
    - ▪ Advanced inoperable cancer
  - o Should be suspected in patient over 60 years of age with moderate constant pain in right hypochondrium associated with recent weight loss
  - o 10% of GBC is confined to organ wall at diagnosis
    - ▪ Liver involvement in 59%
    - ▪ Lymph node involvement in 45%

Demographics
- Age: Peak incidence in 6th and 7th decades
- Gender: Female predominance (M:F = 1:3)

Natural History & Prognosis
- Most patients present with regional or metastatic disease, with poor prognosis
- Median survival with metastatic disease: 2-4 months
- Overall 5 year survival 15-20%
- Stage IB patients treated with extended cholecystectomy have 5 year survival 70-90%
- Stage IA disease cured with cholecystectomy
- Dismal prognosis due to aggressiveness of local invasion and high rate of implantation along peritoneal surfaces and surgical wounds

Treatment
- Simple or radical cholecystectomy is the only curative approach
- Radical cholecystectomy involves regional lymph node dissection and partial hepatectomy
- Contraindication to surgical management is cancer involvement beyond gastrohepatic ligament (stage IVB)
- Any invasive procedure involves risk of tumor seeding along path of entry
- Chemoradiation has very limited efficacy

DIAGNOSTIC CHECKLIST

Image Interpretation Pearls
- Easy to overlook direct liver extension, infiltration along bile ducts, and portal lymphadenopathy
- PET/CT valuable to avoid misinterpretation of misregistered bowel activity onto liver or gallbladder as disease

SELECTED REFERENCES

1. Corvera CU et al: 18F-fluorodeoxyglucose positron emission tomography influences management decisions in patients with biliary cancer. J Am Coll Surg. 206(1):57-65, 2008
2. Maldjian PD et al: Adenomyomatosis of the gallbladder: another cause for a "hot" gallbladder on 18F-FDG PET. AJR Am J Roentgenol. 189(1):W36-8, 2007
3. Miller G et al: The use of imaging in the diagnosis and staging of hepatobiliary malignancies. Surg Oncol Clin N Am. 16(2):343-68, 2007
4. Nishiyama Y et al: Dual-time-point 18F-FDG PET for the evaluation of gallbladder carcinoma. J Nucl Med. 47(4):633-8, 2006
5. Oe A et al: Distinguishing benign from malignant gallbladder wall thickening using FDG-PET. Ann Nucl Med. 20(10):699-703, 2006
6. Petrowsky H et al: Impact of integrated positron emission tomography and computed tomography on staging and management of gallbladder cancer and cholangiocarcinoma. J Hepatol. 45(1):43-50, 2006
7. Ramia JM et al: Gallbladder tuberculosis: false-positive PET diagnosis of gallbladder cancer. World J Gastroenterol. 12(40):6559-60, 2006
8. Rehani B et al: Gallbladder metastasis from malignant melanoma: diagnosis with FDG PET/CT. Clin Nucl Med. 31(12):812-3, 2006
9. Rodríguez-Fernández A et al: Application of modern imaging methods in diagnosis of gallbladder cancer. J Surg Oncol. 93(8):650-64, 2006
10. Shukla HS: Gallbladder cancer. J Surg Oncol. 93(8):604-6, 2006
11. Balan KK: Visualization of the gall bladder on F-18 FDOPA PET imaging: a potential pitfall. Clin Nucl Med. 30(1):23-4, 2005
12. Chander S et al: PET imaging of gallbladder carcinoma. Clin Nucl Med. 30(12):804-5, 2005
13. Persley KM: Gallbladder Polyps. Curr Treat Options Gastroenterol. 8(2):105-108, 2005
14. Anderson CD et al: Fluorodeoxyglucose PET imaging in the evaluation of gallbladder carcinoma and cholangiocarcinoma. J Gastrointest Surg. 8(1):90-7, 2004
15. Rodríguez-Fernández A et al: Positron-emission tomography with fluorine-18-fluoro-2-deoxy-D-glucose for gallbladder cancer diagnosis. Am J Surg. 188(2):171-5, 2004
16. Koh T et al: Differential diagnosis of gallbladder cancer using positron emission tomography with fluorine-18-labeled fluoro-deoxyglucose (FDG-PET). J Surg Oncol. 84(2):74-81, 2003
17. Tasaki K et al: Successful treatment of lymph node metastases recurring from gallbladder cancer. J Hepatobiliary Pancreat Surg. 10(1):113-7, 2003
18. Koh T et al: Possibility of Differential Diagnosis of Small Polypoid Lesions in the Gallbladder Using FDG-PET. Clin Positron Imaging. 3(5):213-218, 2000

GALLBLADDER CARCINOMA

CT Findings: Primary

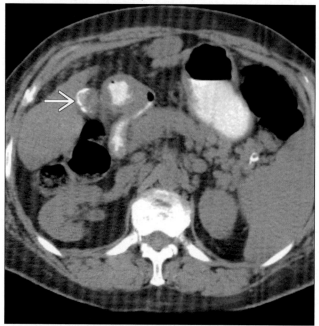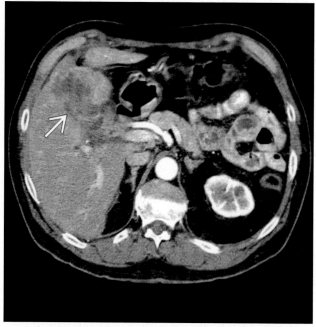

(Left) Axial NECT shows a calcified "porcelain" gallbladder ➡ in this patient without known gallbladder carcinoma. Because of the increased risk for carcinoma of the gallbladder, the patient was referred for resection. *(Right)* Axial CECT shows indistinct margins of the gallbladder with heterogeneity of the adjacent liver parenchyma ➡, corresponding to gallbladder carcinoma invading the liver by direct extension.

CT Findings: Primary

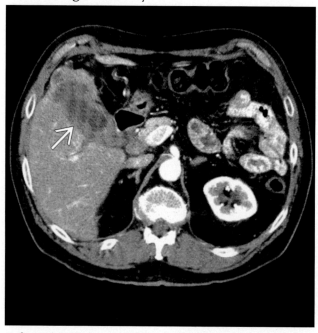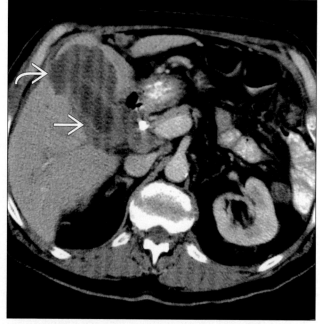

(Left) Axial CECT shows gallbladder wall thickening with irregularity at the fundus that extends to the adjacent liver parenchyma ➡, compatible with gallbladder carcinoma. *(Right)* Axial CECT shows gallbladder wall thickening ➡ with hypoattenuation in the adjacent liver parenchyma, which is concerning for gallbladder carcinoma with direction invasion ➡.

GALLBLADDER CARCINOMA

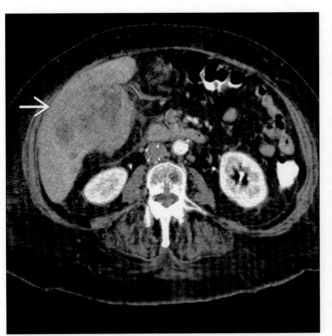 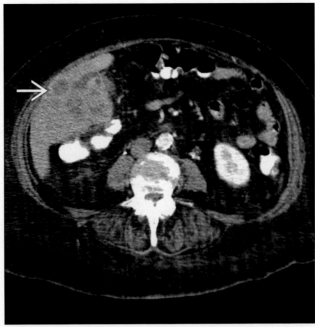

(Left) Axial CECT shows a large heterogeneous mass with indistinct margins that involves segments 5 and 4B of the liver ➡. *(Right)* Axial CECT in the same patient more inferiorly shows the extent of tumor involvement ➡.

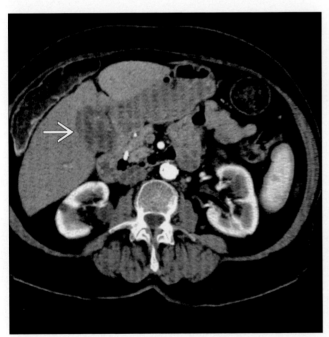 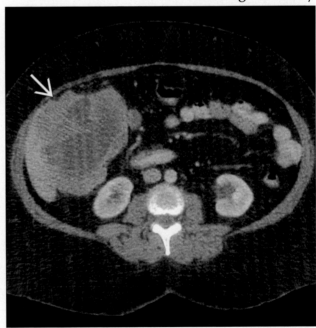

(Left) Axial CECT shows a heterogeneously enhancing lesion involving the gallbladder ➡. *(Right)* Axial CECT shows an enlarged, irregularly marginated mass arising in the gallbladder fossa ➡ in this patient with a recent biopsy that showed gallbladder carcinoma.

GALLBLADDER CARCINOMA

CT Findings: Metastases

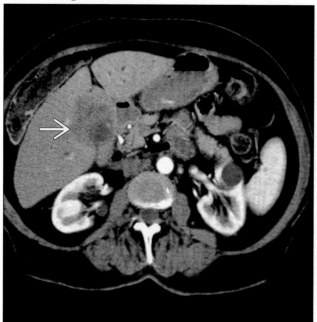 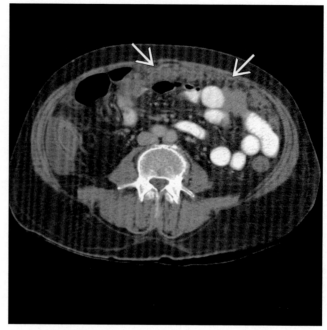

(Left) Axial CECT shows a necrotic hepatic lesion ➡, corresponding to a metastasis. *(Right)* Axial CECT shows omental "caking" ➡, compatible with metastatic disease from the patient's known gallbladder carcinoma.

PET/CT Findings: Primary

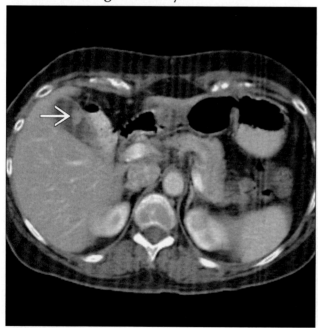 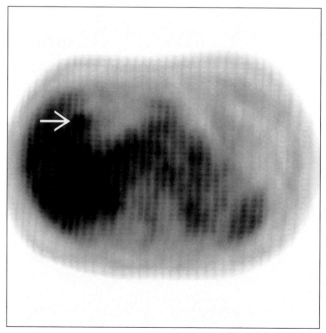

(Left) Axial CECT shows a polypoid lesion ➡ within the gallbladder lumen. *(Right)* Axial PET shows increased FDG uptake ➡ that corresponds to the polypoid gallbladder lesion in the previous image, suggesting malignancy. Subsequent cholecystectomy showed carcinoma of the gallbladder.

GALLBLADDER CARCINOMA

PET/CT Findings: Primary

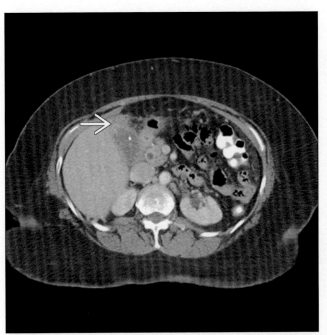
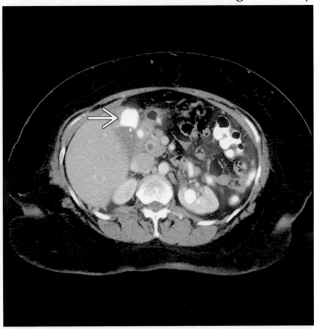

(Left) Axial CECT shows a subtle mass along the peripheral border of the gallbladder ➡, worrisome for gallbladder carcinoma. *(Right)* Axial fused PET/CT shows intense FDG activity correlating to the gallbladder mass ➡, compatible with gallbladder carcinoma.

CT and PET/CT Findings: Metastases

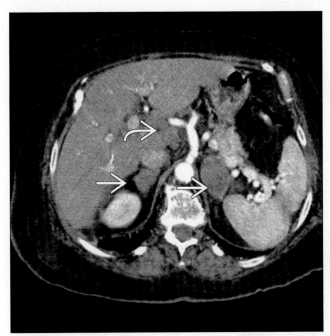
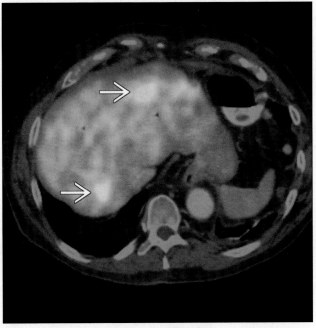

(Left) Axial CECT shows bilateral adrenal metastases ➡ and adenopathy in the celiac and porta hepatis regions ➡. *(Right)* Axial fused PET/CT shows at least two hypermetabolic lesions in the liver ➡. Biopsy confirmed them as gallbladder metastases.

HEPATOCELLULAR CARCINOMA

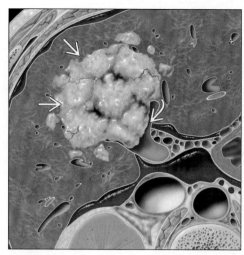

Graphic shows a heterogeneous mass in the liver ➡ with invasion into the portal vein ⮩, compatible with hepatocellular carcinoma.

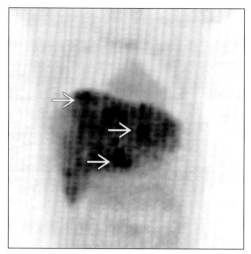

Coronal PET shows multiple lesions within the liver ➡ in this patient with recently diagnosed multifocal hepatocellular carcinoma.

TERMINOLOGY

Abbreviations and Synonyms
- Hepatocellular carcinoma (HCC)
- Hepatoma
- Fibrolamellar hepatocellular carcinoma
- Primary liver cancer
- Alpha-fetoprotein (AFP)
- Orthotopic liver transplant (OLTx)
- Portal vein tumor thrombus (PVTT)

Definitions
- Hepatocellular tumor arising in cirrhotic liver
- In most cases, due to hepatitis C virus (HCV) infection or alcoholism

IMAGING FINDINGS

General Features
- Best diagnostic clue
  - Morphologic imaging
    - Large hypervascular mass
    - Heterogeneous internal architecture

- Often with portal vein invasion
  - CT
    - Vascular or large necrotic mass in the setting of abnormal liver with elevated AFP
    - Highly suggestive of HCC
  - FDG PET
    - Well-differentiated HCC: FDG uptake similar to normal liver parenchyma
    - High grade undifferentiated HCC: FDG avid
- Location
  - **Solitary**
    - Solitary mass in right lobe most common
  - **Multifocal**
    - Presents in both lobes as small nodular multicentric disease
  - **Diffuse**
    - Presents with diffuse infiltration throughout liver
  - Vascular invasion is common
    - Portal vein invasion very common
    - Biliary invasion uncommon
  - Most common metastatic sites include
    - Lung (18-55%)
    - Lymph nodes (26.7-53%)
    - Bone (5.8-38%)

DDx: FDG Activity in the Liver Mimicking HCC

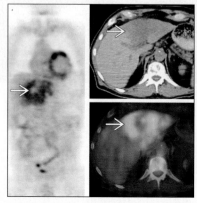

Cholangiocarcinoma

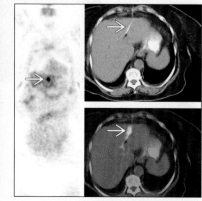

Inflammation around PTC

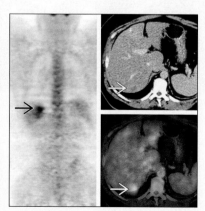

Metastatic Disease

HEPATOCELLULAR CARCINOMA

Key Facts

Terminology
- Most common primary malignant liver tumor usually arising in cirrhotic liver due to chronic viral hepatitis (HBV/HCV) or alcoholism

Imaging Findings
- CECT/MR: Large heterogeneous hypervascular mass with portal vein invasion
- FDG PET
  - Well-differentiated iso-/hypometabolic relative to normal liver
  - High grade undifferentiated-hypermetabolic
- CECT: 90% sensitivity
  - Hepatic arterial phase (HAP) scan: Heterogeneous enhancement
- Portal venous phase (PVP) scan: Decreased attenuation with heterogeneous areas of contrast accumulation
- Contrast CT markedly improves detection rate of PVTT, especially in smaller branches of portal vein
- PET
  - Variable FDG avidity; low general sensitivity 50% (compared to 90% for CT)
  - Well-differentiated tumors may be similar to normal liver

Top Differential Diagnoses
- Cholangiocarcinoma (Peripheral)
- Nodular Regenerative Hyperplasia

Diagnostic Checklist
- HCC: Hypervascular mass invading portal vein

- Size: Large tumor defined as > 4 cm
- Morphology
  - Growth patterns of HCC
    - Solitary
    - Multifocal
    - Diffuse

Imaging Recommendations
- Best imaging tool
  - CT with well-timed dual- or triple-phase enhancement has 60-70% sensitivity
  - FDG PET to
    - Assess degree of differentiation
    - Stage less well-differentiated tumors
  - MR can assist in differentiating cirrhotic nodules from small HCC
- Protocol advice
  - CT imaging of hepatic arterial and portal venous phases and delayed contrast images
    - Important to use high injection rates and appropriate bolus timing

CT Findings
- CT most useful for delineation of anatomical boundaries among tumor masses and normal tissues
  - Affords detail of small lesions
- **Most common enhancement patterns**
  - Noncontrast
    - Isoattenuating
  - Arterial phase
    - Hyperattenuating
  - Venous phase
    - Isoattenuating
  - Regenerative and dysplastic nodules may demonstrate same pattern
- **Non-cirrhotic liver findings**
  - Encapsulated HCC
    - Round
    - Well-defined
    - Hypodense
  - Solitary HCC
    - Large hypodense mass

- Variable necrosis, fat, and calcification
- Commonly in right lobe
  - Multifocal HCC
    - Multiple hypodense lesions in all lobes with occasional central necrosis
    - Dominant mass with lower attenuation satellite lesions = common pattern
- **Cirrhotic liver findings**
  - Diffuse regenerative/dysplastic nodularity
  - HCC mass may be iso- or hypoattenuating to liver
  - Often accompanied by ascites and varices
- **Hepatic arterial phase**
  - Mass typically demonstrates heterogeneous enhancement
  - HCC relies on arterial blood flow only and thus is highly attenuating during arterial phase
    - Large tumors with central necrosis demonstrate central hypoattenuation during this phase
  - Small HCC shows hyperattenuation early and no enhancement during arterial portography
  - Inconspicuous lesions may be revealed by presence of neovascularity
  - Wedge-shaped areas of hyperattenuation may represent increased arterial flow
    - Secondary to portal vein occlusion by tumor thrombus
- **Portal venous phase**
  - HCC lesions demonstrate decreased attenuation with heterogeneous areas of contrast accumulation
  - Normal liver increases in attenuation
    - Can make small lesions that are iso- or hypodense difficult to see
  - Larger lesions with central necrosis remain hypodense
- **Delayed scan**
  - HCC becomes hypodense to surrounding liver
  - May show a tumor capsule, which is a specific sign of HCC
- **Extension/metastasis**
  - Portal vein tumor thrombus detection is markedly improved with contrast enhancement
    - Particularly in smaller portal vein branches

HEPATOCELLULAR CARCINOMA

- o Bone metastases are usually osteolytic, such that they are evident on CT only in advanced disease

Nuclear Medicine Findings

- **FDG PET and PET/CT**
  - o Patient management affected by FDG PET imaging in 28% of patients
  - o HCC demonstrates variable FDG avidity
    - FDG PET has low general sensitivity of 50% (compared to 90% for CT)
    - Well-differentiated tumors may have similar FDG avidity to liver
    - Normal regenerating nodules often show more FDG uptake than HCC lesions
    - Low FDG avidity in well-differentiated HCC due in part to low expression of glut-1 and high levels of glucose-6-phosphatase
    - Higher grade tumors generally demonstrate at least 2:1 intensity of FDG uptake to liver
  - o High background activity is seen in liver parenchyma
    - Due to high glucose metabolism and abundant expression of glut-1 and hexokinase II
    - Delayed PET/CT imaging has been useful for overcoming this dilemma
    - Retention of FDG in malignant cells is the most important factor in delayed lesion detection
    - Also allows for further clearance of blood pool activity
    - In one study, 2-hour delayed images saw ↑ in the SUV tumor-to-noise ratio (86% ↑) and diagnostic sensitivity
    - Revealed new lesions in 17% of patients and identified extrahepatic sites of metastasis not seen on CECT in 20% of patients
    - Produced slight decrease in mean SUV of normal liver tissue
- **Initial diagnosis**
  - o Larger tumors of greater metastatic potential generally show greater FDG uptake
    - PET is more sensitive for these lesions
    - PET will detect ~ 1/3 of primary tumors ≤ 2 cm
    - Positive uptake will be seen in ~ 1/3 of stage I HCC tumors
- **Staging**
  - o Sensitivity shown to be as high as 88% when primary tumor is FDG avid
  - o Baseline study needed to assess inherent FDG avidity
  - o Added anatomic detail of PET/CT is beneficial to describe small lymph node metastases at edges of solid organs or in interspace of tissues
  - o FDG PET/CT for detection of malignant portal vein tumor thrombosis (PVTT)
    - Portal invasion is present in 34-40% of patients
    - PET/CT is reliable for evaluating veins of portal system thrombus
    - Contrast three-phase liver CT in PET/CT system recommended when PVTT suspected
    - False positives are seen with benign hepatic and bile duct epithelial cell uptake in portal vein blood thrombi
  - o False positives in lung commonly caused by

- Infection, e.g., tuberculosis, mycobacterium avium intracellulare, pneumonic consolidation
- Artifacts caused by diaphragmatic motion
  - o Post-OLTx patients benefit from PET/CT imaging for accurate assessment of tumor residue
  - o PET/CT advantageous in the detection of extrahepatic metastasis
    - Allows accurate pre-operative assessment for OLTx candidacy
- **Restaging**
  - o Elevated AFP in the setting of post-transplant high-grade HCC patient is highly suspicious for recurrence
  - o Up to 73% of patients may benefit from localization of recurrence with PET/CT
- **Alternative radiotracers**
  - o C-11 or F-18 choline may show better performance than FDG for HCC
    - Investigational
    - C-11 acetate accumulates preferentially in well-differentiated HCC
    - Complements FDG-18, which shows uptake in poorly-differentiated HCC mostly
    - HCC tumors not seen with FDG PET are often seen with C-11 acetate
    - C-11 acetate is relatively specific for HCC
    - Not accumulated in pure cholangiocarcinoma or metastatic liver tumors from other primary malignancies
    - When primary tumor is C-11 acetate positive, FDG PET sensitivity 67%
    - Negative predictive value less than 50% for single-tracer
    - Therefore, a negative single-tracer study cannot reliably exclude metastatic HCC
    - Not adequate for identifying candidates for curative therapy

DIFFERENTIAL DIAGNOSIS

Cholangiocarcinoma (Peripheral)
- Capsular retraction
- Volume loss
- Bile duct obstruction
- Variably FDG avid
- Demonstrates delayed CT contrast enhancement

Nodular Regenerative Hyperplasia
- Small nodules may not be visualized
- Large nodules (1-4 cm) enhance homogeneously on CT
- Typically have moderate FDG avidity

Hypervascular Metastases
- FDG avidity varies according to primary malignancy
- May mimic small nodular or multifocal HCC
- Portal vein invasion less common than HCC

Focal Nodular Hyperplasia
- Enhancing, homogeneous mass
- Presence of central scar suggests diagnosis
- Generally isodense to liver on nonenhanced and delayed CT

HEPATOCELLULAR CARCINOMA

- Typically brisk enhancement during arterial phase

Small Hepatic Hemangioma
- FDG avidity equal to normal liver
- Spherical mass
- Smooth, well-defined border
- Isoattenuating to blood
  - May demonstrate "flash filling" on CECT
- Usually hyperechoic on ultrasound

PATHOLOGY

General Features
- General path comments
  - Fibrolamellar subtype
    - Typically arises within normal liver
    - Has distinct imaging and histologic characteristics from typical HCC
    - Clear cell variant distinguished by extension fatty infiltration
- Genetics
  - Hepatitis B virus (HBV) integrates viral genome into host DNA
    - May begin malignant transformation
  - Active and latent genetic carriers of acute hepatic porphyrias are at risk for HCC
- Etiology
  - Most common causes in western hemisphere
    - Alcoholic cirrhosis
    - Hemochromatosis
    - Steroid use
  - Cirrhosis
    - 60-90% of HCC patients have liver cirrhosis
    - Secondary to chronic viral hepatitis or alcohol abuse
  - Carcinogens associated with HCC
    - Aflatoxin
    - Siderosis
    - Thorotrast
    - Androgens
  - Metabolic disease
    - Alpha-1-antitrypsin deficiency
    - Hemochromatosis
    - Wilson disease
    - Tyrosinosis
- Epidemiology
  - 350,000 new cases reported annually worldwide
  - > 400,000 deaths worldwide annually
  - Hepatitis C and HCC
    - United States: 30-50% of cases due to HCV
    - Japan: 70% of cases due to HCV
  - High incidence in Asia and Africa
    - Due to high prevalence of aflatoxin and hepatitis B
    - Highest incidence worldwide is in Japan (4-5%)
  - Lowest incidence in western hemisphere (4 per 100,000)
    - 40% of HCC in North America presents in non-cirrhotic livers
  - Second to hepatoblastoma as most common malignant liver tumor in children

Gross Pathologic & Surgical Features
- Soft tumor mass with variable amounts of
  - Necrosis
  - Hemorrhage
  - Calcification
  - Fatty infiltration
  - Vascular invasion

Microscopic Features
- HCC cells resemble normal hepatocytes
  - Solid or acinar
  - May have increased fat and glycogen in cytoplasm
  - Well-differentiated types may produce bile
- Can produce alpha-fetoprotein

CLINICAL ISSUES

Presentation
- Most common signs/symptoms
  - Fever of unknown origin
  - Abdominal pain
  - Hepatomegaly
  - Weight loss
  - Uncommonly jaundice
- Other signs/symptoms
  - In high incidence areas, presentation more commonly aggressive
    - Bleeding
    - Hepatic rupture
    - Hemoperitoneum
- Clinical Profile
  - Elderly patient with history of the following
    - Cirrhosis
    - Ascites
    - Weight loss
    - RUQ pain
    - Elevated serum AFP

Demographics
- Age
  - Western hemisphere: 50-60 years
  - Asia and western Africa: 30-45 years
- Gender
  - Western hemisphere: M:F = 2.5:1
  - Asia and western Africa: M:F = 8:1

Natural History & Prognosis
- Median survival = 6 months
  - With PVTT = 2.7 months
    - PVTT causes acute portal hypertension, acute upper GI hemorrhage, and refractory ascites
    - Ultimately acute liver failure
    - Macroscopic tumor thrombi in portal vein appear to occur during terminal stage of HCC
- 5 year survival = 30%
- SUV appears to be significantly correlated with recurrence-free survival rate
- Extrahepatic recurrence occurs in about 30-50% of patients after treatment
  - Multiple tumor nodules, venous invasion, and impaired liver function associated with recurrence

3

HEPATOCELLULAR CARCINOMA

Treatment

- Small isolated tumors may be treated with alcohol/radiofrequency ablation
- Multifocal unresectable tumor may respond to intra-arterial chemoembolization
  - Intrahepatic arterial Y-90 microspheres (TheraSphere, SIRSphere)
  - TACE
    - Injection of chemotherapy agent into hepatic artery supplying tumor, followed by embolization
    - More beneficial post-op than pre-op
- Surgical resection
  - Resection of isolated extrahepatic HCC advocated for possibility of long-term survival
  - Extrahepatic resection relies heavily on accurate restaging
  - Hepatic resection of HCC > 10 cm at stage II/III is safe and effective for selected patients without liver cirrhosis
  - Limited by inadequate hepatic reserve
    - Overall incidence of post-operative complications is 39%
- Orthotopic liver transplant prerequisites
  - Small, low grade lesions (unresectable)
  - Advanced cirrhosis
  - No extrahepatic metastatic disease or major blood vessel involvement
- Long-term use of immunosuppressants following transplant increases risk of HCC recurrence

DIAGNOSTIC CHECKLIST

Image Interpretation Pearls

- HCC
  - Hypervascular mass invading portal vein
- FDG PET
  - HCC may have similar uptake as normal liver
  - Baseline study important to document FDG avidity
- Regenerating liver nodules may be hypermetabolic on FDG PET

SELECTED REFERENCES

1. He YX et al: Clinical applications and advances of positron emission tomography with fluorine-18-fluorodeoxyglucose (18F-FDG) in the diagnosis of liver neoplasms. Postgrad Med J. 84(991):246-51, 2008
2. Kawamura E et al: Clinical role of FDG-PET for HCC: relationship of glucose metabolic indicator to Japan Integrated Staging (JIS) score. Hepatogastroenterology. 55(82-83):582-6, 2008
3. Kuehl H et al: Mid-term outcome of positron emission tomography/computed tomography-assisted radiofrequency ablation in primary and secondary liver tumours--a single-centre experience. Clin Oncol (R Coll Radiol). 20(3):234-40, 2008
4. Paudyal B et al: Clinicopathological presentation of varying 18F-FDG uptake and expression of glucose transporter 1 and hexokinase II in cases of hepatocellular carcinoma and cholangiocellular carcinoma. Ann Nucl Med. 22(1):83-6, 2008
5. Saar B et al: Radiological diagnosis of hepatocellular carcinoma. Liver Int. 28(2):189-99, 2008
6. Sun L et al: Highly metabolic thrombus of the portal vein: 18F fluorodeoxyglucose positron emission tomography/computer tomography demonstration and clinical significance in hepatocellular carcinoma. World J Gastroenterol. 14(8):1212-7, 2008
7. Yamamoto Y et al: Detection of Hepatocellular Carcinoma Using 11C-Choline PET: Comparison with 18F-FDG PET. J Nucl Med. 49(8):1245-1248, 2008
8. Camaggi V et al: Recent advances in the imaging of hepatocellular carcinoma. From ultrasound to positron emission tomography scan. Saudi Med J. 28(7):1007-14, 2007
9. Cheng MF et al: Whole-body F-18 FDG PET for hepatocellular carcinoma patients after interventional treatment. Neoplasma. 54(4):342-7, 2007
10. Ho CL et al: Dual-tracer PET/CT imaging in evaluation of metastatic hepatocellular carcinoma. J Nucl Med. 48(6):902-9, 2007
11. Salem N et al: Quantitative evaluation of 2-deoxy-2[F-18]fluoro-D-glucose-positron emission tomography imaging on the woodchuck model of hepatocellular carcinoma with histological correlation. Mol Imaging Biol. 9(3):135-43, 2007
12. Sun L et al: Positron emission tomography/computed tomography with (18)F-fluorodeoxyglucose identifies tumor growth or thrombosis in the portal vein with hepatocellular carcinoma. World J Gastroenterol. 13(33):4529-32, 2007
13. Sun L et al: Positron emission tomography/computer tomography in guidance of extrahepatic hepatocellular carcinoma metastasis management. World J Gastroenterol. 13(40):5413-5, 2007
14. Yoon KT et al: Role of 18F-fluorodeoxyglucose positron emission tomography in detecting extrahepatic metastasis in pretreatment staging of hepatocellular carcinoma. Oncology. 72 Suppl 1:104-10, 2007
15. Hatano E et al: Preoperative positron emission tomography with fluorine-18-fluorodeoxyglucose is predictive of prognosis in patients with hepatocellular carcinoma after resection. World J Surg. 30(9):1736-41, 2006
16. Nagaoka S et al: Value of fusing PET plus CT images in hepatocellular carcinoma and combined hepatocellular and cholangiocarcinoma patients with extrahepatic metastases: preliminary findings. Liver Int. 26(7):781-8, 2006
17. Talbot JN et al: PET/CT in patients with hepatocellular carcinoma using [(18)F]fluorocholine: preliminary comparison with [(18)F]FDG PET/CT. Eur J Nucl Med Mol Imaging. 33(11):1285-9, 2006
18. Yang SH et al: The role of (18)F-FDG-PET imaging for the selection of liver transplantation candidates among hepatocellular carcinoma patients. Liver Transpl. 12(11):1655-60, 2006
19. Lee JD et al: Different glucose uptake and glycolytic mechanisms between hepatocellular carcinoma and intrahepatic mass-forming cholangiocarcinoma with increased (18)F-FDG uptake. J Nucl Med. 46(10):1753-9, 2005
20. Gharib AM et al: Molecular imaging of hepatocellular carcinoma. Gastroenterology. 127(5 Suppl 1):S153-8, 2004
21. Hain SF et al: Recent advances in imaging hepatocellular carcinoma: diagnosis, staging and response assessment: functional imaging. Cancer J. 10(2):121-7, 2004
22. Sugiyama M et al: 18F-FDG PET in the detection of extrahepatic metastases from hepatocellular carcinoma. J Gastroenterol. 39(10):961-8, 2004
23. Teefey SA et al: Detection of primary hepatic malignancy in liver transplant candidates: prospective comparison of CT, MR imaging, US, and PET. Radiology. 226(2):533-42, 2003

HEPATOCELLULAR CARCINOMA

CT Findings: Primary

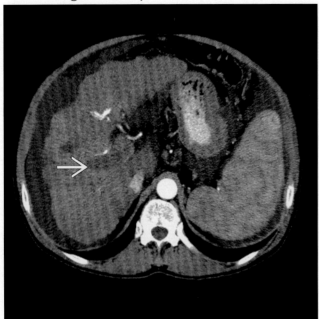
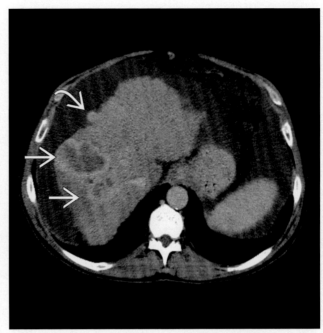

(Left) Axial CECT shows thrombus ➡ in the main right portal vein on the arterial phase. Expansion of the portal vein, in addition to its proximity to the lesion (shown on later images), suggests that it represents tumor thrombus. *(Right)* Axial CECT shows lesions ➡ with continuous rings of peripheral enhancement in a background cirrhotic liver, consistent with HCC. A second exophytic lesion ➡ with enhancement greater than background is also noted.

CT Findings: Primary

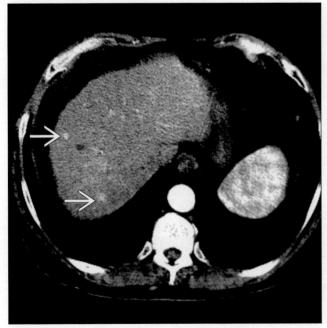
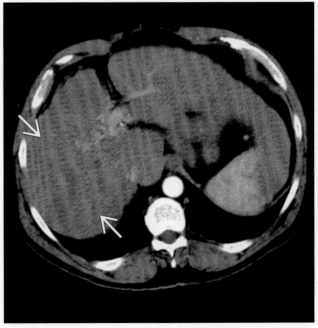

(Left) Axial CECT shows tiny hypervascular lesions ➡ in a cirrhotic liver that are nonspecific but worrisome for HCC. *(Right)* Axial CECT shows heterogeneous, vague enhancement in the posterior segment of the right hepatic lobe ➡.

HEPATOCELLULAR CARCINOMA

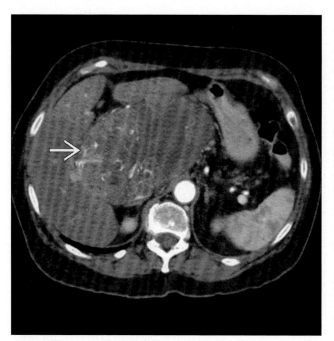 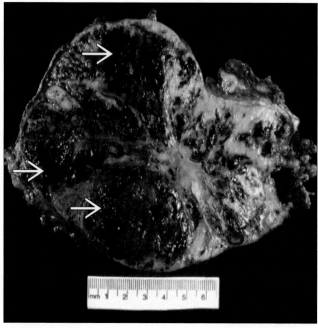

(Left) Axial CECT shows a large heterogeneous lesion on arterial phase with central necrosis and peripheral neovascularity ➡, compatible with hepatocellular carcinoma. *(Right)* Gross pathology, section of the same large lesion shows areas of hemorrhage and necrosis ➡, findings that are characteristic of larger HCC.

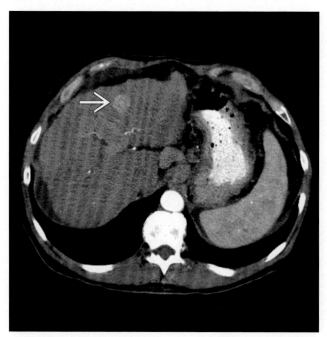 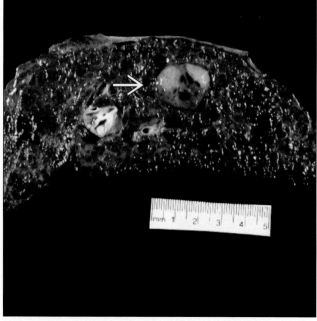

(Left) Axial CECT shows a hypervascular lesion ➡ in the left hepatic lobe on arterial phase imaging, consistent with HCC. *(Right)* Gross pathology following explantation of the liver confirms the small HCC ➡ in the left lobe of the liver.

HEPATOCELLULAR CARCINOMA

CT Findings: Primary

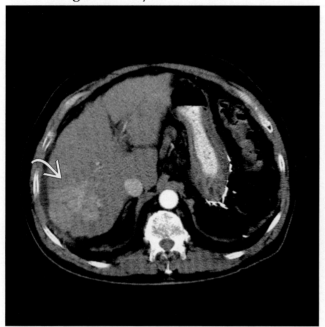
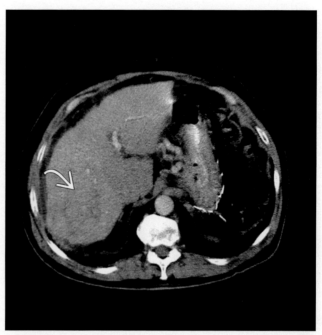

(Left) Axial CECT shows a hypervascular lesion ➔ in segment 7 of the liver, consistent with HCC. *(Right)* Axial CECT shows the same lesion ➔ on portal venous phase imaging. It subtly enhances heterogeneously compared to the background liver but is less apparent than on the arterial phase.

CT Findings: Primary

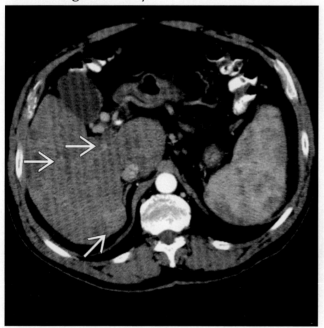
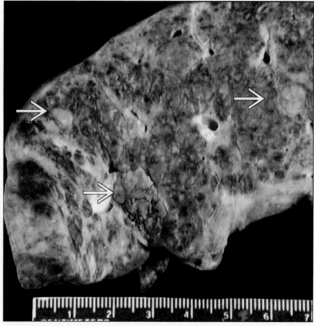

(Left) Axial CECT shows multiple hypervascular lesions ➔ in the right hepatic lobe in this patient with known HCC. *(Right)* Gross pathology shows multiple tan-colored lesions ➔ in the liver, compatible with multifocal HCC within a background cirrhotic liver.

HEPATOCELLULAR CARCINOMA

PET/CT Findings: Primary

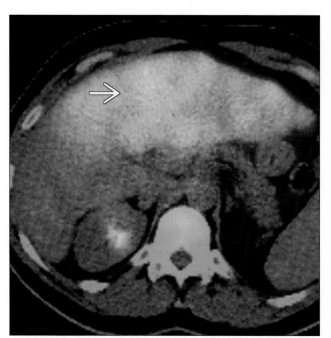
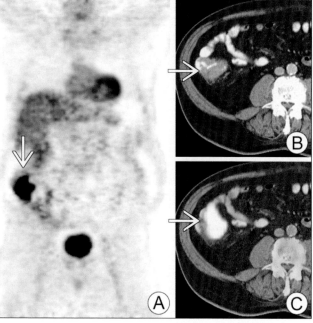

(Left) Axial fused PET/CT shows almost complete replacement of the left hepatic lobe ➡ with tumor in this patient with hepatocellular carcinoma. Approximately 50% of hepatocellular carcinoma primary lesions may not be FDG avid. *(Right)* Coronal PET (A), axial CT (B) and fused PET/CT (C) demonstrate intense activity in the descending colon ➡, compatible with colorectal carcinoma. The next two images are from the same patient, demonstrating a hepatic lesion.

PET/CT Findings: Primary

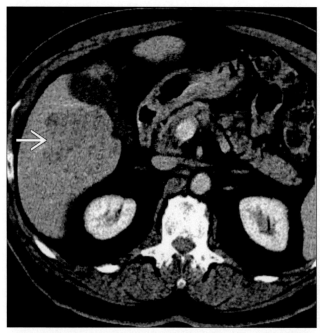
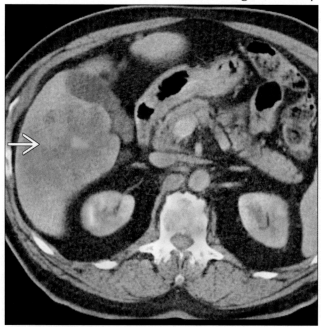

(Left) Axial CECT shows a heterogeneously enhancing mass in the right lobe of the liver ➡, biopsy-proven to be hepatocellular carcinoma. *(Right)* Axial fused PET/CT, in the same patient with carcinoma of unknown primary and subsequent diagnosis of colorectal carcinoma (previous figures), shows mildly increased FDG activity in the hepatic mass ➡. The primary colonic lesion has much greater FDG uptake than the hepatic lesion, suggesting a second primary neoplasm. Subsequent biopsy proved to be hepatocellular carcinoma. This amount of FDG activity is characteristic of hepatocellular carcinoma.

HEPATOCELLULAR CARCINOMA

PET/CT Findings: Primary

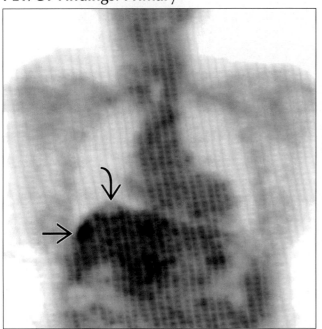
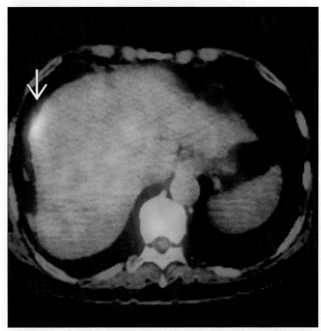

(Left) *Coronal PET shows focal intense activity along the lateral border of the liver* ➡️, *compatible with a recent biopsy specimen showing HCC. Note a successfully radiofrequency-ablated lesion near the hepatic dome* ➡️ *with no increased metabolic activity.* *(Right)* *Axial NECT shows focal intense activity along the peripheral aspect of the anterior right hepatic lobe* ➡️, *compatible with an additional area of malignancy.*

PET/CT Findings: Metastases

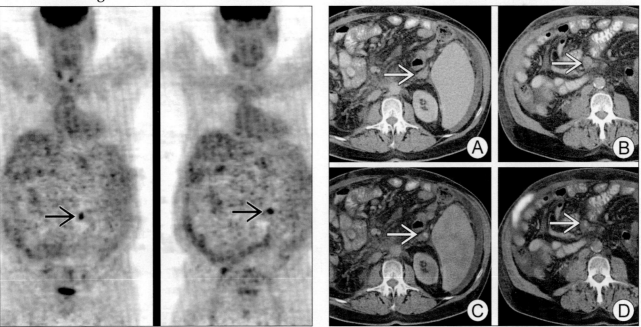

(Left) *Coronal PET images show a couple of intense foci of FDG activity in the abdomen* ➡️ *in this patient with a history of hepatocellular carcinoma. These findings are worrisome for malignancy.* *(Right)* *Axial CT (A, B) and fused PET/CT (C, D) show several foci of nodular mesenteric metastases* ➡️. *The administration of oral contrast helps to differentiate mesenteric lesions from loops of bowel.*

GASTRIC CARCINOMA

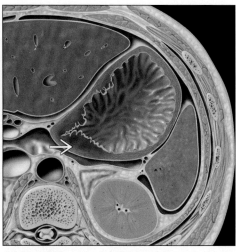

Axial graphic shows focal thickening of the gastric mucosa ➡, compatible with early gastric adenocarcinoma.

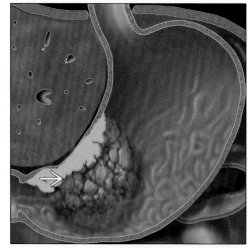

Graphic shows a large mass ➡ arising from the lesser curvature of the stomach, compatible with a large adenocarcinoma of the stomach.

TERMINOLOGY

Abbreviations and Synonyms
- Gastric adenocarcinoma, early/advanced gastric carcinoma (EGC/AGC), gastric cancer, stomach cancer

Definitions
- Adenocarcinoma arising from gastric mucosa
  - Malignant pathway: Gastritis → gastric atrophy → metaplasia → dysplasia → cancer
  - Most common primary tumor to metastasize to ovaries, usually bilaterally (Krukenberg tumors)

IMAGING FINDINGS

General Features
- Best diagnostic clue
  - FDG PET
    - Hypermetabolic FDG activity in primary gastric tumor, regional lymph nodes (LN), peritoneum, distant metastases
  - CT
    - Polypoid mass ± ulceration

- Focal wall thickening with mucosal irregularity, ulceration
- Regional LN > 8 mm: Suspicious for metastatic disease
- Peritoneal dissemination: Peritoneal caking, nodularity, beaded thickening, malignant ascites
- Location
  - Fundus and cardia: 40%
  - Body: 30%
  - Antrum: 30%
  - Most likely sites of recurrence post-gastrectomy: Gastric bed, peritoneal dissemination, liver
  - Large proportion of non-FDG-avid, non-intestinal subtype tumors found in distal 2/3 of stomach
  - Tumor commonly invades directly into
    - Pancreas via lesser sac
    - Transverse colon via gastrocolic ligament
    - Liver via gastrohepatic ligament
  - 60% of carcinoma of cardia will spread to distal esophagus
  - 5-20% of antral carcinoma will involve duodenum
- Size: Often very large before tumor becomes symptomatic
- Morphology

DDx: Gastric FDG Activity

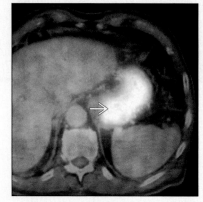

Gastritis

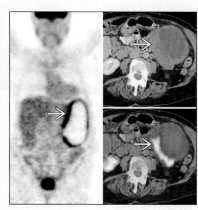

Gastrointestinal Stromal Tumor

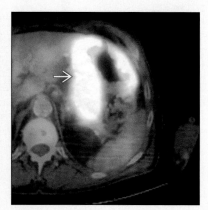

Gastric Lymphoma

GASTRIC CARCINOMA

Key Facts

Terminology
- Adenocarcinoma arising from gastric mucosa

Imaging Findings
- Hypermetabolic FDG activity in primary gastric tumor, regional lymph nodes (LN), peritoneum, distant metastases
- Regional LN > 8 mm: Suspicious for metastatic disease
- Peritoneal dissemination: Peritoneal caking, nodularity, beaded thickening, malignant ascites
- No method currently available capable of staging N disease accurately enough to enable decision making based on the extent of surgical lymph node dissection
- PET/CT for staging, recurrence, response to therapy
- CECT: Focal gastric wall thickening or mass lesion with enhancement
- PET sensitivity for primary tumor depends on extent

- PET and CT similar sensitivity for primary (94% vs. 93%), PET higher specificity (92% vs. 62%)
- Lymphadenopathy: PET insensitive for N1 disease (56%), equally sensitive for N2-3 disease as CT (78%)
- Mucinous and signet-ring cell adenocarcinoma: Low FDG avidity 2° to high mucus, lack of glut-1 transporters

Top Differential Diagnoses
- Gastric Ulcer
- Gastrointestinal Stromal Tumor (GIST)
- Gastric Lymphoma
  - Variable PET activity
- Gastritis
  - Usually mild activity; nonfocal
- Physiologic FDG Activity

- Type I: Elevated, protrude > 5 mm into lumen
- Type II: Superficial lesions that are elevated (IIa), flat (IIb), depressed (IIc)
- Type III: Early gastric cancers that are shallow, irregular ulcers surrounded by nodular, clubbed mucosal folds

Imaging Recommendations
- Best imaging tool
  - PET/CT for staging, recurrence, response to therapy
    - No modality is currently sensitive enough to confidently guide surgical planning
  - CECT to determine whether tumor is resectable
  - Barium X-ray screening is effective but has low sensitivity
    - Side effects include constipation and mis-swallowing of barium into trachea
- Protocol advice
  - PET sensitivity for recurrent disease post-gastrectomy may be ↑ by water ingestion (~ 300 cc) to distend remnant stomach
  - FDG uptake secondary to insulin release associated with food intake can be avoided by feeding at 120 minute time point after FDG administration
  - CT evaluation also aided by negative contrast ingestion (water or gas)

CT Findings
- **General features**
  - Mucosal irregularity
  - Enhancing focal gastric wall thickening
    - Gastric distention important for accurate assessment
  - Enhancing mass lesion
    - Normal gastroesophageal junction may be mistaken for mass
  - Polypoid mass ± ulceration
  - Gas-filled ulcer crater within mass
  - Tumor depth difficult to assess
- **Primary by type**
  - Infiltrating type: Loss of normal rugal folds over thickened wall

- Scirrhous type: Thickened wall with marked contrast enhancement
- Mucinous type: Wall thickening and calcification with decreased attenuation due to mucin content
- Cardia tumor: Lobulated mass with irregular soft tissue thickening
- **Extension/metastasis**
  - CT can delineate fat pad between tumor and organ to determine resectability
    - May normally be absent between stomach and left lobe of liver
    - Inflammation can obscure fat plane between tumor and pancreas
    - Cachexia results in loss of fat planes, producing potential false positive for organ invasion
  - Can often detect peritoneal carcinomatosis
    - Valuable for avoiding futile laparotomies
    - Tiny deposits may be overlooked
  - Extension into perigastric fat appears as wisp-like perigastric soft tissue stranding
- **Lymph nodes**
  - Subcentimeter lymph nodes may harbor malignancy
  - Enlarged lymph nodes may be nonmalignant (inflammation, infection)
  - Perigastric nodes are best visualized when stomach is fully distended

Nuclear Medicine Findings
- **General**
  - False positives
    - Normal stomach uptake
    - Gastritis
    - Inflammatory regional lymph nodes
    - Cholecystitis can produce false positives in liver
  - Water or food ingestion may decrease false positive from 31% to 8%
    - Food has advantage of slower emptying from stomach
    - Misregistration artifacts can occur because of shifting gas/fluid volumes between CT and PET acquisition

GASTRIC CARCINOMA

- Additional single-field PET/CT acquisition can avoid misinterpretation
- **Initial diagnosis**
  - FDG PET sensitivity for primary tumor
    - Early GC: 47%
    - Advanced GC: 98%
    - In general, better sensitivity for more advanced disease
  - PET and CT similar sensitivity for primary (94% vs. 93%)
    - PET has higher specificity (92% vs. 62%)
  - In general, well-differentiated gastric adenocarcinomas tend to take up less FDG than poorly differentiated ones
  - Exceptions
    - Poorly differentiated tubular adenocarcinomas show an especially wide spectrum of FDG uptake, from low to intense
    - Mucinous and signet-ring cell adenocarcinoma: Low FDG avidity 2° to high mucus, lack of glut-1 transporters
- **Staging**
  - Pre-treatment staging is essential to determine potential curability and to plan optimal therapy
  - Lymphadenopathy
    - PET and CT have similar sensitivity for detection of local and distant lymphadenopathy
    - Overall lymph node evaluation: PET less sensitive than CT (56% vs. 78%) but more specific (92% vs. 62%)
    - PET alone has low sensitivity for N1 disease (56%)
    - N1 insensitivity less important because all patients with AGC will undergo at least D1 dissection
    - PET and CT have high specificity for N1 disease
    - Positive findings may change endoscopic mucosal resection to more aggressive surgical approach in patients with EGC
    - Almost all PET-positive lymph nodes prove to be involved in patients with AGC
    - PET and CT equally sensitive for N2-3 disease (about 80%)
    - N2/N3 status determination important: Can change extent of lymph node dissection and, in the case of N3 disease, curative potential
  - Peritoneal dissemination: PET has low sensitivity and CT low specificity, but similar accuracy overall
  - FDG avidity of primary tumor predictive of long-term survival in patients undergoing complete resection of primary
- **Response to therapy**
  - Post-therapy change in tumor SUV predicts both response to therapy and long-term survival with 77% sensitivity, 86% specificity
  - Decreased tumor uptake by > 35% of baseline allowed accurate prediction of response 14 days after initiation of cisplatin-based polychemotherapy
    - Overall accuracy of 83%
    - 1/3 of patients initially have insufficient FDG uptake for quantification
    - Initially low FDG uptake probably correlates with tumors in which chemotherapy has limited effectiveness

- **Other radiotracers**
  - 18F-fluorothymidine sensitive for locally advanced gastric cancers with improved detection of tumors with signet ring cells or mucinous contents

DIFFERENTIAL DIAGNOSIS

Gastric Ulcer
- Benign ulcer
- Crater margin sharply defined and smooth en face, symmetric, confluent with healthy mucosa, mucosal folds radiate from ulcer edge
- Most located in lesser curve or posterior wall of antrum, body of stomach

Gastrointestinal Stromal Tumor (GIST)
- Well-demarcated, spherical, intramural masses that arise from muscularis propria; often project exophytically, intraluminally
- May have overlying mucosal ulceration
- Larger GISTs often outgrow vascular supply → necrosis and hemorrhage

Gastric Lymphoma
- Usually correlative gastric wall thickening
- May be diffuse throughout stomach
- Variable PET activity

Gastritis
- Usually mild to moderate FDG activity
- No associated signs of malignancy on CT

Physiologic FDG Activity
- Usually mild activity; nonfocal

Crohn Disease
- Rarely affects stomach
- Abscess, fistula, small-bowel disease, mesenteric fibrofatty proliferation
- Hypermetabolic PET activity in active disease

PATHOLOGY

General Features
- General path comments
  - ~ 95% of all malignant gastric neoplasms are adenocarcinoma
    - Remaining 5%: Lymphoma, leiomyosarcoma, carcinoid, sarcoma
- Genetics
  - 10% of cases are familial
  - Hereditary syndromes with increased risk of gastric cancer
    - Hereditary nonpolyposis colorectal cancer
    - Li-Fraumeni syndrome
    - Familial adenomatous polyposis
    - Peutz-Jeghers syndrome
- Etiology
  - H. pylori is the strongest risk factor for gastric cancer
    - Infection with H. pylori may be beneficial prognostic factor in patients with EGC
  - Large amounts of dietary salt, smoked meats, and nitrates

GASTRIC CARCINOMA

o Smoking increases risk ~ 1.5x
o Hypochlorhydria
- Epidemiology
  o Incidence decreasing
    - 33 cases per 100,000 population in 1930
    - 3.7 cases per 100,000 population in 1990
  o Worldwide, second only to lung cancer for cancer deaths
  o Mass screening programs with barium studies or endoscopy have contributed to detection of gastric cancer at earlier stages
    - EGC accounts for up to 20% of gastric cancers
- Associated abnormalities: Chronic atrophic gastritis, pernicious anemia, previous partial gastrectomy, Ménétrier disease, and adenomatous polyps

Staging, Grading, or Classification Criteria
- T Classification
  o Tis: Carcinoma in situ, intraepithelial tumor
  o T1: Tumoral extension to submucosa
  o T2: Tumoral extension to the muscularis propria or subserosa
  o T3: Tumoral penetration of the serosa
  o T4: Tumoral invasion of the adjacent organs

CLINICAL ISSUES

Presentation
- Most common signs/symptoms
  o Early stage is generally asymptomatic
  o Most patients present with the following symptoms, which indicate advanced disease
    - Dysphagia, early satiety, anorexia, weight loss
    - Nausea, vomiting
    - Epigastric pain
    - Bloating
- Other signs/symptoms: Signs of upper GI bleeding (hematemesis, melena, iron deficiency anemia, positive fecal occult blood test)

Demographics
- Age: Peak incidence 50-70 years
- Gender: M:F = 2:1
- Ethnicity: 1.5-2.5x more common in African-American, Hispanic, American Indian than Caucasian

Natural History & Prognosis
- 40-60% of patients have advanced disease at time of diagnosis, and recurrences are common after resection
- Poor prognosis due to advanced disease at presentation
  o Overall 5 year survival rate < 20%
  o Median survival 7-10 months
- Prognosis of EGC excellent with radical gastrectomy: 5 year survival > 95%, regardless of lymphadenopathy
- No survival benefit proven for total or subtotal gastrectomy
- When tumor recurs in remnant stomach, palliation is the only meaningful treatment approach

Treatment
- 30-40% of patients show measurable clinical or histopathologic response after neoadjuvant treatment

- Surgical resection is the only curative treatment for localized disease
- Important factors for determining surgical resectability
  o Adjacent organ involvement
  o Peritoneal carcinomatosis
  o LN metastases
  o Distant metastases
- Inoperable obstructing gastric carcinomas can be treated with stent to avoid palliative surgery in frail patients
- Extended D2 dissection of patients with N2 disease associated higher intra-operative complications but substantially improved overall long term survival
  o D2 dissection alone may be more effective than limited D1 lymph node dissection with adjuvant chemotherapy
  o At least D2 dissection needed to achieve curative resection when N2 disease is evident on PET

DIAGNOSTIC CHECKLIST

Consider
- PET/CT valuable
  o For most complete pre-operative staging
  o To evaluate response to therapy
  o To identify recurrence

Image Interpretation Pearls
- PET
  o May miss LN metastases adjacent to primary tumor
  o Has high accuracy for N2, visceral, distant metastases
  o Has limited sensitivity for peritoneal metastases due to small size, resolution limits of equipment

SELECTED REFERENCES

1. Conybeare A et al: PET scanning in the detection of occult gastric metastases from lung carcinoma. Eur J Surg Oncol. 33(2):252-3, 2007
2. Di Fabio F et al: The predictive value of 18F-FDG-PET early evaluation in patients with metastatic gastric adenocarcinoma treated with chemotherapy plus cetuximab. Gastric Cancer. 10(4):221-7, 2007
3. Jensen EH et al: Preoperative staging and postoperative surveillance for gastric cancer. Surg Oncol Clin N Am. 16(2):329-42, 2007
4. Lordick F et al: PET to assess early metabolic response and to guide treatment of adenocarcinoma of the oesophagogastric junction: the MUNICON phase II trial. Lancet Oncol. 8(9):797-805, 2007
5. Pinto C et al: Phase II study of cetuximab in combination with FOLFIRI in patients with untreated advanced gastric or gastroesophageal junction adenocarcinoma (FOLCETUX study). Ann Oncol. 18(3):510-7, 2007
6. Sun L et al: Epidermal growth factor receptor antibody plus recombinant human endostatin in treatment of hepatic metastases after remnant gastric cancer resection. World J Gastroenterol. 13(45):6115-8, 2007
7. van Vliet EP et al: Detection of distant metastases in patients with oesophageal or gastric cardia cancer: a diagnostic decision analysis. Br J Cancer. 97(7):868-76, 2007

GASTRIC CARCINOMA

CT Findings

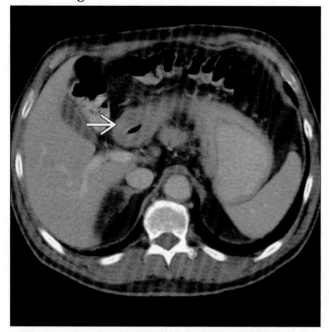
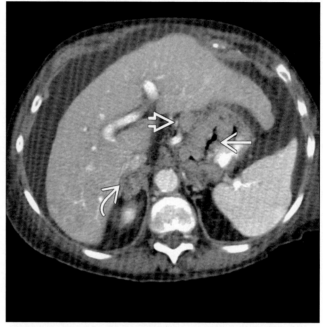

(Left) Axial CECT shows smooth antral wall thickening ➡ that is nonspecific, but subsequent endoscopic biopsy showed adenocarcinoma of the stomach. *(Right)* Axial CECT shows wall thickening of the stomach, mostly along the lesser curvature ➡, a right adrenal lesion ➚, and an enlarged gastrohepatic ligament lymph node ➡.

CT Findings

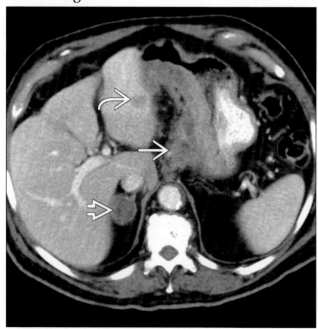
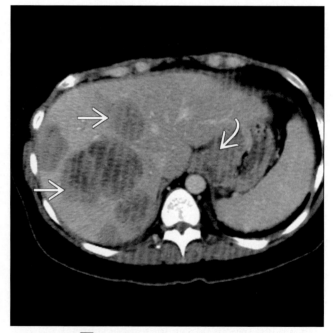

(Left) Axial CECT shows irregular wall thickening just below the esophagogastric junction ➡, a hypodense focus in the lateral segment of the liver ➚, and a right adrenal metastasis ➡. *(Right)* Axial CECT shows numerous hepatic metastases ➡ and thickening just at and below the esophagogastric junction ➚.

GASTRIC CARCINOMA

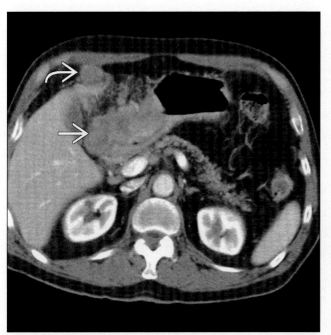 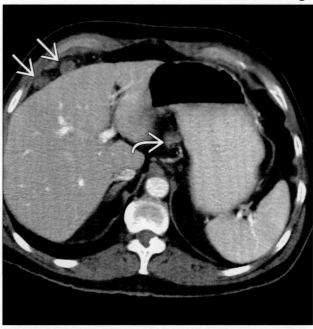

(Left) Axial CECT shows irregular wall thickening at the antrum ➡, corresponding to gastric carcinoma, and a soft tissue metastatic omental implant ➡. *(Right)* Axial CECT of the same patient reveals more omental implants ➡ and an enlarged gastrohepatic ligament lymph node ➡.

PET/CT Findings: Primary

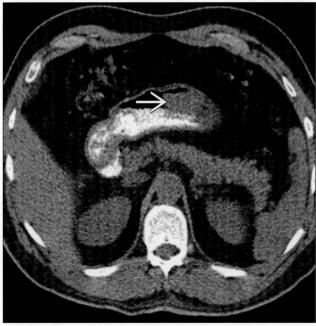 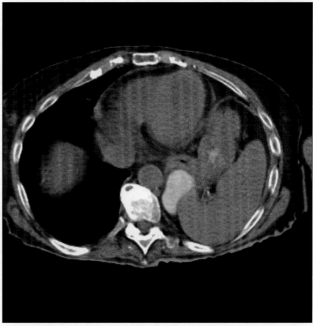

(Left) Axial NECT shows a questionable mass arising from the anterior gastric wall ➡. *(Right)* Axial NECT shows no obvious abnormalities.

GASTRIC CARCINOMA

PET/CT Findings: Primary

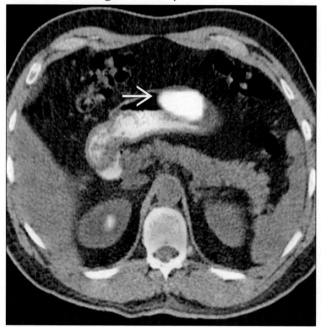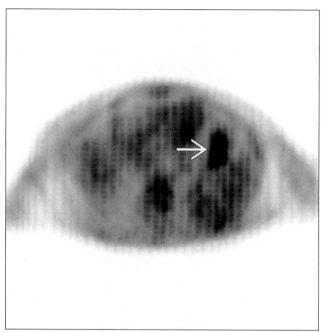

(Left) Axial fused PET/CT shows focal intense FDG activity within the anterior gastric wall mass ➔, compatible with malignancy. This was an incidental PET/CT finding, and a subsequent endoscopy was performed, verifying newly diagnosed adenocarcinoma of the stomach. *(Right)* Axial PET shows focal intense FDG activity ➔ correlating with the stomach in this patient who subsequently underwent endoscopy.

PET/CT Findings: Primary

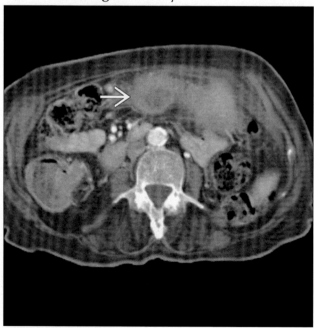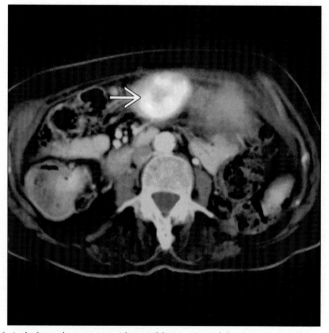

(Left) Axial CECT shows a mass lesion with enhancing walls extending inferiorly from the antrum with possible invasion of the transverse colon ➔. *(Right)* Axial fused PET/CT shows focal intense FDG activity within the wall of the antrum mass ➔, compatible with the patient's known gastric adenocarcinoma.

GASTRIC CARCINOMA

PET/CT Findings: Primary

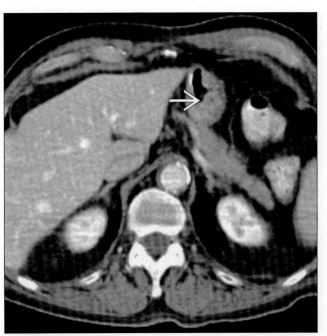 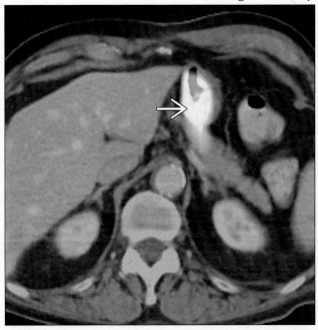

(Left) Axial CECT shows questionable thickening in the stomach ➔ in this patient newly diagnosed with gastric adenocarcinoma. *(Right)* Axial fused PET/CT shows intense activity correlating with the questionable area of thickening in the stomach ➔. Given the patient's history of recently diagnosed adenocarcinoma, this most likely represents the primary lesion.

PET/CT Findings: Primary

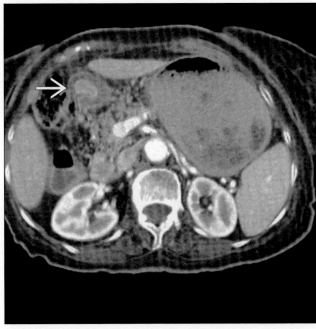 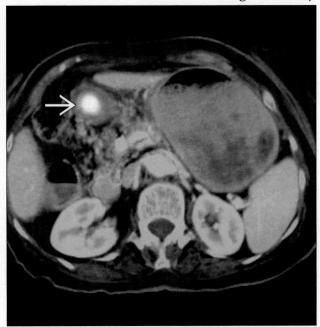

(Left) Axial CECT shows antral wall thickening with mucosal enhancement ➔. *(Right)* Axial fused PET/CT shows intense FDG uptake in the region of antral wall thickening ➔ shown on the previous image.

GASTRIC CARCINOMA

PET/CT Findings: Primary with Metastasis

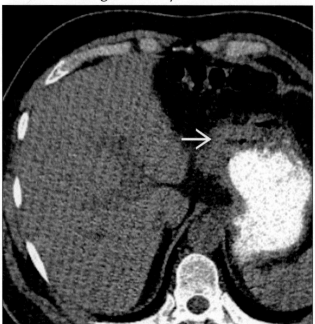 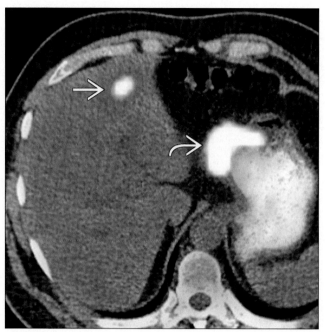

(Left) Axial NECT shows no definite abnormality in this patient with newly diagnosed adenocarcinoma of the stomach. Subtle thickening of the distal gastric mucosa ➡ is questionable for cancer. *(Right)* Axial fused PET/CT shows intense metabolic activity, correlating with the questionable thickening in the gastric mucosa ➡, as well as a focal area of intense FDG activity in the left hepatic lobe ➡, compatible with a metastatic lesion.

PET/CT Findings: Primary with Metastasis

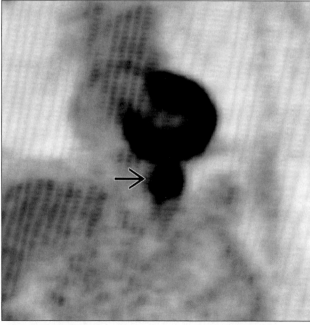 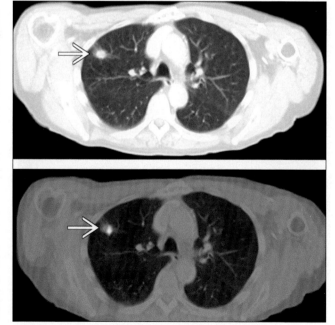

(Left) Coronal PET shows nonspecific intense FDG activity in the area of the stomach ➡. The metabolic activity within the stomach is variable, ranging from almost none to very intense. Therefore, the presence of metabolic activity without a correlative CT abnormality is nonspecific. *(Right)* Axial CT (top) and fused PET/CT (bottom) demonstrate a hypermetabolic pulmonary lesion ➡ in a patient newly diagnosed with adenocarcinoma. The differential diagnosis includes primary lung carcinoma vs. metastatic disease from the known gastric carcinoma.

GASTRIC CARCINOMA

PET/CT Findings: Primary with Metastasis

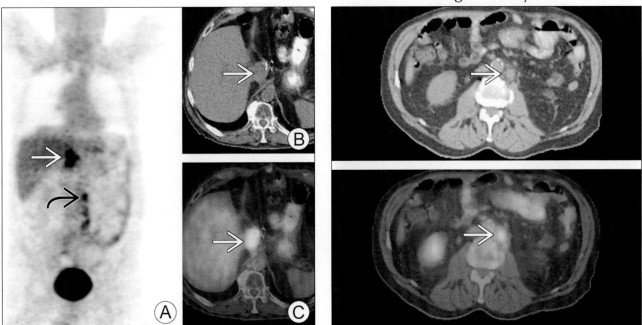

(Left) Coronal PET (A) and axial CT (B) and fused PET/CT (C) demonstrate metastatic disease in this patient with gastric carcinoma to the right adrenal gland ➡ and retroperitoneal lymph nodes ➡. *(Right)* Axial CT (top) and fused PET/CT (bottom) show a moderately hypermetabolic and mildly enlarged left periaortic retroperitoneal lymph node ➡ in a patient with newly diagnosed gastric carcinoma, compatible with metastatic lymphadenopathy.

Restaging

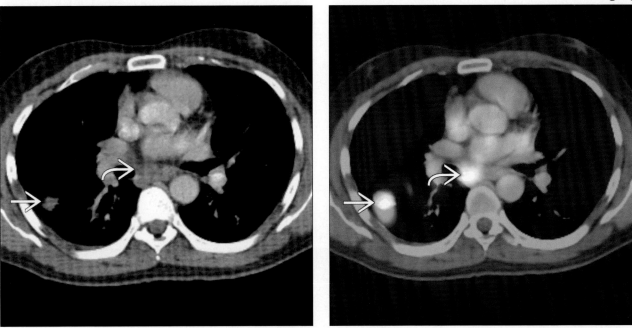

(Left) Axial CECT in a patient with gastric adenocarcinoma shows a new lung lesion ➡ and enlarged mediastinal nodes ➡. *(Right)* Axial fused PET/CT shows intense metabolic activity in both the lung lesion ➡ and subcarinal adenopathy ➡, compatible with metastases.

3

PANCREATIC CARCINOMA

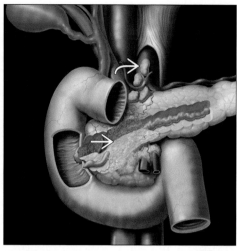

Graphic shows pancreatic adenocarcinoma ➡ with metastatic periceliac nodes ➡.

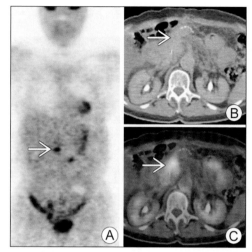

Coronal PET (A), axial (B) and fused PET/CT (C) show typical adenocarcinoma ➡ in a patient with a history of chronic pancreatitis.

TERMINOLOGY

Abbreviations and Synonyms
- Pancreatic cancer (PC)
- Pancreatic ductal carcinoma
- Superior mesenteric artery (SMA)
- Superior mesenteric vein (SMV)

Definitions
- Adenocarcinoma of ductal epithelium of exocrine pancreas
- Less common additional malignancies of exocrine pancreas include
  - Giant cell carcinoma
  - Adenosquamous carcinoma
  - Microadenocarcinoma
  - Mucinous carcinoma
  - Papillary cystic carcinoma
  - Cystadenocarcinoma

IMAGING FINDINGS

General Features
- Best diagnostic clue
  - Hypoattenuating pancreatic mass
    - Eccentric and lobulated
    - Varying degrees of FDG uptake
    - Typically the more well-differentiated the tumor, the lower the FDG activity
    - Also mucinous primaries may be less FDG avid
  - FDG uptake indicates invasion of lymph nodes and adjacent vessels
  - Distal pancreatic ductal dilatation
  - Encasement of vessels
    - SMA/SMV, celiac vessels, portal vein, and splenic vein
  - Loss of peripancreatic fat
- Location
  - Most (65-75%) located in head of pancreas
  - 60% have liver metastases at presentation
- Size
  - Size is nonspecific

DDx: FDG Uptake in Pancreas Mimicking Adenocarcinoma

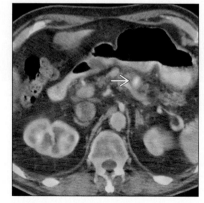

Metastasis

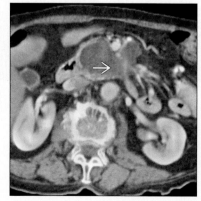

Mucinous Cystic Tumor

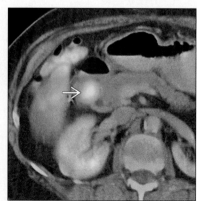

Neuroendocrine Tumor

PANCREATIC CARCINOMA

Key Facts

Terminology
- Pancreatic cancer, pancreatic ductal carcinoma

Imaging Findings
- Poorly enhancing pancreatic mass with increased FDG uptake
- Hypermetabolic activity in regional lymph nodes, metastatic sites
- Initial diagnosis: Endoscopic ultrasound for pancreatic head; CECT for body and tail
- Staging: PET/CT with CECT correlation; current reimbursement limitations
- CECT predicts resectability with ~ 70-80% accuracy; many patients later found unresectable at surgery
- Vascular encasement key to determining resectability
- Variable appearance, may only see contour deformity or area of enlargement

- Direct invasion of adjacent organs, commonly duodenum or stomach
- Moderate to marked increased FDG uptake in pancreatic mass
- PET tumor diagnosis: Sensitivity 90-95%, specificity 82-100%

Top Differential Diagnoses
- Pancreatitis
- Islet Cell Tumor
- Cystic Pancreatic Neoplasm
- Periampullary Tumors
- Nonepithelial Tumors

Diagnostic Checklist
- PET/CT for optimal staging
- CECT to determine resectability

- Diffuse enlargement may be due to chronic pancreatitis
- Normal pancreatic head size with atrophy of remaining pancreas is suggestive of malignancy
- Pancreatic head masses often present at smaller size due to obstruction
- Tail lesions may reach 10 cm before presentation
- Morphology
  - Normal sharp margins may become blurred
  - Ductal dilation common in the setting of pancreatic head tumor
  - May present with focal lobulated mass
  - Often infiltrative mass
  - Small pancreatic head masses may not be visualized on CT

Imaging Recommendations
- Best imaging tool
  - Initial diagnosis in symptomatic patients usually done with ultrasound
    - Ductal dilation
    - Enlargement
  - PET/CECT for diagnosis, staging, and restaging
    - Valuable for surgical planning
    - Current reimbursement limitations
  - ERCP for localization of duct stricture and therapeutic relief
- Protocol advice
  - No caloric intake 6 hours before scan
  - Blood glucose > 200 requires rescheduling
  - Keep patient relaxed and warm to minimize muscle and brown fat uptake
  - Administer 370-555 MBq FDG and image in 60-120 minutes
  - Negative bowel contrast improves interpretation (water, oral contrast)
  - CECT as part of the PET/CT may be helpful

CT Findings
- **Primary lesion**
  - Sensitivity for detection very high ~ 95%

- May miss small head/uncinate process/ periampullary lesions
  - Isodense mass without hemorrhage or calcification
  - Poorly enhancing heterogeneous composition
  - Infiltration of surrounding fat
  - May appear only as enlargement or contour deformity
  - Atrophy of parenchyma distal to tumor
  - If large, central necrosis is common
- **Ductal dilation**
  - Pancreatic duct may dilate distal to mass
  - Benign vs. malignant obstruction
    - Ex: Obstruction stone
    - Abrupt interruption of duct (vs. smooth taper) favors malignancy
  - Double duct sign
    - Common bile duct (CBD) obstruction → ductal dilation
    - Secondary to invasion of porta hepatis or mass effect
- **Vascular invasion**
  - Major determinant of surgical resectability
  - Tumor may encase or invade mesenteric root and branches
  - More than 50% or 180° of tumor contact with vessel = unresectable
  - Dilated collateral mesenteric/splanchnic veins = unresectable
  - Venous involvement more commonly presents as altered shape ("teardrop-shaped" SMV) or thrombosis
- **Metastasis**
  - Insensitive for liver metastases when unsuspected
  - Direct invasion with contiguous organs (duodenum, stomach, and mesenteric root)
  - Local invasion into porta hepatis and splenic hilum
  - Distant invasion
  - Common metastatic locations
    - Liver, regional lymph nodes, and peritoneum
  - Rare metastatic locations
    - Bone, lung, pleura, and adrenals
- **Contrast enhancement**

PANCREATIC CARCINOMA

- o Contrast enhancement depends heavily on good technique and administration dynamics
- o Primary pancreatic carcinoma usually heterogeneous and hypoattenuating after arterial phase
- o Hypoattenuating due to abundant fibrous stroma and hypovascularity
- o Vascular involvement evaluation on arterial phase
- Pancreatitis
  - o Chronic pancreatitis characterized by cystic and necrotic areas and calcifications
  - o Appearance is nonspecific for malignant vs. benign disease
    - PET/CT may be helpful for differentiating chronic tumefactive pancreatitis vs. pancreatic carcinoma
  - o In the setting of known malignancy, pancreatitis may lead to staging overestimation

Nuclear Medicine Findings

- General
  - o PET/CT
    - Sensitivity 85-100%
    - Specificity 67-99%
    - Accuracy 85-93%
  - o Dual modality imaging exceptionally useful due to complex anatomy and normal background FDG uptake
    - Normal pancreatic bed has relatively high tumor:background ratio
- Initial diagnosis
  - o FDG uptake is a sensitive tool to distinguish benign from malignant disease
    - Especially useful for liver lesions
  - o Common cutoff SUV for malignancy is 2.5
    - Most malignant tumors show higher uptake
    - Tumors with mucin production (e.g., mucinous adenocarcinoma) may have variable SUV
- Staging/restaging
  - o Extension to adjacent organs and vascular invasion are more accurately diagnosed with PET/CT
    - Nonenlarged and distant lesions may be detected
    - Staging changed in 10-20% and management altered in 15-50%
  - o Has shown value in detection of recurrent tumor and evaluation of response to therapy

DIFFERENTIAL DIAGNOSIS

Pancreatitis

- Acute: May present false positive due to increased FDG uptake
- Chronic
  - o Often indistinguishable from cancer on morphologic imaging
  - o Reliably differentiated by FDG PET: Sensitivity and specificity 85-89% and 55-93%, respectively
  - o Common findings include gland enlargement &/or atrophy, calcification, ductal dilation, pseudocyst, and vascular abnormalities

Islet Cell Tumor

- Often low FDG uptake

- Correlate with clinical features of secretory neuroendocrine tumor
- Hypervascular enhancement and vascular encasement are rare findings

Cystic Pancreatic Neoplasm

- Types
  - o Intraductal papillary mucinous tumor (IPMT)
  - o Mucinous cystic neoplasm
    - Formerly known as macrocystic adenoma, mucinous cystadenoma, cystadenocarcinoma
  - o Microcystic adenoma or serous cystadenoma
    - Benign lesion associated with von Hippel-Lindau disease
- As a group these tumors show little FDG uptake due to hypocellularity

Periampullary Tumors

- Adenocarcinoma of duodenum and ampulla
- Whipple procedure is standard of care
- Survival better than for pancreatic adenocarcinoma

Nonepithelial Tumors

- Very rare primary pancreatic lymphoma and sarcoma may be seen
  - o More often, these tumors indicate disease elsewhere
- Metastatic disease from breast, melanoma, lung, and GI tumors

Pancreatic Metastases

- Often more well-rounded, but may be indistinguishable
- Common malignancies that metastasize to pancreas
  - o Lung, breast, kidney, gastrointestinal tract, thyroid, melanoma, hepatocellular carcinoma, and osteosarcoma

PATHOLOGY

General Features

- Genetics
  - o 40% of pancreatic adenocarcinoma is hereditary
    - K-ras and other genetic mutations play a role
    - Many cases due to hereditary form of chronic pancreatitis
    - Acquired pancreatitis has weak association with pancreatic cancer
- Etiology
  - o Overall risk is doubled in the presence of cigarette smoking and diabetes mellitus
  - o High protein & fat diet and industrial carcinogens also implicated
- Epidemiology
  - o Roughly equal incidence and death rate, accounting for ~ 30,000 cases/year in USA
  - o 11th most common cancer and 5th leading cause of cancer death
  - o Only 5-15% of tumors are resectable at presentation
- Associated abnormalities: Portal vein tumor thrombus (PVTT) marks dismal prognosis for clinical outcome and survival

PANCREATIC CARCINOMA

Gross Pathologic & Surgical Features
- Tumors of exocrine pancreas often demonstrate mucin production and fibrosis
  - Usually decreased SUV on PET compared to non-mucinous subtypes

Microscopic Features
- Biopsy is highly sensitive and specific, but obtaining tissue sample may be difficult
  - Biopsy needle tract bears small risk of tumor seeding and fistula formation

CLINICAL ISSUES

Presentation
- Most common signs/symptoms
  - Presents with a constellation of vague symptoms
    - Weakness, malaise, anorexia, &/or weight loss
    - Pancreatic head tumors may present earlier due to obstruction
    - Tail and body tumors present later with systemic symptoms
  - Most common symptom at diagnosis: Abdominal pain
    - Extension to the back is a poor prognostic indicator, implying retroperitoneal invasion
  - Classic presentation is painless jaundice
    - Courvoisier sign: Palpable gallbladder with painless jaundice
- Other signs/symptoms
  - 60% of patients at presentation have
    - Liver metastasis, malignant ascites, or other evidence of tumor spread
- Clinical profile
  - CA19-9 and CEA tumor markers may be elevated
  - Consider PET/CT when rising tumor markers

Demographics
- Age
  - Age of presentation: Mean 55 years, median 65-70 years
  - Earlier presentation in hereditary forms
- Gender: Slight male predominance
- Ethnicity: African Americans > Caucasians

Natural History & Prognosis
- Mean survival with unresectable tumor is 4-6 months
- Patients who survive Whipple procedure have overall 5 year survival of 20%
  - Very few patients are candidates for surgery at presentation
  - As many as 30% of patients have unsuspected mets at surgery
  - As many as 70% have early recurrence 6-12 months after surgery
- Overall 3 year survival of 2%

Treatment
- Surgical resection is the only treatment shown to improve survival
- Standard of care is pancreaticoduodenectomy (Whipple procedure)
  - Patients with R0 resection in the setting of localized disease may achieve long-term survival
- Palliative treatment modalities include chemoradiotherapy and selective neurolysis

DIAGNOSTIC CHECKLIST

Image Interpretation Pearls
- Consider PET/CT for differentiation of chronic pancreatitis vs. carcinoma
- Consider PET/CT when rising tumor markers

SELECTED REFERENCES

1. Quon A et al: Initial evaluation of 18F-fluorothymidine (FLT) PET/CT scanning for primary pancreatic cancer. Eur J Nucl Med Mol Imaging. 35(3):527-31, 2008
2. Sahani DV et al: Radiology of pancreatic adenocarcinoma: current status of imaging. J Gastroenterol Hepatol. 23(1):23-33, 2008
3. Singer E et al: Differential diagnosis of benign and malign pancreatic masses with 18F-fluordeoxyglucose-positron emission tomography recorded with a dual-head coincidence gamma camera. Eur J Gastroenterol Hepatol. 19(6):471-8, 2007
4. Bang S et al: The clinical usefulness of 18-fluorodeoxyglucose positron emission tomography in the differential diagnosis, staging, and response evaluation after concurrent chemoradiotherapy for pancreatic cancer. J Clin Gastroenterol. 40(10):923-9, 2006
5. Hamer OW et al: How useful is integrated PET and CT for the management of pancreatic cancer? Nat Clin Pract Gastroenterol Hepatol. 3(2):74-5, 2006
6. Mansour JC et al: The utility of F-18 fluorodeoxyglucose whole body PET imaging for determining malignancy in cystic lesions of the pancreas. J Gastrointest Surg. 10(10):1354-60, 2006
7. Miura F et al: Diagnosis of pancreatic cancer. HPB (Oxford). 8(5):337-42, 2006
8. Pakzad F et al: The role of positron emission tomography in the management of pancreatic cancer. Semin Nucl Med. 36(3):248-56, 2006
9. Ruf J et al: Impact of FDG-PET/MRI image fusion on the detection of pancreatic cancer. Pancreatology. 6(6):512-9, 2006
10. Borbath I et al: Preoperative assessment of pancreatic tumors using magnetic resonance imaging, endoscopic ultrasonography, positron emission tomography and laparoscopy. Pancreatology. 5(6):553-61, 2005
11. Goh BK et al: Utility of fusion CT-PET in the diagnosis of small pancreatic carcinoma. World J Gastroenterol. 11(24):3800-2, 2005
12. Heinrich S et al: Positron emission tomography/computed tomography influences on the management of resectable pancreatic cancer and its cost-effectiveness. Ann Surg. 242(2):235-43, 2005
13. Lytras D et al: Positron emission tomography does not add to computed tomography for the diagnosis and staging of pancreatic cancer. Dig Surg. 22(1-2):55-61; discussion 62, 2005
14. Nishiyama Y et al: Contribution of whole body FDG-PET to the detection of distant metastasis in pancreatic cancer. Ann Nucl Med. 19(6):491-7, 2005
15. Sahani DV et al: Detection of liver metastases from adenocarcinoma of the colon and pancreas: comparison of mangafodipir trisodium-enhanced liver MRI and whole-body FDG PET. AJR Am J Roentgenol. 185(1):239-46, 2005

3

PANCREATIC CARCINOMA

CT Findings: Pancreatic Adenocarcinoma

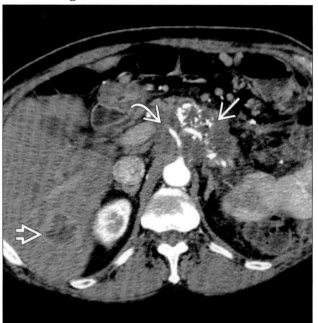 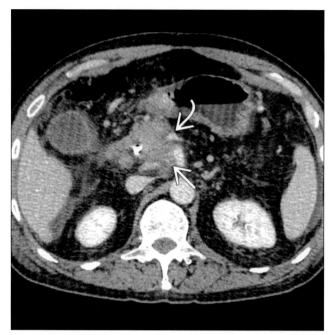

(Left) Axial CECT shows a soft tissue mass that envelopes the pancreatic body and celiac artery at the trifurcation ➡. This soft tissue cuff extends along the common hepatic artery ➡. Additionally, there is a hepatic metastasis ➡. *(Right)* Axial CECT shows subtle soft tissue infiltration at the uncinate process. It also abuts the right aspect of the superior mesenteric artery ➡ and attenuates the porto-systemic confluence ➡, concerning for pancreatic adenocarcinoma.

CT Findings: Pancreatic Adenocarcinoma

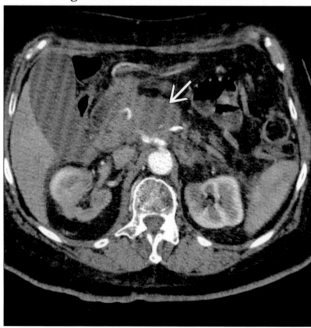 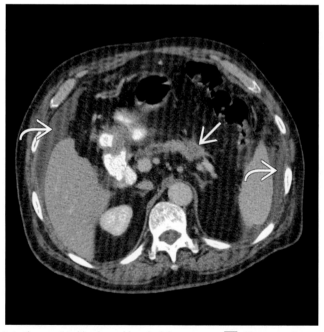

(Left) Axial CECT shows an infiltrative soft tissue mass with central necrosis in the proximal body and head of the pancreas ➡. The necrosis encases the celiac at its trifurcation and the gastroduodenal artery. *(Right)* Axial CECT shows a small spiculated pancreatic tail mass ➡, subsequently shown to be an adenocarcinoma. Note the perihepatic and perisplenic ascites ➡.

PANCREATIC CARCINOMA

CT Findings: Pancreatic Adenocarcinoma

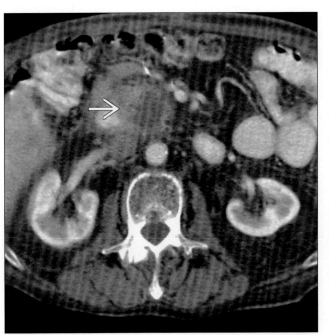 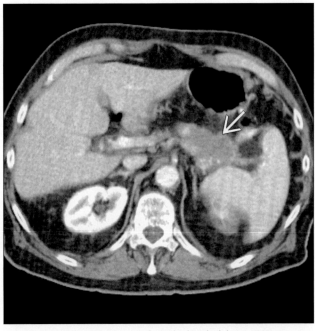

(Left) Axial CECT shows a large heterogeneously enhancing mass ➡️ *with areas of central necrosis arising from the head of the pancreas, compatible with pancreatic adenocarcinoma. (Right) Axial CECT shows a soft tissue mass in the distal body and tail of the pancreas* ➡️*.*

PET/CT Findings: Staging

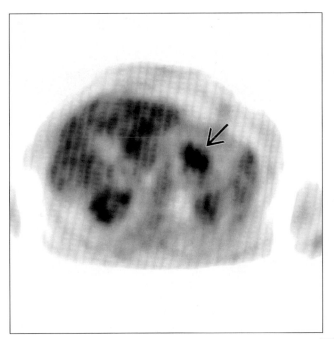 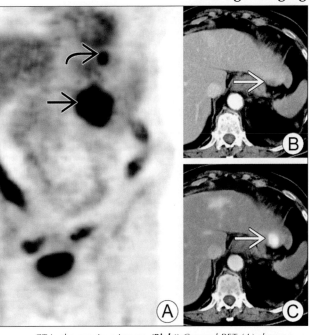

(Left) Axial PET shows increased FDG uptake in the pancreatic lesion ➡️ *seen on CT in the previous image. (Right) Coronal PET (A) shows a large primary adenocarcinoma of the pancreas* ➡️ *with a focal area of intense activity* ➡️ *that is difficult to localize. Axial CT (B) and fused PET/CT (C) show a subtle hepatic metastasis* ➡️*.*

PANCREATIC CARCINOMA

PET/CT Findings: Staging

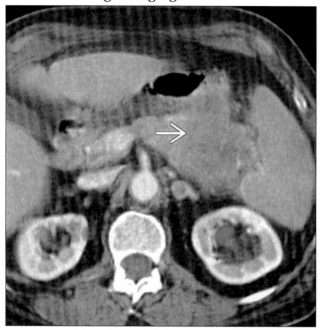 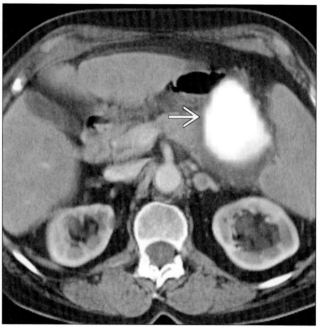

(Left) Axial CECT shows an infiltrative mass in the distal body and tail of the pancreas ➔. *(Right)* Axial fused PET/CT shows marked FDG uptake in the pancreatic lesion ➔, compatible with the subsequent diagnosis of adenocarcinoma.

PET/CT Findings: Staging

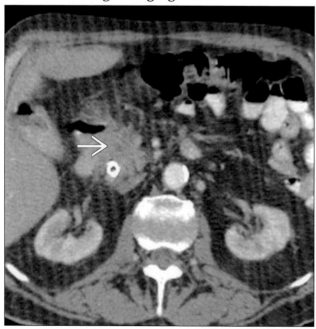 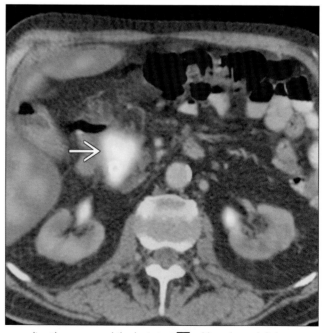

(Left) Axial CECT shows "fullness" in the region of the pancreatic head surrounding the common bile duct stent ➔, although no definite mass is identified. *(Right)* Axial fused PET/CT of the same patient reveals that the region of "fullness" corresponds to a metabolically active tumor ➔. The placement of the common bile duct stents may obscure the lesion secondary to streak artifact. Localization, in this instance, was easy to confirm.

PANCREATIC CARCINOMA

PET/CT Findings: Staging

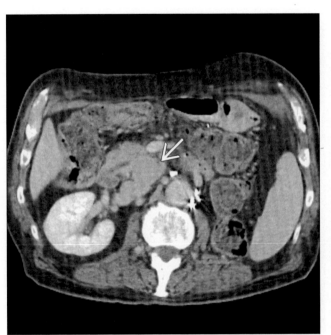 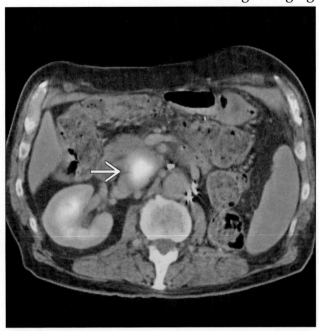

(Left) Axial CECT shows an exophytic, homogeneously enhancing lesion ➡ arising from the uncinate process, worrisome for malignancy. *(Right)* Axial fused PET/CT confirms the presence of a hypermetabolic lesion ➡, later identified as adenocarcinoma.

PET/CT Findings: Staging

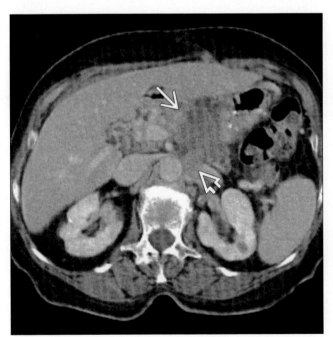 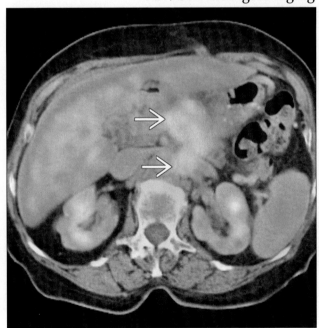

(Left) Axial CECT shows an infiltrative mass ➡, consistent with pancreatic adenocarcinoma and a left para-aortic nodal metastasis ➡. *(Right)* Axial fused PET/CT of the same patient shows only mild metabolic activity of the primary tumor and the nodal metastasis ➡.

3

PANCREATIC CARCINOMA

PET/CT Findings: Staging

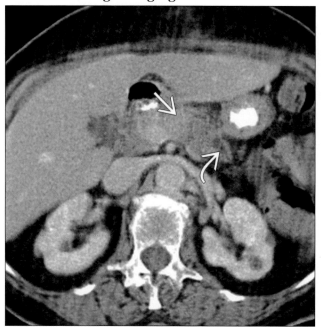 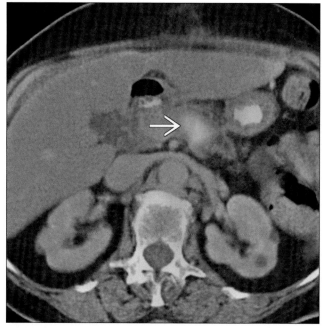

(Left) Axial CECT shows a slightly hypodense lesion in the pancreatic body ➡ with distal ductal dilation and atrophy ➡. (Right) Axial fused PET/CT of the same patient demonstrates increased metabolic activity ➡, consistent with pancreatic adenocarcinoma.

PET/CT Findings: Staging

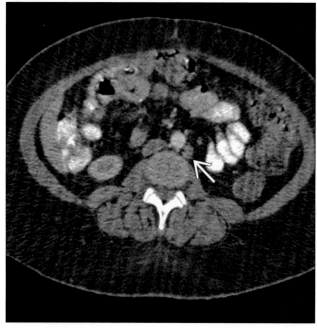 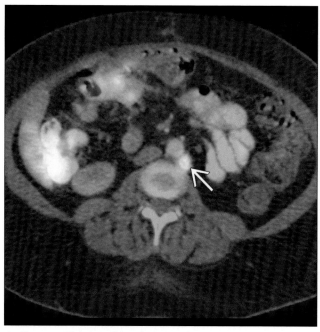

(Left) Axial CECT shows a small para-aortic node ➡ of uncertain clinical significance. (Right) Axial fused PET/CT shows an FDG-avid para-aortic node ➡ that is normal in size but metabolically abnormal. One of the added benefits of PET/CT is the detection of normal-sized but malignant nodes, particularly those in the 6-10 mm range.

PANCREATIC CARCINOMA

PET/CT Findings: Restaging

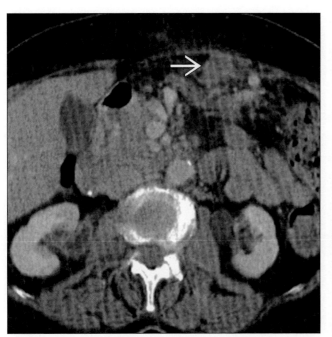 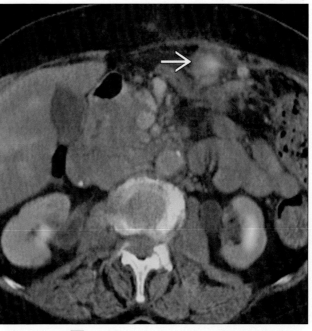

(Left) Axial CECT shows a ring-enhancing, partially necrotic lesion involving the omentum ➡ and worrisome for metastatic disease in this patient with a history of pancreatic adenocarcinoma. (Right) Axial fused PET/CT shows mild to moderate FDG activity within the omental lesion ➡, compatible with metastatic disease. Some well-differentiated adenocarcinomas, including those that are mucinous, may demonstrate less FDG activity than lesions that are poorly differentiated.

PET/CT Findings: Restaging

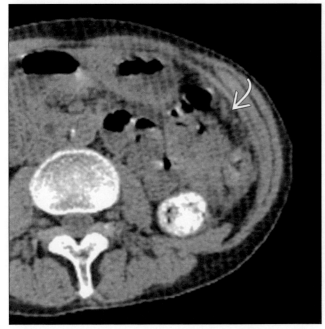 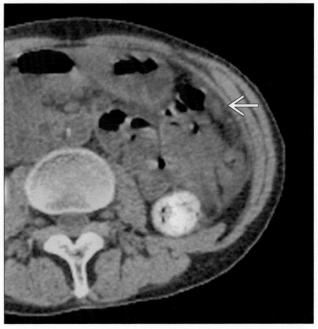

(Left) Axial NECT shows nodularity in the omentum ➡ in a patient with known pancreatic adenocarcinoma. (Right) Axial fused PET/CT of the same patient reveals increased metabolic activity within the omental metastases ➡.

PANCREATIC CARCINOMA

PET/CT Findings: Restaging

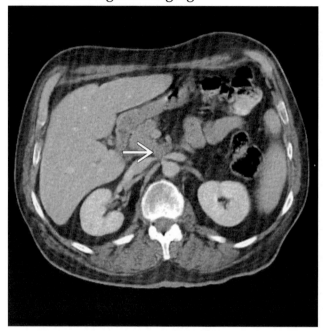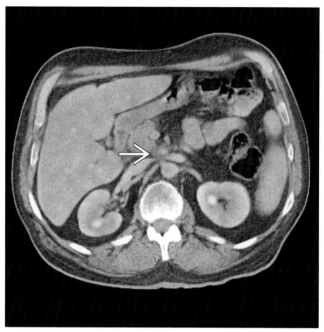

(Left) Axial CECT shows a nodal metastasis ➡ in a patient who is status post distal pancreatectomy for adenocarcinoma. *(Right)* Axial fused PET/CT of the same patient confirms that the lesion is hypermetabolic ➡ and is consistent with metastatic disease.

PET/CT Findings: Restaging

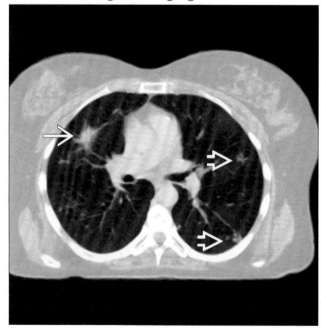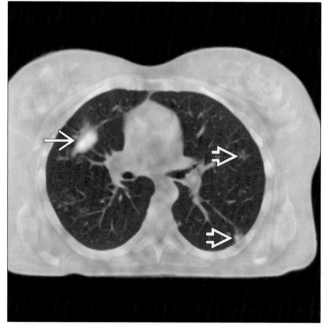

(Left) Axial CECT shows a spiculated nodule in the right upper lobe ➡. This was proven to be metastatic; however, the same appearance could also represent a second primary neoplasm. Smaller clusters of nodules ➡ in the left upper lobe and superior segment of the left lower lobe are related to airway disease. Note the "tree-in-bud" pattern. *(Right)* Axial fused PET/CT shows marked increased FDG uptake in the right upper lobe metastasis ➡ and more moderate activity in the regions of inflammation ➡.

PANCREATIC CARCINOMA

PET/CT Findings: Restaging

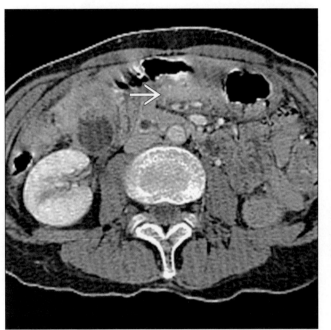 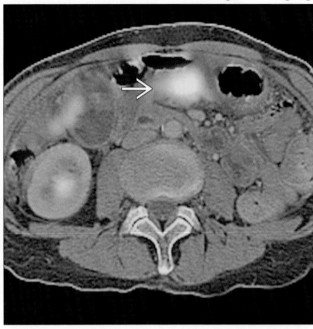

(Left) Axial CECT in this patient who is status post distal pancreatectomy for adenocarcinoma shows thickening of the posterior gastric wall ➡. *(Right)* Axial fused PET/CT confirms the increased metabolic activity within the metastasis ➡.

PET/CT Findings: Restaging

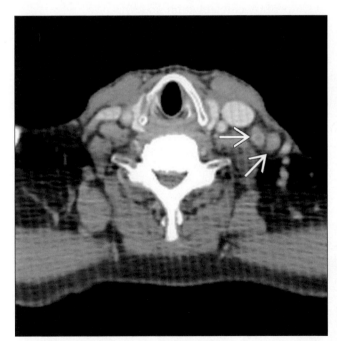 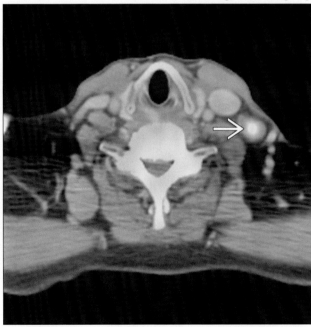

(Left) Axial CECT shows two borderline enlarged left supraclavicular lymph nodes ➡ in a patient with a history of pancreatic adenocarcinoma and metastatic disease. *(Right)* Axial fused PET/CT shows focal intense FDG activity ➡, worrisome for metastasis. Subsequent biopsy showed adenocarcinoma, likely from the pancreas, although this is an atypical location for pancreatic metastases.

CARCINOID

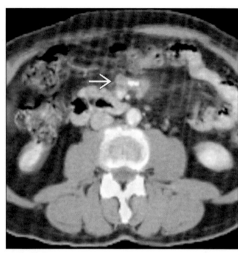

Axial CECT shows a slightly spiculated mass in the small bowel mesentery with areas of calcifications ➡, most compatible with carcinoid.

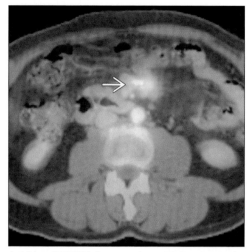

Axial fused PET/CT shows moderate FDG activity in the mesenteric mass ➡, compatible with carcinoid.

TERMINOLOGY

Abbreviations and Synonyms
- Carcinoid, carcinoid syndrome (CS), carcinoid tumor
  - May indicate malignant or benign disease

Definitions
- Neuroendocrine tumors arising from enterochromaffin cells of Kulchitsky

IMAGING FINDINGS

General Features
- Best diagnostic clue
  - Variably calcified soft tissue mass in abdomen with spiculation and desmoplastic reaction
    - Often asymptomatic
  - Tumors of liver or lung in patients with carcinoid syndrome
  - Mass within bronchus with varying degrees of post-obstructive pneumonia
- Location
  - Abdominal carcinoid common, specifically in large intestine and appendix
    - Primary carcinoids of bowel are often not seen with CT
    - Metastases are frequent from midgut tumor but rare from appendiceal primary
  - Thoracic carcinoid most commonly found within bronchial lumen
    - Also seen in lung parenchyma and peribronchiolar lymph nodes
    - Peripheral lung tumor may represent atypical pulmonary carcinoid, half of which show lymph node involvement or distant metastases
- Size
  - May become bulky, up to 25 cm
  - Size generally correlates with malignant behavior
    - Tumors < 1 cm metastasize in 2% of cases
    - Tumors 1-2 cm in 50% of cases
    - Tumors > 2 cm in 85% of cases
  - Volume may not change following treatment despite good clinical response
- Morphology
  - Thoracic carcinoid highly vascular with no characteristic calcification distribution

DDx: FDG-Avid Lesions in the Mesentery/Retroperitoneum

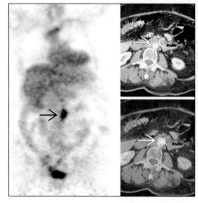

Retroperitoneal Fibrosis (Early)

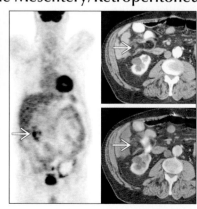

Torsed Omental Infarct (Early)

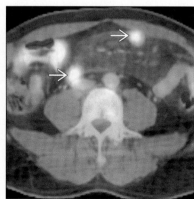

Non-Hodgkin Lymphoma

CARCINOID

Key Facts

Terminology
- Neuroendocrine tumor derived from enterochromaffin cells
- Carcinoid, carcinoid syndrome (CS), carcinoid tumor

Imaging Findings
- Primary bowel lesion with spiculated soft tissue mass in abdomen ± desmoplastic reaction ± calcifications
- Hepatic or lung tumors in patient with CS
- Chest mass: Endobronchial lesion with or without post-obstructive pneumonia
- FDG PET: Sensitivity 75%
  - Generally low FDG uptake among neuroendocrine tumors
- Atypical carcinoid can appear as a small pulmonary nodule with extensive hilar or mediastinal lymph node enlargement

- Carcinoids tend to be vascular and can exhibit considerable enhancement
  - Helpful for differentiating tumor from obstructive atelectasis and adjacent mucous plugs
- Whole-body morphologic imaging and somatostatin receptor scintigraphy best combination

Top Differential Diagnoses
- Lymphoma
- Other Neuroendocrine Tumors
- Mesenteritis
- Liver Metastases

Diagnostic Checklist
- FDG PET or PET/CT may show only mild to moderate FDG activity within lesions

---

- Atypical carcinoid: Small peripheral nodule surrounded by extensive hilar/mediastinal lymphadenopathy
- Abdominal carcinoid typically manifests as homogeneous mesenteric mass with spiculation and variable calcification
  - Primary bowel lesion often not identified
  - Thickened neurovascular bundles may present as stellate or curvilinear fibrosis radiating from lesion and distorting surrounding bowel

Imaging Recommendations
- Best imaging tool
  - Whole-body morphologic imaging and somatostatin receptor scintigraphy
  - SUV on FDG PET generally correlates with aggressiveness of tumor
- Protocol advice
  - Somatostatin receptor imaging (SRI)
    - Administer 6 mCi (222 MBq) In-111 pentetreotide IV
    - Image with 173 keV and 247 keV photopeaks of In-111
    - Administer mild bowel cathartic to decrease colon accumulation in patients not experiencing diarrhea
    - Urinary bladder should be emptied prior to imaging to avoid obscuring pelvic findings

CT Findings
- **General**
  - CT has shown superiority to octreotide scan for characterization of primary tumor and liver metastases
  - Benign and malignant disease cannot reliably be differentiated with CT
    - Half of indeterminate lesions are benign on biopsy
  - Carcinoid tumor highly vascular
    - Distinguishable from obstructive atelectasis and mucous plugs on contrast-enhanced images
- **Chest**

- Small pulmonary nodule with extensive hilar/ mediastinal lymphadenopathy is classic finding for atypical carcinoid
- Central carcinoids more commonly have variable calcification (~ 1/3 of cases)
  - No pathognomonic pattern of calcium distribution known
  - Less commonly seen in peripheral tumors
- **CECT**
  - Typical carcinoid
    - Homogeneous, smooth-bordered lesion
    - Highly vascular tumor with intense contrast enhancement
  - Atypical carcinoid
    - Generally larger tumors
    - May show central necrosis and be associated with hilar lymphadenopathy
- **Abdomen**
  - Submucosal lesions
    - Vascular lesions enhance intensely
    - Mural nodules more clearly visualized with water contrast
    - Well-defined morphology
  - Small bowel carcinoid
    - Masses are soft-tissue attenuation of variable size
    - Radiating stranding and border spiculation common
    - Retractile mesenteritis and treated lymphoma may share appearance, with calcification and desmoplastic reaction
    - Bowel loop ischemia may present as wall thickening and submucosal edema
  - Extension to mesentery
    - Homogeneous or heterogeneous ill-defined mass with spiculations and variable calcification
    - Desmoplastic reaction presents with finger-like extension into adjacent mesentery
    - Variable encasement and narrowing of mesenteric vessels
    - Fibrosis and desmoplastic reaction leads to fixation and obstruction of small bowel
    - Some tumors demonstrate cystic density

CARCINOID

o Metastasis to liver
- Hypoattenuating on NECT
- Strongly enhancing on CECT
- Delayed images may show lesion isodense to liver
- Often multiple

o Colonic extension
- Extraluminal mass common and better delineated on CT
- Colon carcinoid has similar CT findings to adenocarcinoma, including a discrete mass or focal wall thickening

Nuclear Medicine Findings

- Metabolic activity related to carcinoid in abdomen may be evaluated with several radionuclides: In-111 pentetreotide (Octreoscan), I-123/I-131 MIBG, FDG PET
- **FDG uptake generally low among carcinoid (and other neuroendocrine tumors)**
  o May help differentiate pulmonary carcinoid from primary lung cancer
  o High suspicion for carcinoid in patients with clinical suspicion and low-uptake pulmonary nodule
  o SUV shown to correlate with aggressiveness of tumor; uptake correlates with mitotic figure and tumor proliferation
  o Overall PET/CT sensitivity 75%; specificity very low unless classic carcinoid syndrome is present
  o PET most beneficial when detection of extrahepatic disease, bone metastases, and overall tumor load leads to changes in surgical or radiotherapy management
- **Somatostatin receptor imaging**
  o Radiotracer commonly used is In-111 pentetreotide (Octreoscan)
  o Sensitivity 88-96%; specificity 80-95%
  o Tumor to background ratio increases with passage of time
  o Good overall accuracy in ruling out distant metastases
  o Limited in detection of small masses, especially on background of normal uptake
  o Mandatory in cases where patient is considered for radiopeptide treatment
  o Prone to false positives in inflammatory areas of lung and LNs
- **Additional nuclear medicine imaging options**
  o I-131 or I-123 metaiodobenzylguanidine (MIBG)
  - Sensitivity 55-75%; specificity 95%

DIFFERENTIAL DIAGNOSIS

Lymphoma

- Somatostatin receptor imaging may be positive in lymphoma
- Lymphomatous involvement seen in lymph nodes as well as lung, liver, and bowel
- Can be distinguished with biopsy and laboratory testing

Other Neuroendocrine Tumors

- Gastrinoma

- Vasoactive intestinal polypeptide-secreting tumors (VIPomas)
- Insulinoma
- Pheochromocytoma
- Medullary carcinoma of thyroid

Mesenteritis

- Can also present as spiculated mass in mesentery

Liver Metastases

- Majority are hypovascular/hypoattenuating compared to surrounding parenchyma
- Nonenhanced scans useful for detection of calcified metastases
- Accuracy of contrast-enhanced scans depends on timing of acquisition, with optimal portal venous phase of 60 seconds

PATHOLOGY

General Features

- General path comments
  o Generally indolent tumor arising from neuroendocrine cells
  o As with other neuroendocrine tumors, carcinoid is commonly secretory
  - Serotonin is produced and metabolized to 5-hydroxyindoleacetic acid (5-HIAA)
  - Other substances produced include ACTH, histamine, bradykinin, kallikrein
  o Variable mitotic figure and tumor proliferation correlates with aggressiveness and glucose/FDG uptake
  o Subclassified by malignant potential
  - Low: Typical carcinoid
  - Intermediate: Atypical carcinoid
  - High: Small cell and giant cell neuroendocrine tumors
  o Incidence ratio of typical to atypical carcinoid is 9:1
- Genetics
  o Occasionally attributed to MEN-1 syndrome (< 1%)
  o Relative risk of 3.6 when 1st-degree family member is affected
- Etiology: Excessive serotonin production causes carcinoid syndrome
- Epidemiology
  o 1-2 new cases per 100,000 per year
  o Likelihood of symptomatic disease increases with age
  o Typical carcinoid demonstrates metastasis in 10-15% of newly diagnosed cases
  o Small bowel carcinoid found at autopsy in asymptomatic individuals in 97 of 14,852 (0.7%)
  o Overall 3rd most frequent pulmonary tumor is bronchial carcinoid, representing 1-2% of all lung cancer
  - Usually located in hilar/perihilar area
- Associated abnormalities
  o Deposition of fibrous tissue in the cardiac valves may occur in carcinoid syndrome
  - Right heart and endocardium more commonly affected

CARINOID

- Tricuspid stenosis/insufficiency may result in right heart failure
- Left-sided valves may be affected, with loss of trabeculation of ventricle secondary to fibrosis
- Left-heart disease more common with pulmonary carcinoid

Gross Pathologic & Surgical Features
- Firm, ovoid, yellow soft tissue mass in submucosa

Microscopic Features
- Low number of mitoses in typical carcinoid corresponds to low aggressiveness
- Cellular growth pattern may be insular, trabecular, glandular, or diffuse
- Specificity improved with immunohistochemistry and silver stain analysis
- Cells are small with round, uniform nuclei, stippled chromatin, and absence of prominent nucleoli

CLINICAL ISSUES

Presentation
- Most common signs/symptoms
  - Most carcinoids are clinically silent
  - Symptomatic disease may be present several years before tumor is diagnosed
  - Flushing and diarrhea most common (85% and 80% respectively)
  - Pain or intestinal obstruction
  - Most patients presenting with carcinoid syndrome have liver metastases from a bowel primary
  - Palpable mass may be due to massive hepatomegaly
  - Cardiac symptoms present in 35-40%
- Other signs/symptoms
  - Elevations in
    - Urinary 5-HIAA (sens/spec 73%/100%)
    - Serum chromogranin A (sens 80%)
    - Catecholamine metabolites
  - Gastrointestinal bleed

Demographics
- Age
  - Most occur in patients age 50 and older
  - Appendiceal carcinoids in patients 20-40 years (reported as young as 3 years)
- Gender: M:F = 2:1

Natural History & Prognosis
- Survival of 10-15 years is not uncommon
- Tumor aggressiveness correlates with size
- Severe carcinoid syndrome connotes worse prognosis
- GI carcinoid diagnosed without liver or lymph node metastasis has excellent prognosis
- **Survival (5 year)**
  - Typical: > 95%
  - Atypical: 60% s/p resection
  - Untreated severe CS: 20-50%

Treatment
- Options include curative/debulking surgery, radiopeptide therapy, and medical treatment with somatostatin analogues and interferon

- Surgery
  - Smaller tumors may be completely resected
    - If local disease is removed completely, resection usually curative
    - Resection of appendiceal tip tumor often adequate treatment
  - Larger masses are debulked for comfort/palliation
    - Palliation often brief and associated with considerable morbidity
    - May reduce systemic symptoms caused by liver invasion
    - Hepatic transplant has been performed but is still under study
- Angiographic embolization
  - Reduces tumor mass
  - Involves hepatic artery infusion of 5-FU or doxorubicin combined with embolization
  - May reduce tumor burden as much as 50%
  - Adverse effects of embolization are frequent and often severe
- Sandostatin
  - Somatostatin receptor blocker
  - May reduce flushing and other endocrine symptoms
  - Tumor size rarely reduced, but growth rate may slow
  - In-111 pentetreotide-avid tumors most likely to respond

DIAGNOSTIC CHECKLIST

Consider
- Diarrhea is frequent in carcinoid patients, and new constipation should prompt evaluation for bowel obstruction
- Bowel and bladder collection of radiotracer can obscure somatostatin receptor imaging (SRI)

Image Interpretation Pearls
- SRI often demonstrates normal uptake in kidneys, bladder, liver, bowel, and especially spleen
- Thyroid and pituitary normally have low uptake but may show increased uptake in presence of MTC or pituitary adenoma
- FDG PET or PET/CT may show only mild to moderate FDG activity within lesions

SELECTED REFERENCES

1. Gustafsson BI et al: Neuroendocrine tumors of the diffuse neuroendocrine system. Curr Opin Oncol. 20(1):1-12, 2008
2. Jager PL et al: 6-L-18F-fluorodihydroxyphenylalanine PET in neuroendocrine tumors: basic aspects and emerging clinical applications. J Nucl Med. 49(4):573-86, 2008
3. Koopmans KP et al: Improved staging of patients with carcinoid and islet cell tumors with 18F-dihydroxy-phenyl-alanine and 11C-5-hydroxy-tryptophan positron emission tomography. J Clin Oncol. 26(9):1489-95, 2008
4. Suemitsu R et al: Pulmonary typical carcinoid tumor and liver metastasis with hypermetabolism on 18-fluorodeoxyglucose PET: a case report. Ann Thorac Cardiovasc Surg. 14(2):109-11, 2008
5. Yeung YP et al: Primary hepatic carcinoid tumour: a detailed account of imaging findings. Hepatogastroenterology. 55(82-83):663-5, 2008

CARCINOID

Bronchial Carcinoid

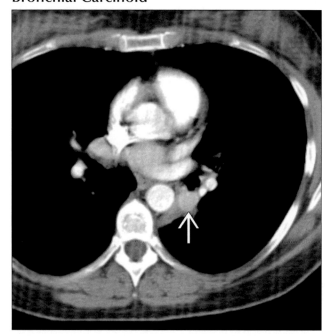 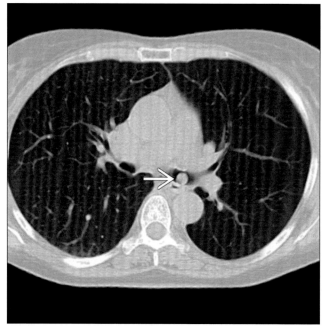

(Left) Axial CECT shows an enhancing nodule/node in the left hilar region ➔. The hypervascularity of the nodule is one of the characteristics of neuroendocrine neoplasms such as carcinoid. *(Right)* Axial NECT shows an endobronchial smooth lesion in the left main bronchus ➔. Carcinoid is among the top diagnostic considerations for lesions within the airway.

Bronchial Carcinoid

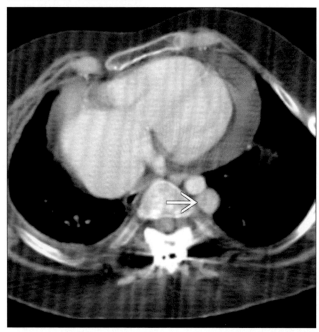 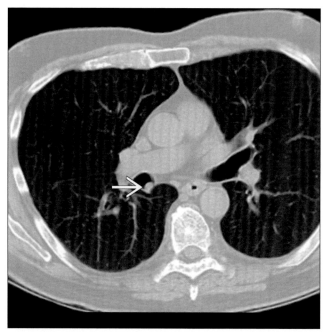

(Left) Axial CECT shows an enhancing nodule adjacent to the aorta ➔, suggestive of carcinoid. It is imperative to exclude a vascular lesion prior to considering any type of tissue sampling. *(Right)* Axial NECT shows a soft tissue nodule in the proximal bronchus intermedius ➔ in this patient who had subsequent bronchoscopic confirmation of carcinoid.

CARCINOID

Typical Carcinoid

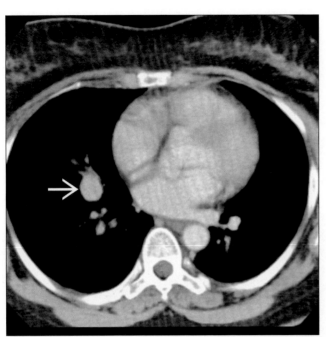

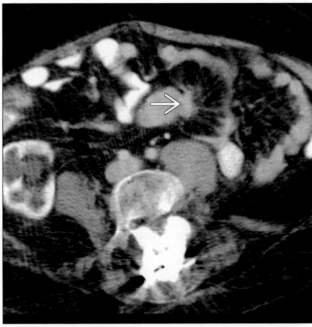

(Left) Axial CECT shows an enhancing nodule ⇒ in another patient with known carcinoid. Enhancement comparable to blood pool should be viewed with caution to ensure that the "lesion" is not an aneurysm or pseudoaneurysm. (Right) Axial CECT shows a soft tissue nodule in the mesentery ⇒ with surrounding desmoplastic response. The differential diagnostic considerations are few and include both carcinoid and fibrosing mesenteritis.

Mesenteric Carcinoid

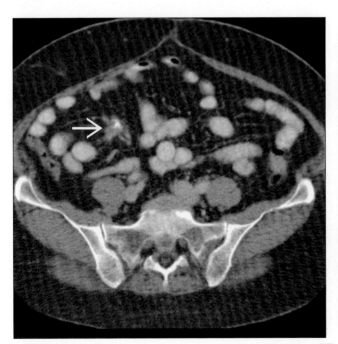

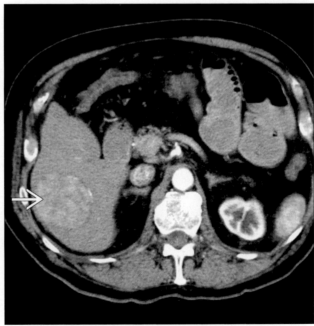

(Left) Axial CECT shows a partially calcified nodule in the mesentery ⇒, which suggests carcinoid. (Right) Axial CECT shows a heterogeneously enhancing liver lesion that is hypervascular ⇒ on the arterial phase of imaging in this patient with carcinoid.

CARCINOID

Mesenteric Carcinoid

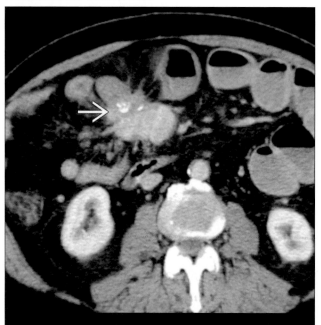 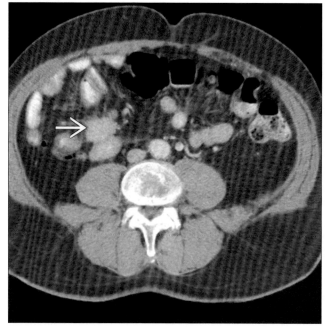

(Left) Axial CECT shows a partially calcified mesenteric mass ➡ characteristic of carcinoid. Note the soft tissue in the adjacent small bowel loop, which corresponds to the site of the primary lesion. *(Right)* Axial CECT shows an enhancing soft tissue mesenteric lesion that has smooth borders and does not have a surrounding desmoplastic response ➡. Given the lack of desmoplastic response, desmoid tumor would also be high in the differential diagnosis list.

Metastatic Abmoninal Carcinoid

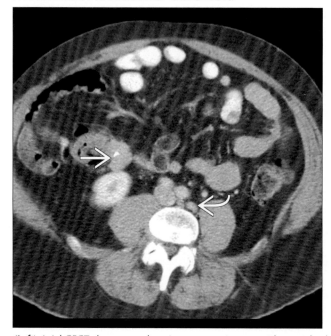 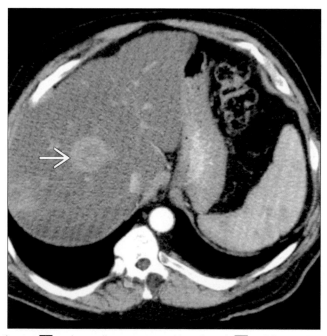

(Left) Axial CECT shows an enhancing mesenteric mass with central calcification ➡ and a small retroperitoneal lymph node ➡. *(Right)* Axial CECT shows a hypervascular lesion with continuous peripheral enhancement on arterial phase imaging ➡.

CARCINOID

PET/CT: Abdominal Carcinoid

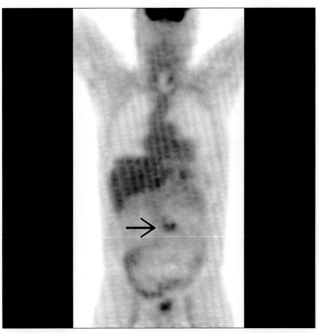
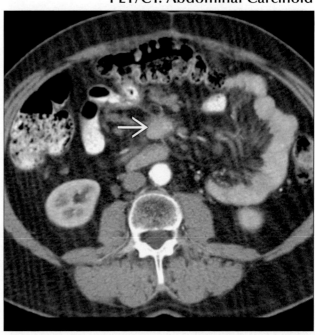

(Left) Coronal PET shows mild to moderate focal FDG activity in the mid-abdomen ➔ in this patient with carcinoid. *(Right)* Axial CECT shows a mesenteric mass with a mild desmoplastic response ➔.

PET/CT: Bronchial Carcinoid

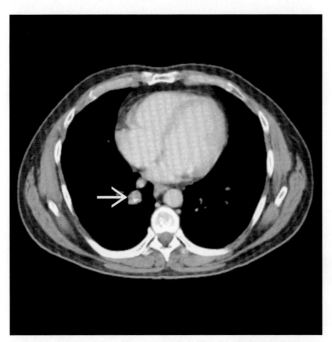
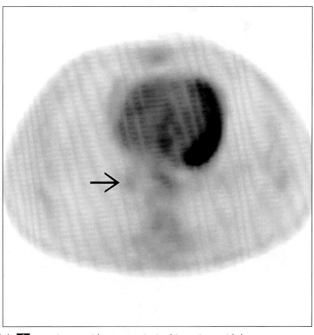

(Left) Axial CECT shows a partially calcified, partially enhancing lung nodule ➔, consistent with metastasis, in this patient with known carcinoid. *(Right)* Axial PET shows no FDG activity of the pulmonary nodule ➔. Carcinoid and neuroendocrine tumors may not be very FDG avid.

GIST

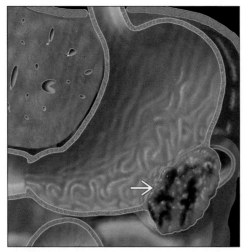

Graphic shows a heterogeneous exophytic mass arising from the greater curvature of the stomach ➔, compatible with a gastrointestinal stromal tumor.

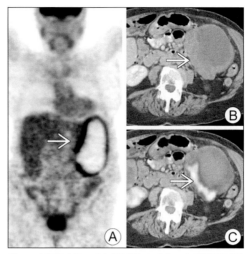

Coronal PET (A), axial CT (B) and fused PET/CT (C) show a large heterogeneous mass arising from the greater curvature of stomach with areas of central necrosis ➔, compatible with a GIST.

TERMINOLOGY

Abbreviations and Synonyms
- Gastrointestinal stromal tumor (GIST)

Definitions
- Distinct group of mesenchymal tumors derived from the muscularis propria of the esophageal/gastric/intestinal wall
- Constitute 80% of mesenchymal tumors of the gastrointestinal tract
- Identified immunohistochemically by c-KIT positivity

IMAGING FINDINGS

General Features
- Best diagnostic clue
  - Spherical mass with varying degrees of central necrosis arising from muscularis propria of GI wall and projecting intraluminally or exophytically
  - Intense FDG uptake is typical, although uptake may be variable
- Location
  - Primary tumor location by frequency
    - Stomach (60-70%)
    - Small intestine (20-25%)
    - Colon/rectum (5%)
    - Esophagus (< 5%)
  - Metastases
    - Liver and peritoneum most common
    - Less common: Lymph nodes, lungs, and pleurae
  - Second primary tumors not uncommon in GIST patients
- Size
  - From several millimeters to over 30 cm
  - Size does not always correlate with malignancy
  - Larger tumors always outgrow blood supply and are identified by regions of necrosis and hemorrhage
  - Tumors with positive response to imatinib mesylate (Gleevec) may enlarge or remain same size during therapy
- Morphology
  - Spherical with smooth margins
  - Larger tumors demonstrate necrosis and hemorrhage
  - Usually exophytic and adjacent to organ periphery
    - Sometimes intraluminal &/or pedunculated

DDx: FDG Uptake in Stomach

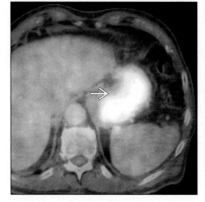

Gastritis

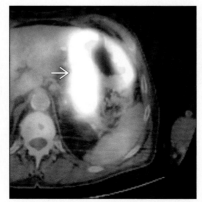

Gastric Lymphoma

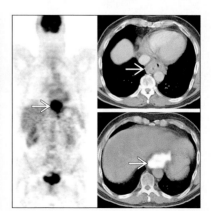

Hiatal Hernia

GIST

Key Facts

Terminology
- Most common mesenchymal tumors of gastrointestinal (GI) tract
- Positivity of c-KIT on immunohistochemistry is sine qua non for diagnosis of GIST

Imaging Findings
- FDG PET: Primary staging
  - Look carefully at liver for metastatic deposits that could be missed on CT scan
- Response to treatment
  - FDG PET can detect early responders to systemic therapy
  - Treated tumors may show decreased HU on CT
  - Prompt decrease in FDG uptake in tumor, before anatomic changes

- Decreased FDG avidity often detected within one week
- NECT: Calcifications in 25% of cases
- Combination of functional and anatomic imaging most accurate

Top Differential Diagnoses
- Gastric Carcinoma
- Lymphoma
- Metastases
- Leiomyosarcoma, Other Gastric Wall Tumors

Diagnostic Checklist
- Bulky abdominal soft tissue mass without lymphadenopathy = common GIST presentation
- Central necrosis/hemorrhage common
- Usually highly FDG avid tumor

- Enhancing FDG-avid nodule within tumor mass is a sensitive sign of recurrence and progression

Imaging Recommendations
- Best imaging tool
  - FDG PET highly sensitive for primary and metastatic disease
  - CT is ideal for delineating tumor extent and identifying metastatic disease
  - MR offers improved tissue contrast for identification of lesions within GI tract
  - US useful for guiding biopsy for tissue diagnosis
    - Concern for seeding needle tract with tumor
- Protocol advice
  - Oral contrast media recommended for improved bowel delineation
  - Pre-treatment FDG PET imaging may be useful for determining response to therapy (controversial)
- Additional nuclear medicine imaging options
  - Bone scan rarely performed, in part due to rarity of bone metastases

CT Findings
- CT has overall sensitivity of 87% for GIST
- **Early GIST**
  - Smaller lesions
  - Homogeneous submucosal/intramural mass with sharply-defined, smooth borders
  - Uniform or rim-like contrast enhancement
  - Calcification may appear as dense foci in 25% of cases
- **Advanced GIST**
  - Large, complex intestinal mass
  - Liver lesions
    - Hypervascular
    - Multilocular cystic structures with fluid-fluid levels
  - Absence of significant lymphadenopathy
  - Necrosis alters morphology
    - Heterogeneous internal architecture with central areas of fluid, air, or oral contrast attenuation

- Enhancement of borders reveals variable thickness and irregularity
  - Local extension and mucosal ulceration
- **Post-treatment**
  - Successful treatment may not be evident as macroscopic structural change for weeks to months
  - Enhancement may be reduced in treated lesions
    - Responders showed decrease in target lesion enhancement (HU) of more than 25% within target lesions
    - Nonresponders showed increased or unchanged enhancement
    - Interpretation of HU among studies depends on consistent quantity of administered IV contrast
  - Single CECT following treatment not useful for providing prognostic information
  - Previous surgical intervention alters anatomy and further reduces ability of CT to diagnose recurrence

Nuclear Medicine Findings
- FDG PET
  - **General**
    - FDG uptake may correlate with quantity of malignant cells or aggressiveness of solid tumors
    - Possible to find lesions with very high, moderate, or no uptake at all in the same patient, possibly due to origination from different cell clones
    - Patients with clinically active disease but no FDG-avid lesions should nevertheless be candidates for imatinib therapy
  - **Initial diagnosis**
    - Small primary tumors may appear to have lower FDG uptake and can be obscured by the physiologic activity in adjacent bowel or stomach
    - Larger lesions often demonstrate central necrosis with corresponding decrease in FDG uptake
  - **Staging**
    - Malignant lesions generally have SUV greater than that of normal tissue
    - Liver deposits are often missed on CT but may be detected on PET as FDG-avid foci

GIST

- PET imaging of pulmonary and upper abdominal lesions often obscured by motion artifact and partial-volume averaging
- CT portion of PET/CT requires careful scrutiny in these anatomic regions
- More lesions are identified with CECT alone than with FDG PET alone, but FDG-avid lesions appear to be more clinically relevant
- IV contrast is beneficial for CT portion of exam and has not been shown to adversely affect image interpretation
  - **Response to therapy**
    - FDG PET can detect early responders to systemic therapy
    - Metabolic response
    - Occurs much earlier than morphologic regression in treated lesions
    - May be a useful prognostic indicator of progression-free survival
    - Decreased FDG avidity often detected within one week
    - Single post-treatment scan provides accurate prognostic information on overall survival and time to progression
    - Pre-treatment scan is unnecessary
    - Alternative therapy can be instituted for patients who do not show response within days or weeks after initiation of treatment

DIFFERENTIAL DIAGNOSIS

Gastric Carcinoma
- May be indistinguishable from a GIST
- Large centrally necrotic exophytic lesion favors GIST

Lymphoma
- Can present as large soft tissue mass adjacent to GI wall
- GIST rarely presents with lymphadenopathy, which is hallmark of lymphoma

Metastases
- Presence of lymphadenopathy lowers suspicion for GIST
- Melanoma may mimic GIST, presenting as a cavitary small bowel lesion

Leiomyosarcoma, Other Gastric Wall Tumors
- Represent 20% of GI mesenchymal tumors
- Lack c-KIT on immunohistochemistry
- May arise in same region and have same FDG avidity as GIST

PATHOLOGY

General Features
- General path comments
  - Sine qua non of GIST is identification of mutant c-KIT receptor on immunohistochemistry (90% of cases)
  - Prior to immunohistochemistry, GIST was separated into the following subcategories
    - Leiomyomas, leiomyoblastomas, leiomyosarcomas, neurofibromas, and schwannomas
  - Believed to arise from stem cells that differentiate toward interstitial cells of Cajal
  - GIST of any size or morphology may be malignant and should be treated
- Genetics
  - May be inherited due to rare autosomal dominant disorder resulting in KIT germline mutation
  - Association with neurofibromatosis type 1 is due to a different cellular mechanism
    - Multiple small intestinal GISTs
  - Sporadic mutation of c-KIT (CD117) or PDGFR
    - Tyrosine kinase growth factor receptor
    - Mutation releases cell from growth inhibition
- Etiology: No risk factor has been identified
- Epidemiology: 10-20 per million new cases/year in United States

Gross Pathologic & Surgical Features
- Classic features include submucosal tumor mass with central umbilication and ulceration
- Mucosal ulceration &/or central necrosis in large tumors

Microscopic Features
- Cell types by frequency
  - Spindle cell (70%)
  - Epithelioid (20%)
  - Mixed epithelioid and spindle cell (10%)
- Immunohistochemical
  - 90-95% CD117+ (c-KIT+)

CLINICAL ISSUES

Presentation
- Most common signs/symptoms
  - 40-65% of patients present with hematemesis or melena due to upper GI bleed related to mucosal ulceration
  - Physical examination usually nonspecific
  - Symptoms depend on tumor size and location
- Other signs/symptoms
  - Abdominal pain
  - Early satiety, anorexia
  - Nausea, vomiting

Demographics
- Age
  - Any age
  - Most common past 6th decade
- Gender: No clear gender predominance

Natural History & Prognosis
- Primary predictors for prognosis include
  - Resectability of tumor
  - Tumor size
  - Tumor grade
- Long-term survival following resection strongly correlates with tumor size and grade

- Large disparity in survival between local and metastatic disease at presentation (5 years vs. 10 months)
- 5 year survival rate after complete resection with negative margins roughly 60%
- Survival improved with introduction of imatinib mesylate (Gleevec)
- Most common sites of recurrence after resection are liver and peritoneum
  - Extra-abdominal sites (e.g., lungs) are infrequent, in contrast to other soft tissue sarcomas

Treatment

- For primary localized disease, surgical resection may be curative
  - High recurrence with subsequent repeat resection common
- Standard chemotherapy and radiotherapy have poor success rates
- Imatinib mesylate (Gleevec)
  - First drug that was effective against GIST progression
  - Tyrosine kinase inhibitor
  - Standard care after surgical resection
  - Primary therapy in non-resectable disease
  - 70% of patients with metastatic disease live more than 2 years with oral therapy
  - Recommended as lifelong therapy
  - Sunitinib malate is alternative in patients resistant to imatinib

DIAGNOSTIC CHECKLIST

Consider

- Absence of lymphadenopathy in a bulky abdominal soft tissue mass should prompt suspicion of GIST

Image Interpretation Pearls

- Look for small nodular areas of viable tumor in areas of necrosis on F-18 FDG PET
- Liquefaction of hepatic metastases following therapy may pose interpretation problems
  - Previously inapparent isodense lesions may be unmasked and impress the observer as newly developed lesions

SELECTED REFERENCES

1. Choi H: Response evaluation of gastrointestinal stromal tumors. Oncologist. 13 Suppl 2:4-7, 2008
2. Cichoz-Lach H et al: Gastrointestinal stromal tumors: epidemiology, clinical picture, diagnosis, prognosis and treatment. Pol Arch Med Wewn. 118(4):216-21, 2008
3. Davies AR et al: Port site metastasis following diagnostic laparoscopy for a malignant Gastro-intestinal stromal tumour. World J Surg Oncol. 6:55, 2008
4. Shinto A et al: Early response assessment in gastrointestinal stromal tumors with FDG PET scan 24 hours after a single dose of imatinib. Clin Nucl Med. 33(7):486-7, 2008
5. Van den Abbeele AD: The lessons of GIST--PET and PET/CT: a new paradigm for imaging. Oncologist. 13 Suppl 2:8-13, 2008
6. Benjamin RS et al: We should desist using RECIST, at least in GIST. J Clin Oncol. 25(13):1760-4, 2007
7. Blum MG et al: Surgical considerations for the management and resection of esophageal gastrointestinal stromal tumors. Ann Thorac Surg. 84(5):1717-23, 2007
8. Choi H et al: Correlation of computed tomography and positron emission tomography in patients with metastatic gastrointestinal stromal tumor treated at a single institution with imatinib mesylate: proposal of new computed tomography response criteria. J Clin Oncol. 25(13):1753-9, 2007
9. Desai J et al: Clonal evolution of resistance to imatinib in patients with metastatic gastrointestinal stromal tumors. Clin Cancer Res. 13(18 Pt 1):5398-405, 2007
10. Fang FC et al: Surgical treatment of gastrointestinal stromal tumor in the esophagus: report of three cases. Z Gastroenterol. 45(12):1252-6, 2007
11. Holdsworth CH et al: CT and PET: early prognostic indicators of response to imatinib mesylate in patients with gastrointestinal stromal tumor. AJR Am J Roentgenol. 189(6):W324-30, 2007
12. Kurzrock R: Studies in target-based treatment. Mol Cancer Ther. 6(5):1477, 2007
13. Ludvigsen L et al: Successful resection of an advanced duodenal gastrointestinal stromal tumor after down-staging with imatinib: report of a case. Surg Today. 37(12):1105-9, 2007
14. Mandalà M et al: Neoadjuvant imatinib in a locally advanced gastrointestinal stromal tumour (GIST) of the rectum: a rare case of two GISTs within a family without a familial GIST syndrome. Eur J Gastroenterol Hepatol. 19(8):711-3, 2007
15. Sevinc A et al: The diagnosis of C-kit negative GIST by PDGFRA staining: clinical, pathological, and nuclear medicine perspective. Onkologie. 30(12):645-8, 2007
16. Yamada M et al: Gastric GIST malignancy evaluated by 18FDG-PET as compared with EUS-FNA and endoscopic biopsy. Scand J Gastroenterol. 42(5):633-41, 2007
17. Bümming P et al: Use of 2-tracer PET to diagnose gastrointestinal stromal tumour and pheochromocytoma in patients with Carney triad and neurofibromatosis type 1. Scand J Gastroenterol. 41(5):626-30, 2006
18. De Chiara A et al: Primary gastrointestinal stromal tumor of the liver with lung metastases successfully treated with STI-571 (imatinib mesylate). Front Biosci. 11:498-501, 2006
19. Goh BK et al: Pathologic, radiologic and PET scan response of gastrointestinal stromal tumors after neoadjuvant treatment with imatinib mesylate. Eur J Surg Oncol. 32(9):961-3, 2006
20. Tarn C et al: Therapeutic effect of imatinib in gastrointestinal stromal tumors: AKT signaling dependent and independent mechanisms. Cancer Res. 66(10):5477-86, 2006
21. Trent JC et al: Early effects of imatinib mesylate on the expression of insulin-like growth factor binding protein-3 and positron emission tomography in patients with gastrointestinal stromal tumor. Cancer. 107(8):1898-908, 2006
22. Barnes G et al: A review of the surgical management of metastatic gastrointestinal stromal tumours (GISTs) on imatinib mesylate (Glivec). Int J Surg. 3(3):206-12, 2005
23. Chang WC et al: Gastrointestinal stromal tumor (GIST) of the esophagus detected by positron emission tomography/ computed tomography. Dig Dis Sci. 50(7):1315-8, 2005
24. Goerres GW et al: The value of PET, CT and in-line PET/ CT in patients with gastrointestinal stromal tumours: long-term outcome of treatment with imatinib mesylate. Eur J Nucl Med Mol Imaging. 32(2):153-62, 2005

GIST

CT Findings: Primary

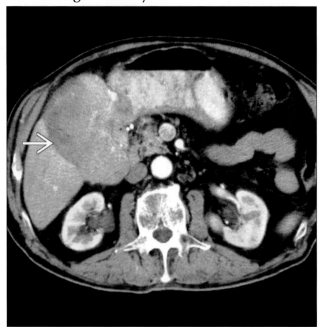 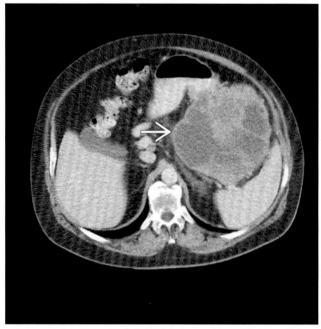

(Left) Axial CECT shows a large heterogeneously enhancing mass that arises from the gastric antrum ➡, suggestive of a GIST. *(Right)* Axial CECT shows a large heterogeneous mass that arises from the gastric fundus and that is largely centered in the region of the gastrosplenic ligament ➡. The large areas of central necrosis and large septations are suggestive of a GIST.

CT Findings: Primary

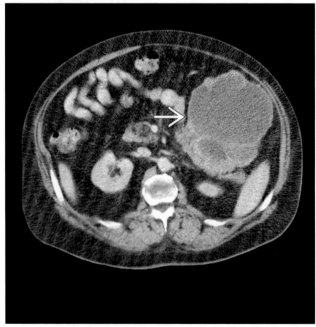 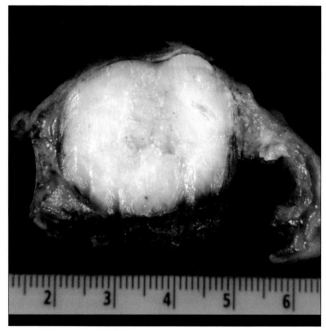

(Left) Axial CECT shows the same lesion more inferiorly ➡ with a larger area of central low attenuation (necrosis). *(Right)* Gross pathology specimen shows a 4 cm, whitish resected GIST.

GIST

CT Findings: Primary

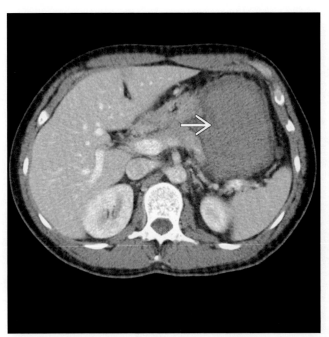 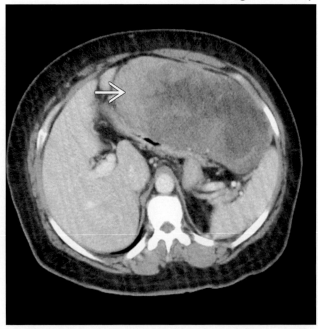

(Left) Axial CECT shows a centrally necrotic mass ➜ arising from the gastric wall in a patient with recently diagnosed GIST. *(Right)* Axial CECT shows a large, well-circumscribed, heterogeneously enhancing mass ➜ arising from the greater curvature of the stomach, compatible with a GIST.

CT Findings: Primary

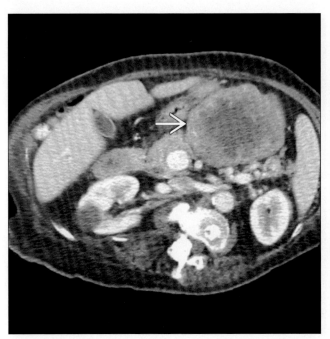 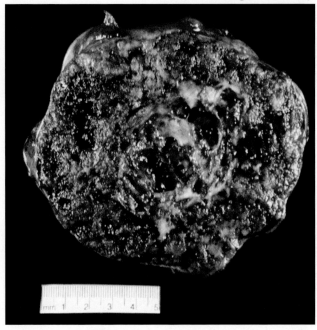

(Left) Axial CECT shows a large necrotic mass arising from the inferior margin of the stomach ➜, subsequently confirmed to be a GIST. *(Right)* Gross pathology shows a reddish-brown, approximately 10 cm tumor with areas of blood products and necrosis, representing the pathologic specimen from the same patient as the previous image.

GIST

CT Findings: Primary

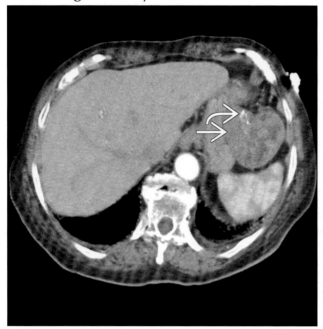
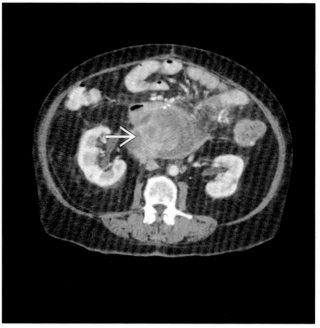

(Left) Axial CECT shows a heterogeneously enhancing mass ➡ arising from the lateral gastric fundus, subsequently resected and shown to be a GIST. Also note a few calcifications ➡ within the tumor. *(Right)* Axial CECT shows a necrotic mass ➡ in the region of the duodenal sweep and near the ligament of Treitz, compatible with a duodenal GIST.

CT Findings: Mestastases

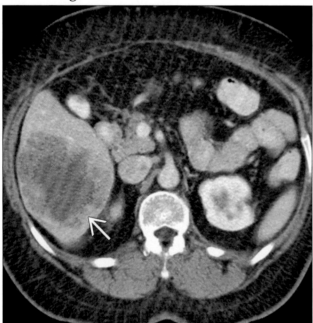
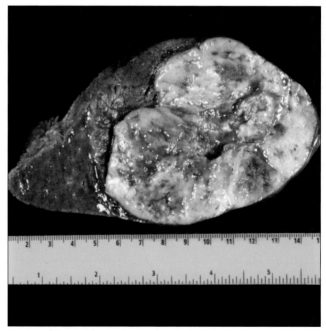

(Left) Axial CECT shows large necrotic hepatic GIST metastasis ➡. *(Right)* Gross pathology shows the hepatic lesion following surgical resection from the same patient as the previous image.

GIST

CT Findings: Mestastases

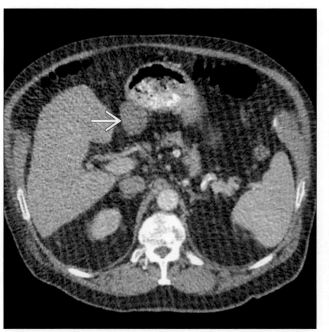 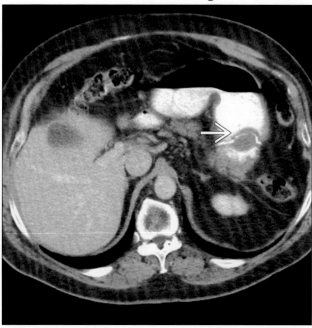

(Left) Axial CECT shows a more solid appearing smaller GIST than the previous examples, arising from the gastric antrum ➡. *(Right)* Axial CECT shows a soft tissue lesion ➡ along a suture resection margin, compatible with recurrent GIST.

PET/CT Findings: Primary and Response to Therapy

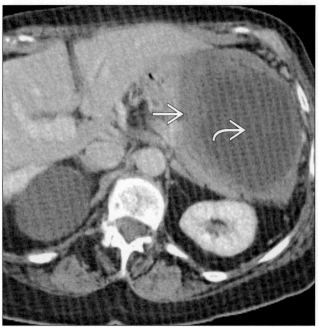 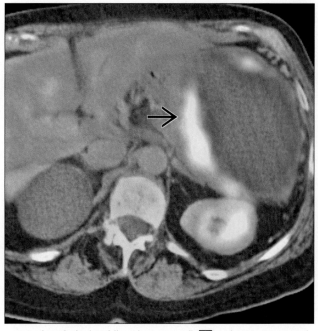

(Left) Axial CECT shows a large mass arising from the lateral portion of the stomach with thick mildly enhancing walls ➡ and extensive central necrosis ➡, compatible with a GIST. *(Right)* Axial fused PET/CT shows a large necrotic tumor in the upper abdomen with nodular ring-like FDG uptake ➡, compatible with a viable tumor, in patient with GIST before chemotherapy.

3

GIST

PET/CT Findings: Primary and Response to Therapy

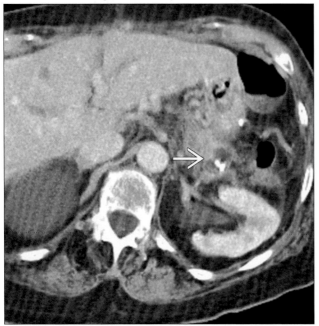 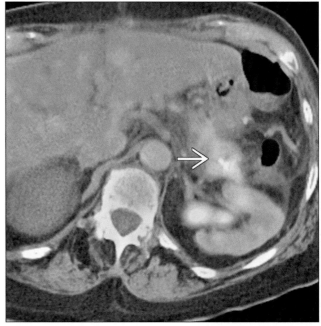

(Left) Axial CECT following 3 cycles of chemotherapy demonstrates marked interval reduction in size of the large necrotic tumor ➡ shown in the previous image. *(Right)* Axial fused PET/CT shows mildly persistent FDG activity corresponding to the shrunken tumor ➡, likely indicating a positive therapeutic response.

PET/CT Findings: Primary and Response to Therapy

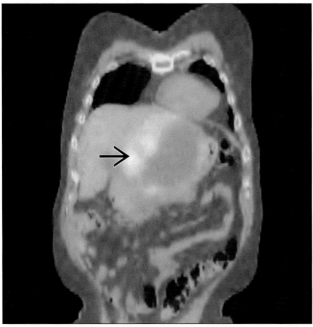 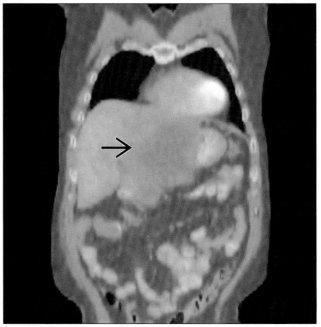

(Left) Coronal fused PET/CT shows a large necrotic tumor in the upper abdomen ➡ with nodular FDG uptake, compatible with a viable tumor in a patient with GIST. *(Right)* Coronal fused PET/CT in the same patient after one month of chemotherapy shows that areas of peripheral FDG uptake ➡ have resolved, consistent with a positive response to therapy. Overall tumor size was not significantly changed.

GIST

PET/CT Findings: Restaging

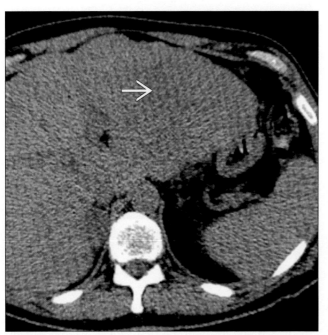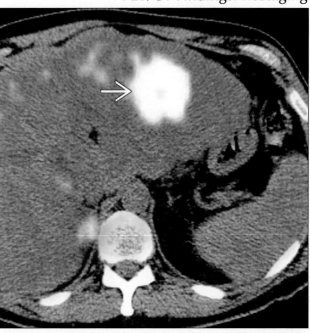

(Left) Axial NECT shows subtle area of slightly decreased attenuation ➡ in the left hepatic lobe. However, this noncontrast evaluation of the liver is suboptimal. *(Right)* Axial fused PET/CT shows focal intense metabolic activity ➡ corresponding to the questionable area of low attenuation in the left hepatic lobe, compatible with metastatic GIST.

PET/CT Findings: Restaging

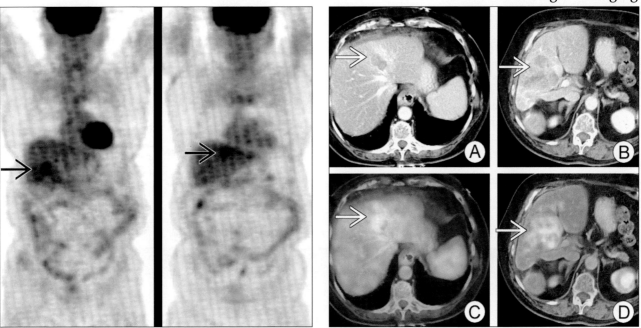

(Left) Coronal PET shows two areas of moderately increased FDG activity in the liver ➡ in this patient with a history of GIST. *(Right)* Axial CT (A, B) and fused PET/CT (C, D) demonstrate two large heterogeneously enhancing hepatic masses ➡ with moderately increased FDG activity, compatible with metastatic disease in this patient with known GIST.

ANAL CARCINOMA

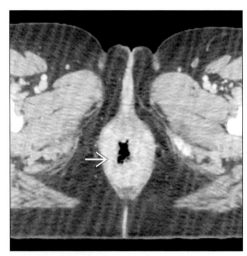
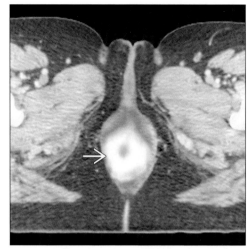

Axial CECT shows massive diffuse thickening of the anal mucosa ➡ in this patient with recently diagnosed squamous cell carcinoma of the anus.

Axial fused PET/CT shows correlative circumferential intense FDG activity corresponding to the anal mucosal thickening ➡.

TERMINOLOGY

Abbreviations and Synonyms
- Squamous cell carcinoma (SCCA) of the anus
- Anal carcinoma
- Anal cancer

Definitions
- Carcinoma arising from tissue of the anal canal or anal margin
  - Subclassified as transitional and cloacogenic

IMAGING FINDINGS

General Features
- Best diagnostic clue
  - Usually diagnosed by physical exam
  - Best imaging features include focal intense FDG activity on a PET/CT scan with a correlative CT abnormality ± inguinal/iliac nodes
- Location
  - Most lesions arise in anal canal

- Anatomic area extends from anorectal ring to zone approximately halfway between pectinate (dentate) line and the anal verge
  - Carcinomas arising proximal to pectinate line (transitional zone between glandular mucosa of rectum and squamous epithelium of distal anus)
    - Basaloid, cuboidal, or cloacogenic tumors
    - About 1/3 of anal cancers have this histology
  - Malignancies distal to pectinate line are of squamous histology
    - Account for 55% of all anal cancers
    - Ulcerate more frequently
  - Dentate line and extending approximately 1 cm proximally
    - Transitional zone of epithelium that connects squamous cell epithelium of anoderm with columnar epithelium of rectum
    - Transitional zone includes columnar, cuboidal, transitional, and squamous epithelial cells
    - Represents the source for a variety of malignancies that arise in the anal canal
  - WHO divides anal canal into 2 regions for grading malignancies

DDx: Focal FDG Activity in Anal/Perianal Area

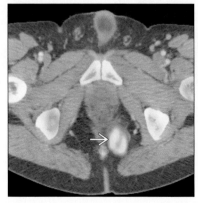
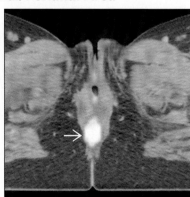
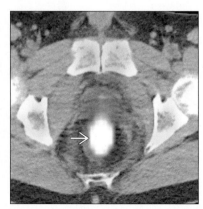

Metastasis

Physiologic Anorectal Activity

Rectal Carcinoma

ANAL CARCINOMA

Key Facts

Terminology
- Anal cancer, squamous cell carcinoma (SCCA) of the anus

Imaging Findings
- Most lesions arise in anal canal
- Consider PET/CT for staging
- MR and endoluminal US commonly used to assist in determining depth of penetration and local spread
- Post-treatment PET/CT results are more predictive of survival outcome than pre-treatment factors such as T-stage and nodal status
- Patient with partial metabolic response, i.e., persistent FDG uptake in irradiated region, have 2 year progression-free survival rate of 22%

- Best imaging features include focal intense FDG activity on a PET/CT scan with a correlative CT abnormality ± inguinal/iliac nodes
- Focal intense FDG activity is usually identified within the primary lesion if large enough (> 6 mm)
- Regional lymph nodes including inguinal, perirectal, and iliac nodes may be involved

Top Differential Diagnoses
- Physiologic FDG Activity at the Anorectal Junction
- Metastatic Disease
- Distal Colonic Adenocarcinoma
- Rectovaginal Fistula
- Inflammation of the Anus

Diagnostic Checklist
- FNA of inguinal adenopathy helpful to establish histologic proof of metastasis

---

- Anal canal portion: Proximal to dentate line and including transitional zone
- Anal margin: Anoderm distal to dentate line
- Anal canal malignancies metastasize to
  - Mesenteric lymph nodes and portal circulation
  - Regional inguinal nodes and via systemic circulation
- Nodal dissemination pathways commonly target perirectal, iliac, and inguinal basins
- Distant spread frequently involves liver and lung
  - Metastases to spine and musculoskeletal system are rare
- Size: Variable, ranging from subcentimeter to several centimeters

Imaging Recommendations
- Best imaging tool
  - MR and endoluminal US are commonly used to assist in determining depth of penetration and local spread
  - Consider PET/CT for regional and distant staging
- Protocol advice
  - Immediate voiding prior to PET is recommended to minimize FDG activity in the bladder
  - Scan from bottom to top to minimize FDG accumulation in the bladder during the exam

Nuclear Medicine Findings
- PET
  - Focal intense FDG activity is usually identified within primary lesions > 6 mm
  - Regional lymph nodes including inguinal, perirectal, and iliac nodes may be involved
    - Usually FDG avid unless small
- FDG PET for prognosis
  - Complete metabolic response was associated with significantly improved progression-free and cause-specific survival compared with partial response
    - Patients with complete metabolic response had 2 year progression-free rate of 95%

- Patients with partial metabolic response, i.e., persistent FDG uptake in irradiated region, have 2 year progression-free survival rate of 22%, regardless of presenting T-stage
- Post-treatment PET/CT results were more predictive of survival outcome than pre-treatment factors such as T-stage and nodal status

DIFFERENTIAL DIAGNOSIS

Physiologic FDG Activity at the Anorectal Junction
- Very common and the most likely alternative diagnosis
- No correlative CT abnormality

Metastatic Disease
- Rare
- Occasionally seen with melanoma or local metastases from cervical, ovarian, or other pelvic malignancies

Distal Colonic Adenocarcinoma
- May involve the anus

Rectovaginal Fistula
- Associated with pelvic irradiation

Inflammation of the Anus
- Indistinguishable from small malignancy or physiologic activity on PET and PET/CT

PATHOLOGY

General Features
- General path comments
  - Squamous cancers make up majority of anal malignancies
  - Anal margin neoplasms include Bowen disease, squamous cell carcinoma, basal cell carcinoma, and Paget disease

ANAL CARCINOMA

- Lower grade malignant potential and slow to metastasize
  - o Anal canal neoplasms include primarily adenocarcinoma of glands and ducts that tend to metastasize early and have poor prognoses
- Etiology
  - o HPV detected in 80% of cases, suggesting the virus as a causal factor
  - o Combination of HIV and HPV markedly increases risk
  - o HPV infection may lead to anal warts, which progress to anal intraepithelial neoplasia and onto squamous cell carcinoma
- Epidemiology
  - o Accounts for 1-2% of cancers of the anus and large intestine
  - o Increased incidence among those practicing receptive anal intercourse and those with history of other STDs
  - o Increased in individuals with HIV
  - o Over the last 30 years, annual incidence of anal carcinoma has increased 160% in men and 78% in women

CLINICAL ISSUES

Presentation
- Most common signs/symptoms
  - o Bleeding, pain, and local tumor are the most common symptoms
    - ▪ Lesions are often confused with hemorrhoids and other common anal disorders
  - o At diagnosis, patients may experience
    - ▪ Bleeding, pain, sensation of perianal mass, and pruritus
  - o Early anal canal malignancies
    - ▪ Present with pruritus, pain, bleeding admixed with stool, sensation and presence of lump in anal canal
  - o Symptoms of more advanced disease
    - ▪ Anorexia, weight loss, diarrhea, constipation, and narrowing caliber of stool
  - o 30-50% of patients present with advanced stage malignancy at presentation with palpable inguinal adenopathy
- Other signs/symptoms
  - o May produce partial rectal prolapse
  - o Hemorrhoidal dilation and prolapse may also occur
  - o More advanced malignancies may present as perirectal abscesses or fistulas

Natural History & Prognosis
- Tumors tend to become annular, invade sphincter, and spread upward via lymphatics into perirectal mesenteric lymph nodes
- 5 year survival following radical surgery
  - o 60-70% for localized tumor
  - o 25% for metastatic stage IV disease
- Prognosis for patients with basaloid and squamous cell carcinoma of anus are identical when corrected for tumor size and nodal spread

- Squamous cell carcinoma of anal canal has poorer prognosis than anal margin counterpart
- Tumor size and nodal metastasis are the key prognostic factors for the clinical outcome of anal SCCA

Treatment
- Depends heavily on stage
- Small (< 3 cm) and superficial lesions of perianal skin may be treated with wide local excision
- Squamous cell cancer of anal canal and large perianal tumors invading sphincter and rectum
  - o Treated with combined-modality therapy including external beam radiation and chemotherapy
  - o Local control achieved in 80% of patients with initial lesions < 3 cm
  - o Tumor recurrence in fewer than 10% of patients, so up to 70% of patients with anal cancers can be cured with non-operative treatment
- Radical surgery includes abdominal-perineal resection with lymph node sampling and permanent colostomy

DIAGNOSTIC CHECKLIST

Consider
- FNA of inguinal adenopathy is helpful to establish histologic proof of metastasis

SELECTED REFERENCES

1. Schwarz JK et al: Tumor response and survival predicted by post-therapy FDG-PET/CT in anal cancer. Int J Radiat Oncol Biol Phys. 71(1):180-6, 2008
2. Anderson C et al: PET-CT fusion in radiation management of patients with anorectal tumors. Int J Radiat Oncol Biol Phys. 69(1):155-62, 2007
3. Nguyen BD et al: F-18 FDG PET/CT imaging of anal canal squamous cell carcinoma. Clin Nucl Med. 32(3):234-6, 2007
4. Cotter SE et al: FDG-PET/CT in the evaluation of anal carcinoma. Int J Radiat Oncol Biol Phys. 65(3):720-5, 2006
5. Niederkohr RD et al: F-18 FDG PET/CT imaging of extramammary Paget disease of the perianal region. Clin Nucl Med. 31(9):561-3, 2006
6. Piperkova E et al: Impact of PET/CT on initial staging, restaging and treatment management of anal cancer: a clinical case with literature review. J BUON. 11(4):523-7, 2006
7. Trautmann TG et al: Positron Emission Tomography for pretreatment staging and posttreatment evaluation in cancer of the anal canal. Mol Imaging Biol. 7(4):309-13, 2005
8. Trautmann TG et al: Positron Emission Tomography for pretreatment staging and posttreatment evaluation in cancer of the anal canal. Mol Imaging Biol. 7(4):309-13, 2005
9. Berry JM et al: Anal cancer and its precursors in HIV-positive patients: perspectives and management. Surg Oncol Clin N Am. 13(2):355-73, 2004
10. Lonneux M et al: Positive F-18 FDG positron emission tomography in the perineum after anorectal reconstruction. Clin Nucl Med. 27(5):363-4, 2002
11. Stoker J et al: Imaging of anorectal disease. Br J Surg. 87(1):10-27, 2000

ANAL CARCINOMA

Initial Diagnosis

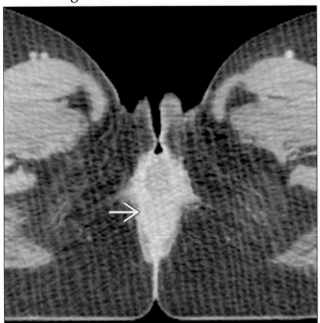 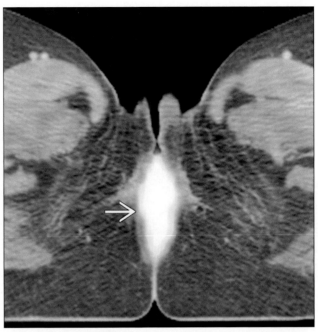

(Left) Axial CECT shows no obvious abnormality. There is questionable anal mucosal thickening ➡ in retrospect. *(Right)* Axial fused PET/CT shows intense FDG activity correlating to the area of anal mucosal thickening in this patient with newly diagnosed squamous cell carcinoma of the anus ➡.

Initial Diagnosis

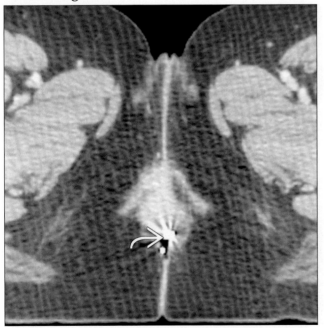 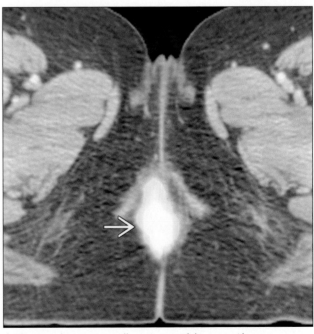

(Left) Axial CECT shows no obvious abnormality in this patient with recently diagnosed squamous cell carcinoma of the anus. Also note surgical clip from recent pathologic tissue sampling ➡. *(Right)* Axial fused PET/CT shows intense FDG activity ➡, compatible with carcinoma of the anus.

3

ANAL CARCINOMA

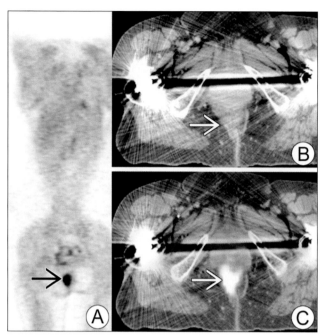 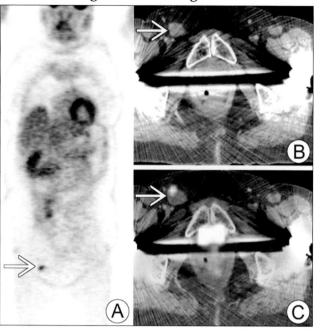

(Left) Coronal PET (A) demonstrates focal FDG activity in the area of the anorectal junction ➡. Axial CT (B) and fused PET/CT (C) localizes the activity to the anorectal junction ➡. (Right) Coronal PET (A), axial CT (B) and fused PET/CT (C) show a hypermetabolic right inguinal lymph node ➡ in this patient with newly diagnosed anal carcinoma.

Staging

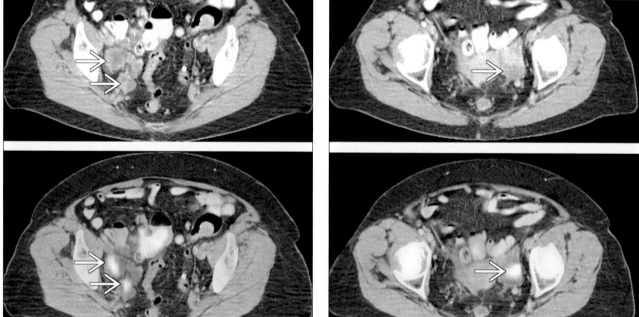

(Left) Axial CT (top) and fused PET/CT (bottom) demonstrate multiple partially necrotic right pelvic lymph node metastases ➡. (Right) Axial CT (top) and fused PET/CT (bottom) demonstrate a left-sided pelvic metastasis ➡ in this patient with newly diagnosed anal carcinoma.

ANAL CARCINOMA

Staging

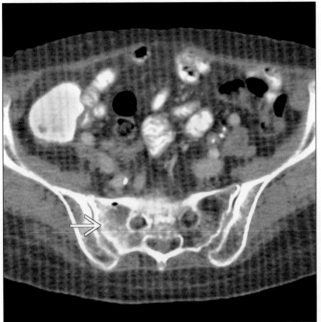 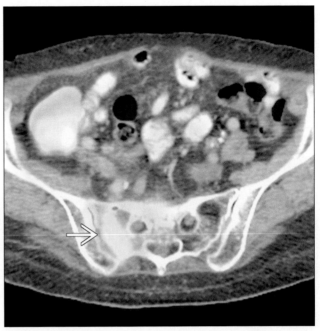

(Left) Axial CECT shows no obvious abnormality except some questionable subtle sclerotic change of the right side of the sacrum ➡. Conversely, subtle increased lucency of the left side of the sacrum could have a similar appearance. *(Right)* Axial fused PET/CT shows intense FDG activity correlating with the area of minimally increased sclerotic change ➡ in this patient with newly diagnosed squamous cell carcinoma of the anus.

Staging

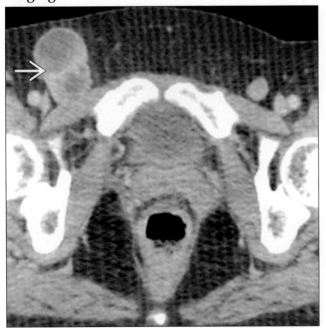 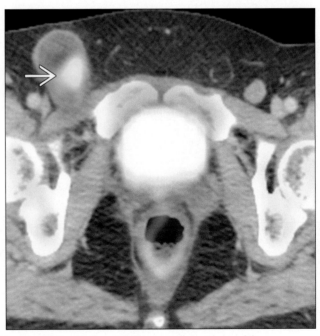

(Left) Axial CECT shows bilobar-shaped right inguinal metastases ➡ in this patient with a history of squamous cell carcinoma of the cervix. *(Right)* Axial fused PET/CT shows intense FDG activity ➡ correlating with the right inguinal metastasis.

ANAL CARCINOMA

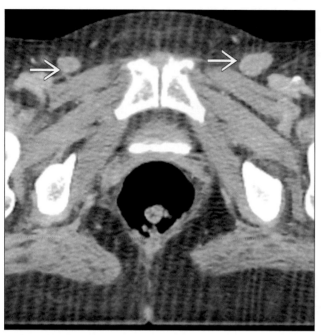 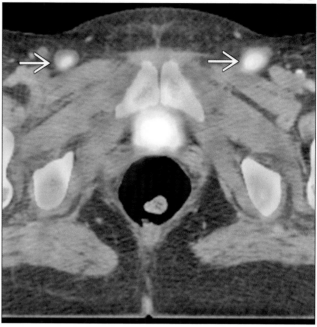

(Left) Axial CECT shows borderline enlarged bilateral inguinal nodes ➡ that are not clearly malignant. *(Right)* Axial fused PET/CT shows bilateral intense inguinal FDG activity ➡, compatible with metastatic nodes.

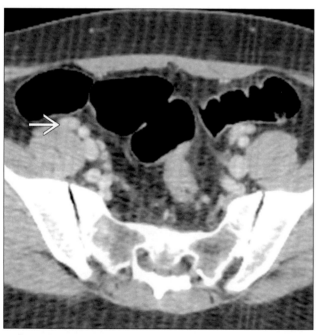 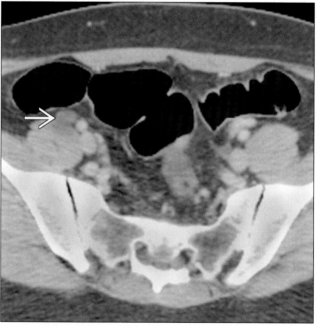

(Left) Axial CECT shows a single borderline enlarged right external iliac lymph node ➡. *(Right)* Axial fused PET/CT shows minimally increased FDG activity ➡ correlating with the small lymph node called equivocal on PET/CT. Subsequent biopsy showed metastatic disease.

ANAL CARCINOMA

Restaging

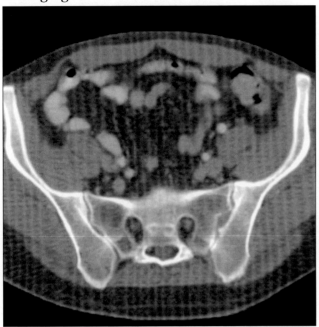 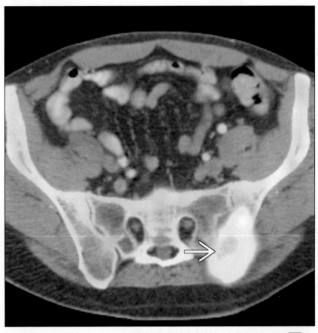

(Left) Axial CECT shows no obvious abnormalities. *(Right)* Axial fused PET/CT shows intense FDG activity correlating to the left iliac bone ➡ in this patient with a history of anal carcinoma, compatible with metastatic disease.

Restaging

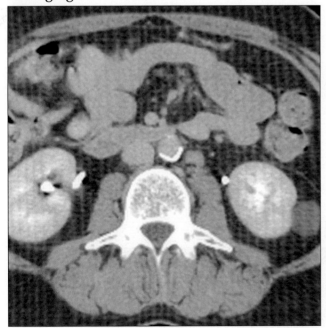 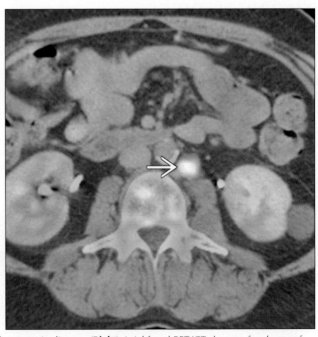

(Left) Axial CECT shows no obvious enlarged nodes or other evidence of metastatic disease. *(Right)* Axial fused PET/CT shows a focal area of intense FDG activity ➡ correlating with a lesion just anterior to the left psoas muscle, compatible with malignancy.

RENAL CELL CARCINOMA

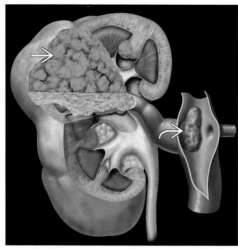

Graphic shows a typical appearance of a large renal cell carcinoma ➡ with invasion of the renal vein and inferior vena cava ➡.

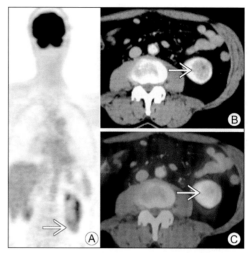

Coronal PET (A), axial CT (B) and fused PET/CT (C) show a relatively non-FDG-avid renal cell carcinoma ➡.

TERMINOLOGY

Abbreviations and Synonyms
- Renal cell carcinoma (RCC), clear cell carcinoma, hypernephroma, renal cancer

Definitions
- Carcinoma of renal tubular epithelium

IMAGING FINDINGS

General Features
- Best diagnostic clue
  - Iso- or hypermetabolic renal mass ± lymphadenopathy, metastases on FDG PET
  - Presents most commonly as incidental solid tumor on imaging
  - Enhancing solitary mass on CT highly suspicious for RCC
    - Necrosis, hemorrhage, septae more likely in large masses
- Location
  - Usually renal cortex
  - Often exophytic
  - Rarely bilateral (2%) or multicentric (more common in von Hippel-Lindau)
- Size: Variable depending on time of diagnosis
- Morphology
  - 10% calcified, often irregular
  - 2-5% cystic

Imaging Recommendations
- Best imaging tool
  - Combination of CT, ultrasound
    - CECT often shows enhancing lesion; hyperdense benign cysts will not enhance
    - US indicated in patients with nonenhancing hyperdense renal lesions to differentiate cyst from mass
    - If contraindication to contrast, MR superior to CT
  - FDG PET and PET/CT not currently covered by Medicare, but may be helpful for staging and restaging
- Protocol advice
  - For CT: Noncontrast and CECT, thin sections (2.5-5.0 mm), during both corticomedullary and nephrographic phases

DDx: Renal Mass Encountered on PET or PET/CT

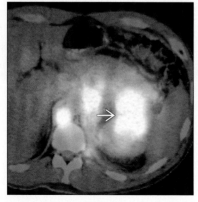

Lymphoma

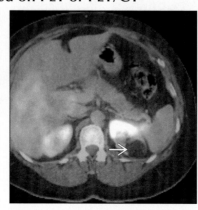

Angiomyolipoma

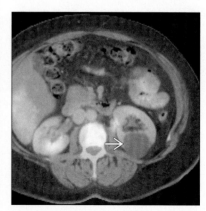

Hyperdense Cyst

RENAL CELL CARCINOMA

Emerging Clinical Applications of PET/CT

Key Facts

Terminology
- Renal cell carcinoma (RCC), clear cell carcinoma, hypernephroma, renal cancer

Imaging Findings
- Iso- or hypermetabolic renal mass ± lymphadenopathy, metastases on FDG PET
- Presents most commonly as incidental solid tumor on imaging
- Enhancing solitary mass on CT highly suspicious for RCC
- Hypervascular mass with enhancement (HU increase by > 20) compared to noncontrast
- Enhancement often heterogeneous, particularly larger lesions
- FDG PET and RCC
  - FDG uptake by RCC, metastases variable

- Sensitivity 60%, specificity ~ 100% for evaluating primary RCC
- 80-100% specific for bony metastases

Top Differential Diagnoses
- Angiomyolipoma (AML)
- Renal Oncocytoma
- Hemorrhagic Renal Cyst
- Transitional Cell Carcinoma (TCC)
- Rare Parenchymal TCC (Indistinguishable from RCC)
- Lymphoma
- Renal Infection or Abscess
- Metastatic Disease

Diagnostic Checklist
- FDG PET for staging, evaluation of bony metastases
- RCC has variable uptake on FDG PET

- For PET CT: If only single phase obtained, use later nephrographic phase of contrast enhancement
- Corticomedullary phase (25-70 seconds post-injection)
  - Better visualization of renal vessels; evaluate for renal vein/IVC thrombosis or tumor extension
  - Limited detection of small renal lesions
  - Centrally located tumors commonly mistaken for normal hypoattenuating medulla
- Nephrographic phase (80-180 seconds post-injection)
  - Best imaging of renal medulla masses

CT Findings
- NECT
  - Solid-tissue-density mass, which distorts normal kidney contour and typically is in the 30-50 HU range
  - Can be hyperdense, isodense, or hypodense to surrounding normal kidney
  - Heterogeneous mass (hemorrhage and necrosis); high (acute hemorrhage) or low attenuation (chronic)
    - ± Calcifications (10% of cases); amorphous internal (most common), curvilinear (peripheral or central), dense or diffuse calcification
  - High density rim may separate mass from adjacent renal tissue (pseudocapsule)
  - Rarely contains small areas of fat (-50 to -150 HU)
  - Combination of fat and calcification suggests RCC, not renal angiomyolipoma
  - Cystic RCC
    - Uni- or multilocular cystic mass with a thick calcification of septa or tumor capsule
    - Septa may enhance on CECT
- CECT
  - Hypervascular mass with enhancement (HU increase by > 20) compared to noncontrast
    - Enhancement often heterogeneous, particularly larger lesions
  - Tumor extension or thrombus in renal vein (23%), inferior vena cava (7%)

- Local extension common
  - Nodal spread typically to para-aortic or aortocaval lymph nodes
- Most common metastatic locations include lung, liver, bone, adrenal, and opposite kidney
- Usually solid, and decreased attenuation suggestive of necrosis often present
- Sometimes presents as predominantly cystic mass with thick septa and wall nodularity
- Nephrographic phase is most sensitive for tumor detection, especially for masses smaller than 3 cm
- Corticomedullary phase required for tumor extension into renal veins
  - Evaluation for hypervascular metastases
- Helical CT improves diagnosis and eliminates respiratory misregistration

Nuclear Medicine Findings
- FDG PET and PET/CT for RCC
  - Iso- or hypermetabolic renal mass ± lymphadenopathy, metastases
  - FDG uptake by primary RCC and metastases is somewhat variable; therefore, PET and PET/CT are more helpful when positive
    - Negative study may represent either a non-FDG-avid RCC or truly negative disease
  - Sensitivity 60%, specificity ~ 100% for evaluating primary RCC
  - Excretory FDG in collecting system can mask small RCCs adjacent to collecting system
  - 80-100% specific for bony metastases

DIFFERENTIAL DIAGNOSIS

Angiomyolipoma (AML)
- Fat attenuation (-30 to -150 HU) fairly specific for this neoplasm
- Low FDG uptake
- Reliably distinguished from malignancy by CT characteristics

3

145

RENAL CELL CARCINOMA

Renal Oncocytoma
- Central scar on CT/MR and spoke-wheel pattern of vessels on angiograms suggest oncocytoma; not entirely specific
- Cannot confidently differentiate from RCC by PET

Hemorrhagic Renal Cyst
- > Water attenuation on CT (~ 30-70 HU)
- Should not enhance when comparing noncontrast and CE series

Transitional Cell Carcinoma (TCC)
- Renal pelvis filling defect, narrowing
- Urothelial thickening or involvement
- Rare parenchymal TCC indistinguishable from RCC

Lymphoma
- Typically more diffusely infiltrative than discrete mass

Renal Infection or Abscess
- Focal nephritis can appear mass-like
  - Short term follow-up helpful
- Clinical history and urine analysis often helpful

Metastatic Disease
- History essential
- Common primary cancers include lung, breast, colon, melanoma, pancreatic
- Typically only hypervascular metastases mistaken for RCC

PATHOLOGY

General Features
- General path comments
  - Staging
    - Stage I: Solid mass ≤ 7 cm, confined to kidney
    - Stage II: > 7 cm but still organ confined; spread to perinephric fat
    - Stage III: Invasion of renal vein or vena cava, involvement of ipsilateral adrenal gland &/or perinephric fat, or spread to one local lymph node
    - Stage IV: Invasion of adjacent organs, more than one local node, or distant metastases
- Genetics: Associated with von Hippel-Lindau syndrome (autosomal dominant)
- Etiology
  - Arise from tubular epithelium
  - Bilateral lesions associated with von Hippel-Lindau syndrome, tuberous sclerosis, chronic dialysis
  - Other risk factors: Smoking, chemical exposure (diethylstilbestrol and fluoroacetamide)
- Epidemiology
  - Approximately 2% of adult malignancies (30,000/year in USA)
  - Undiagnosed small RCCs found at autopsy even more frequently

Gross Pathologic & Surgical Features
- Solid to cystic components with necrosis, hemorrhage, and rarely fat

Microscopic Features
- 70% clear cell, 13% papillary, 7% granular, 10% other

CLINICAL ISSUES

Presentation
- Most common signs/symptoms
  - Usually a combination of hematuria (50%), flank pain (40%), &/or flank mass (35%)
  - Nearly half of RCCs discovered incidentally
- Other signs/symptoms
  - Fever, nausea, weight loss
  - Rarely, humoral factors such as erythropoietin, renin, parathyroid hormone, or prolactin may cause symptoms

Demographics
- Age: Generally 50-70 years, with wide distribution
- Gender: M > F, 2:1

Natural History & Prognosis
- 5 year survival
  - Stage I: 67%, stage II: 51%, stage III: 33.5%, stage IV: 13.5%
- Prognosis worse for larger, marginated, or necrotic tumors, which tend to be ↑ grade

Treatment
- Complete surgical resection only curative treatment
- Occasionally offer nephron sparing resection or RFA

DIAGNOSTIC CHECKLIST

Consider
- FDG PET for staging, evaluation of bony metastases
- Noncontrast CT followed by CECT for primary evaluation
- US to differentiate hyperdense cyst from mass if CT unclear

Image Interpretation Pearls
- RCC has variable uptake on FDG PET
- Excretory FDG in collecting system can mask adjacent small RCCs

SELECTED REFERENCES

1. Coll DM et al: Update on radiological imaging of renal cell carcinoma. BJU Int. 99(5 Pt B):1217-22, 2007
2. Mueller-Lisse UG et al: Staging of renal cell carcinoma. Eur Radiol. 17(9):2268-77, 2007
3. Powles T et al: Does PET imaging have a role in renal cancers after all? Lancet Oncol. 8(4):279-81, 2007
4. Tsakiris P et al: Imaging in genitourinary cancer from the urologists' perspective. Cancer Imaging. 7:84-92, 2007
5. Zhang J et al: Imaging of kidney cancer. Radiol Clin North Am. 45(1):119-47, 2007
6. Dilhuydy MS et al: PET scans for decision-making in metastatic renal cell carcinoma: a single-institution evaluation. Oncology. 70(5):339-44, 2006
7. Francis IR: Detection, staging and surveillance in renal cell carcinoma. Cancer Imaging. 6:168-74, 2006

RENAL CELL CARCINOMA

CT Findings: Primary

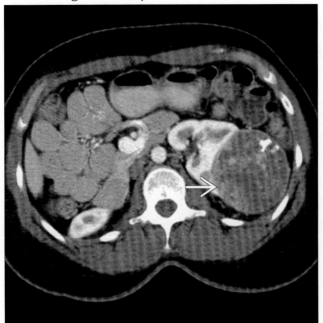
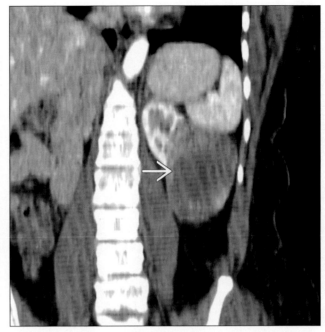

(Left) Axial CECT shows a large heterogeneously enhancing lesion that contains coarse calcifications ⇒ in the posterior aspect of the left kidney. *(Right)* Coronal CECT shows the same mass ⇒ as the previous image.

CT Findings: Primary

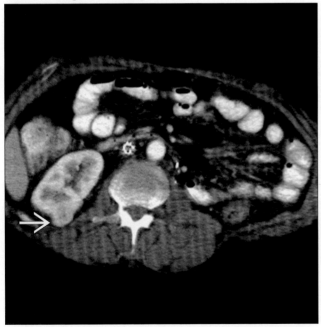
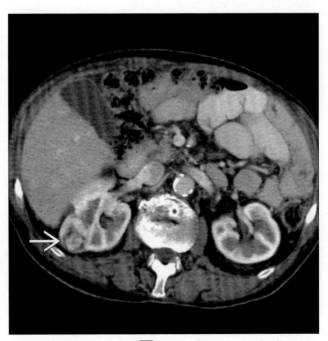

(Left) Axial CECT shows a heterogeneously enhancing lesion off the posterior aspect of the right kidney ⇒, compatible with a renal cell carcinoma. *(Right)* Axial CECT shows a heterogeneously enhancing lesion in the posterior aspect of the right kidney ⇒, compatible with a renal cell carcinoma.

RENAL CELL CARCINOMA

CT Findings: Primary

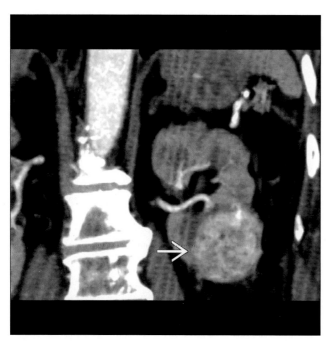
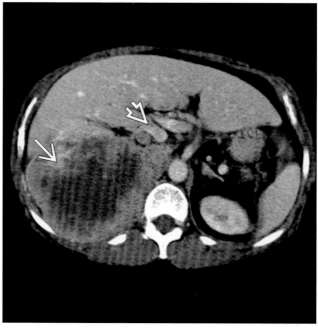

(Left) Coronal CECT shows another hypervascular lesion in the lower pole of the left kidney ➡, consistent with renal cell carcinoma. *(Right)* Axial CECT shows a large centrally necrotic mass ➡ invading the posterior margin of the liver. The mass completely engulfs the adrenal gland and has invaded the entire perirenal and pararenal spaces. The IVC ➡ is not invaded but displaced anteriorly.

CT Findings: Atypical Primary with Metastases

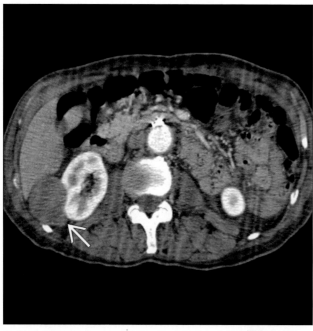
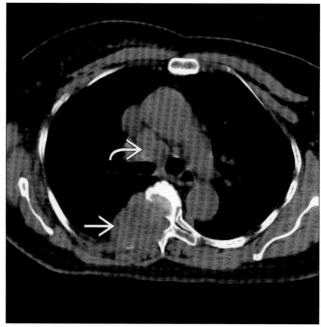

(Left) Axial CECT shows a mildly enhancing renal mass ➡. Papillary subtypes of renal cell carcinoma may show very mild enhancement on more delayed phases of imaging that are not always apparent on early phases of imaging. *(Right)* Axial NECT in the same patient approximately 1 month later shows enlarged mediastinal nodes ➡ and a destructive soft tissue lesion that invades the epidural space and encroaches on the thecal sac ➡.

RENAL CELL CARCINOMA

CT Findings: Metastases

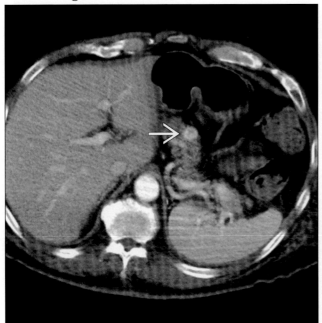
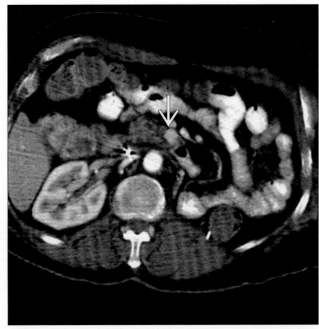

(Left) Axial CECT shows a hypervascular lesion in the body of the pancreas ➡, consistent with metastasis in this patient with known renal cell carcinoma. *(Right)* Axial CECT shows another hypervascular lesion in the body of the pancreas ➡, consistent with metastasis in this patient with known renal cell carcinoma.

PET/CT Findings: Primary

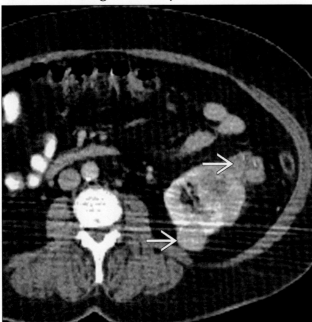
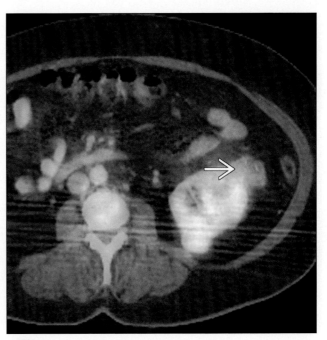

(Left) Axial CECT shows heterogeneously enhancing exophytic renal masses ➡ off the left kidney, compatible with renal cell carcinoma. *(Right)* Axial fused PET/CT shows very little FDG activity within the more anteriorly enhancing renal mass ➡. This amount of FDG activity should not rule out the diagnosis of renal cell carcinoma, as carcinomas often may have only mild to moderate FDG activity.

RENAL CELL CARCINOMA

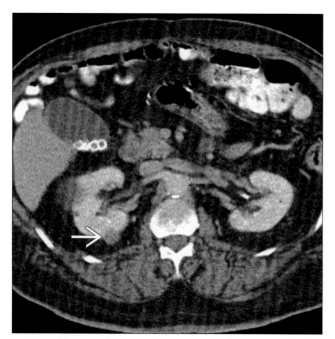 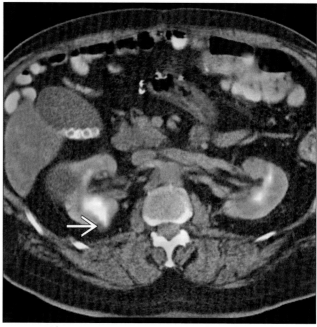

(Left) Axial CECT shows a small enhancing mass ➡ in the posterior aspect of the right kidney. *(Right)* Axial fused PET/CT shows increased metabolic activity within the small mass off the posterior aspect of the right kidney ➡, worrisome for renal cell carcinoma. Incidentally, this patient also had a prior left-sided renal cell carcinoma that was treated with a partial nephrectomy.

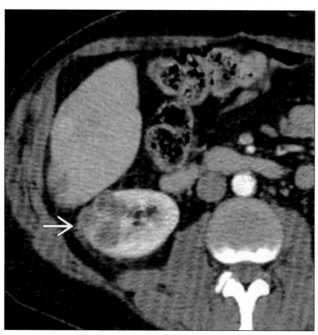 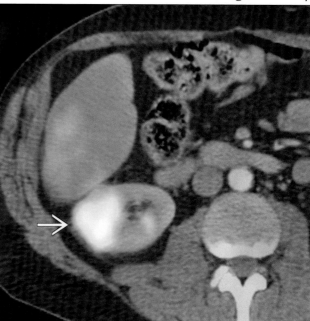

(Left) Axial CECT shows a complex cystic lesion ➡ in the right kidney. *(Right)* Axial fused PET/CT of the same patient shows the complex cystic lesion ➡ to be hypermetabolic. It was subsequently pathologically identified as renal cell carcinoma.

RENAL CELL CARCINOMA

PET/CT Findings: Primary

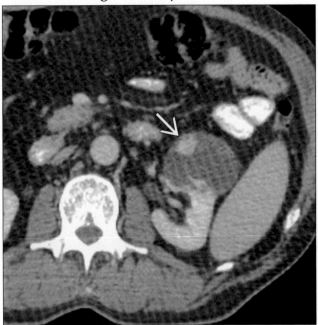 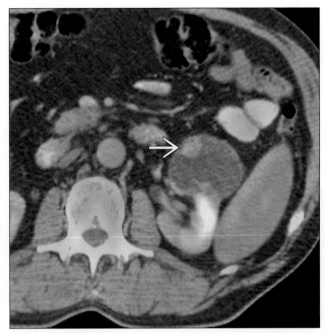

(Left) Axial CECT shows a predominantly cystic lesion with enhancing mural nodularity ➡. *(Right)* Axial fused PET/CT shows minimally increased metabolic activity in the enhancing mural nodule ➡ within the left renal lesion, subsequently pathologically proven to be a cystic renal cell carcinoma.

PET/CT Findings: Primary

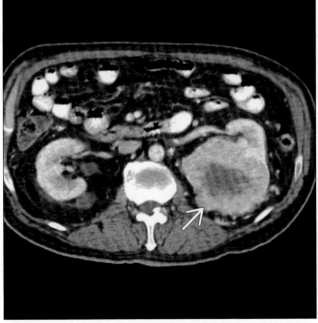 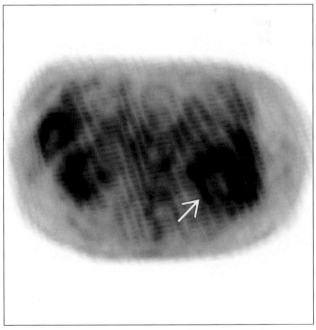

(Left) Axial CECT shows a large centrally necrotic renal mass on the left ➡, consistent with renal cell carcinoma. *(Right)* Axial PET shows the same left renal mass with intense FDG uptake ➡.

RENAL CELL CARCINOMA

PET/CT Findings: Primary with Regional Nodes

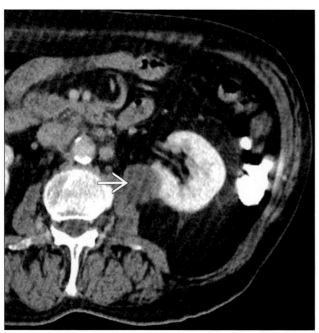 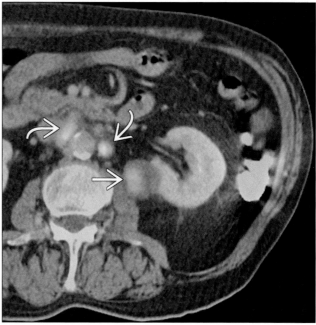

(Left) Axial contrast enema shows a low attenuation mass ➡ arising from the medial aspect of the left kidney. *(Right)* Axial fused PET/CT shows mild to moderate increased FDG activity within the left renal mass ➡ with moderately hypermetabolic retroperitoneal adenopathy ➡. The overall appearance is compatible with renal cell carcinoma and regional metastases.

PET/CT Findings: Staging

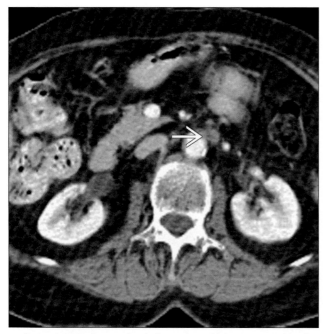 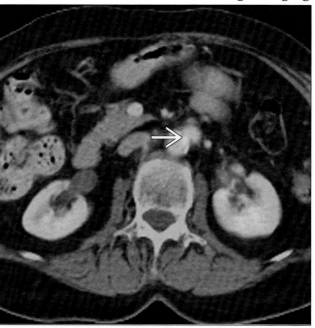

(Left) Axial CECT shows a borderline enlarged left para-aortic lymph node ➡ in this patient with newly diagnosed renal cell carcinoma. *(Right)* Axial fused PET/CT shows intense metabolic activity within the left para-aortic lymph node ➡, compatible with regional metastases.

RENAL CELL CARCINOMA

PET/CT Findings: Staging

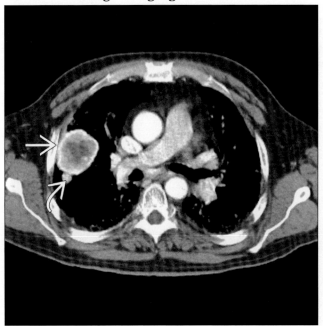
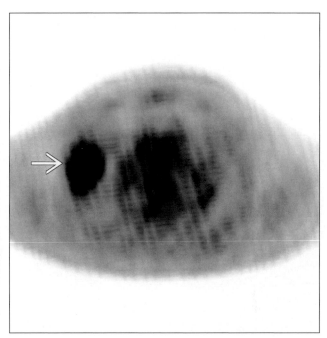

(Left) Axial CECT shows a necrotic mass in the right upper lobe ➡ with an adjacent enhancing satellite lesion ➡, consistent with renal cell carcinoma metastases. *(Right)* Axial PET reveals intense FDG uptake in the renal cell metastasis ➡.

PET/CT Findings: Staging

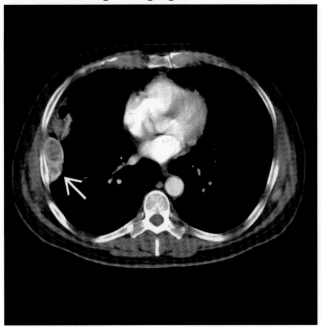
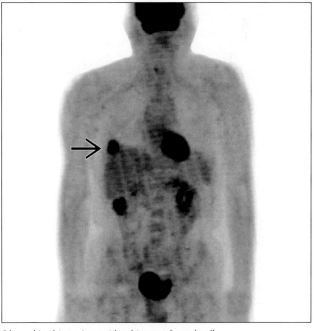

(Left) Axial CECT shows a hypervascular enhancing mass ➡ that is pleural based in this patient with a history of renal cell carcinoma. *(Right)* Coronal PET shows intense FDG activity within the pleural-based metastasis ➡ that was subsequently resected. Final pathology revealed metastatic renal cell carcinoma.

RENAL CELL CARCINOMA

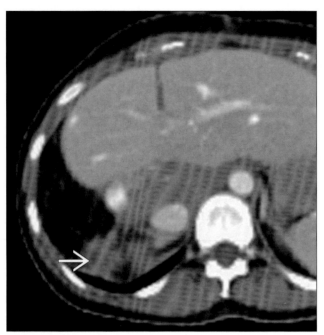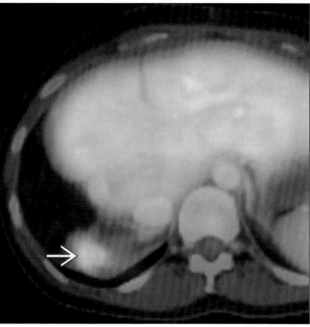

(Left) Axial CECT shows nonspecific equivocal soft tissue within the right nephrectomy bed ➡. This patient had a nephrectomy for renal cell carcinoma approximately 6 months earlier. *(Right)* Axial fused PET/CT shows moderately increased FDG activity correlating to the surgical bed soft tissue ➡, very worrisome for recurrent disease.

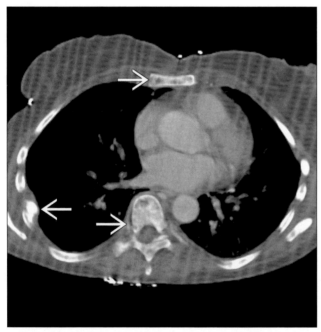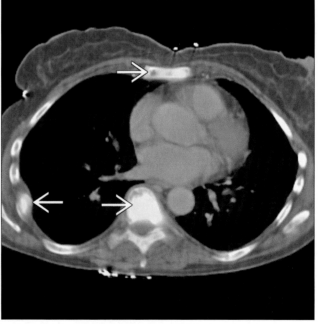

(Left) Axial CECT shows several sclerotic bony lesions ➡ in the spine, right rib, and sternum. The sclerotic nature of the lesions is characteristic of renal cell carcinoma. *(Right)* Axial fused PET/CT of the same patient shows that the bony lesions ➡ are all hypermetabolic, consistent with metastases.

RENAL CELL CARCINOMA

PET/CT Findings: Restaging

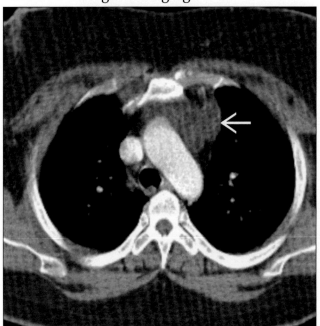 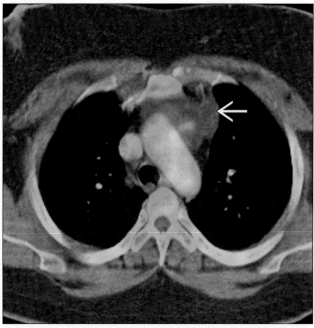

(Left) Axial CECT shows nodal tissue in the anterior mediastinum ➜. *(Right)* Axial fused PET/CT of the same patient does not show any increased FDG uptake in the enlarged prevascular nodes ➜, which was subsequently biopsy-proven to be renal cell carcinoma recurrence.

PET/CT Findings: Restaging Atypical

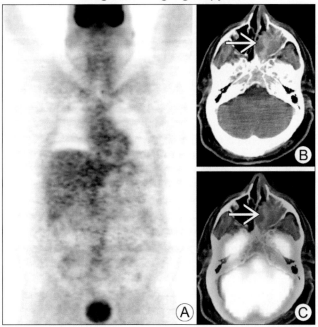 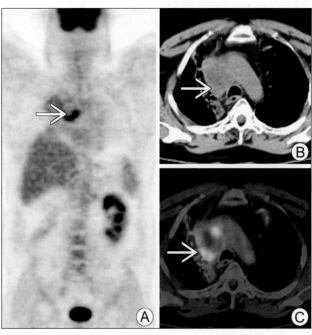

(Left) Coronal PET (A), axial CT (B) and fused PET/CT (C) demonstrate a very atypical case of biopsy-confirmed metastatic renal cell carcinoma to the left maxillary sinus ➜ in this patient with a history of a large renal cell carcinoma. Note the absence of increased metabolic activity. *(Right)* Coronal PET (A), axial CT (B) and fused PET/CT (C) demonstrate mediastinal metastases ➜ for renal cell carcinoma with variably increased FDG activity.

BLADDER CARCINOMA

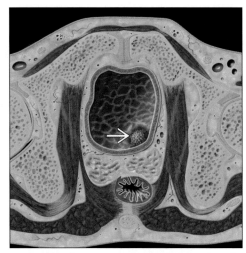

Axial graphic demonstrates a focal mass arising from the posterior aspect of the bladder near the left ureterovesical junction ➡️*.*

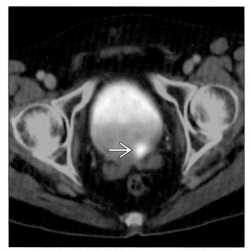

Axial fused PET/CT in a patient scanned in the prone position shows a focal area of activity ➡️*, compatible with known bladder cancer.*

TERMINOLOGY

Abbreviations and Synonyms
- Bladder carcinoma, urothelial carcinoma, transitional cell carcinoma (TCC)

Definitions
- Malignancy of the urinary bladder

IMAGING FINDINGS

General Features
- Best diagnostic clue
  - PET/CT: Focal increased FDG activity in primary tumor, ± in regional and distant lymph nodes, lung, liver, bone
  - CT: Enhancing focal/asymmetric mass in the urinary bladder
- Location
  - Usually arises in the bladder wall
  - Can be multifocal
  - Local invasion

- Detrusor muscle, prostate, uterus, vagina, seminal vesicles, rectum
  - Lymphatic spread (30% of tumors that only involve bladder wall; 60% of those with extravesicular invasion)
    - Regional (pelvic) lymph nodes (LN)
    - Distant LN
  - Hematogenous spread
    - Lung > > liver, bone
  - Recurrences of superficial bladder cancer remain confined to bladder wall in 70-80% of patients
    - Remaining 20-30% may become muscle-invasive and lead to metastatic disease
  - Common metastatic sites include pelvic and retroperitoneal lymph nodes, lungs, liver, and bones
- Size: Varies from undetectable on CT to large enhancing mass
- Morphology
  - Superficial: Most common representing 70-80%
    - Confined to mucosa and lamina propria
    - Project into bladder lumen (papillary)
    - Usually low grade
  - Invasive: Less common, representing 20-30%
    - Detrusor muscle involvement

DDx: FDG Activity in the Pelvis in or near Bladder

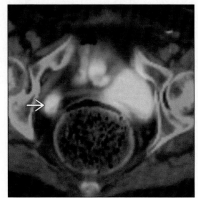

Bladder Diverticulum

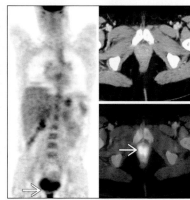

Incontinence

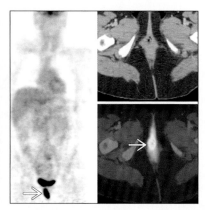

Menstruation

BLADDER CARCINOMA

Key Facts

Imaging Findings

- CT: Enhancing focal/asymmetrical mass in the urinary bladder
  - Can be multifocal
  - Lymphatic spread (30% of tumors that only involve bladder wall; 60% of those with extravesicular invasion)
  - Common metastatic sites include pelvic and retroperitoneal lymph nodes, lungs, liver, and bones
- Initial workup: Cystoscopy and biopsy; CT or MR for evaluation of primary tumor, LN metastases
- PET/CT: Valuable for pre-operative staging, response to therapy, distinguishing post-surgical change from recurrence

- CT findings nonspecific, diagnosis usually based on biopsy
  - Focal or diffuse bladder wall thickening
  - Mass projecting into bladder ± enhancement

Pathology

- ~ 90% transitional cell carcinomas (TCC); often multifocal

Clinical Issues

- Hydronephrosis, renal obstruction, particularly with lesions near UVJ

Diagnostic Checklist

- Bladder cancer may have variable FDG uptake; baseline PET/CT useful to confirm FDG avidity
- Immediate post-void imaging, retrograde bladder irrigation with normal saline, IV Lasix administration with parenteral hydration have been recommended

---

- Solid, more infiltrating
- Usually high grade

Imaging Recommendations

- Best imaging tool
  - Initial workup: Cystoscopy and biopsy; CT or MR for evaluation of primary tumor and LN metastases
    - CT: Reported accuracy in detecting LN involvement 70-90% with false negative rates 25-40%
    - MR: 73-98% reported accuracy for determining nodal metastases
  - PET/CT
    - Utility mostly for pre-operative staging, distinguishing post-surgical change from recurrence
    - Minimally useful for evaluation of primary tumor, usually obscured by excretory FDG
  - Bone scan: Helpful if there is clinical suspicion of bone metastases
  - CT/MR tend to overestimate degree of extension through bladder wall but underestimate presence of pelvic lymph node metastases
- Protocol advice
  - PET/CT: 10-15 mCi (370-555 MBq) F18-FDG IV, start imaging at pelvis to avoid FDG filling bladder
  - PET/CT: Excreted FDG in urinary bladder can mask pelvic pathology
    - Techniques include Immediate post-void imaging, retrograde bladder irrigation with normal saline, IV Lasix administration with parenteral hydration
    - Prone positioning may be useful for visualization of posteriorly located lesions
  - Urinary excretion of FDG leads to pooled activity in bladder, making evaluation of bladder wall lesions difficult to impossible with standard protocol
    - Furosemide injected at least 2 hours after radiotracer injection provides excellent urinary radiotracer washout, reducing bladder activity to background levels
    - Oral hydration aids in diuresis

- Full bladder is required to avoid artifactual thickening of the walls
- Protocol not satisfactory in patients with cystectomy because urinary diversions show higher residual activities, but recurrence is extremely rare in bladder diversion walls

CT Findings

- CT findings of primary usually nonspecific (diagnosis often based on biopsy performed during cystoscopy)
  - Focal or diffuse bladder wall thickening
  - Mass projecting into bladder ± enhancement
- Occasionally calcifications
- Hydronephrosis 2° to tumor near vesicoureteric junction
- Extravesicular extension: Nodules, irregularity of outer bladder wall, stranding of perivesicular fat
- T status of tumor most often determined by biopsy
- Causes of circumferential bladder thickening that can mimic bladder cancer include
  - Previous biopsy, inflammation, radiotherapy, systemic chemotherapy, and intravesical agents like Bacille Calmette-Guérin (BCG)
- Sessile or pedunculated soft tissue mass projecting into the lumen; similar density to bladder wall
- ± Enlarged (> 10 mm) metastatic lymph nodes; extravesical tumor extension
- Fine punctate calcifications with tumor; may suggest mucinous adenocarcinoma
- Ring pattern of calcification; may suggest pheochromocytoma
- Inability to distinguish tumors from bladder wall hypertrophy, local inflammation, and fibrosis
- Unable to differentiate Ta-T3a, invasion of dome/base of bladder or local organ (due to partial volume effect), nonenlarged lymph nodes
- Also consider urachal adenocarcinoma
  - Midline abdominal mass ± calcification
  - Solitary lobulated tumor arising from dome of bladder on ventral surface

BLADDER CARCINOMA

MR Findings
- T1WI: Isointense to muscle
- T2WI: Hyperintense to muscle
- Superior to CT for assessing deep muscle involvement, invasion of adjacent organs

Nuclear Medicine Findings
- Focal increased FDG activity in primary tumor, regional and distant LN, lung, liver, bone
  - Bladder cancer may have variable uptake of FDG
  - Baseline PET/CT useful for confirmation of FDG avidity
  - Max SUV may range from 5-10 in typical hypermetabolic bladder lesions
- Primary tumor may be masked by excreted FDG in urine
  - FDG is not resorbed as glucose and is excreted in the urine
  - With delayed imaging, ratio of tumor:bladder FDG uptake was 13:1 in one study
- False positives: Bladder diverticula and urinary leak
  - CT portion of PET/CT essential for ruling out such pitfalls
  - CT also useful for precise separation of uptake foci in the bladder wall vs. lymph nodes adjacent to bladder
  - One study showed 3 month period post-resection was sufficient to heal inflammatory reactions and reduce false positives
- C-11-choline PET/CT radiotracer does not collect in urinary tract, but its value for lesion staging has not been shown superior to conventional methods
- Bone scan: Bone metastases classically appear as multiple, scattered foci of increased activity, axial > appendicular skeleton

DIFFERENTIAL DIAGNOSIS

Cystitis
- Usually more diffuse thickening of the bladder wall
- Chronic urinary tract infection, fungus
- Radiation- or chemotherapy-induced
- Hemorrhagic cystitis

Hematoma
- Trauma
- Iatrogenic

Cystitis Cystica
- Degeneration of urothelial cells in Brunn nests

Other Neoplasm
- Endometriosis
- Metastases

PATHOLOGY

General Features
- General path comments
  - ~ 90% transitional cell carcinomas (TCC); often multifocal
  - 5-10% squamous cell (chronic inflammation)
  - < 5% mixed TCC and squamous cell
  - 2-3% adenocarcinoma (persistent urachal remnant)
  - < 1% rare types (e.g., leiomyomas, lymphoma, melanoma)
- Etiology
  - Risk factors
    - Cigarette smoking
    - Exposure to aniline, aromatic amines, diesel fumes
    - Phenacetin use (once used as analgesic, now often mixed with cocaine)
    - Infection: Chronic urinary tract infection, schistosomiasis
- Epidemiology
  - Most common tumor of urinary tract
    - More than 90% are transitional cell carcinoma
  - Men: Fourth most common cancer
    - 7% of all malignancies in men
  - Women: Tenth most common cancer
    - 2% of all malignancies in women

Staging, Grading, or Classification Criteria
- Preinvasive
  - TNM: To, Tis, Ta
  - Jewett-Strong-Marshall (JSM): 0
- Submucosal invasion
  - TNM: T1
  - JSM: A
- Superficial muscle invasion
  - TNM: T2a
  - JSM: B1
- Deep muscle invasion
  - TNM: T2b, T3a
  - JSM: B2
- Extravesicular spread
  - TNM: T3b
  - JSM: C
- Fixed to or invading prostate, uterus, vagina; pelvic lymph nodes
  - TNM: T4a, T4b; N1 (1 pelvic LN < 2 cm); N2 (1 pelvic LN 2-5 cm; multiple LN < 5 cm); N3 (LN > 5 cm)
  - JSM: D1
- Extrapelvic LN or distant metastases
  - TNM: M1
  - JSM: D2

CLINICAL ISSUES

Presentation
- Most common signs/symptoms
  - 80-90% have painless gross hematuria
  - Urination problems
    - Dysuria
    - Urgency
    - Frequency
- Other signs/symptoms: Hydronephrosis, renal obstruction (particularly with lesions near UVJ)

Demographics
- Age: Peak incidence 50-60 years
- Gender: M:F = 4:1
- Ethnicity: Caucasians:African-Americans = 2:1

BLADDER CARCINOMA

Natural History & Prognosis
- Most patients with metastatic disease die within 2 years
- High local recurrence rate
- Low grade tumors
  - Usually superficial
  - Confined to epithelial or transitional cell layer of bladder
  - Low potential for metastatic spread
- High grade tumors
  - Invade deeper layers of bladder wall
  - Much greater potential for metastatic spread
- At least 50% of high grade tumors may have occult metastases at initial diagnosis and gross metastases within 2 years of diagnosis despite prompt aggressive regional intervention

Treatment
- Surgery
  - Early stage: Transurethral resection, segmental cystectomy
  - Later stages: Radical cystectomy, pelvic LN dissection
- Chemotherapy
  - Intravesicular
  - Systemic
- Radiation
  - Early stage: Radiation implants
  - Later stages: External beam radiation
- Immunotherapy
  - Intravesicular biologic therapy (BCG)

DIAGNOSTIC CHECKLIST

Consider
- At diagnosis, 75-85% have superficial tumors and 15-25% have lymph node metastases
- As many as 50% of patients who have invasive cancer will have occult metastases that present within 5 years of diagnosis
- Use PET/CT for optimal pre-operative staging (N, M), evaluating response to therapy, detecting recurrence
- Bladder cancer may have variable FDG uptake; baseline PET/CT useful to confirm FDG avidity

Image Interpretation Pearls
- Primary bladder cancer often obscured by excreted FDG in urinary bladder (PET not useful for primary tumor evaluation)
- Immediate post-void imaging, retrograde bladder irrigation with normal saline, IV Lasix administration with parenteral hydration
  - Decrease amount of FDG in urinary bladder on PET
  - Decrease rate of false negatives (small adjacent LN) in pelvis due to high FDG activity in bladder
- Excreted bladder FDG may be displaced anteriorly by denser iodinated IV contrast, leading to anterior layering of radiotracer
  - May occasionally help unmask an FDG-avid posterior bladder malignancy

SELECTED REFERENCES
1. Bouchelouche K et al: Positron emission tomography and positron emission tomography/computerized tomography of urological malignancies: an update review. J Urol. 179(1):34-45, 2008
2. Bouchelouche K et al: Recent developments in urologic oncology: positron emission tomography molecular imaging. Curr Opin Oncol. 20(3):321-6, 2008
3. Jadvar H et al: [F-18]-Fluorodeoxyglucose PET and PET-CT in diagnostic imaging evaluation of locally recurrent and metastatic bladder transitional cell carcinoma. Int J Clin Oncol. 13(1):42-7, 2008
4. Anjos DA et al: 18F-FDG PET/CT delayed images after diuretic for restaging invasive bladder cancer. J Nucl Med. 48(5):764-70, 2007
5. Fanti S et al: PET in genitourinary tract cancers. Q J Nucl Med Mol Imaging. 51(3):260-71, 2007
6. Machtens S et al: Positron emission tomography (PET) in the urooncological evaluation of the small pelvis. World J Urol. 25(4):341-9, 2007
7. Powles T et al: Molecular positron emission tomography and PET/CT imaging in urological malignancies. Eur Urol. 51(6):1511-20; discussion 1520-1, 2007
8. Rinnab L et al: 11C-choline positron-emission tomography/computed tomography and transrectal ultrasonography for staging localized prostate cancer. BJU Int. 99(6):1421-6, 2007
9. Setty BN et al: State-of-the-art cross-sectional imaging in bladder cancer. Curr Probl Diagn Radiol. 36(2):83-96, 2007
10. Tsakiris P et al: Imaging in genitourinary cancer from the urologists' perspective. Cancer Imaging. 7:84-92, 2007
11. Zhang J et al: Imaging of bladder cancer. Radiol Clin North Am. 45(1):183-205, 2007
12. Iagaru A et al: F-18 FDG PET imaging of urinary bladder oat cell carcinoma with widespread osseous metastases. Clin Nucl Med. 31(8):476-8, 2006
13. Liu IJ et al: Evaluation of fluorodeoxyglucose positron emission tomography imaging in metastatic transitional cell carcinoma with and without prior chemotherapy. Urol Int. 77(1):69-75, 2006
14. Saksena MA et al: New imaging modalities in bladder cancer. World J Urol. 24(5):473-80, 2006
15. Sharir S: Update on clinical and radiological staging and surveillance of bladder cancer. Can J Urol. 13 Suppl 1:71-6, 2006
16. Drieskens O et al: FDG-PET for preoperative staging of bladder cancer. Eur J Nucl Med Mol Imaging. 32(12):1412-7, 2005
17. Hain SF: Positron emission tomography in uro-oncology. Cancer Imaging. 5(1):1-7, 2005
18. Lin WY et al: A pitfall of FDG-PET image interpretation: accumulation of FDG in the dependent area of the urinary bladder after bladder irrigation--the usefulness of the prone position. Clin Nucl Med. 30(9):638-9, 2005
19. Schöder H et al: Positron emission tomography for prostate, bladder, and renal cancer. Semin Nucl Med. 34(4):274-92, 2004
20. Hain SF et al: Positron emission tomography for urological tumours. BJU Int. 92(2):159-64, 2003
21. Jichlinski P: New diagnostic strategies in the detection and staging of bladder cancer. Curr Opin Urol. 13(5):351-5, 2003
22. van der Heijden AG et al: Future strategies in the diagnosis, staging and treatment of bladder cancer. Curr Opin Urol. 13(5):389-95, 2003
23. de Jong IJ et al: Visualisation of bladder cancer using (11)C-choline PET: first clinical experience. Eur J Nucl Med Mol Imaging. 29(10):1283-8, 2002

3

BLADDER CARCINOMA

CT Findings: Primary

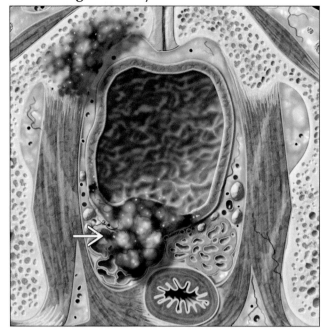
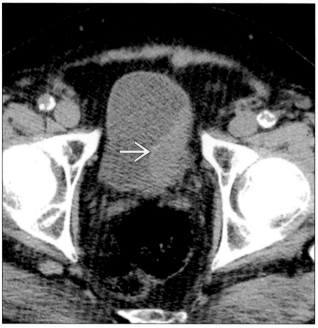

(Left) Graphic shows an exophytic mass arising from the inferior aspect of the bladder ➡, compatible with transitional cell carcinoma. *(Right)* Axial CECT shows asymmetric soft tissue attenuation in the left posterolateral aspect of the bladder ➡ in this patient with newly diagnosed transitional cell carcinoma of the bladder.

CT Findings: Primary

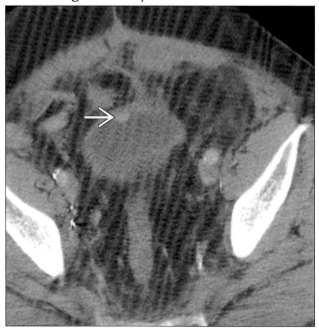
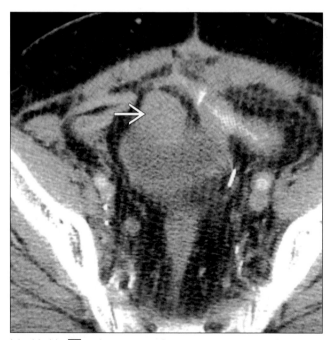

(Left) Axial CECT shows soft tissue nodule in the nondependent portion of the bladder ➡ in this patient with a recent cystoscopy and biopsy positive for transitional cell carcinoma. *(Right)* Axial CECT shows soft tissue lesion ➡ in the nondependent aspect of the bladder wall anteriorly. It appears to extend beyond the margins of the bladder wall, compatible with carcinoma of the bladder.

BLADDER CARCINOMA

CT Findings: Primary

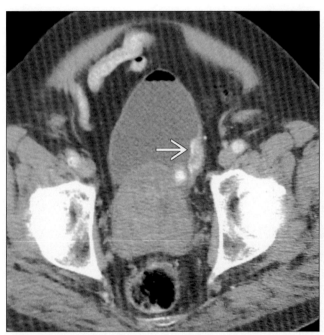

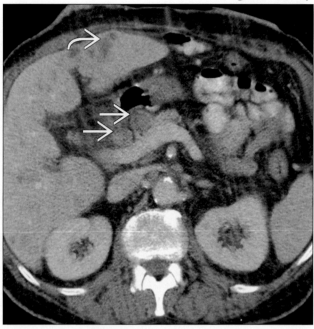

(Left) Axial CECT shows enhancing lesions along the left lateral border of the urinary bladder ➡, compatible with the patient's recent diagnosis of transitional cell carcinoma. *(Right)* Axial CECT shows peripancreatic/porta-hepatis lymph nodes ➡ and hypoattenuating lesions in the liver ➡, compatible with malignancy.

CT Findings: Metastastic

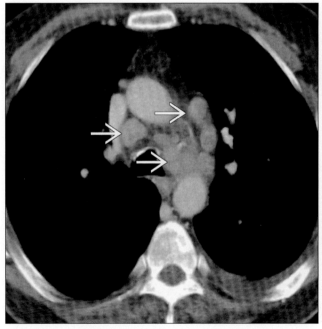

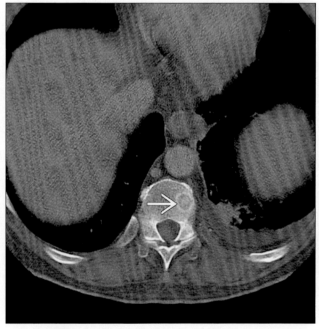

(Left) Axial CECT demonstrates enlarged mediastinal, partially necrotic lymph nodes ➡, compatible with malignancy. *(Right)* Axial CECT shows lytic lesion ➡ within the left lateral aspect of the vertebral body.

BLADDER CARCINOMA

CT Findings: Metastatic

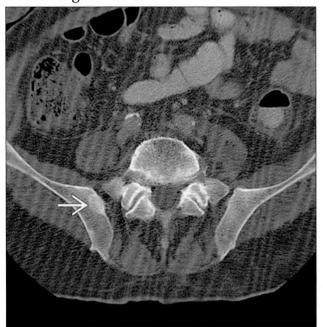
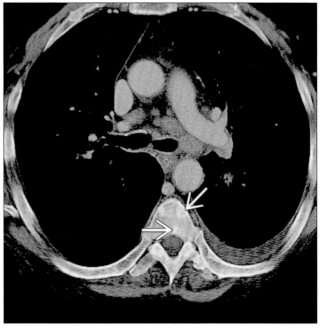

(Left) Axial CECT shows mixed lytic and sclerotic lesion ➡ in the right iliac bone. *(Right)* Axial CECT shows partially sclerotic vertebral metastases ➡. Transitional cell carcinoma often has sclerotic type osseous metastases.

CT Findings: Primary

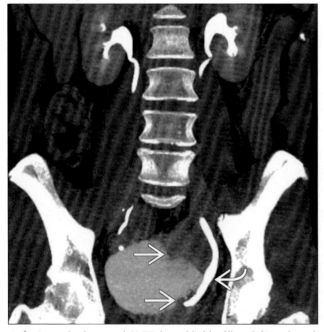
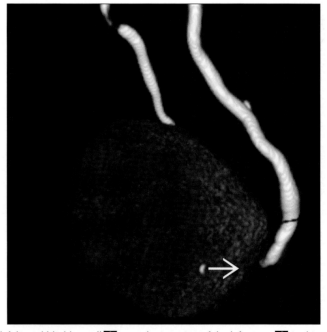

(Left) Coronal reformatted CECT shows bladder filling defects along the left lateral bladder wall ➡ near the insertion of the left ureter ➡ in this patient with newly diagnosed transitional cell carcinoma. *(Right)* 3D reformatted image of the ureters and urinary bladder shows mass effect near the insertion of the left ureter ➡ in this patient with transitional cell carcinoma of the bladder.

BLADDER CARCINOMA

PET/CT Findings: Primary

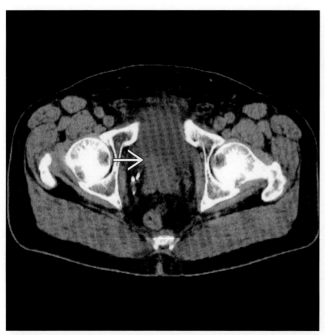 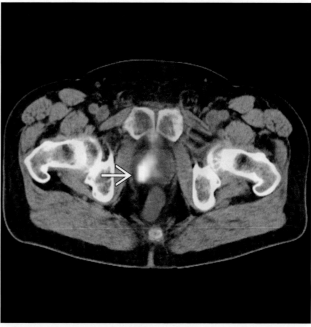

(Left) Axial NECT shows a focal area of thickening along the right posterior lateral aspect of the bladder ➔, compatible with this patient's known history of primary transitional cell carcinoma. *(Right)* Axial fused PET/CT shows an asymmetrical focus of FDG activity correlating with the patient's primary transitional cell carcinoma ➔. Note slight misregistration of the images caused by filling of the urinary bladder during the PET portion of the exam.

PET/CT: Staging

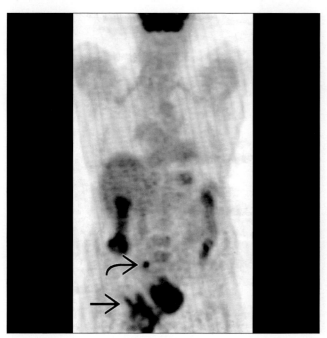 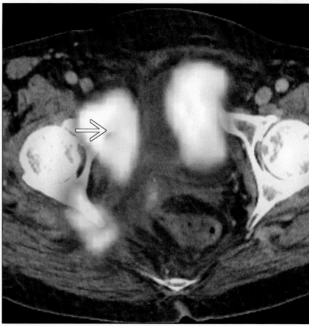

(Left) Coronal PET shows intense FDG activity correlating to the patient's primary transitional cell carcinoma of the bladder ➔. An additional focal area of intense activity ➔ is present along the right common iliac nodal chain, compatible with metastatic lymphadenopathy. *(Right)* Axial fused PET/CT shows intense FDG activity ➔ correlating to the patient's primary mass, compatible with transitional cell carcinoma.

BLADDER CARCINOMA

PET/CT: Staging

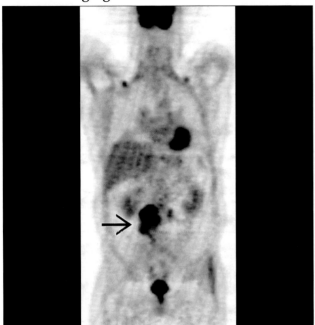 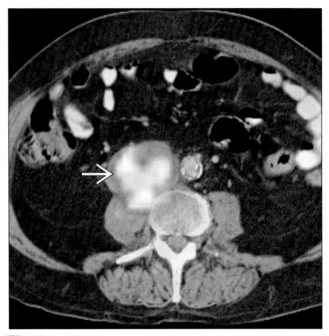

(Left) Coronal PET shows intense FDG activity in the right periaortic area ⮕ in this patient with newly diagnosed transitional cell carcinoma. *(Right)* Axial fused PET/CT shows intense FDG activity ⮕ corresponding to the metastatic adenopathy.

PET/CT Findings: Restaging

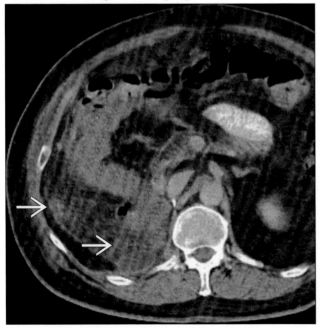 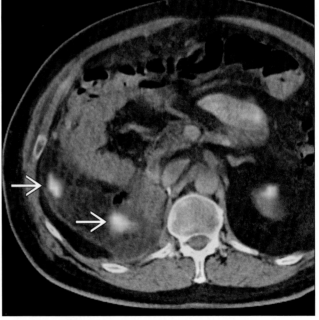

(Left) Axial CECT shows nodularity along the posterior aspect of the peritoneal surfaces ⮕ in this patient with newly diagnosed transitional cell carcinoma of the bladder. Metastatic disease involving the mesenteric and peritoneal surfaces are unusual manifestations of metastatic transitional cell carcinoma. *(Right)* Axial fused PET/CT shows areas of increased metabolic activity ⮕, compatible with malignant transitional cell carcinoma involving peritoneal surfaces as seen on the previous CT image.

BLADDER CARCINOMA

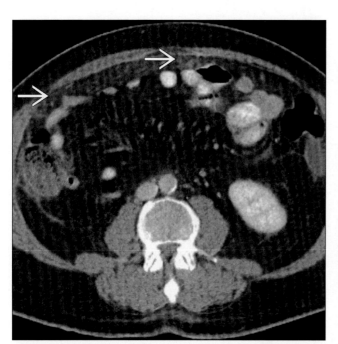 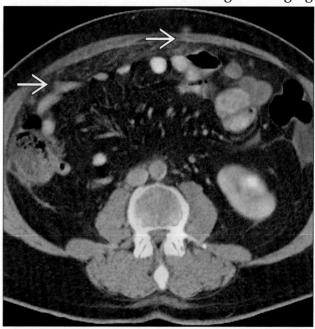

(Left) Axial CECT shows nodularity along the omentum ➔ in this patient with transitional cell carcinoma, compatible with metastatic disease. *(Right)* Axial fused PET/CT shows areas of mild to moderately increased FDG activity corresponding to the areas of omental nodularity ➔. The metabolic activity is not significantly increased, a common finding of omental/mesenteric carcinomatosis on PET.

PET/CT Findings: Restaging

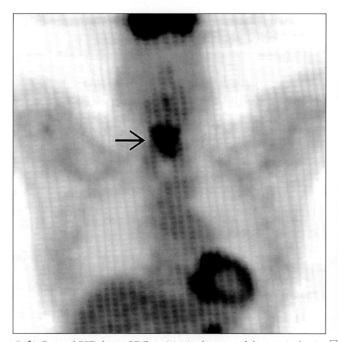 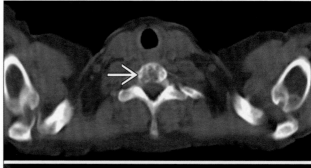 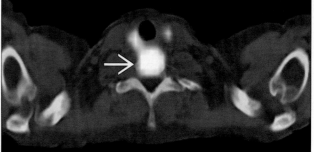

(Left) Coronal PET shows FDG activity in the area of the cervical spine ➔ in this patient with a history of transitional cell carcinoma. *(Right)* Axial NECT (top) and fused PET/CT (bottom) images demonstrate a lytic lesion in the cervical spine vertebral body ➔ with intense FDG activity, compatible with metastatic lesion.

TESTICULAR CARCINOMA

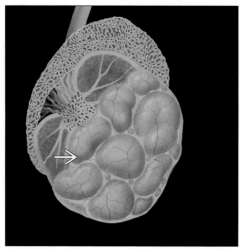

Graphic shows a large heterogeneous testicular mass ➡, compatible with testicular carcinoma.

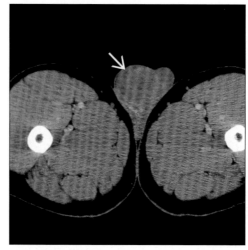

Axial CECT shows a near water density mass in the right scrotum ➡, a nonspecific finding that was diagnosed as testicular carcinoma.

TERMINOLOGY

Abbreviations and Synonyms
• Germ cell tumors (GCT): 95% of testicular carcinomas
• Non-germ cell tumors also referred to as
  ○ Gonadal stromal tumors
  ○ Interstitial cell tumors
  ○ Sex cord tumors

Definitions
• Germ cell tumors (GCT): Malignancy arising from germ cell elements
  ○ Seminomas
  ○ Teratoma/teratocarcinoma (embryonal cell)
  ○ Choriocarcinoma
• Non-germ cell tumors: Neoplasm arising from non-germ cell elements
  ○ Leydig cell tumors (LCT): From interstitial cells
  ○ Sertoli cell tumors (SCT): From sustentacular cells lining seminiferous tubules
  ○ Granulosa cell tumors: Rare, benign tumors
  ○ Gonadoblastomas: Contain both stromal and germ cell elements

IMAGING FINDINGS

General Features
• Best diagnostic clue: Palpable, intratesticular, homogeneous or mixed consistency hypoechoic mass on US
• Location
  ○ Germ cell tumors
    ▪ Local: Testis, epididymis, spermatic cord
    ▪ Regional: Retroperitoneal lymph nodes
    ▪ Distant: Supradiaphragmatic nodes or visceral sites
    ▪ Most common site of recurrence is retroperitoneum
  ○ Non-germ cell tumors: 90% local (benign), 10% metastasize
  ○ Rarely bilateral
• Size: > 5 cm indicates high stage disease
• Morphology
  ○ Germ cell tumors: Solid mass with internal heterogeneity
  ○ Non-germ cell tumors: Round, lobulated, well-circumscribed mass

DDx: Mimics of Testicular Carcinoma

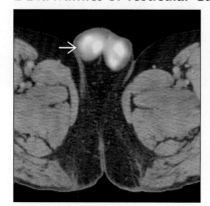

Normal Physiologic Activity

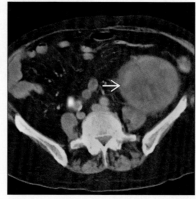

Sarcoma Metastasis

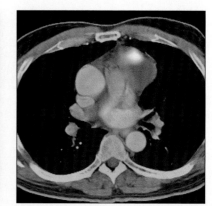

Cystic Thymic Carcinoid

TESTICULAR CARCINOMA

Key Facts

Terminology
- Germ cell tumors (GCT)
- Non-germ cell tumors
- Gonadal stromal tumors
- Interstitial cell tumors
- Sex cord tumors

Imaging Findings
- CT or MR for initial staging
- FDG PET/CT: Therapeutic response; restaging
- For seminoma, sensitivity/specificity of FDG PET are 100% and 80%, of CT are 74% and 70%
- FDG PET demonstrates PPV and NPV of 91% and 62% in differentiating tumor from non-tumor lesions in patients with non-seminomatous GCT

- FDG PET is the modality of choice to determine therapeutic response/restaging in malignant germ cell tumors
- Ultrasonography to localize mass and determine internal structure

Top Differential Diagnoses
- Epidermoid Cyst
- Lymphoma, Leukemia, Metastases
- Focal Orchitis

Diagnostic Checklist
- US for primary diagnosis
- CT or MR for initial staging
- FDG PET/CT for therapeutic response/restaging
- Testicular neoplasms may not be FDG avid
  - May lead to false negative PET; always correlate with CT

- Teratoma and choriocarcinoma often demonstrate calcification, necrosis, hemorrhage, and cystic elements

Imaging Recommendations
- Best imaging tool
  - Ultrasonography to localize mass and determine internal structure
  - CT or MR for initial staging
    - For stage I, GCT CXR may be used at diagnosis and for follow-up
  - FDG PET/CT: Restaging and response to therapy
- Protocol advice
  - High frequency linear array US including both testes

CT Findings
- CT indicated for staging of metastasis in retroperitoneum, lymph nodes, and mediastinum/lungs
  - Insensitive for undiagnosed testicular lesions
  - Especially useful when metastatic disease in thorax is suspected
- Lymphoma and metastatic testicular cancer may have similar appearance
  - Obtain tissue sample from abnormal testicle
- Lymph nodes
  - Typical locations for malignant involvement include left renal hilus and retrocaval area
  - Low attenuation, poorly enhancing nodes in these regions suspicious even when small
- Residual low attenuation masses after treatment
  - Lesions > 3 cm 4 weeks after chemotherapy have 30% chance of harboring viable tumor
  - Surgical resection recommended > 3 cm
- Recurrence most common in retroperitoneum; CT may identify "growing teratoma" syndrome

Nuclear Medicine Findings
- **Initial diagnosis**
  - Limited data on FDG PET evaluation of malignant non-germ cell tumors is available
  - Sensitivity/specificity for seminoma
    - FDG PET: 100% and 80%

- CT: 74% and 70%
  - SUV > 3 used as cutoff for suspicion of malignancy in primary testicular tumor
- **Staging**
  - For initial staging of testicular germ cell tumors, FDG PET offers no statistical advantage over CT
  - FDG PET demonstrates positive predictive value (PPV) and negative predictive value (NPV) of 91% and 62% in differentiating tumor from non-tumor lesions in patients with non-seminomatous GCT
    - Negative FDG PET studies may not exclude presence of disease (due largely to presence of teratoma)
    - Residual masses with negative FDG PET usually still require surgical resection
    - Additional FDG PET exams are without benefit in cases of elevated tumor markers and tumor progression diagnosed by CT
  - FDG PET useful for identifying stage IIA in clinical stage I non-seminomatous GCT patients
- **Restaging**
  - Anterior mediastinum: Normal thymic uptake may be mistaken for disease recurrence
  - Tumor marker elevation in the absence of CT changes should prompt PET scan for possibility of salvage surgery
  - Overall, FDG PET is the best predictor of viable seminoma in residual masses after chemotherapy
    - Also useful in non-seminomatous GCT patients
    - Masses with residual malignancy may appear negative on PET 10-14 days after chemotherapy ("stunned" tumor)
  - Post-therapy non-seminomatous GCT
    - Difficult to differentiate mature teratoma from necrosis or scar
    - Both entities have low FDG uptake
    - Non-standard dynamic imaging: Kinetic parameter for FDG transport in mature teratoma higher than those for necrosis/scar
  - Longitudinal follow-up required for late relapse patients, even with negative FDG PET scan

TESTICULAR CARCINOMA

o In complicated multiple-relapse seminoma patients, use of FDG PET has been shown to change decision on therapy in 57% of cases
• **Response to therapy**
  o FDG PET is the modality of choice for determining therapeutic response/restaging in malignant germ cell tumors
    ▪ Best predictor of viable residual seminoma in post-chemotherapy masses
  o Negative FDG PET excludes presence of viable tumor for lesions > 3 cm
    ▪ Sensitivity 80%, specificity 100%, PPV 100%, NPV 96%
    ▪ Compares to 74%, 70%, 34%, 92% for CT
    ▪ Lesions < 3 cm: Sensitivity/specificity 25% and 100%
  o FDG PET predicts response to therapy of germ cell tumors
    ▪ Mean SUV of nonresponders: 2.7
    ▪ Mean SUV of responders: 1.8
    ▪ PPV/NPV of FDG PET in patients with raised tumor markers and negative CT: 92% and 50%
    ▪ PPV/NPV for patients with residual mass: 96% and 90%

DIFFERENTIAL DIAGNOSIS

Focal Orchitis
• FDG uptake due to infection/inflammation
• Presents with pain/tenderness

Subacute Hematoma
• FDG uptake seen due to inflammatory response in subacute setting
• Correlates with history of trauma
• Associated hematocele with no flow on color Doppler

Epidermoid Cyst
• Concentric rings of hypoechogenicity and hyperechogenicity on US ("onion ring" appearance)
• Cystic cavity lined by stratified squamous epithelium with variable peripheral calcification
• Normally no FDG uptake

Sarcoidosis
• 100x higher risk of sarcoidosis in patients with testicular cancer
• Classic finding is enlargement of bilateral hilar lymph nodes
• Granulomatous disease may be positive on FDG PET scans

Lymphoma, Leukemia, Metastases
• Often have intense FDG uptake compared to testicular tumors
  o Otherwise indistinguishable from primary testicular cancer
• High incidence of bilateral disease (~ 50%)
• Most common testicular cancer in men > age 60 years
• Look for flow on color Doppler

PATHOLOGY

General Features
• General path comments
  o Germ cell tumor accounts for 95% of testicular cancer
    ▪ 40-50% seminomas
    ▪ 35% multiple subtypes
    ▪ 25% embryonal cell (teratocarcinoma)
    ▪ 5-10% teratoma
  o Non-germ cell tumor accounts for 4-5% of testicular cancer
    ▪ In children it accounts for 10-30% of testicular cancer
  o Leydig cell tumors
    ▪ Generally benign (90%)
    ▪ Presence of metastases indicates more aggressive disease
    ▪ May produce testosterone
  o Sertoli cell tumors
    ▪ Generally benign (85-90%)
    ▪ May produce estrogen or Müllerian inhibiting factors
• Genetics
  o Histologic discordance among sibling pairs is greater than discordance among identical twins
    ▪ Suggests familial grouping
  o Mutations in 12p chromosomal segment associated with malignant development
• Etiology
  o Infection
    ▪ Epstein-Barr, human T-cell leukemia virus type 1, hepatitis C virus
    ▪ Helicobacter pylori associated with development of primary GI lymphoma
  o Environmental factors: Industrial chemicals (pesticides, solvents, hair dye), chemotherapy, and radiation
  o Congenital immunodeficiency states: SCID, Wiskott-Aldrich, AIDS
  o Autoimmune disorders (2° inflammation): Sjögren, Hashimoto thyroiditis
  o Cryptorchidism: 10-40x higher risk
  o Testicular microlithiasis (> 5 microcalcifications within a testicle): Risk of malignancy unclear
• Epidemiology
  o Germ cell tumors
    ▪ Account for majority of cancer in males age 15-35
    ▪ Comprise 1% of all cancers in men
  o Seminoma occurs most commonly between ages 35-39
    ▪ Rare before age 10
    ▪ Pure seminoma comprises 60% of all GCTs
    ▪ Incidence of seminoma has doubled in last 30 years
  o Non-germ cell tumors: Age 30-60 years; 25% before puberty
    ▪ Patients aged 30-60 years
    ▪ 25% occur before puberty
  o Lymphoma: Most common testicular tumor over age 50
• Associated abnormalities

TESTICULAR CARCINOMA

- o Germ cell tumors
  - Gynecomastia (choriocarcinoma)
  - Prepubescent virilization
- o Non-germ cell tumors
  - Prepubescent virilization
  - Feminization

Staging, Grading, or Classification Criteria

- International Germ Cell Cancer Collaborative Group staging system
  - o Based on sites of disease and serum tumor marker levels (alpha-fetoprotein [AFP], beta HCG, LDH)
- **Stage I (A):** Tumor confined to testis
- **Stage II (B):** Metastatic to nodes below diaphragm
- **Stage IIA (B1):** Retroperitoneal node mets < 2 cm (5 cm^3)
- **Stage IIB (B2):** Retroperitoneal node mets 2-5 cm (10 cm^3)
- **Stage IIC (B3):** Retroperitoneal node mets > 5 cm
- **Stage III (C):** Mets to lymph nodes above diaphragm
- **Stage IIIA (C1):** Mets confined to lymphatic system
- **Stage IIIB (IV):** Extranodal mets
- Definition of true stage I disease in non-seminomatous GCT is extremely important
  - o True stage I can undergo surveillance only
  - o FDG PET has a clear role in these patients

CLINICAL ISSUES

Presentation

- Most common signs/symptoms
  - o Primary disease: Painless testicular mass (present with pain in 30-40%)
  - o Metastatic disease: Back pain, cough, hemoptysis
- Other signs/symptoms
  - o GCT: Tumor markers include AFP, beta-HCG, and LDH
    - Used for diagnosis, staging, prognosis, and response to therapy
    - AFP: Secreted only by non-seminomatous tumor
    - Beta-HCG: Associated with gynecomastia, nipple tenderness
    - LDH: Levels correlate with aggressiveness of tumor

Demographics

- Age
  - o Malignant LCT seen only in adults
  - o SCT may occur in all ages (1/3 < 12 years)
- Ethnicity: Caucasian > > African-American

Natural History & Prognosis

- Surgery and radiotherapy provide cure for 97% of stage I seminoma patients
- Introduction of cisplatin-based chemotherapy regimens in the 1970s improved cure rate dramatically
- Modern imaging detects residual masses in up to 80% of patients 1 month after completion of chemotherapy
  - o Following treatment of primary disease, up to 30% of patients have residual masses
  - o In non-seminomatous GCT, these may contain tumor, fibrosis/necrosis, or mature teratoma

Treatment

- **Germ cell tumors**
  - o Inguinal/radical orchiectomy
  - o High rate of occult retroperitoneal involvement in stage I disease → retroperitoneal nodal dissection
  - o Chemoradiotherapy for metastatic disease
    - Seminoma: Para-aortic radiotherapy with chemo
    - Cisplatin, etoposide, and bleomycin
    - ~ 35% of patients who undergo chemotherapy for GCT become sterile, and sperm-banking is offered
- **Non-germ cell tumors**
  - o Orchiectomy or testis-sparing surgery
  - o Treatment of metastases similar to GCT

DIAGNOSTIC CHECKLIST

Consider

- Primary diagnosis: US
- Initial staging: CT or MR
- Baseline PET/CT will help establish FDG avidity of the primary tumor
- Restaging and response to therapy: PET/CT
- Patients are often over- or understaged with seminoma; accurate staging is crucial for appropriate treatment

Image Interpretation Pearls

- Testicular neoplasms may not be FDG avid
  - o May lead to false negative PET; always correlate with CT

SELECTED REFERENCES

1. Haba Y et al: Stage migration and pilot studies of reduced chemotherapy supported by positron-emission tomography findings suggest new combined strategies for stage 2 nonseminoma germ cell tumour. BJU Int. 101(5):570-4, 2008
2. Hinz S et al: The role of positron emission tomography in the evaluation of residual masses after chemotherapy for advanced stage seminoma. J Urol. 179(3):936-40; discussion 940, 2008
3. Huddart RA et al: 18fluorodeoxyglucose positron emission tomography in the prediction of relapse in patients with high-risk, clinical stage I nonseminomatous germ cell tumors: preliminary report of MRC Trial TE22--the NCRI Testis Tumour Clinical Study Group. J Clin Oncol. 25(21):3090-5, 2007
4. Bridges B et al: Testicular germ cell tumors. Curr Opin Oncol. 18(3):271-6, 2006
5. Dalal PU et al: Imaging of testicular germ cell tumours. Cancer Imaging. 6:124-34, 2006
6. Lewis DA et al: Positron emission tomography scans in postchemotherapy seminoma patients with residual masses: a retrospective review from Indiana University Hospital. J Clin Oncol. 24(34):e54-5, 2006
7. Becherer A et al: FDG PET is superior to CT in the prediction of viable tumour in post-chemotherapy seminoma residuals. Eur J Radiol. 54(2):284-8, 2005
8. De Giorgi U et al: FDG-PET in the management of germ cell tumor. Ann Oncol. 16 Suppl 4:iv90-94, 2005
9. Hussain A: Germ cell tumors. Curr Opin Oncol. 17(3):268-74, 2005

TESTICULAR CARCINOMA

CT Findings: Primary

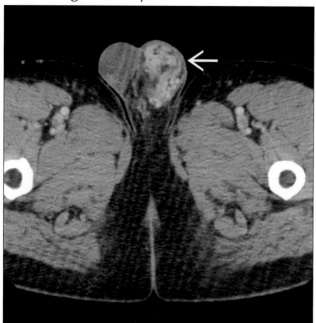 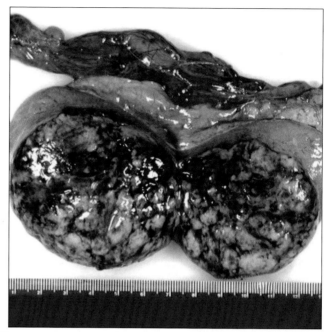

(Left) Axial CECT shows a complex enhancing mass in the left scrotum →, compatible with testicular carcinoma. *(Right)* Gross pathology from the mass in the previous image shows the irregular appearance of testicular carcinoma.

CT Findings: Regional Metastases

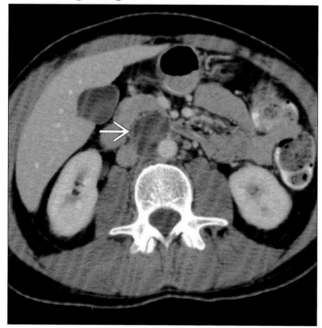 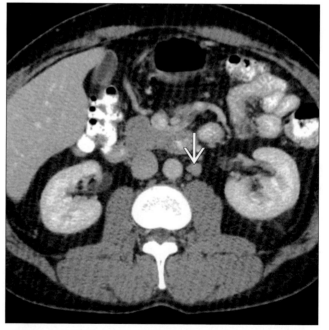

(Left) Axial CECT shows a necrotic nodal mass → in the aortocaval region. *(Right)* Axial CECT shows a borderline enlarged lymph node → at the level of the right renal hilum. Following retroperitoneal dissection, the node was shown to represent metastatic testicular cancer.

TESTICULAR CARCINOMA

CT Findings: Metastases

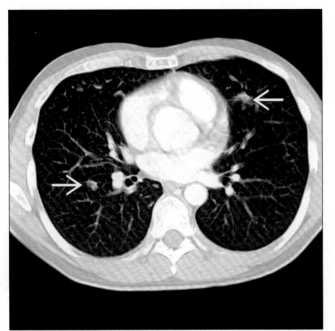 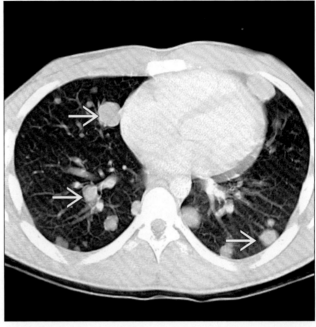

(Left) Axial CECT shows pulmonary nodules in both lungs ➡, consistent with metastatic disease. *(Right)* Axial CECT shows increase in the size of the pulmonary nodules ➡, compatible with worsening disease.

CT Findings: Metastases

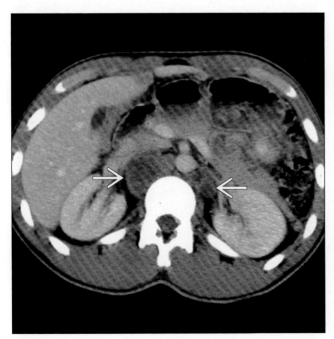 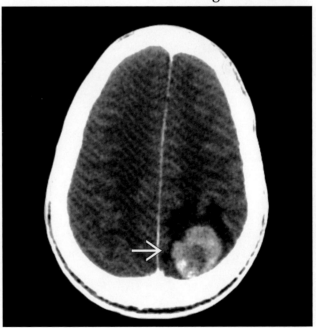

(Left) Axial CECT shows large retroperitoneal nodes, which are partly necrotic in the retrocaval and peri-aortic regions ➡, characteristic of testicular carcinoma metastases. *(Right)* Axial CECT of the head reveals a large left parietal metastasis with surrounding vasogenic edema ➡ in this patient with a brain metastasis from testicular carcinoma.

TESTICULAR CARCINOMA

PET/CT Findings: Staging

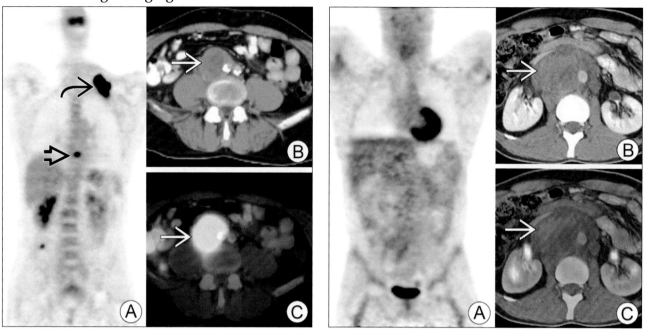

(Left) Coronal PET (A), axial CT (B) and fused PET/CT (C) in a patient recently diagnosed with testicular carcinoma show a left supraclavicular lesion ➔, a paraspinal metastasis ➔, and extensive retroperitoneal hypermetabolic metastases ➔. *(Right)* Coronal PET (A), axial CT (B) and PET/CT (C) in a patient with recently diagnosed germ cell tumor show large retroperitoneal metastases ➔ with only minimally increased FDG activity, a characteristic finding on FDG PET.

PET/CT Findings: Staging

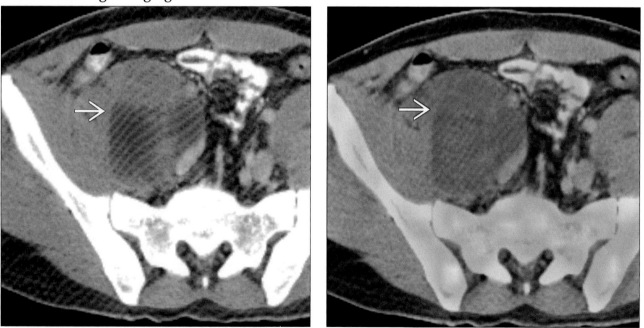

(Left) Axial CECT shows large heterogeneously enhancing right pelvic metastasis ➔ with central necrosis in a patient with newly diagnosed germ cell malignancy of the testis. *(Right)* Axial fused PET/CT shows only minimally increased FDG activity ➔ within the non-necrotic areas. Testicular neoplasms may demonstrate only mild to moderately increased FDG activity.

TESTICULAR CARCINOMA

PET/CT Findings: Restaging

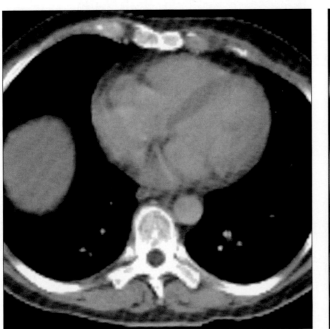 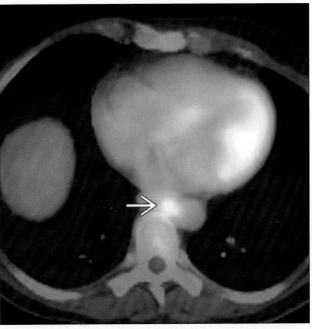

(Left) Axial CECT shows no definite abnormality to suggest metastatic disease in this patient with a history of testicular carcinoma. (Right) Axial fused PET/CT shows a focal area of intense FDG activity in the left posterior mediastinum ➡, compatible with metastatic disease.

Typical

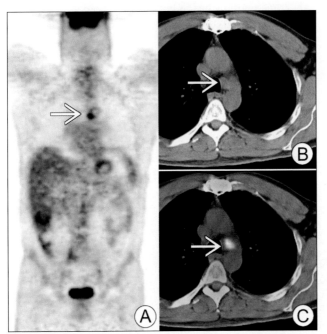 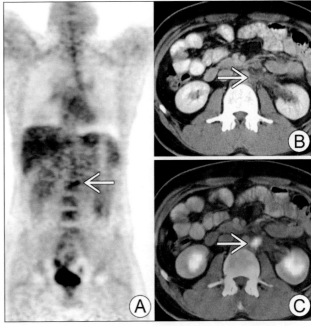

(Left) Coronal PET (A), axial CT (B) and fused PET/CT (C) in a patient with known testicular germ cell tumor show a new focus of intense FDG activity ➡ in the AP window, interpreted as suspicious for metastatic disease. Subsequent thoracotomy and resection confirmed metastatic disease. (Right) Coronal PET (A), axial CT (B) and fused PET/CT (C) of a patient with a history of testicular seminoma show borderline enlarged, but recurrent, malignant left para-aortic lymph nodes ➡.

OVARIAN CARCINOMA

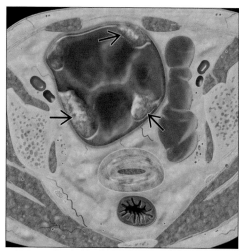

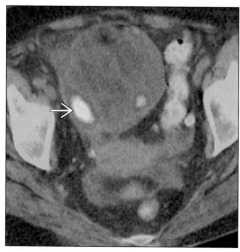

Axial graphic shows a heterogeneous pelvic mass with areas of central necrosis and peripheral areas of nodularity ⟹, compatible with ovarian carcinoma.

Axial fused PET/CT shows the areas of peripheral nodularity ⟹ with intense activity.

TERMINOLOGY

Abbreviations and Synonyms
- Ovarian carcinoma, carcinoma of the ovary, ovarian cancer

Definitions
- Primary malignancy of ovary
  - Epithelial (90%)
    - Arises from germinal epithelium on outside of ovary
  - Stromal (6%)
    - Arises from connective tissue
    - Low rate of metastasis
  - Germ cell (3%)
    - Teens/young women
    - Highly curable
- Staging of ovarian cancer
  - Stage I: Confined to one or both ovaries
  - Stage II: Spread to uterus/fallopian tube, within pelvis
  - Stage III: Lymph nodes, abdominal cavity
  - Stage IV: Outside abdomen, intrahepatic metastases

IMAGING FINDINGS

General Features
- Best diagnostic clue: Solid or complex cystic mass arising from ovary ± ascites
- Location
  - Primary generally found in ovary
  - Metastases most common to peritoneum, omentum
  - Rare intrahepatic metastases
  - Three main routes of lymphatic spread
    - Accompanying ovarian blood vessels cranially to para-aortic and paracaval nodes
    - Following subovarian plexus in broad ligament to obturator and pelvic nodes
    - Following round ligament to external iliac and inguinal nodes
- Size
  - Variable
    - However, most ovarian carcinoma detected late, so tumors tend to be large

Imaging Recommendations
- Best imaging tool

DDx: FDG-Avid Pelvic Mass

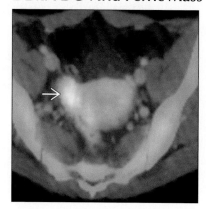

Physiologic

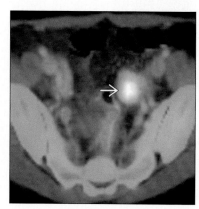

Corpus Luteal Cyst

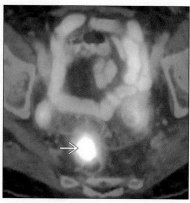

Metastasis

OVARIAN CARCINOMA

Key Facts

Terminology
- Ovarian cancer, carcinoma of the ovary

Imaging Findings
- Solid or complex cystic mass arising from ovary ± ascites
- Metastases most common to peritoneum, omentum
- Primary lesion usually complex cystic mass with mural nodularity
- In general, malignancy suggested by thickness and irregularity of cavity walls, septae, enhancing nodules
- Sensitivity 92% for peritoneal metastases
- Pure mucinous adenocarcinoma more likely to be falsely negative by standard SUV criteria due to low cellularity and better differentiation properties
- PET limited in detecting lymph node micrometastases

- In one study, PET/CT failed to identify microscopic disease in 59% of pathologically positive lymph nodes
- PET/CT: Sensitivity > 95%, specificity 80-93%, and positive predictive value of 83-94% for detection of recurrence

Top Differential Diagnoses
- Pelvic Inflammatory Disease
- Tubo-Ovarian Abscess
- Complex Functional Cysts
- Benign Ovarian Tumors
- Borderline Ovarian Tumors

Diagnostic Checklist
- PET/CT valuable in patient with rising CA-125, negative anatomic imaging

---

- o Most common: Transvaginal ultrasound followed by MR &/or CT for evaluation of metastasis
  - Risk of malignancy index (RMI) calculated using transvaginal ultrasound results, CA-125 blood level, menopausal status
- o Consider PET/CT for most complete staging
  - Especially use PET/CT for suspected recurrence, particularly with mild rise in CA-125
- Protocol advice: Consider using contrast-enhanced CT as part of the PET/CT scan

CT Findings
- Primary lesion usually complex cystic mass with mural nodularity
- In general, malignancy suggested by thickness and irregularity of cavity walls, septae, enhancing nodules
- Sensitivity 92% for peritoneal metastases
- GI contrast especially helpful for distinguishing pelvic viscera from intestinal tract
- Primary use of CT scanning is to evaluate metastatic disease, not ovarian mass
  - o For evaluation of the ovarian mass, ultrasonography and MR are more valuable
- CT scanning is helpful in diagnosing cystic teratomas, 93% of which contain fat and 56% of which are calcified
  - o If a large (> 10 cm) soft tissue mass is present, malignant transformation should be suspected
- Serous cystadenoma has an attenuation similar to that of water
  - o But mucinous cystadenoma has an attenuation closer to that of soft tissue
- CT imaging has much greater sensitivity than techniques used previously
  - o Detects 2-3 mm lesions in the lungs and solid viscera
- Scans with contrast yield high-quality information about retroperitoneal lymph nodes and ureters
- Low contrast between peritoneal tumors and adjacent soft tissues limits overall sensitivity
  - o MR sensitivity in this case 91%

- But limited in depiction of small calcified peritoneal implants, which are common in patients with serous carcinoma
- NECT
  - o Cystic adnexal mass with septations and soft tissue density papillary projections
- CECT
  - o Solid mural nodules demonstrate enhancement
  - o May facilitate detection of peritoneal implants and distant metastases
- CT angiogram: Can be used to assess vascular invasion

Nuclear Medicine Findings
- **Initial diagnosis**
  - o FDG PET almost never used to evaluate an adnexal mass or to evaluate for primary ovarian carcinoma
  - o Pure mucinous adenocarcinoma more likely to be falsely negative by standard SUV criteria, due to low cellularity and better differentiation properties
- **Staging**
  - o Not currently covered by Medicare
  - o Three lymph node stations with high rate of false positives: Axillary, inguinal, hilar
  - o PET limited in detecting lymph node micrometastases
    - In one study, PET/CT failed to identify microscopic disease in 59% of pathologically positive lymph nodes
  - o Also limited for differentiating peritoneal tumors from adjacent soft tissue or bowel activity
- **Restaging**
  - o PET/CT: Sensitivity > 95%, specificity 80-93%, and positive predictive value of 83-94% for detection of recurrence
  - o PET has 6-8 mm limit of resolution
    - Limited in detection of small disseminated lesions (e.g., peritoneal carcinosis and mesenteric or omental recurrences)
  - o Degenerative change in pelvis, such as sacroiliac arthritis, has been mistaken for recurrence
    - Active degenerative change in bone can have ↑ FDG activity

OVARIAN CARCINOMA

○ For detection of ovarian cancer recurrence mean sensitivity, specificity, and accuracy each 83%
○ In one study of patients with primarily subcentimeter lesions, sensitivity of FDG PET for recurrence was only 10%
  ▪ With mean lesion size of 1.1 cm, patient-based sensitivity 81%
- **Response to therapy**
  ○ Paucity of studies in the literature; not currently covered or recommended for evaluating response to therapy

DIFFERENTIAL DIAGNOSIS

Pelvic Inflammatory Disease
- CT findings nonspecific
- Disrupted fat planes
- Thickened fascial planes

Tubo-Ovarian Abscess
- Commonly depicted as regular mass with debris similar to that seen with endometrioma or hemorrhagic cyst

Complex Functional Cysts
- May have intense FDG activity

Benign Ovarian Tumors
- Includes cystadenoma, dermoid tumors

Borderline Ovarian Tumors
- Pathologically difficult to differentiate between benign and malignant
- Low malignant potential

Normal Physiologic FDG Activity
- Mostly in younger premenopausal women
- Helpful if bilateral physiologic activity present
- Look for CT findings of corpus luteal cyst: Rind of enhancement in an otherwise normal-appearing ovary

PATHOLOGY

General Features
- General path comments
  ○ Ovarian cancer spreads primarily intraperitoneally as well as to lymph nodes
    ▪ Peritoneal fluid flows upward from pelvis to paracolic gutters and subphrenic regions, carrying tumor cells that implant on abdominal viscera
  ○ Common sites of metastatic implantation
    ▪ Pelvis
    ▪ Right hemidiaphragm
    ▪ Perihepatic
    ▪ Right paracolic gutter
    ▪ Bowel
    ▪ Omentum
  ○ Distant lymph nodes are involved in approximately 7% of cases of serous ovarian adenocarcinoma
- Genetics
  ○ 10% of patients with ovarian cancer appear to have genetic predisposition

○ These patients may develop cancer early, between ages 30 and 50
○ One study suggested patients with BRCA gene have 60% risk of developing ovarian cancer
- Etiology
  ○ Unknown
  ○ Number of reproductive cycles appears to be related to risk
  ○ Ovulation suppression may decrease cancer incidence
- Epidemiology
  ○ Leading cause of death among women with gynecological malignancies
  ○ Third most common cancer of female reproductive organs

Microscopic Features
- Most common histologies are papillary serous adenocarcinoma and endometrioid type
- Serous adenocarcinoma comprises 40% of epithelial ovarian cancers
- Psammoma bodies may be present
  ○ Ovarian cancer with multiple psammoma bodies may have better prognosis

CLINICAL ISSUES

Presentation
- Most common signs/symptoms
  ○ Early stage: Nonspecific, pelvic pain
    ▪ Often attributed to other causes (e.g., menstruation, irritable bowel syndrome)
  ○ With metastases: Abdominal/pelvic bloating, pain, pressure, early satiety, nausea/vomiting, frequent urination, feeling similar to pregnancy
- Other signs/symptoms
  ○ CA-125 has accuracy of 79-95% for recurrence; increase precedes apparent recurrence by 3-6 months
  ○ Doubling of CA-125 above normal limit has been shown to have sensitivity of 85.9% and specificity of 91.3% for detection of recurrence

Demographics
- Age: Average age at diagnosis 57 years
- Ethnicity: More common among Caucasians than African-Americans

Natural History & Prognosis
- Most patients asymptomatic until disease is in advanced stage
- In 75-80% of patients, cancer has spread beyond ovary at diagnosis
- Overall survival approximately 35%
- Despite clinical advances and improved surgery, overall survival has not changed because the disease presents at advanced stage
  ○ 75% of patients are diagnosed in stage III/IV, and in this group the 5 year survival rate is 17%
- Up to 85% of women ultimately relapse
- Well-known that patients with advanced ovarian cancer have better outcome when neoadjuvant chemotherapy is performed before surgery

OVARIAN CARCINOMA

- Up to 24% of ovarian tumors in premenopausal women are malignant and up to 60% in postmenopausal women

Treatment
- Surgery, chemotherapy, radiation therapy; depends on stage of disease, institution where treated
  - Surgery for earlier stages: Total abdominal hysterectomy, bilateral oophorectomy, omentectomy, biopsy of lymph nodes/tissues
  - Surgery for later stages: Early stage surgery plus tumor debulking
  - Chemotherapy: Paclitaxel &/or platinum-based drugs
  - Radiation therapy: Stage II
- Exploratory laparotomy done for high suspicion of malignancy
  - Only 1 ovarian cancer detected for every 8-9 benign cyst operations
- Benefit of optimal primary cytoreductive debulking surgery is well established
- Following debulking surgery, stage IV patients have same median survival as stage III patients
- 75% of women have complete clinical response, but the majority of these will experience recurrence

DIAGNOSTIC CHECKLIST

Consider
- Benign increased FDG uptake in ovaries can mimic ovarian primary malignancy
  - Look for other signs of ovarian malignancy (ascites, peritoneal implants, lymphadenopathy)
- PET/CT valuable in patient with rising CA-125, negative anatomic imaging
  - Some claim PET is as valuable for detection of recurrence as second-look surgery and may be substituted as noninvasive option
- PET/CT valuable to distinguish post-surgical change from recurrence

Image Interpretation Pearls
- Serous adenocarcinoma may contain microcalcifications that can be confused with old granulomatous disease
- Incidence of groin metastases less than 3%; isolated inguinal nodal metastasis without other nodal involvement very rare

SELECTED REFERENCES

1. Hillner BE et al: Impact of positron emission tomography/computed tomography and positron emission tomography (PET) alone on expected management of patients with cancer: initial results from the National Oncologic PET Registry. J Clin Oncol. 26(13):2155-61, 2008
2. Reinhardt MJ: Gynecologic tumors. Recent Results Cancer Res. 170:141-50, 2008
3. Risum S et al: Prediction of suboptimal primary cytoreduction in primary ovarian cancer with combined positron emission tomography/computed tomography--a prospective study. Gynecol Oncol. 108(2):265-70, 2008
4. Sebastian S et al: PET-CT vs. CT alone in ovarian cancer recurrence. Abdom Imaging. 33(1):112-8, 2008
5. Soussan M et al: Impact of FDG PET-CT imaging on the decision making in the biologic suspicion of ovarian carcinoma recurrence. Gynecol Oncol. 108(1):160-5, 2008
6. Castellucci P et al: Diagnostic accuracy of 18F-FDG PET/CT in characterizing ovarian lesions and staging ovarian cancer: correlation with transvaginal ultrasonography, computed tomography, and histology. Nucl Med Commun. 28(8):589-95, 2007
7. Cho SM et al: 18F-fluorodeoxyglucose positron emission tomography in patients with recurrent ovarian cancer: in comparison with vascularity, Ki-67, p53, and histologic grade. Eur Radiol. 17(2):409-17, 2007
8. Chung HH et al: Role of [18F]FDG PET/CT in the assessment of suspected recurrent ovarian cancer: correlation with clinical or histological findings. Eur J Nucl Med Mol Imaging. 34(4):480-6, 2007
9. Fanti S et al: PET in genitourinary tract cancers. Q J Nucl Med Mol Imaging. 51(3):260-71, 2007
10. Gadducci A et al: Surveillance procedures for patients treated for epithelial ovarian cancer: a review of the literature. Int J Gynecol Cancer. 17(1):21-31, 2007
11. García-Velloso MJ et al: Diagnostic accuracy of FDG PET in the follow-up of platinum-sensitive epithelial ovarian carcinoma. Eur J Nucl Med Mol Imaging. 34(9):1396-405, 2007
12. Goonewardene TI et al: Management of asymptomatic patients on follow-up for ovarian cancer with rising CA-125 concentrations. Lancet Oncol. 8(9):813-21, 2007
13. Iyer RB et al: PET/CT and cross sectional imaging of gynecologic malignancy. Cancer Imaging. 7 Spec No A:S130-8, 2007
14. Ju W et al: Discrepancy between magnetic resonance and 18F-fluorodeoxyglucose positron emission tomography imaging in a case of borderline ovarian tumor. Int J Gynecol Cancer. 17(5):1031-3, 2007
15. Kim CK et al: Detection of recurrent ovarian cancer at MRI: comparison with integrated PET/CT. J Comput Assist Tomogr. 31(6):868-75, 2007
16. Lai CH et al: Positron emission tomography imaging for gynecologic malignancy. Curr Opin Obstet Gynecol. 19(1):37-41, 2007
17. Lutz AM et al: 2-deoxy-2-[F-18]fluoro-D-glucose accumulation in ovarian carcinoma cell lines. Mol Imaging Biol. 9(5):260-6, 2007
18. Mangili G et al: Integrated PET/CT as a first-line re-staging modality in patients with suspected recurrence of ovarian cancer. Eur J Nucl Med Mol Imaging. 34(5):658-66, 2007
19. Mironov S et al: Ovarian cancer. Radiol Clin North Am. 45(1):149-66, 2007
20. Risum S et al: The diagnostic value of PET/CT for primary ovarian cancer--a prospective study. Gynecol Oncol. 105(1):145-9, 2007
21. Thrall MM et al: Clinical use of combined positron emission tomography and computed tomography (FDG-PET/CT) in recurrent ovarian cancer. Gynecol Oncol. 105(1):17-22, 2007
22. Hama Y: Positron emission tomography with 18F-fluoro-2-deoxyglucose for the detection of recurrent ovarian cancer. Int J Clin Oncol. 11(3):250-1, 2006
23. Yang QM et al: The diagnostic value of PET-CT for peritoneal dissemination of abdominal malignancies. Gan To Kagaku Ryoho. 33(12):1817-21, 2006
24. Yen TC et al: Positron emission tomography in gynecologic cancer. Semin Nucl Med. 36(1):93-104, 2006
25. Ames J et al: 18F-FDG uptake in an ovary containing a hemorrhagic corpus luteal cyst: false-positive PET/CT in a patient with cervical carcinoma. AJR Am J Roentgenol. 185(4):1057-9, 2005

OVARIAN CARCINOMA

CT Findings

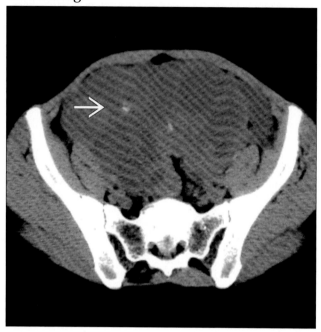 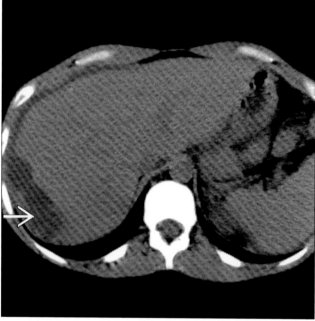

(Left) Axial NECT shows an irregular mixed cystic and solid mass ➡ with thickened septae and foci of calcification, a typical appearance of metastatic ovarian carcinoma. *(Right)* Axial NECT shows low attenuation material ➡ adjacent to the lateral margin of the liver, compatible with metastatic disease.

CT Findings

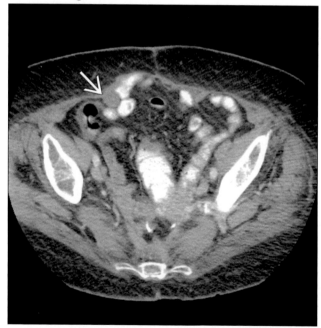 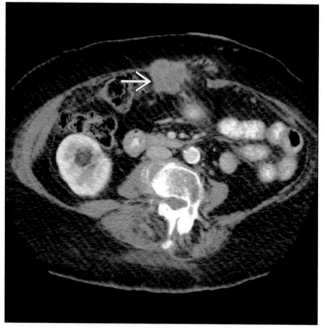

(Left) Axial CECT shows an abnormal nodular density ➡ in the right lower quadrant, consistent with ovarian carcinoma metastasis. *(Right)* Axial CECT shows an irregular peripherally enhancing mass at the ventral aspect of the abdominal wall ➡, consistent with metastasis.

OVARIAN CARCINOMA

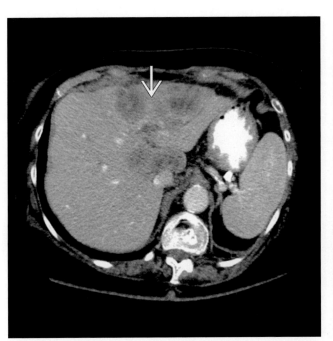 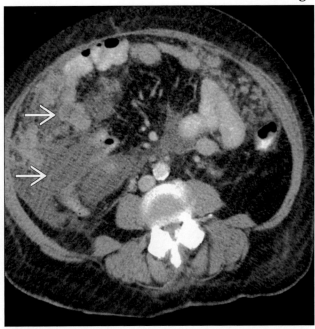

(Left) Axial CECT demonstrates a heterogeneously enhancing hepatic mass ➡, shown in this patient to be metastatic ovarian carcinoma. *(Right)* Axial CECT shows gelatinous ascites and a nodular metastases ➡ in the right abdomen, consistent with omental metastasis and pseudomyxoma peritonei from ovarian cancer.

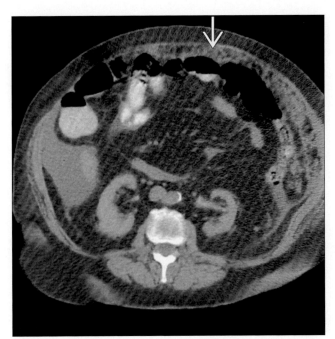 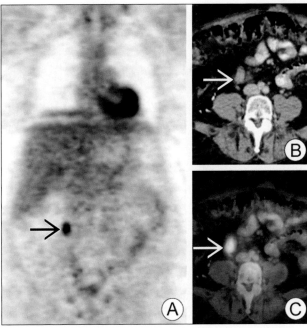

(Left) Axial NECT shows "omental caking" ➡, a characteristic finding of ovarian carcinoma metastases. *(Right)* Coronal PET (A) shows focal intense activity ➡ localized to a borderline enlarged retroperitoneal lymph node ➡ on axial CT (B) and fused PET/CT (C) in this patient with a history of ovarian carcinoma.

OVARIAN CARCINOMA

Restaging

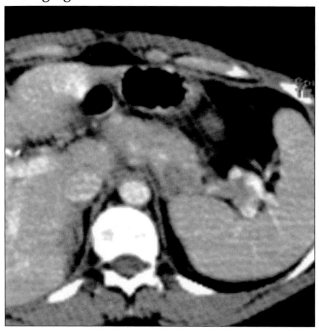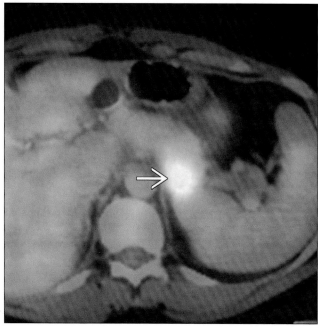

(Left) Axial CECT of a patient with a mild rise in CA-125 shows no definite evidence for malignancy. *(Right)* Axial fused PET/CT shows focal intense activity ➡ along the gastrosplenic ligament, very worrisome for recurrent ovarian carcinoma.

Restaging

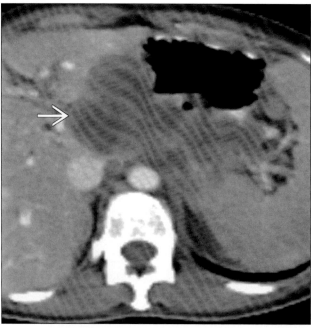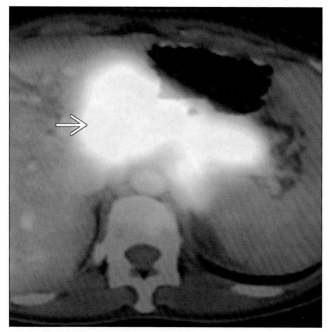

(Left) Axial CECT performed approximately 8 months later in the same patient as the previous two images shows extensive mesenteric/peritoneal disease ➡. *(Right)* Axial fused PET/CT shows diffusely increased intense metabolic activity throughout the large mesenteric/peritoneal mass ➡, compatible with recurrent ovarian carcinoma.

OVARIAN CARCINOMA

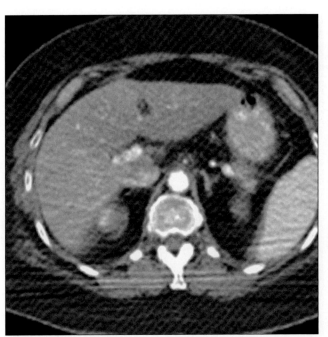 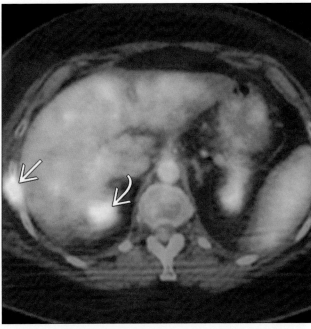

(Left) Axial CECT shows no obvious evidence for recurrent disease. *(Right)* Axial fused PET/CT shows a focal area of intense FDG activity in the right posterolateral abdominal wall musculature, compatible with recurrent disease. Also visible on this image is the superior pole ➡ of the right kidney ➡.

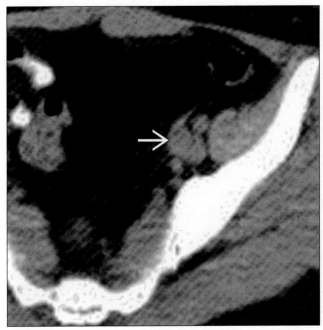 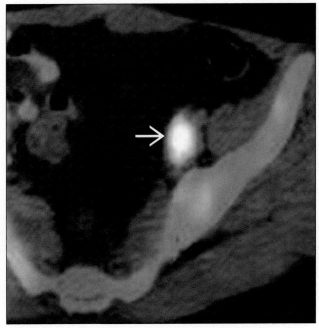

(Left) Axial NECT shows a borderline enlarged left pelvic lymph node ➡ in this patient with a mild rising tumor marker. *(Right)* Axial fused PET/CT shows focal intense activity correlating with the borderline enlarged equivocal node ➡ in the left hemipelvis, compatible with malignancy.

OVARIAN CARCINOMA

Restaging

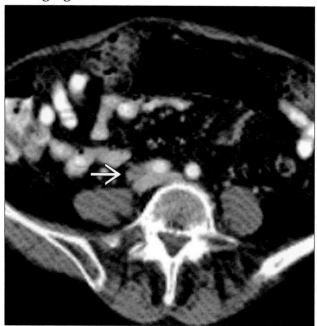 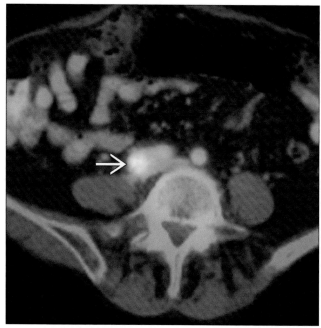

(Left) Axial CECT shows a subtle borderline enlarged right common iliac lymph node ➔, interpreted as equivocal on a recent CT scan (not shown). *(Right)* Axial fused PET/CT shows focal intense activity correlating with the right common iliac lymph node ➔, raising the confidence level of the interpreting physician.

Restaging

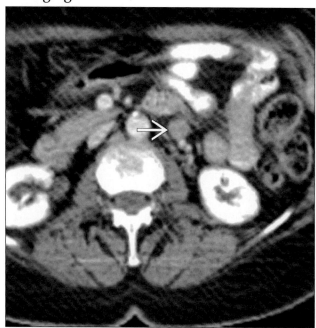 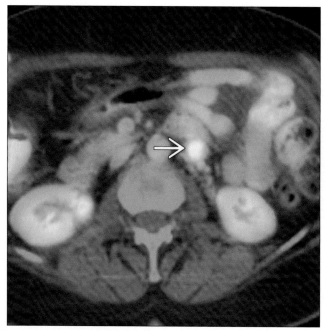

(Left) Axial CECT shows a mildly enlarged left para-aortic lymph node ➔ in a patient with a history of ovarian carcinoma with no other evidence of recurrent disease. *(Right)* Axial fused PET/CT shows focal intense FDG activity corresponding to the left para-aortic lymph node ➔, compatible with recurrent disease.

OVARIAN CARCINOMA

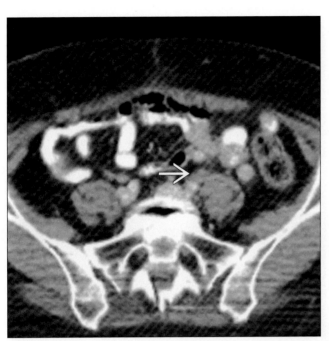 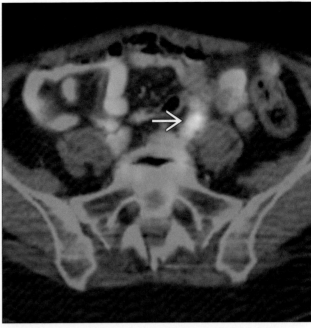

(Left) Axial CECT shows a normal-sized left common iliac lymph node ➡, not identified prospectively on CT. *(Right)* Axial fused PET/CT shows focal intense FDG activity correlating with a small lymph node ➡, compatible with recurrent malignancy.

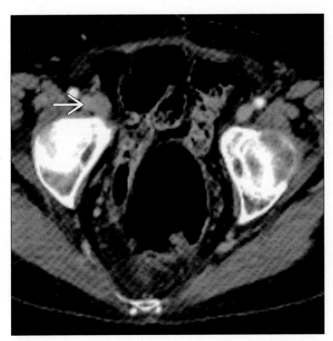 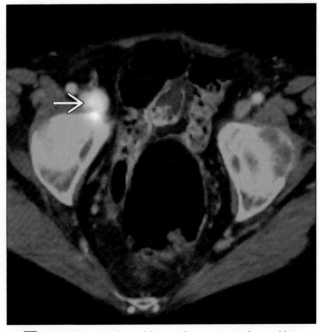

(Left) Axial CECT shows a borderline enlarged right external iliac lymph node ➡ in this patient with a mild rise in her tumor marker and history of ovarian cancer. *(Right)* Axial fused PET/CT shows focal intense FDG activity in the borderline enlarged right external iliac lymph node ➡, compatible with malignancy.

OVARIAN CARCINOMA

Restaging

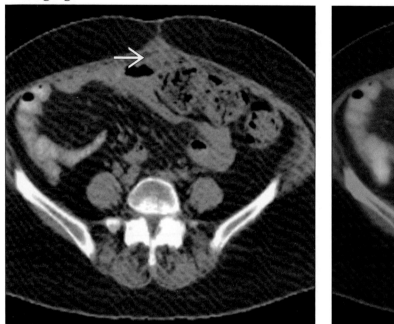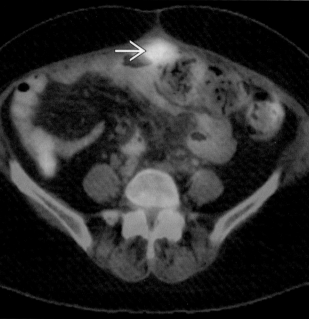

(Left) Axial NECT shows questionable infiltration of the omentum. On this noncontrast examination, it is difficult to separate unopacified bowel from the omental nodularity ➡. *(Right)* Axial fused PET/CT shows focal intense FDG activity corresponding to the omental nodularity ➡, compatible with recurrent disease.

Restaging

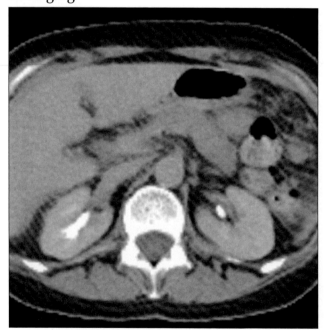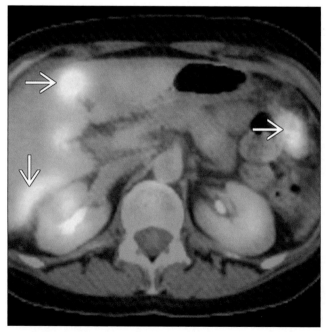

(Left) A late phase CECT shows no definite evidence for malignancy. *(Right)* Axial fused PET/CT shows at least 3 hypermetabolic lesions ➡. Two of them line the peritoneal surfaces, and one is in the liver, adjacent to the falciform ligament.

OVARIAN CARCINOMA

Restaging

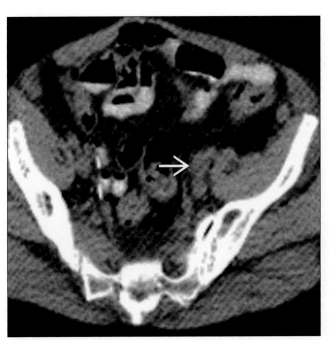 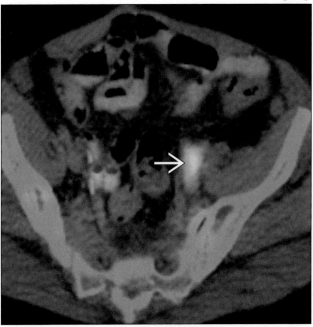

(Left) Axial NECT shows no definite evidence for malignancy. However, a borderline enlarged left pelvic sidewall ➡ should be noted. *(Right)* Axial fused PET/CT shows focal increased FDG activity corresponding to the previously described lymph node ➡, compatible with malignancy.

Restaging

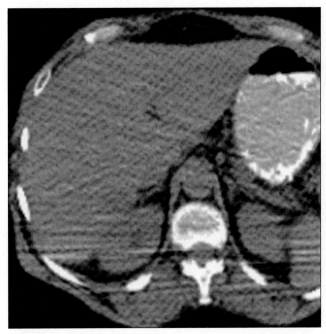 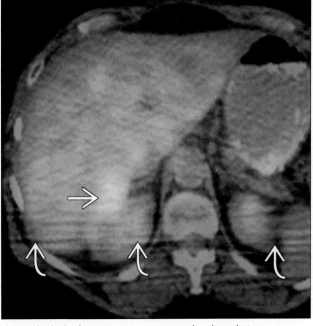

(Left) Axial NECT shows the solid organs. This is a suboptimal evaluation, due to the lack of intravenous contrast, and no large lesions are identified. *(Right)* Axial fused PET/CT shows intense FDG activity correlating with a lesion in the medial aspect of the posterior segment of the liver ➡, compatible with malignancy. The linear streaks ➡ along the posterior aspect of the image are due to the patient's arms being down, causing beam hardening artifact.

OVARIAN CARCINOMA

Restaging

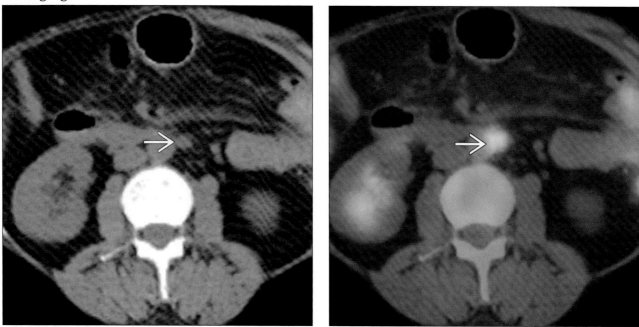

(Left) Axial NECT shows no definite evidence for malignancy in the abdomen. A nonenlarged left periaortic node ➡ is seen. *(Right)* Axial fused PET/CT shows focal intense FDG activity correlating with the normal-sized lymph node ➡, compatible with malignancy. One of the added benefits of PET/CT is detection of normal-sized lymph nodes in the 6-10 mm range.

Restaging

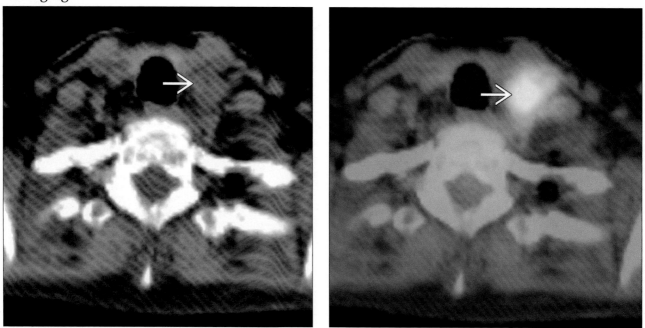

(Left) Axial NECT shows borderline left supraclavicular lymph node enlargement ➡ in this patient with a history of ovarian carcinoma. *(Right)* Axial fused PET/CT shows focal intense FDG activity correlating with the overlying large left supraclavicular lymph node ➡, compatible with recurrent ovarian carcinoma.

OVARIAN CARCINOMA

Restaging

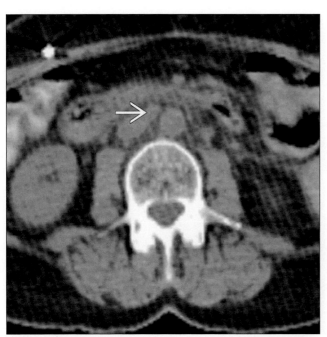 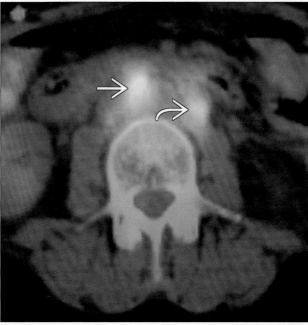

(Left) Axial NECT shows a normal-sized aortocaval lymph node ➡ without any other evidence of metastatic disease. The lymph node was not called prospectively suspicious for malignant involvement. *(Right)* Axial fused PET/CT shows intense FDG activity within the aortocaval lymph node ➡, as well as a small left para-aortic lymph node ➡, compatible with malignancy.

Restaging

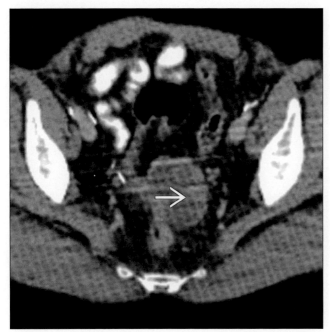 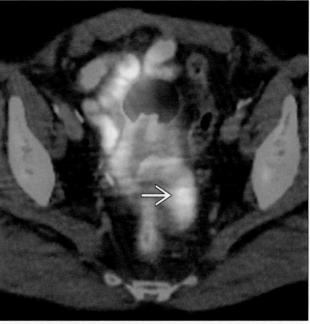

(Left) Axial CECT shows a mixed attenuation pelvic mass with apparent mural nodularity ➡ and central cystic change. *(Right)* Axial fused PET/CT shows focal intense FDG activity along the left lateral border of the pelvic mass ➡, which was subsequently biopsy-proven to be ovarian carcinoma.

OVARIAN CARCINOMA

Restaging

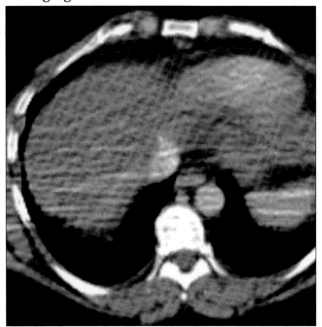 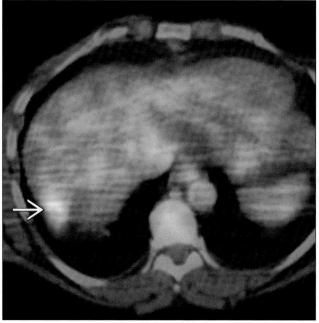

(Left) Axial CECT shows linear beam hardening artifact that obscures anatomical detail of the posterior aspect of the liver. No definite lesions were identified prospectively on this CT. *(Right)* Axial fused PET/CT shows focal intense FDG activity ➔ within the artifact along the lateral peripheral border of the right lobe of the liver, compatible with malignancy.

Restaging

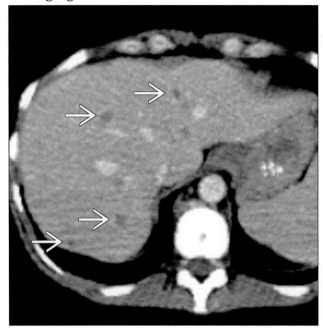 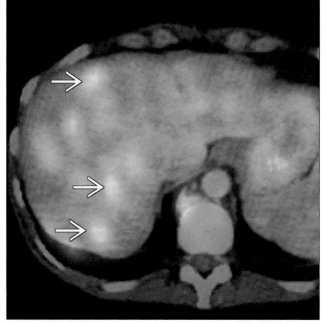

(Left) Axial CECT shows multiple low attenuation lesions ➔ in the liver in this patient with newly diagnosed ovarian carcinoma. Without PET/CT, these lesions, all 1 cm or smaller, may be classified as too small to further characterize. *(Right)* Axial fused PET/CT shows moderate to intense FDG activity within the majority of the low attenuation hepatic lesions ➔, compatible with malignancy.

OVARIAN CARCINOMA

Restaging

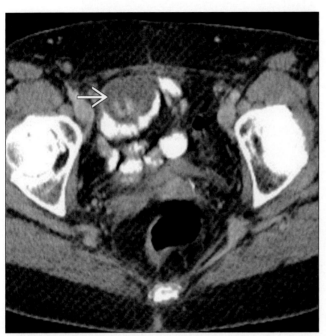 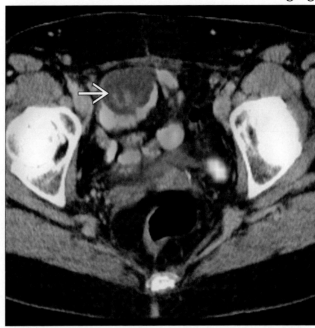

(Left) Axial CECT shows a large low attenuation mass adjacent to a loop of well-opacified small bowel ➡ in this patient with biopsy-confirmed, well-differentiated adenocarcinoma of the ovary. *(Right)* Axial fused PET/CT shows no increased metabolic activity within the previously described mass ➡. Although many ovarian carcinomas are intensely FDG avid, the more well-differentiated or mucinous parotids may not take up much of the tracer.

Restaging

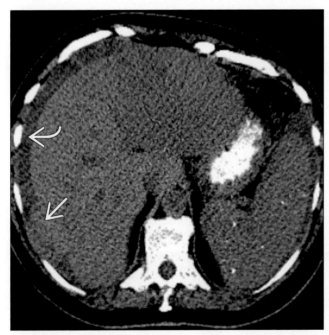 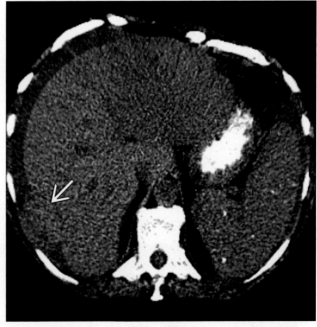

(Left) Axial NECT shows perihepatic ascites ➡ in addition to a subtle mass adjacent to the capsule of the liver ➡ in this patient with a history of ovarian carcinoma. *(Right)* Axial fused PET/CT shows a photopenic defect correlating with the questionable peritoneal mass ➡. Subsequent biopsy showed recurrent well-differentiated mucinous ovarian carcinoma. In general, FDG uptake is lower in the more well-differentiated adenocarcinoma, particularly the mucinous variety.

UTERINE CARCINOMA

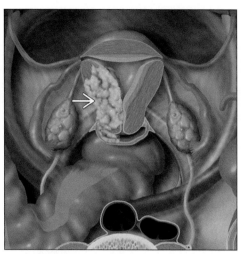

Graphic shows a representation of uterine body carcinoma ➡.

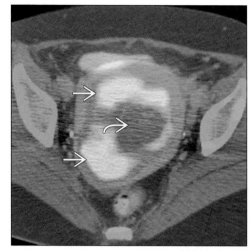

Axial fused PET/CT shows an enlarged uterus with circumferential FDG activity ➡ and central necrosis ➡ in this patient with uterine leiomyosarcoma.

TERMINOLOGY

Abbreviations and Synonyms
- Endometrial carcinoma, uterine sarcoma, uterine carcinosarcoma, leiomyosarcoma

Definitions
- Malignancy of uterine endometrium or uterine body
  - Most common type is endometrioid adenocarcinoma

IMAGING FINDINGS

General Features
- Best diagnostic clue
  - Primary endometrial cancer
    - Thickened endometrium on CT
    - Intense FDG activity on PET corresponding to lesion
  - FDG uptake in metastatic sites
    - Lymphadenopathy
    - Abdominal and distant metastases
- Location

  - Usually glandular component of superior endometrium
    - May spread within endo-/myometrium and from fundus toward isthmus and cervix
    - May arise within an endometrial polyp

Imaging Recommendations
- Best imaging tool
  - CT/MR
    - Evaluate disease extension
    - Provide information for treatment planning
    - Detect lymph node metastases; 18-66% sensitivity and 73-99% specificity
    - Limited in recurrent disease due to anatomic distortion 2° surgery and radiation
  - FDG PET
    - For staging, restaging, early detection, and evaluating response to therapy
    - Incorporation of FDG PET into post-therapy surveillance shown to influence treatment in up to 20% of patients
    - Particularly useful for asymptomatic disease
  - PET/CT useful for anatomic and functional localization of sites of recurrence

DDx: FDG Activity in the Uterus

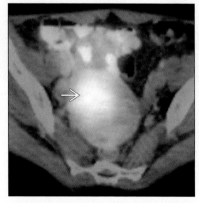

Uterine Fibroid

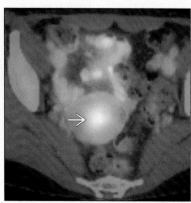

Menstruation

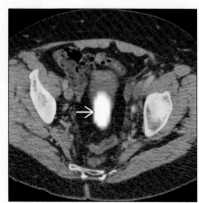

Cervical Carcinoma

UTERINE CARCINOMA

Key Facts

Imaging Findings

- Primary endometrial cancer: Thickened endometrium on CT with intense FDG activity on PET, correlating with mass
- MR/CT used to evaluate disease extension and provide information for treatment planning, ± ultrasound
- FDG PET for staging, restaging, early detection, evaluating response to therapy
- Signs of metastatic disease on PET/CT: Lymphadenopathy with increased FDG, abdominal/distant metastases
- PET/CT useful for anatomic and functional localization of sites of recurrence
- Significant nonmalignant uptake in younger patients who are menstruating

- Sensitivity of PET alone (87%) or plus MR or CT (91%) is higher than MR or CT alone (~ 67% in overall lesion detection)
- PET most useful for detecting distant metastases

Top Differential Diagnoses

- Uterine Leiomyoma
- Endometrial Hyperplasia
- Endometrial Polyp
- Cervical Cancer
- Endometrial Sarcoma

Diagnostic Checklist

- MR or CT for extent of primary tumor
- PET/CT for optimal staging
- Note benign causes of increased FDG activity in endometrium (e.g., menstruation)

- Protocol advice
  - Oral contrast agent for CT
    - Helps better delineate normal bowel activity
    - Demonstrates pathologic intra-abdominal activity (peritoneal implants)
  - IV contrast
    - Differentiates small lymph nodes from vessels, intestine, or the ureter
    - Correctly detects small liver metastases, small peritoneal dissemination, and local recurrence at the vagina

CT Findings

- Inconsistent depiction of endometrium and endometrial thickness
- Findings associated with endometrial carcinoma are nonspecific and similar to other conditions
- Uterine cancer and normal endometrium are often indistinguishable on nonenhanced CT
  - May see diffuse thickening, discrete mass, or polypoid mass within endometrial cavity
  - Cavity may be expanded with fluid
  - Mass may be of uniform or heterogeneous attenuation
  - Usually poorly enhancing relative to myometrium
    - Variable areas of contrast enhancement
- IV contrast also aids in evaluating local invasion by increasing conspicuity of tumor
- Invasion of myometrium suggested by irregular tumor-myometrium border
  - CT limited in ability to delineate deep myometrial invasion and cervical involvement
- CT reasonably sensitive for lymphadenopathy and distant metastases
  - Size cutoff for suspicion of malignancy > 8-10 mm in short axis

MR Findings

- T1WI
  - Endometrium and myometrium have similar signal intensity and cannot readily be distinguished
- T2WI

- Endometrium appears as central zone of high signal intensity
- Myometrium depicted as zone of low signal intensity at its inner aspect and a wider zone of intermediate signal intensity at its outer aspect
- Endometrial thickness varies in menstruating women from 4 mm in early proliferative phase to 13 mm in late secretory phase

Nuclear Medicine Findings

- **General**
  - Sensitivity of PET alone (87%) or plus MR or CT (91%) is higher than MR or CT alone (~ 67% in overall lesion detection)
  - PET has 89% PPV and 91% NPV in patients with endometrial cancer; 87.5% and 97.5% for uterine sarcoma
  - Lesion size-related sensitivity
    - < 4 mm: 16.7%
    - 5-9 mm: 66.7%
  - Mean SUV of true positive lesions in one study
    - 13 for central pelvic lesions
    - 11 for metastases
  - False positives
    - Normal cycle variation of FDG activity in endometrium
    - Significant nonmalignant uptake in younger patients who are menstruating
    - Bone fracture
    - Post-operative changes
- **Staging**
  - Primary benefit of FDG PET is improved staging of distant metastatic disease
    - Has shown clinical impact in 22.2% of patients for primary staging
  - PET/CT superior to conventional imaging for detecting lymph node metastases
    - Sensitivity 60-67%, specificity 94-98%
    - Limited detection of microscopic mets
  - Shown to alter treatment in 35% of patients with endometrial cancer

UTERINE CARCINOMA

o Several groups have found FDG uptake correlates with tumor grade in uterine sarcomas
  ▪ May be useful for indicating most aggressive area for biopsy
- **Restaging**
  o PET has sensitivity 96-100%/specificity 78-88% for post-therapy restaging/surveillance
  o Clinical impact
    ▪ Up to 73% of cases may have a clinical impact when PET is performed for post-therapy surveillance
  o Commonly overlooked sites of recurrence
    ▪ Local disease in retrovesical region
    ▪ Pelvic recurrence
    ▪ Lung metastases
    ▪ Peritoneal dissemination
    ▪ Pelvic lymph node metastases
    ▪ Para-aortic lymph node metastases

DIFFERENTIAL DIAGNOSIS

Cervical Cancer
- Cervical mass on CT
  o Masses up to 3 cm may be normal, benign hypertrophy
- 80-90% of patients experience vaginal bleeding

Uterine Leiomyoma
- Fibroids may be indistinguishable unless calcified or necrotic
- Intramural or exophytic lesions more easy to differentiate

Endometrial Hyperplasia
- May have same findings on US as endometrial carcinoma

Endometrial Polyp
- Can mimic endometrial cancer on CT

Tamoxifen-Related Endometrial Changes
- Prolonged tamoxifen therapy associated with increased risk of endometrial polyps, hyperplasia, and cancer

Endometrial Sarcoma
- Leiomyosarcoma tends to occur in women aged 30-50 years
- Carcinosarcoma and endometrial stromal sarcoma have higher incidence in women > 50 years

PATHOLOGY

General Features
- General path comments
  o Histologic subtypes
    ▪ Endometrioid carcinoma (60-80% of cases)
    ▪ Serous papillary carcinoma (5-10%)
    ▪ Adenosquamous carcinoma (5-6%)
    ▪ Clear cell carcinoma (3-6%)
    ▪ Small cell undifferentiated carcinoma (least common)
  o Uterine sarcoma

▪ Incidence increasing, reportedly 8% in USA
▪ Subtypes in decreasing incidence: Malignant mixed Müllerian tumor, leiomyosarcoma, endometrial stromal sarcoma
▪ Approximately half of patients experience recurrence within 2 years of initial treatment
o Uterine carcinosarcoma (malignant mixed Müllerian tumor)
  ▪ Rare, extremely aggressive, poor prognosis
  ▪ 2-4% of all uterine malignancies
  ▪ 20-55% of patients are upstaged secondary to finding of extrauterine disease
o Uterine prolapse
  ▪ 30% prevalence in ages 20-59 years
  ▪ Most frequent lesion in prolapse specimens is leiomyoma, which shows moderately intense FDG uptake
- Etiology
  o Most common risk factor: Protracted exposure to endogenous or exogenous estrogen unopposed by progesterone
  o Other risk factors
    ▪ Menopause after age 52 years
    ▪ Prolonged reproductive lifespan between menarche and menopause
    ▪ Estrogen replacement therapy
    ▪ Tamoxifen use
    ▪ Endometrial hyperplasia
    ▪ Obesity
    ▪ Nulliparity
- Epidemiology
  o Most common genital malignancy in USA and other developed countries
  o Fourth most common malignancy in women after breast, lung, colorectal
  o Up to 1 in 100 women in USA may develop the disease

Staging, Grading, or Classification Criteria
- FIGO staging defined by results of
  o Exploratory laparotomy, including hysterectomy, bilateral salpingo-oophorectomy, pelvic and para-aortic lymphadenectomy, and peritoneal cytology
- Staging of endometrial cancer
  o **Stage I**: Cancer confined to uterine corpus
    ▪ IA: Tumor limited to endometrium, and CT appearance of uterus may be normal
    ▪ IB: Tumor extends into less than 1/2 the width of the myometrium
    ▪ IC: Tumor extends into 1/2 or more of the myometrial width
  o **Stage II**: Cancer involving corpus and cervix, without extrauterine spread
    ▪ IIA: Cancer extends from uterine corpus into endocervical glandular region of cervix
    ▪ IIB: Fibromuscular stroma of cervix is involved
  o **Stage III**: Cancer extending outside the uterus but confined to the true pelvis
    ▪ IIIA: Extends outside the uterus into parametria, pelvic sidewall, fallopian tube, or ovary
    ▪ IIIB: Vaginal metastases characterize this stage
    ▪ IIIC: Enlarged pelvic &/or para-aortic lymph nodes characterize this stage

UTERINE CARCINOMA

- o **Stage IV**: Cancer invading the bladder or bowel mucosa &/or spreading outside the true pelvis
  - ▪ IVA: Tumor invasion spreads into urinary bladder or bowel mucosa
  - ▪ IVB: Metastases outside the true pelvis characterize this stage, including metastasis into the intra-abdominal &/or inguinal lymph nodes

CLINICAL ISSUES

Presentation
- Most common signs/symptoms
  - o Postmenopausal bleeding
    - ▪ Eventually 80% present with vaginal bleeding, mostly postmenopausal
  - o Early endometrial cancer usually asymptomatic
- Other signs/symptoms
  - o 10% of patients present with purulent vaginal discharge, sometimes tinged with blood
  - o Pelvic pain and pressure usually manifestations of advanced disease
  - o Conventional surveillance for post-operative endometrial cancer patients
    - ▪ Physical exam, pap smear, serum tumor marker levels (CA125, CA 19-9), and imaging studies

Demographics
- Age
  - o Primarily arises in postmenopausal women
    - ▪ Peak incidence 55-65 years
    - ▪ 75% of patients > 50 years
    - ▪ 5% of patients < 40 years
- Ethnicity
  - o Prevalence and survival rates higher in Caucasians than in women of African descent
  - o Uterine sarcoma more common in women of African descent

Natural History & Prognosis
- Most tumors diagnosed at early stages, making them curable by surgery with or without adjuvant therapy
  - o 75% confined to uterine corpus
  - o Significant portion of patients with risk factors nevertheless have recurrence
- Survival rates 84% in USA
- Prognosis depends on
  - o Age
  - o Tumor grade and histology
  - o Depth of muscular invasion
  - o Cervical involvement
  - o Lymph node metastases
- Depth of myometrial invasion important in predicting lymph node metastases
  - o Incidence of lymph node metastases
    - ▪ 3% with superficial myometrial invasion, stage IB
    - ▪ More than 40% with deep myometrial invasion, stage IC

Treatment
- Complete resection includes
  - o Total abdominal hysterectomy
  - o Bilateral salpingo-oophorectomy
  - o Pelvic/para-aortic node sampling

- Radical hysterectomy performed only for unequivocal cervical involvement
- Patients with localized recurrences are classically treated with surgery &/or radiation
- Systemic chemotherapy &/or progesterone therapy advocated for disseminated recurrent disease

DIAGNOSTIC CHECKLIST

Consider
- MR or CT for extent of primary tumor
- PET/CT for optimal staging
  - o Stage IIIC: Lymphadenopathy
  - o Stage IVB: Distant metastases
- Note benign causes of increased FDG activity in endometrium (e.g., menstruation)

SELECTED REFERENCES

1. Akcaer M et al: Imaging of endometrioid adenocarcinoma of the uterus metastatic to the ciliary body. Ophthalmic Surg Lasers Imaging. 39(3):246-9, 2008
2. Chung HH et al: The clinical impact of [(18)F]FDG PET/CT for the management of recurrent endometrial cancer: correlation with clinical and histological findings. Eur J Nucl Med Mol Imaging. 35(6):1081-8, 2008
3. Kitajima K et al: Accuracy of 18F-FDG PET/CT in detecting pelvic and paraaortic lymph node metastasis in patients with endometrial cancer. AJR Am J Roentgenol. 190(6):1652-8, 2008
4. Kitajima K et al: Performance of FDG-PET/CT in the diagnosis of recurrent endometrial cancer. Ann Nucl Med. 22(2):103-9, 2008
5. Nayot D et al: Does preoperative positron emission tomography with computed tomography predict nodal status in endometrial cancer? A pilot study. Curr Oncol. 15(3):123-5, 2008
6. Oshiro H et al: Endometrial adenocarcinoma without myometrial invasion metastasizing to the pancreas and masquerading as primary pancreatic neoplasm. Pathol Int. 58(7):456-61, 2008
7. Tsujikawa T et al: Uterine tumors: pathophysiologic imaging with 16alpha-[18F]fluoro-17beta-estradiol and 18F fluorodeoxyglucose PET--initial experience. Radiology. 248(2):599-605, 2008
8. Akin O et al: Imaging of uterine cancer. Radiol Clin North Am. 45(1):167-82, 2007
9. Iyer RB et al: PET/CT and cross sectional imaging of gynecologic malignancy. Cancer Imaging. 7 Spec No A:S130-8, 2007
10. Lai CH et al: Positron emission tomography imaging for gynecologic malignancy. Curr Opin Obstet Gynecol. 19(1):37-41, 2007
11. Sironi S et al: Post-therapy surveillance of patients with uterine cancers: value of integrated FDG PET/CT in the detection of recurrence. Eur J Nucl Med Mol Imaging. 34(4):472-9, 2007
12. Suzuki R et al: Validity of positron emission tomography using fluoro-2-deoxyglucose for the preoperative evaluation of endometrial cancer. Int J Gynecol Cancer. 17(4):890-6, 2007
13. Yoshida Y et al: The positron emission tomography with F18 17beta-estradiol has the potential to benefit diagnosis and treatment of endometrial cancer. Gynecol Oncol. 104(3):764-6, 2007
14. Kaneta T et al: Prolapsed endometrial cancer: FDG PET/CT findings. Clin Nucl Med. 31(3):180, 2006

3

UTERINE CARCINOMA

CT Findings: Metastases

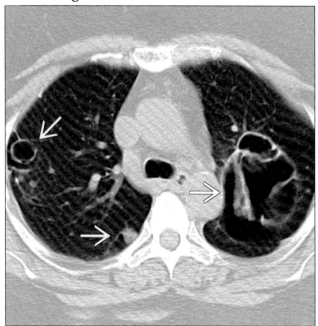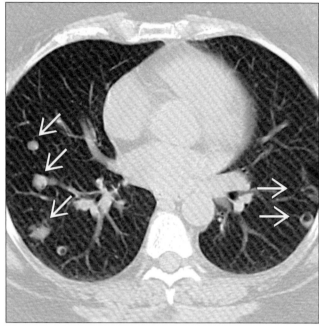

(Left) Axial CECT shows multiple bilateral pulmonary metastases ➡ in a patient with a uterine sarcoma. *(Right)* Axial CECT shows additional bilateral pulmonary metastases ➡.

PET/CT Findings: Primary

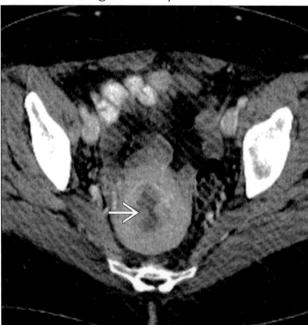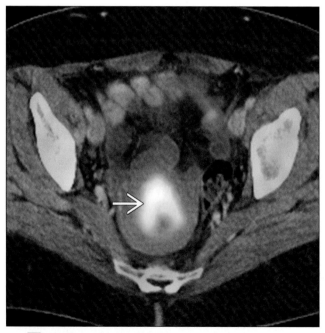

(Left) Axial CECT in a postmenopausal woman shows thickened endometrium ➡. *(Right)* Axial fused PET/CT shows intense FDG activity corresponding to the thickened endometrium ➡. A scan in a menstruating premenopausal woman may have a similar appearance. However, intense FDG activity in a postmenopausal woman typically represents endometrial carcinoma, as in this patient.

UTERINE CARCINOMA

PET/CT Findings: Staging

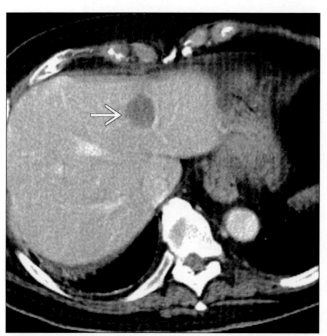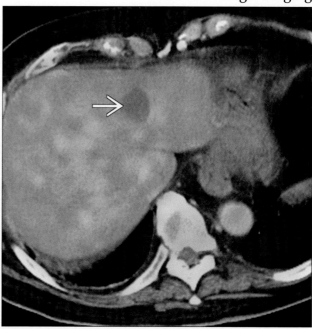

(Left) Axial CECT shows a low attenuation lesion in the left hepatic lobe ➔ in this patient with a history of uterine leiomyosarcoma. However, the attenuation measured above water attenuation, suggesting that this lesion is not a hepatic cyst. *(Right)* Axial fused PET/CT shows no increased metabolic activity ➔. Subsequent ultrasound-guided biopsy showed metastatic disease. Low FDG activity is characteristic of many sarcomas.

PET/CT Findings: Staging

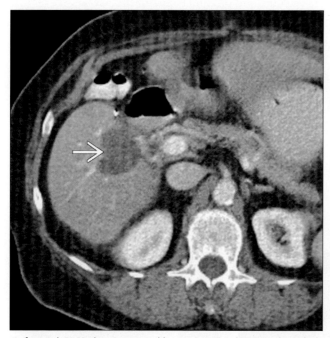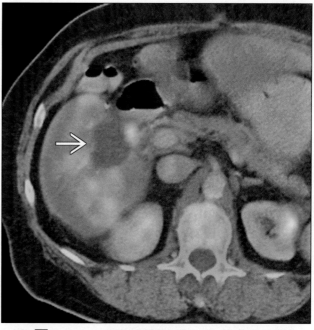

(Left) Axial CECT shows a second low attenuation lesion in the right hepatic lobe ➔ in this patient with a history of uterine leiomyosarcoma. However, the attenuation measured above water attenuation, suggesting this lesion is not a hepatic cyst. *(Right)* Axial fused PET/CT shows no increased metabolic activity ➔. Subsequent ultrasound-guided biopsy showed metastatic disease. Low FDG activity is characteristic of many sarcomas.

3

PROSTATE CARCINOMA

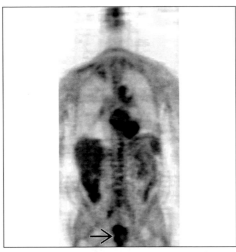

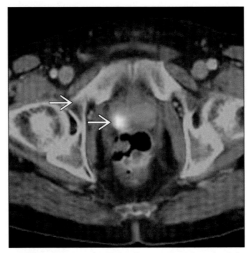

Coronal PET shows focal intense FDG activity inferior to the bladder ⇨, subsequently confirmed to be prostate carcinoma.

Axial fused PET/CT shows focal intense activity in the right side of the prostate gland ⇨.

TERMINOLOGY

Abbreviations and Synonyms
- Prostate cancer, prostate carcinoma, adenocarcinoma of the prostate

Definitions
- Malignancy arising from glandular tissue of the prostate

IMAGING FINDINGS

General Features
- Best diagnostic clue
  - **Primary tumor**
    - FDG PET and CT are both limited in detection of primary disease
  - **Local extension**
    - Obliteration of periprostatic fat plane and abnormally enhancing contiguous neurovascular bundle
    - MR with endorectal coil helpful for looking at primary tumor and local extension
  - **Bone invasion**
    - Sclerotic lesions on CT with areas of uptake on bone scan
- Location
  - ~ 70% occur in posterior region of peripheral zone
  - ~ 30% in transitional and central zones
  - Bone metastasis most commonly seen in pelvis and lower vertebrae
  - Common sites of bone metastasis
    - Axial and proximal appendicular skeleton
    - Often spares distal appendicular skeleton and skull ("legless and headless")
- Size: Mets may range from small and focal to confluent

Imaging Recommendations
- Best imaging tool
  - Conventional imaging and standard digital rectal examination both have been shown to understage disease localized to the prostate
  - FDG PET
    - Not routinely used in prostate cancer
    - May be helpful in more aggressive pathologic subtypes

DDx: Mimics of Prostate Bone Metastases

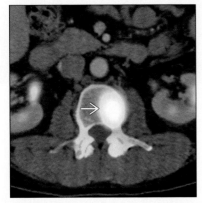

Other Bone Metastases: Breast

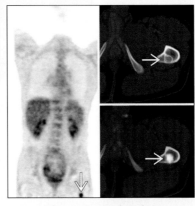

Fibrous Cortical Defect

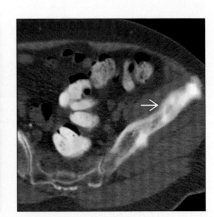

Paget Disease

PROSTATE CARCINOMA

Key Facts

Terminology
- Prostate cancer, prostate carcinoma, adenocarcinoma of the prostate

Imaging Findings
- Multiple areas of uptake on bone scan with sclerotic lesions on CT, plain radiograph
- Whole body bone scan sensitive for detecting bone metastases
- Plain radiograph, CT: Sclerotic mets, lytic with more poorly differentiated tumor
- FDG PET does not have an important role in primary diagnosis or staging of prostate cancer due to low metabolic glucose metabolism
- **FDG PET**
  - Not routinely used in prostate cancer

- May be helpful in more aggressive pathologic subtypes
  - Sensitive for diffuse bony involvement
- **Bone scan**
  - FDG PET and CT are both limited in detection of primary disease

Top Differential Diagnoses
- Occult Fracture in the Elderly
- Osteoarthritis
- Paget Disease
- Other Metastases

Diagnostic Checklist
- Consider baseline PET/CT with patients newly diagnosed with prostate carcinoma and a high Gleason score

---

  - Useful for detection of distant metastases in hormone-refractory disease
  - PPV 98% for untreated mets in viscera (not lymph nodes)
  - **Bone scan**
    - Sensitive for diffuse bony involvement
    - Usually more sensitive than FDG PET for detecting sclerotic/blastic bone metastases
  - **CT**
    - Generally inaccurate for detection of T1 or T2 cancer within the prostate gland
    - May also be used to depict soft tissue metastases elsewhere in the body
    - Detects sclerotic and more aggressive lytic mets in bone
    - Does not provide sufficient accuracy in localizing recurrent disease
  - **MR**
    - Best for evaluation of extracapsular tumor growth and seminal vesicle invasion
    - Endorectal MR for most accurate local staging, but may still understage in up to 30% of cases
- Protocol advice
  - Empty urinary bladder immediately before commencing scanning with FDG PET
  - Scan from bottom to top to avoid accumulation of FDG in bladder

CT Findings
- **Local invasion**
  - T3 tumor invasion into periprostatic fat or seminal vesicles can be demonstrated, although MR more sensitive
  - With overt capsular breach, there should be clear deformity of the outline of the prostate
  - Microscopic spread through prostatic capsule is not detected by CT, which leads to understaging
    - Particularly difficult to detect at base and apex of gland
- **Extracapsular extension may demonstrate**
  - Loss of fat plane surrounding prostate

  - Abnormal enhancement of contiguous neurovascular bundle
  - Invasion of rectum and urinary bladder
  - Signs of lymph node involvement
    - Early disease usually subcentimeter and may be overlooked
    - Sensitivity/specificity for LN metastases: Range from 25-78% and 77-98% respectively
- **Arterial phase contrast enhancement**
  - Helps differentiate between PZ and TZ regions
  - Cannot demonstrate intraprostatic pathology
  - May be helpful in detecting nodal involvement

Nuclear Medicine Findings
- **Bone scan**
  - Fairly intense bony uptake in multiple areas
    - Mostly in axial, proximal appendicular skeleton
  - Solitary hot spots are more likely benign
    - Even if known extraosseous malignancy
  - Secondary/complicated findings
    - Flare response rarely occurs later than 6 months after treatment
    - Can result in transient worsening of bone scan with chemo or hormone therapy
    - Typically regresses in 2-3 months
- **FDG PET**
  - FDG PET has little role in primary diagnosis or staging of prostate cancer
    - Low metabolic glucose metabolism
    - Urinary FDG excretion may mask pathologic uptake
    - Excreted FDG accumulates in prostatic urethra and subsequently the prostatic parenchyma
    - Inflammatory processes such as prostatitis may be confused for malignancy
  - FDG PET/CT has not been shown to improve on results of FDG PET alone
  - 11-C choline PET/CT (investigational)
    - Theoretically, a better tracer for visualization of prostate carcinoma using PET imaging
    - Advantages include minimal urinary excretion and increased prostatic choline metabolism

3

PROSTATE CARCINOMA

- 11-C choline is a controversial tracer
- So far failed to show significant correlation between uptake and tumor grade or Gleason score
- For detection of primary has shown sensitivity of 86.5% and specificity of 61.9%
- For metastatic spread, 81.8% and 100%
  - **Initial diagnosis**
    - Tumor grows relatively slowly and shows low or absent FDG uptake vs. other cancers
    - Difficult to differentiate prostate cancer from benign prostatic hypertrophy (BPH) and prostatitis
    - Limited use of PET for initial diagnosis
    - However, focal intense FDG activity should be correlated with serum prostate specific antigen (PSA)
  - **Staging**
    - Major use is for detection and localization of distant mets in hormone-refractory prostate cancer
    - PPV of 98% for untreated visceral and nodal metastases
  - **Restaging**
    - Interpretation of recurrence after radical prostatectomy or radiation therapy is difficult unless large mass lesions are present

DIFFERENTIAL DIAGNOSIS

Occult Fracture in the Elderly
- Particularly vertebral compression fractures or insufficiency fractures of the sacrum
- Clinical correlation with laboratory markers may aid in diagnosis

Osteoarthritis
- May appear as inflammatory foci with variable FDG uptake
- Look for contour of osteophytes projecting beyond expected location of vertebral body
- Pedicle disease found at level of vertebral body
- Benign facet disease found at level of disc space

Paget Disease
- Cortical thickening and coarse thickened trabeculae can be demonstrated on plain film

Other Metastases
- Other malignancies that manifest with blastic metastases can be indistinguishable

Other Benign Osseous Lesions
- Fibrous cortical defects and other benign osseous lesions may have increased metabolic activity

PATHOLOGY

General Features
- Genetics
  - Risk of prostate cancer doubled if patient has affected brother or father
  - Human prostate cancer gene (X chromosome)

- Chromosome 1
  - Hereditary prostate cancer 1 gene (HPC1)
  - Predisposing for cancer of the prostate gene (PCAP)
- Etiology
  - High fat diets have been implicated
    - Diets high in soy may be protective
- Epidemiology
  - Incidence
    - ~ 186,000 new cases in USA in 2008
    - Approximately 26,000 men in the USA will die of prostate cancer each year
    - Incidence has been decreasing since 1993

Gross Pathologic & Surgical Features
- Firm, fibrotic tissue may appear "gritty"

Microscopic Features
- Gleason score is used to classify histologic characteristics based on degree of differentiation
  - 95% of tumors are adenocarcinoma
  - Well-differentiated cells have uniform epithelium, oval nuclei, pale cytoplasm, and rare mitotic features
  - Poorly differentiated tumor shows sheets of tumor cells with mitoses and cellular atypia
- Bone lesions are primarily osteoblastic, but in more aggressive forms osteolytic lesions are seen

Staging, Grading, or Classification Criteria
- **Jewett-Whitmore & TNM staging**
  - A & T1: Clinically localized (tumor not palpable on digital rectal exam)
    - A1 & T1a: Focal tumor or low grade
    - A2 & T1b: Diffuse tumor or high grade
  - B & T2: Clinically localized (tumor palpable)
    - B1 T2a: Tumor involves < 1/2 lobe
    - B2 & T2b: Tumor involves > 1/2 lobe
  - C & T3: Locally invasive beyond prostatic capsule (tumor palpable)
    - C1 & T3a: Unilateral extracapsular extension
    - C1 & T3b: Bilateral extracapsular extension
    - C1 & T3c: Seminal vesicle invasion
  - C2 & T4: Invades adjacent tissues
    - e.g., bladder, rectum, levator ani
  - D & N/M: Lymph node & distant metastases (bones, lung, liver, & brain)

CLINICAL ISSUES

Presentation
- Most common signs/symptoms
  - Half of patients are asymptomatic at presentation since advent of PSA screening
  - Most common presenting symptoms overlap with BPH
    - Urinary frequency
    - Decreased urine stream
  - Symptoms of advanced disease include weight loss, anorexia, bone pain
- Other signs/symptoms: Back pain should prompt further investigation, even with negative initial workup

3

PROSTATE CARCINOMA

Demographics
- Age
  - Uncommon finding in patients younger than 50 years
  - Latent prostate carcinoma found at autopsy in greater than 50% of men over age 70
- Ethnicity
  - African-American men have ~ 60% higher incidence than Caucasians
    - Correlates with higher levels of testosterone
  - Mortality rates for African Americans are twice that for Caucasians

Natural History & Prognosis
- For all but stage IV disease, 5 year survival nearly 100%
- ~ 16% chance of acquiring disease in lifetime
- Rate of PSA recurrence after radical prostatectomy greater than 50%
  - Most common in patients with > T3 disease and positive resection margins
- Many instances of prostate cancer demonstrate slow growth, such that survival is prolonged even with distant metastases

Treatment
- Absence of overall consensus on optimal treatment strategies
- Treatment strategies are based on risk of intra- vs. extraprostatic disease
- **Current treatment approaches**
  - **Brachytherapy**: Radioactive seeds implanted in prostate with recurrence free rates 75-95%
  - **Chemotherapy**: Used for advanced disease or disease that has stopped responding to hormonal therapy; mostly palliative
  - **Cryotherapy**: Minimally invasive procedure that applies freezing gases to prostate
  - **Hormone therapy**: May slow tumor growth and contribute to effectiveness of other therapies
  - **Radiotherapy**: Used with good long-term success for local disease
  - **Surgery**: Transabdominal, transperineal, laparoscopic, robotic resection of prostate

DIAGNOSTIC CHECKLIST

Consider
- PSA
  - Upper limit of normal defined as 4 ng/mL
  - Not entirely reliable for detection of disease recurrence
  - Rate of rise can be good indicator of tumor aggressiveness
  - Nonpalpable cancers account for 75% of newly diagnosed disease
- Consider baseline PET/CT with patients newly diagnosed with prostate carcinoma and a high Gleason score

Image Interpretation Pearls
- FDG uptake in weight-bearing areas in patients with prostate carcinoma may be indicator of impending pathologic fracture

SELECTED REFERENCES

1. Colabufo NA et al: PB183, a sigma receptor ligand, as a potential PET probe for the imaging of prostate adenocarcinoma. Bioorg Med Chem Lett. 18(6):1990-3, 2008
2. Ho L et al: High-grade urothelial carcinoma of the prostate on FDG PET-CT. Clin Nucl Med. 32(9):746-7, 2007
3. Kwee SA et al: Cancer imaging with fluorine-18-labeled choline derivatives. Semin Nucl Med. 37(6):420-8, 2007
4. Powles T et al: Molecular positron emission tomography and PET/CT imaging in urological malignancies. Eur Urol. 51(6):1511-20; discussion 1520-1, 2007
5. Schuster DM et al: Initial experience with the radiotracer anti-1-amino-3-18F-fluorocyclobutane-1-carboxylic acid with PET/CT in prostate carcinoma. J Nucl Med. 48(1):56-63, 2007
6. Maeda T et al: Distant metastasis of prostate cancer: early detection of recurrent tumor with dual-phase carbon-11 choline positron emission tomography/computed tomography in two cases. Jpn J Clin Oncol. 36(9):598-601, 2006
7. Reske SN et al: Imaging prostate cancer with 11C-choline PET/CT. J Nucl Med. 47(8):1249-54, 2006
8. Rubens DJ et al: Image-guided brachytherapy for prostate cancer. Radiol Clin North Am. 44(5):735-48, viii-ix, 2006
9. Wachter S et al: 11C-acetate positron emission tomography imaging and image fusion with computed tomography and magnetic resonance imaging in patients with recurrent prostate cancer. J Clin Oncol. 24(16):2513-9, 2006
10. Dehdashti F et al: Positron tomographic assessment of androgen receptors in prostatic carcinoma. Eur J Nucl Med Mol Imaging. 32(3):344-50, 2005
11. Farsad M et al: Detection and localization of prostate cancer: correlation of (11)C-choline PET/CT with histopathologic step-section analysis. J Nucl Med. 46(10):1642-9, 2005
12. Malmström PU: Lymph node staging in prostatic carcinoma revisited. Acta Oncol. 44(6):593-8, 2005
13. Schmid DT et al: Fluorocholine PET/CT in patients with prostate cancer: initial experience. Radiology. 235(2):623-8, 2005
14. Tóth G et al: Detection of prostate cancer with 11C-methionine positron emission tomography. J Urol. 173(1):66-9; discussion 69, 2005
15. Sanz G et al: PET and prostate cancer. World J Urol. 22(5):351-2, 2004
16. Schöder H et al: Positron emission tomography for prostate, bladder, and renal cancer. Semin Nucl Med. 34(4):274-92, 2004
17. Hain SF et al: Positron emission tomography for urological tumours. BJU Int. 92(2):159-64, 2003
18. Oyama N et al: 11C-acetate PET imaging of prostate cancer: detection of recurrent disease at PSA relapse. J Nucl Med. 44(4):549-55, 2003
19. de Jong IJ et al: Visualisation of bladder cancer using (11)C-choline PET: first clinical experience. Eur J Nucl Med Mol Imaging. 29(10):1283-8, 2002
20. Price DT et al: Comparison of [18 F]fluorocholine and [18 F]fluorodeoxyglucose for positron emission tomography of androgen dependent and androgen independent prostate cancer. J Urol. 168(1):273-80, 2002

PROSTATE CARCINOMA

Typical

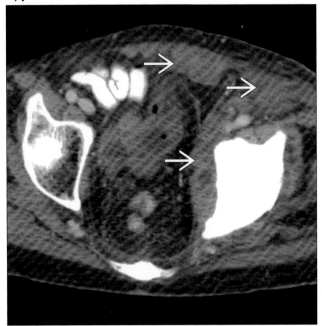 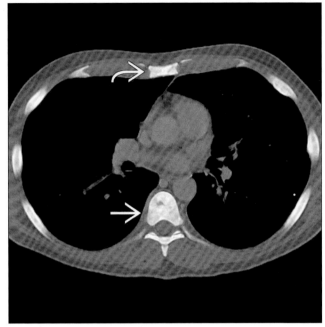

(Left) Axial CECT shows extensive soft tissue metastases ➡ in this patient with metastatic prostate cancer. *(Right)* Axial CECT shows a dense vertebral body ➡ and sternum ➡ in a patient with prostate cancer. These findings are compatible with bone metastases.

Typical

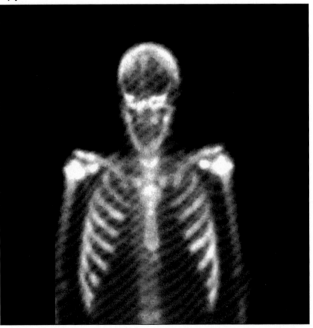 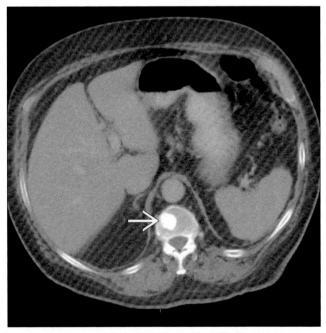

(Left) Coronal bone scan shows uptake of the axial and appendicular skeleton but no tracer activity in the kidneys. These findings are compatible with a "super scan" and usually seen in patients with diffuse bony metastases from prostate or breast cancer. *(Right)* Axial CECT shows a typical blastic vertebral body metastasis ➡ in a patient with prostate carcinoma.

PROSTATE CARCINOMA

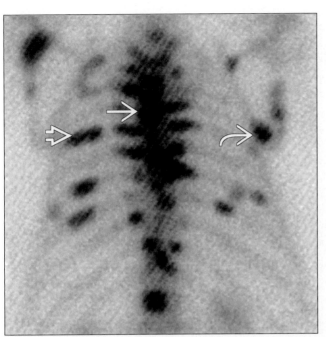
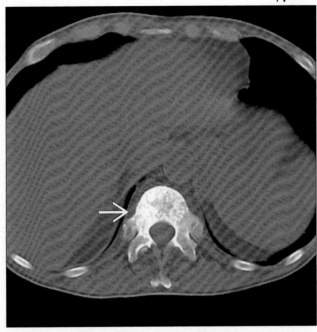

(Left) Coronal bone scan shows intense radiotracer uptake scattered throughout the spine ➜, ribs ➜, and scapulae ➜. *(Right)* Axial NECT shows a blastic vertebral body metastasis ➜, compatible with prostate carcinoma.

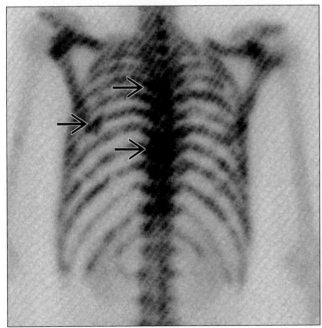
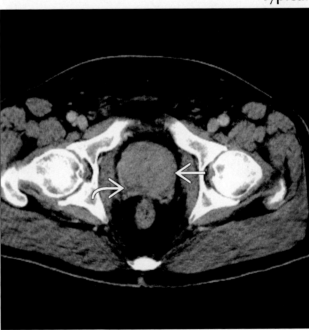

(Left) Coronal bone scan shows diffuse spinal and rib metastases ➜. *(Right)* Axial CECT shows an enlarged prostate ➜ with a questionable small area of low attenuation in the right posterior peripheral zone ➜ of uncertain clinical significance.

PROSTATE CARCINOMA

Typical

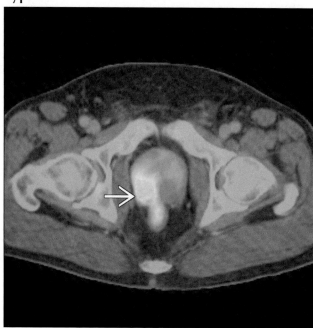 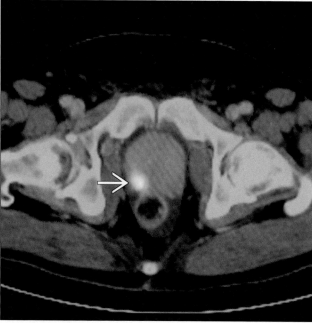

(Left) Axial fused PET/CT in the same patient shows asymmetric increased FDG activity ➡ in the right aspect of the prostate, subsequently proven to be an aggressive prostate carcinoma. *(Right)* Axial fused PET/CT shows a focus of increased FDG uptake ➡ in the posterior right aspect of the prostate, subsequently biopsy-proven to be prostate carcinoma. Many prostate carcinomas may not be FDG avid, but focal intense FDG activity in a patient without a history of prostate cancer should prompt correlation with serum PSA.

Typical

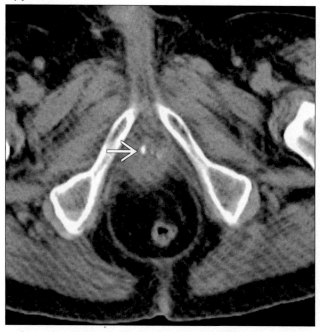 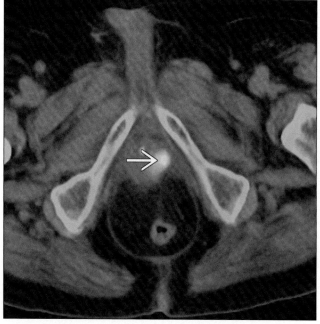

(Left) Axial NECT shows dystrophic calcifications ➡ in the inferior aspect of the prostate gland without definite mass. *(Right)* Axial fused PET/ CT shows focal intense FDG activity ➡ in the left side of the prostate peripherally. Subsequent correlation revealed an elevated PSA, and follow-up biopsy confirmed prostate carcinoma.

PROSTATE CARCINOMA

Typical

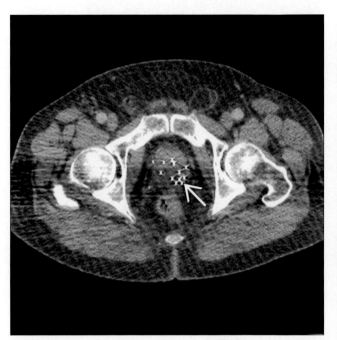
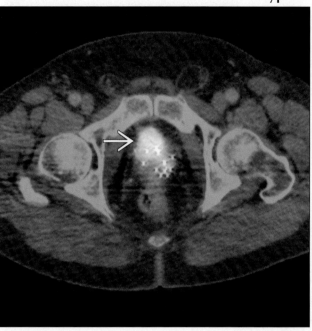

(Left) Axial CECT shows brachytherapy beads ➡ within the prostate. *(Right)* Axial fused PET/CT shows increased FDG activity in the anterior aspect of the prostate ➡ in this patient with prostate carcinoma being treated with brachytherapy seeds.

Typical

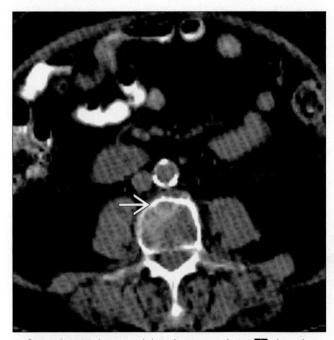
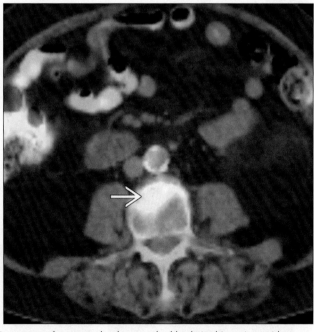

(Left) Axial NECT shows a subtle indeterminate lesion ➡ along the anterior aspect of an upper lumbar vertebral body in this patient with a history of prostate carcinoma and rising PSA. *(Right)* Axial fused PET/CT shows moderately increased FDG activity ➡ that correlates with the subtle lucent lesion within the vertebral body, worrisome for metastatic disease.

3

CARCINOMA OF UNKNOWN PRIMARY

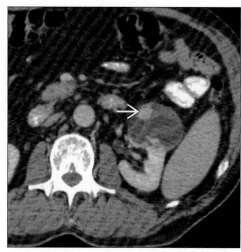 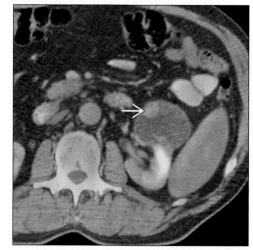

Axial CECT shows a complex cystic left renal mass suggestive of renal cell carcinoma ➡ in this patient with a brain metastasis and no primary.

Axial fused PET/CT shows mildly increased FDG activity corresponding to the mural nodularity ➡, confirmed to be renal cell carcinoma.

TERMINOLOGY

Abbreviations and Synonyms
- Carcinoma of unknown primary (CUP)
- Includes undifferentiated carcinomas in addition to adenocarcinoma

Definitions
- Metastatic cancer without known site of origin
  - Histology inconsistent with known tumors from organ biopsied
- Also defined as presence of metastatic disease for which site of primary lesion remains unidentified
  - Remains unknown despite review of
    - Medical history
    - Physical exam
    - Lab work (CBC, kidney/liver/pancreas function tests, PSA, U/A)
  - Imaging evaluation usually includes CXR, abdominopelvic CT, mammography
  - After common imaging investigation, 20-27% of primaries remain unidentified

IMAGING FINDINGS

General Features
- Best diagnostic clue: Detection of focal intense FDG activity in potential primary organ or site in patient with biopsy-proven carcinoma of unknown primary
- Location
  - Most common site: Upper aerodigestive tract, specifically lung
    - May also have abnormal mediastinal nodes
    - Consider accessible areas for subsequent confirmatory biopsy
  - Gastrointestinal and urogenital tract also common
    - Appear as focal areas of intense FDG activity in bowel rather than linear areas of physiologic activity
    - Look carefully at kidneys as a small renal cell carcinoma may be missed or obscured by physiologic excretory FDG activity
  - Frequency of metastases by location
    - Lymph node (LN) 46.3%
    - Liver 12%
    - Brain 11%

DDx: Common Locations of Primary Lesions in Patients with CUP

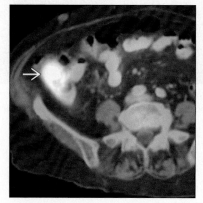 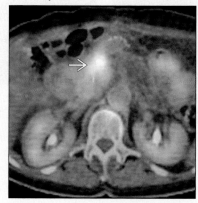 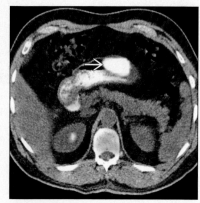

Colon Carcinoma *Pancreatic Carcinoma* *Gastric Carcinoma*

CARCINOMA OF UNKNOWN PRIMARY

Key Facts

Terminology
- Metastatic cancer without known site of origin; histology inconsistent with known tumors from organ biopsied

Imaging Findings
- Most common site: Upper aerodigestive tract, specifically lung
- Gastrointestinal and urogenital tract also common
- Squamous cell: Primary most often in tonsils, nasopharynx
- Adenocarcinoma: Primary most often in thorax, GI tract, urogenital tract
- Likelihood of primary detection with PET/CT: 25-40%; CT: 25%
- FDG PET provides whole-body survey

- PET may commonly reveal "missed primary" rather than unknown primary in true sense, i.e., following complete work-up
- Small study showed PET/CT more sensitive than PET alone, with 53% detection rate for occult cancers missed by other techniques

Top Differential Diagnoses
- Physiologic Activity
- Inflammation
- Infection

Diagnostic Checklist
- In patient with CUP, perform conventional laboratory workup and combination of imaging studies, with consideration of PET/CT

- Bone 11%
- Lung 6%
- Pleura 4%
- Peritoneum 4%
- Other 10%
- Involvement of supraclavicular and low cervical lymph nodes may be suspicious for primary in chest or abdomen
  - Associated with poorer prognosis than metastases of upper neck levels
- Squamous cell
  - Primary most often in tonsils &/or nasopharynx
  - Look for asymmetrical focal intense FDG activity on PET and PET/CT
- Adenocarcinoma
  - Primary most often in thorax, GI tract, or urogenital tract
- Size: Varies from small (< 1 cm) to several centimeters
- Morphology: Range of morphologies, including no obvious findings on CT to a several centimeter mass

Imaging Recommendations
- Best imaging tool
  - Likelihood of primary detection with PET/CT: 25-40%; CT: 25%
  - FDG PET provides whole-body survey
  - Patients with head/neck mets of non-SCCA histology should not be limited to imaging of head/neck area only
    - Whole-body imaging has been proven beneficial
  - Typical workup for patients with SCCA lymph node mets
    - Thorough physical exam including transnasal fibre-endoscopy of nasal cavity, nasopharynx, oropharynx, hypopharynx, larynx
    - CECT or CEMR of neck and PA/Lat CXR
    - Panendoscopy includes rigid esophagoscopy, tracheobronchoscopy, hypopharyngoscopy, laryngoscopy
    - Inspection/palpation of oropharynx and oral cavity, with biopsies taken from suspicious mucosal areas

- Ipsilateral tonsillectomy if no primary detected during panendoscopic random biopsies
- FDG PET often used when all of the above approaches have failed; may also direct biopsies
- Non-SCCA histology has similar workup, with CT of chest and abdomen along with pelvic/prostate examinations
- Mammography very low yield; rarely do patients with CUP have primary mass in breast
- Protocol advice
  - Consider PET/CT evaluation, although currently not routinely used for CUP
  - Contrast-enhanced CT may provide additional benefit
    - Better characterization of focal areas of FDG activity
    - Differentiation of potential bowel lesion from those adjacent to bowel

CT Findings
- CT typically used to help identify primary
  - Low sensitivity (~ 25%)
- CT scanning is the imaging modality of choice in terms of availability, cost effectiveness, quickness, and patient compliance
  - Especially for evaluation of cervical lymphadenopathy and identification of occult primary lesions
- Newer technology and methods of acquisition
  - Better image quality and resolution
  - Better reconstructive capabilities
  - Quicker scans
  - Decreased artifact
- Quicker scans also allow dynamic maneuvers to be used
  - Puffed cheek and modified Valsalva techniques can help open opposed mucosal surfaces in the oral cavity, oropharynx, and hypopharynx
    - May allow easier detection of unknown mucosal primaries

CARCINOMA OF UNKNOWN PRIMARY

o Nonetheless, critical evaluation of the CT scan helps direct biopsies during panendoscopy in the workup of the unknown primary tumor
- For evaluation of cervical lymphadenopathy, a CT scan of the neck is helpful to assess the involvement of vital structures
  o Also provides the clinician with useful data regarding surgical resectability
- CT scan can also be used to evaluate clinically negative cervical lymph node zones
- Radiographic criteria of potential pathological lymph nodes
  o Rounding of the lymph node
  o Size > 1.5 cm in the jugulodigastric region or > 1 cm in other regions
  o Hypodense fluid center of the lymph node that signifies necrosis
  o Mass effect

Nuclear Medicine Findings

- PET
  o FDG PET shown to identify lesion in ~ 25-40% of patients with negative conventional imaging investigations
  o PET may commonly reveal "missed primary"
    ▪ Rather than unknown primary in true sense, i.e., following complete workup
  o False negative may result from
    ▪ Low tumor uptake (e.g., carcinoid) or high background uptake (e.g., liver, high serum glucose level)
  o PET has high specificity for tumors in lung, breast, and pancreas
- Possibly low clinical impact of FDG PET in patients who have already undergone extensive workup with panendoscopy
- Small study showed PET/CT more sensitive than PET alone, with 53% detection rate for occult cancers missed by other techniques
- Criteria for malignancy on FDG PET or PET/CT
  o FDG hypermetabolism at site of pathological changes on CT
  o Marked focal hypermetabolism at sites suggestive of malignancy (liver parenchyma, bone marrow)
    ▪ Despite absence of signs of pathology at those sites on CT
- Identification of primary is more complex than identification of metastatic lesions
  o Patient's history is often helpful
  o Distribution of pathological lesion may be helpful
    ▪ Knowledge of the pattern of spread of different tumors
  o More difficult in cases of generalized disease with many foci in different organs
  o If unable to identify a lesion as the site of primary, may conclude that CUP syndrome was generalized
  o Rate of detection of malignancy in general will be higher than that of primary

DIFFERENTIAL DIAGNOSIS

Physiologic Activity

- Following structures commonly have increased physiologic activity that may mimic that of malignancy
  o Colon: Can be focal, short segment, or linear
  o Cardiac: Usually left ventricular, though all chambers may have increased wall activity in pathologic states
  o Thymus: Seen in younger patients, usually linear if physiologic
  o Glands: Look for symmetry to differentiate physiologic from pathologic activity
  o Lymphoid tissue: May be asymmetrical or symmetrical
  o Muscle: Often linear, helping to establish as physiologic; when focal can look like malignancy; correlate with CT
  o Brown fat: CT showing fat attenuation is diagnostic
- PET/CT helps facilitate differentiation of pathologic from physiologic FDG activity

Inflammation

- Several inflammatory or granulomatous conditions, such as sarcoidosis, may cause focal FDG activity and mimic malignancy

Infection

- Infectious processes such as underlying fungal infection or TB may cause focal activity
- Dental abscesses may cause focal intense FDG activity, mimicking head and neck cancer

Benign Lesion

- Colonic adenomas and thyroid adenomas may have focal FDG activity
- Benign osseous lesions include fibrous cortical defect, osteoradionecrosis, and Paget

Iatrogenic

- Post-operative changes or catheters and ostomies may appear as focal areas of FDG activity, mimicking malignancy

PATHOLOGY

General Features

- General path comments
  o Reasons for low rate of primary detection include
    ▪ Lesion size smaller than spatial resolution of technique
    ▪ Involution of primary mass due to limited angiogenic competence
- Etiology: Variable depending on the actual primary tumor
- Epidemiology
  o High percentage of CUP patients have adenocarcinoma (60-75%)
  o CUP makes up only a small proportion of all cancer at 0.5-6%

CARCINOMA OF UNKNOWN PRIMARY

Microscopic Features
- Adequate biopsy specimen rather than FNA essential for diagnostic purposes
  - Histological workup includes immunohistochemistry techniques to better describe potential origin of primary
    - Complemented by EM, chromosome analysis, and gene microarray analysis
- Diagnosis of adenocarcinoma based on identification of glandular structures formed by neoplastic cells

CLINICAL ISSUES

Presentation
- Most common signs/symptoms
  - Variable depending on site of presenting metastasis
  - GI bleeding with GI primary tumors
  - Hemoptysis with primary lung carcinomas
  - Brain metastasis or neurologic dysfunction often first presenting symptom
- Other signs/symptoms: Occasionally hematuria in a patient with occult renal cell carcinoma

Demographics
- Age: Median age at presentation = 59 years
- Gender: Equal distribution of CUP between men and women

Natural History & Prognosis
- Primary will not be found in majority of cases despite full workup
- 20% of patients still have no identifiable primary site postmortem
- Median survival for CUP is 12 months
  - Detection of primary lesions and initiation of therapy can prolong survival to 23 months

Treatment
- If primary is identified, aggressive chemotherapy or hormonal therapy may be considered

DIAGNOSTIC CHECKLIST

Consider
- In patient with CUP, perform conventional laboratory workup and combination of imaging studies, with consideration of PET/CT
- PET/CT: Image top of skull to feet to identify all possible primary sites
- Perform contrast-enhanced CT as part of the PET/CT exam to maximize the specificity of potential lesions

SELECTED REFERENCES

1. Miller FR et al: Management of the unknown primary carcinoma: long-term follow-up on a negative PET scan and negative panendoscopy. Head Neck. 30(1):28-34, 2008
2. Fencl P et al: Prognostic and diagnostic accuracy of [18F]FDG-PET/CT in 190 patients with carcinoma of unknown primary. Eur J Nucl Med Mol Imaging. 34(11):1783-92, 2007
3. Parini CL et al: Occult metastatic lung carcinoma presenting as locally advanced uterine carcinosarcoma on positron emission tomography/computed tomography imaging. Int J Gynecol Cancer. 17(3):731-4, 2007
4. Paul SA et al: FDG PET and PET/CT for the detection of the primary tumour in patients with cervical non-squamous cell carcinoma metastasis of an unknown primary. Eur Arch Otorhinolaryngol. 264(2):189-95, 2007
5. Sève P et al: The role of 2-deoxy-2-[F-18]fluoro-D-glucose positron emission tomography in disseminated carcinoma of unknown primary site. Cancer. 109(2):292-9, 2007
6. Ambrosini V et al: 18F-FDG PET/CT in the assessment of carcinoma of unknown primary origin. Radiol Med (Torino). 111(8):1146-55, 2006
7. Asakura H et al: Unknown primary carcinoma, diagnosed as inflammatory breast cancer, and successfully treated with trastuzumab and vinorelbine. Int J Clin Oncol. 10(4):285-8, 2005
8. Ghosh L et al: Management of patients with metastatic cancer of unknown primary. Curr Probl Surg. 42(1):12-66, 2005
9. Kolesnikov-Gauthier H et al: FDG PET in patients with cancer of an unknown primary. Nucl Med Commun. 26(12):1059-66, 2005
10. Nanni C et al: Role of 18F-FDG PET-CT imaging for the detection of an unknown primary tumour: preliminary results in 21 patients. Eur J Nucl Med Mol Imaging. 32(5):589-92, 2005
11. Scott CL et al: The utility of 2-deoxy-2-[F-18]fluoro-D-glucose positron emission tomography in the investigation of patients with disseminated carcinoma of unknown primary origin. Mol Imaging Biol. 7(3):236-43, 2005
12. Hawksworth J et al: Surgical and ablative treatment for metastatic adenocarcinoma to the liver from unknown primary tumor. Am Surg. 70(6):512-7, 2004
13. Mintzer DM et al: Cancer of unknown primary: changing approaches. A multidisciplinary case presentation from the Joan Karnell cancer center of pennsylvania hospital. Oncologist. 9(3):330-8, 2004
14. Dittmann H et al: [18F]FLT PET for diagnosis and staging of thoracic tumours. Eur J Nucl Med Mol Imaging. 30(10):1407-12, 2003
15. Fogarty GB et al: The usefulness of fluorine 18-labelled deoxyglucose positron emission tomography in the investigation of patients with cervical lymphadenopathy from an unknown primary tumor. Head Neck. 25(2):138-45, 2003
16. Pavlidis N et al: Diagnostic and therapeutic management of cancer of an unknown primary. Eur J Cancer. 39(14):1990-2005, 2003
17. Peterson JJ et al: Diagnosis of occult bone metastases: positron emission tomography. Clin Orthop Relat Res. (415 Suppl):S120-8, 2003
18. Stoeckli SJ et al: Lymph node metastasis of squamous cell carcinoma from an unknown primary: impact of positron emission tomography. Eur J Nucl Med Mol Imaging. 30(3):411-6, 2003
19. Haas I et al: Diagnostic strategies in cervical carcinoma of an unknown primary (CUP). Eur Arch Otorhinolaryngol. 259(6):325-33, 2002
20. No authors listed: FDG positron emission tomography to manage patients with an occult primary carcinoma and metastasis outside the cervical lymph nodes. TEC Bull (Online). 19(2):14-8, 2002
21. Regelink G et al: Detection of unknown primary tumours and distant metastases in patients with cervical metastases: value of FDG-PET versus conventional modalities. Eur J Nucl Med Mol Imaging. 29(8):1024-30, 2002

CARCINOMA OF UNKNOWN PRIMARY

Use of CT for CUP

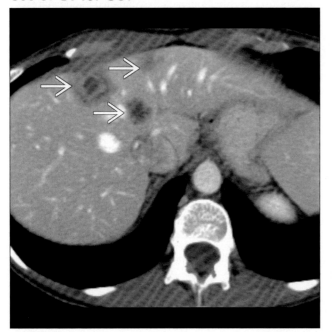 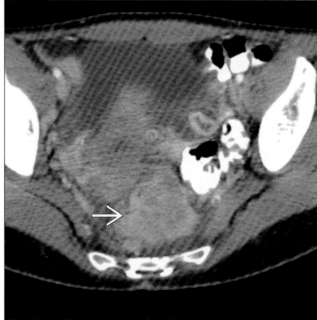

(Left) Axial CECT shows 3 low attenuation hepatic lesions ➡ suggestive of metastatic disease in this patient without a history of malignancy. *(Right)* Axial CECT shows an enhancing presacral mass ➡, subsequently shown to be a large colon carcinoma arising from the distal sigmoid colon.

Use of CT for CUP

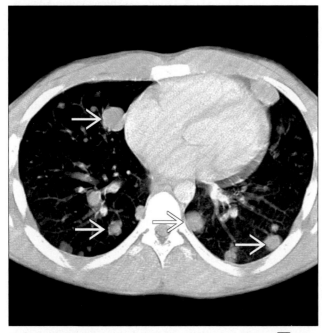 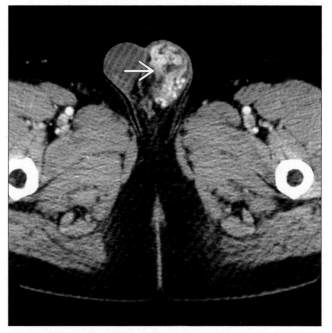

(Left) Axial CECT shows multiple bilateral pulmonary lesions ➡, very worrisome for metastases in this patient without a history of malignancy. *(Right)* Axial CECT in the same patient shows a heterogeneously enhancing mass in the left testis ➡, subsequently proven to be this patient's primary malignancy.

CARCINOMA OF UNKNOWN PRIMARY

Use of PET/CT for CUP

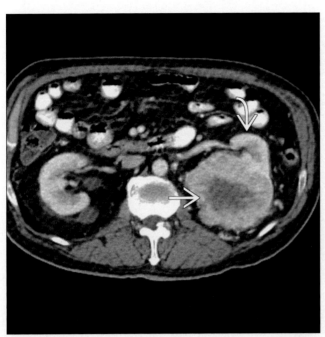
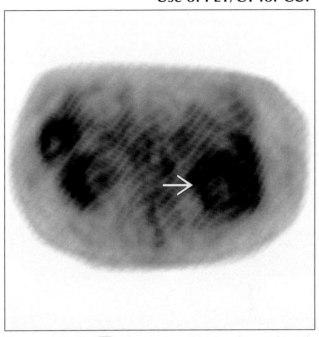

(Left) Axial CECT shows a solid renal mass with central necrosis ➘ arising from the left kidney ➘ in this patient with a recent biopsy of a neck mass showing metastatic carcinoma. *(Right)* Axial PET shows moderate to intense FDG activity in the left renal mass ➘, compatible with renal cell carcinoma.

Use of PET/CT for CUP

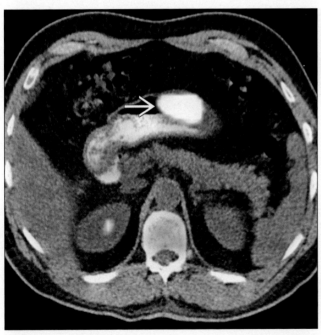
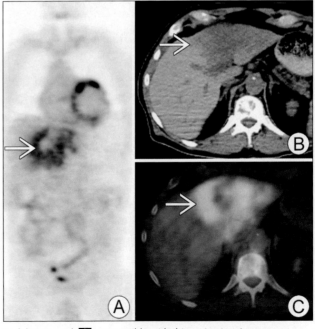

(Left) Axial fused PET/CT shows intense FDG activity in the anterior aspect of the stomach ➙, compatible with this patient's primary malignancy. The patient had a recent biopsy of a lung lesion showing adenocarcinoma, likely from bowel primary. *(Right)* Coronal PET (A), axial CT (B) and fused PET/CT (C) show a large lesion in the left hepatic lobe ➙, suggestive of cholangiocarcinoma in this patient with lung metastases and unknown primary.

CARCINOMA OF UNKNOWN PRIMARY

Use of PET/CT for CUP

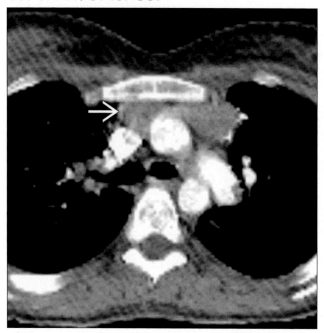 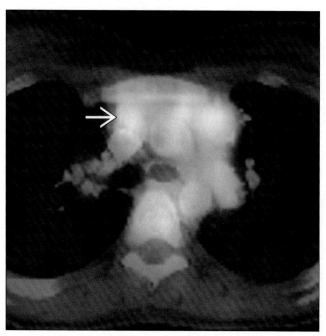

(Left) Axial CECT shows anterior mediastinal mass ➡ biopsy proven to be adenocarcinoma. The patient had no known primary malignancy. *(Right)* Axial fused PET/CT shows moderate to intense FDG activity in the anterior mediastinal mass ➡, compatible with malignancy. Although FDG PET or PET/CT can be helpful in detecting primary malignancies in those with CUP, no primary was identified in this patient.

Use of PET/CT for CUP

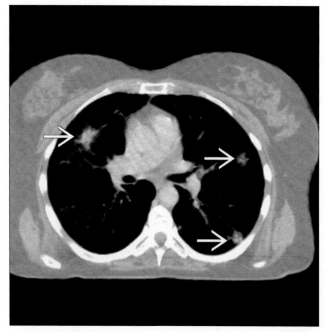 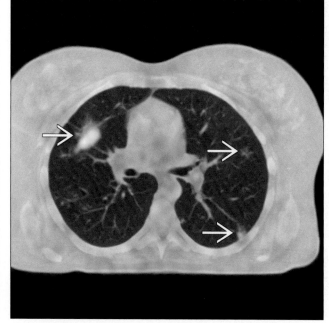

(Left) Axial CECT shows multiple suspicious pulmonary lesions ➡ bilaterally in this patient without a history of malignancy. *(Right)* Axial fused PET/CT shows moderate to intense FDG activity within at least 3 pulmonary lesions ➡, suggestive of metastatic disease in this patient without a history of malignancy.

CARCINOMA OF UNKNOWN PRIMARY

Use of PET/CT for CUP

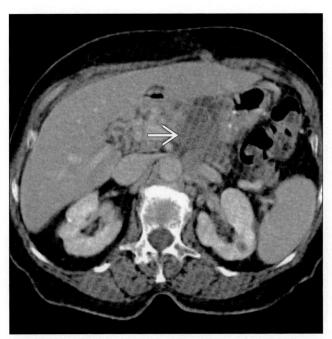 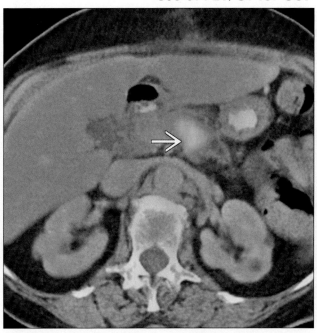

(Left) Axial fused PET/CT shows a heterogeneously enhancing, low attenuation mass in the body/tail of the pancreas ➡️, suggestive of pancreatic carcinoma as the primary malignancy. *(Right)* Axial fused PET/CT shows moderately increased activity corresponding to the pancreatic lesion ➡️, most compatible with pancreatic adenocarcinoma. Subsequent biopsy proved adenocarcinoma of the pancreas.

Use of PET/CT for CUP

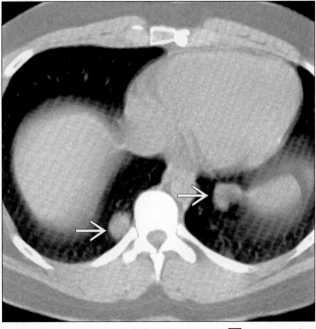 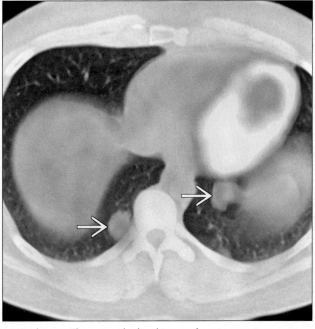

(Left) Axial CECT shows new bilateral lung masses ➡️, worrisome for metastatic disease. The patient had no history of a primary malignancy. *(Right)* Axial fused PET/CT shows mildly increased FDG activity in the pulmonary lesions ➡️. Although the lesions demonstrate only mildly increased FDG activity, it is still worrisome for malignancy, likely a relatively non-FDG-avid malignancy.

3

CARCINOMA OF UNKNOWN PRIMARY

Use of PET/CT for CUP

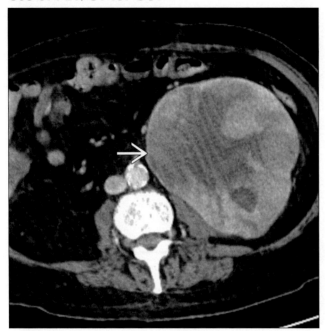
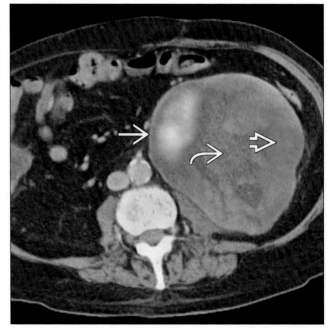

(Left) Axial CECT shows a large mass ➡ centered in the retroperitoneal/mesenteric junction with a large area of central necrosis, worrisome for this patient's primary malignancy. *(Right)* Axial fused PET/CT shows moderately increased FDG activity along the medial border of the mass ➡, no increased activity correlating with the central necrosis ➡, and minimally increased activity correlating with the lateral and posterior borders ➡. The overall appearance and location are very suggestive of a primary sarcoma.

Use of PET/CT for CUP

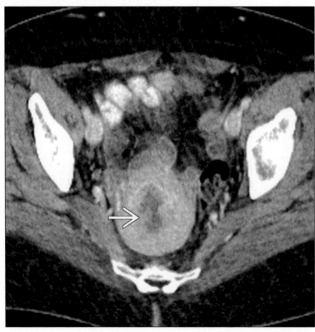
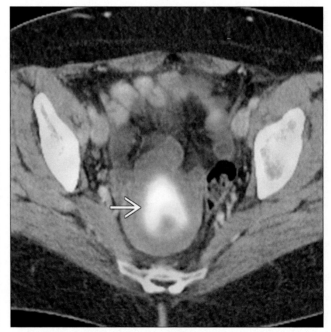

(Left) Axial CECT in this patient without a known primary malignancy shows probable endometrial thickening ➡. Primary consideration would be endometrial carcinoma. *(Right)* Axial fused PET/CT shows intense FDG activity corresponding to the area of endometrial thickening ➡, subsequently proven to be endometrial carcinoma.

CARCINOMA OF UNKNOWN PRIMARY

Use of PET/CT for CUP

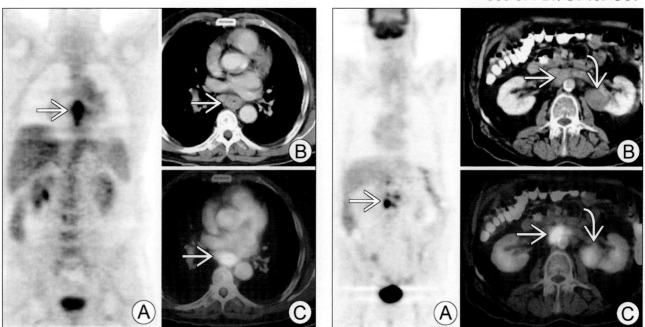

(Left) Coronal PET (A), axial CT (B) and fused PET/CT (C) demonstrate focal intense activity in the mid to distal esophagus ➡. This patient with an unknown primary was subsequently diagnosed with poorly differentiated adenocarcinoma of the esophagus. *(Right)* Coronal PET (A), axial CT (B) and fused PET/CT (C) in a patient with recently diagnosed esophageal carcinoma shows multiple foci of intense FDG activity in the retroperitoneal area ➡. An incidental mass in the mild to moderate FDG activity is also present in the left kidney ➡, compatible with a second renal cell carcinoma with regional metastatic nodes.

Use of PET/CT for CUP

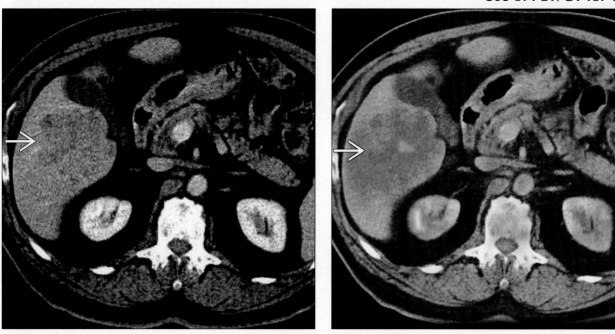

(Left) Axial CECT shows a heterogeneously enhancing mass in the right lobe of the liver ➡, biopsy-proven to be hepatocellular carcinoma in this patient with CUP. *(Right)* Axial fused PET/CT shows mildly increased FDG activity in the hepatic mass ➡ in a patient with carcinoma of unknown primary and subsequent diagnosis of colorectal carcinoma. Subsequent biopsy specimen proved to be a second primary hepatocellular carcinoma. This amount of FDG activity is characteristic of hepatocellular carcinoma.

SECTION 4
Pitfalls and Limitations

Benign Causes of FDG Activity   4-2

BENIGN CAUSES OF FDG ACTIVITY

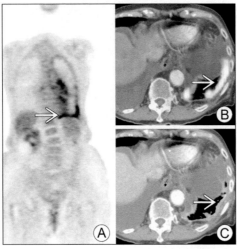

Multiple images (A, B, C) show inflammation ➡ from talc pleurodesis. PET may be positive indefinitely.

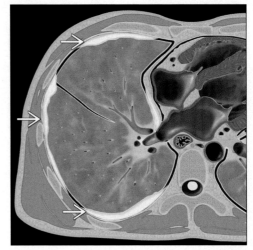

Graphic shows a representation of talc pleurodesis ➡. The talc is often discontinuous.

TERMINOLOGY

Abbreviations and Synonyms
- Nonmalignant areas of increased metabolism

Definitions
- Benign nonphysiologic uptake of FDG may be encountered in as many as 25% of studies
  o As many as 75% of those lesions will be inflammatory

IMAGING FINDINGS

General Features
- Best diagnostic clue
  o FDG activity in a typical distribution suggests a benign process
  o Sarcoidosis, fungal infections, post-radiation, post-surgical and other benign processes may have recognizable patterns of involvement
- Location: Varies

Nuclear Medicine Findings
- **Tuberculoma and tuberculous lymphadenopathy**
  o Tuberculoma well-known cause of intense FDG uptake
  o Appears as discrete nodule or mass with central caseous necrosis and surrounding inflammatory mantle
- **Sarcoidosis**
  o Typical distribution is bilateral hilar and right paratracheal
  o FDG uptake secondary to accumulation of T-lymphocytes and mononuclear phagocytes and noncaseating epithelioid granulomas
  o Intensity of FDG uptake may reflect activity of disease
  o Multisystem disease
  o Easily misinterpreted as malignancy
    ▪ Thus FDG PET most useful for response to treatment and evaluation of extent of disease
- **Cryptococcosis**
  o Caused by Cryptococcus neoformans
  o Infection occurs by inhaling fungus into lung

DDx: Focal Intense FDG Activity

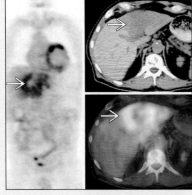

Malignancy

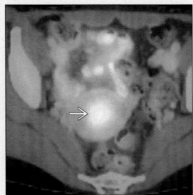

Physiologic: Menstruation

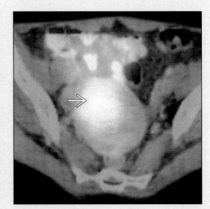

Benign Mass: Fibroid

BENIGN CAUSES OF FDG ACTIVITY

Key Facts

Terminology
- Nonmalignant areas of increased metabolism
- Benign nonphysiologic uptake of FDG may be encountered in as many as 25% of studies
  - As many as 75% of those lesions will be inflammatory

Imaging Findings
- Similar imaging findings may be present for malignant and various benign processes
- History is critical for reducing misinterpretation
- FDG activity in a typical distribution suggests a benign process
- Sarcoidosis, fungal infections, post-radiation, post-surgical, and other benign processes may have recognizable patterns of involvement

Top Differential Diagnoses
- Malignancy
- Benign Masses
- Iatrogenic
- Inflammation
- Infection
- Granulomatous Disease

Pathology
- Activated inflammatory cells have greatly elevated levels of glycolysis

Diagnostic Checklist
- Accurate differentiation between malignant and benign disease can reduce unnecessary surgical explorations

---

- Lung lesions generally demonstrate intense granulomatous inflammation
- Several reports have shown false positives due to high FDG uptake
- **Paragonimiasis**
  - Endemic to southern Asia
  - Parasitic disease with larval damage ultimately in lungs and brain
  - Reported cause of high FDG uptake
- **Abscesses**
  - Glycolytic metabolism elevated in association with leukocytic infiltration
  - Usually has central photopenia secondary to necrosis or pus
- **Pneumocystis**
  - Associated with high FDG uptake
- **Other infections**
  - Sinusitis, pneumonia, radiation-induced pneumonitis, pancreatitis
  - Each may show elevated FDG uptake
- **Radiation pneumonitis/fibrosis**
  - FDG uptake caused by infiltration of leukocytes and macrophages
  - Radiation leads to production of local cytokines including IL-6, TNF, and TGF-beta, which provoke inflammatory morphologic changes
  - Early after radiation to the lung, PET may be positive (up to several months); may not be able to interpret effect on underlying tumor until resolution
- **Pneumoconiosis**
  - Parenchymal reaction to presence of foreign substances in lungs
  - May present with massive fibrosis and associated FDG uptake
- **Peri-tumoral granulation tissue**
  - Granulation tissue surrounding tumor and inflammatory cells within necrotic areas of tumor contribute to FDG uptake in tumors
  - As much of 24% of concentration may be due to non-tumor tissue
- **Chemotherapy**

- FDG uptake generally decreases after chemotherapy, correlating with clinical response
- **Splenic uptake**
  - In the setting of infection, splenic uptake can be intense
  - Spleen has multiple roles in the immune response, reflected in increased FDG activity in patients with infection or inflammation
- **AIDS**
  - This patient group is vulnerable to a wide range of infections and malignancies
  - Difficult to distinguish infection from tumor
  - Toxoplasmosis can be differentiated from lymphoma because it is much less FDG avid, with virtually no overlap in SUV
- **Fever of undetermined origin**
  - Diagnosis entails 3 weeks duration, episodic fever exceeding 38.3° C, and no diagnosis after standard workup
  - Causes include infection, neoplasms, collagen vascular disease, granulomatous disease, pulmonary emboli, CVA, and drug fever
  - FDG PET provides helpful information in 41% of cases
    - Negative FDG PET makes it very unlikely that a morphologic origin of the fever will be identified
  - In spite of normal cardiac uptake, FDG PET aids in identification of sites of infective endocarditis
- **Post-operative uptake**
  - Several weeks should elapse prior to imaging to reduce likelihood of positives due to post-operative changes
  - Good sensitivity for identification of infection in post-operative patients
  - Wound healing, such as tracheostomy and colostomy sites or indwelling stents, commonly show elevated FDG uptake
- **Osteomyelitis**
  - Useful for detection of osteomyelitis
  - Inflammatory arthritis, acute fracture, and normal healing bone may also cause positive signal
- **Prosthetic joint infection**

4

BENIGN CAUSES OF FDG ACTIVITY

- o Commonly seen due to high prevalence of hip and knee arthroplasties
- o Joint infection vs. aseptic loosening is a difficult differentiation
- o FDG PET does not effectively distinguish the two conditions, as they are both inflammatory
- **Bone fractures**
  - o Degree of FDG accumulation usually modest in rib fractures, but may closely mimic malignancy
  - o FDG uptake in healing bone can be present as late as 6 months after the injury
- **Arthritis**
  - o FDG uptake seen especially in acromioclavicular, sternoclavicular, and glenohumeral joints
  - o Uptake can be intense and asymmetric, leading to misinterpretation as neoplasm
- **Spinal osteomyelitis**
  - o Usually confined to vertebral body and intervertebral disk
  - o MR is imaging modality of choice for diagnosis
  - o FDG PET has similarly high sensitivity and specificity
- **Vasculitis**
  - o FDG uptake in giant cell arteritis, Takayasu disease, aortitis, and unspecified large vessel vasculitis has been described
- **Lymph Nodes**
  - o Uptake in lymph nodes is not specific for malignant neoplasm
  - o Granulomatous diseases such as tuberculosis and sarcoidosis may provoke intense FDG uptake in lymph nodes
  - o Necrotic lymph nodes may show poor accumulation

DIFFERENTIAL DIAGNOSIS

Malignancy
- When in doubt, consider short term follow-up exam to differentiate

Benign Masses
- Adenomas can have focal intense FDG activity
- Indistinguishable from malignancy

Iatrogenic
- History is imperative for reducing misinterpretation

Inflammation
- Almost any inflammatory process may cause false positives on FDG PET
- Consider dual-phase PET imaging

Infection
- Clinical symptoms often helpful for differentiating malignancy from benign process

Granulomatous Disease
- Sarcoidosis and other granulomatous processes can often mimic malignancy
- Look for other clues such as distribution, calcifications, and lack of features suggesting malignancy

PATHOLOGY

General Features
- General path comments
  - o Inflammatory cells such as neutrophils and activated macrophages at site of inflammation or injection show increased FDG accumulation
    - Active granulomatous disease, other infectious processes, and active fibrosis may also show FDG uptake and cause false positives
  - o Activated inflammatory cells have greatly elevated levels of glycolysis
    - 20-30x increased in hexose monophosphate shunt, which accounts for high FDG uptake

DIAGNOSTIC CHECKLIST

Consider
- Accurate differentiation between malignant and benign disease can reduce unnecessary surgical explorations
- Dual-phase or delayed-phase PET imaging may be helpful for distinguishing between malignancy and benign processes
- Hyperglycemia promotes greater glucose utilization in inflammatory cells
  - o Leads to more false positives in the setting of elevated blood glucose

SELECTED REFERENCES

1. Chryssikos T et al: FDG-PET imaging can diagnose periprosthetic infection of the hip. Clin Orthop Relat Res. 466(6):1338-42, 2008
2. Chundru S et al: Granulomatous disease: is it a nuisance or an asset during PET/computed tomography evaluation of lung cancers? Nucl Med Commun. 29(7):623-7, 2008
3. Nigg AP et al: Tuberculous Spondylitis (Pott's Disease). Infection. 36(3):293-4, 2008
4. Saleem BR et al: Periaortic endograft infection due to Listeria monocytogenes treated with graft preservation. J Vasc Surg. 47(3):635-7, 2008
5. Balink H et al: Diagnosis of abdominal aortic prosthesis infection with FDG-PET/CT. Vasc Endovascular Surg. 41(5):428-32, 2007
6. Helleman JN et al: Mycotic aneurysm of the descending thoracic aorta. Review and case report. Acta Chir Belg. 107(5):544-7, 2007
7. Inoue K et al: Diagnosing active inflammation in the SAPHO syndrome using 18FDG-PET/CT in suspected metastatic vertebral bone tumors. Ann Nucl Med. 21(8):477-80, 2007
8. Kang K et al: Positron emission tomographic findings in a tuberculous brain abscess. Ann Nucl Med. 21(5):303-6, 2007
9. Maldonado F et al: Focal organizing pneumonia on surgical lung biopsy: causes, clinicoradiologic features, and outcomes. Chest. 132(5):1579-83, 2007
10. Sheehy N et al: Acute varicella infection mimics recurrent Hodgkin's disease on F-18 FDG PET/CT. Clin Nucl Med. 32(10):820-1, 2007
11. Lustberg MB et al: FDG PET/CT Findings in Acute Adult Mononucleosis Mimicking Malignant Lymphoma. Eur J Haematol. (In Press)

BENIGN CAUSES OF FDG ACTIVITY

Benign Causes of FDG Uptake in the Neck

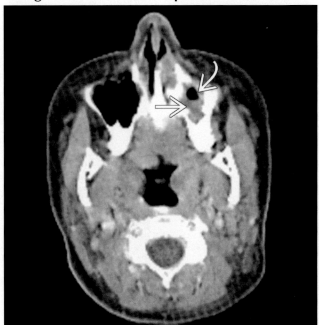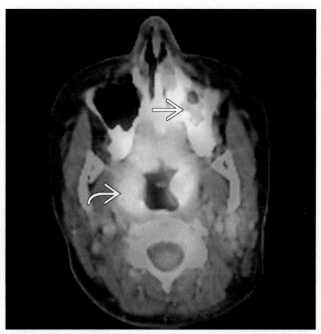

(Left) Axial CECT shows left maxillary sinus mucosal thickening ➡ and a subtle air-fluid level ➡, compatible with acute sinusitis. *(Right)* Axial fused PET/CT shows mild to moderately increased FDG activity within the left maxillary sinus ➡, compatible with sinusitis. Also note physiologic FDG activity within both palatine tonsils ➡.

Benign Causes of FDG Uptake in the Neck

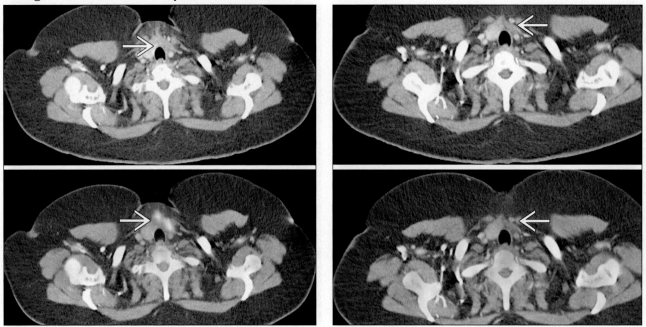

(Left) Axial CECT (top) and PET/CT (bottom) show moderately increased FDG activity ➡ in the thyroidectomy bed in a patient who had a left hemithyroidectomy approximately 3 weeks prior to this scan. *(Right)* Axial CT (top) and fused PET/CT (bottom), 16 weeks following thyroidectomy, show resolution of the inflammatory activity in the thyroidectomy bed ➡.

BENIGN CAUSES OF FDG ACTIVITY

Benign Causes of FDG Uptake in the Neck

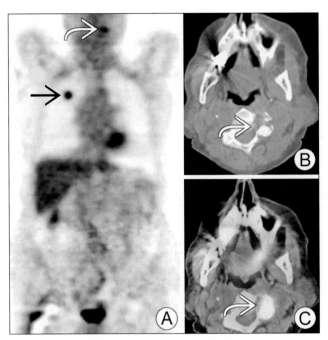

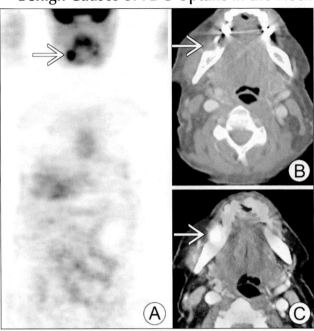

(Left) Coronal PET (A), axial CT (B) and fused PET/CT (C) demonstrate a hypermetabolic right upper lobe mass ➡, compatible with primary lung cancer, and an incidental focal area of moderately increased FDG activity ➡, corresponding to facet arthrosis in the cervical spine. *(Right)* Coronal PET (A), axial CT (B) and fused PET/CT (C) demonstrate focally increased FDG activity ➡ in the right maxillary molar, compatible with patient's history of a dental abscess.

Benign Causes of FDG Uptake in the Neck

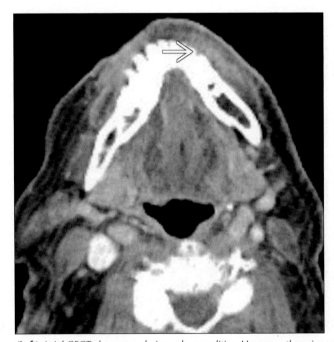

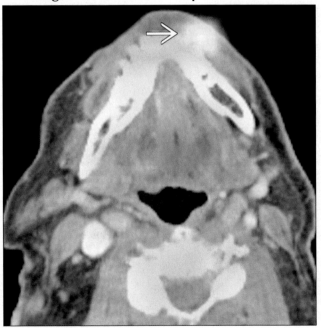

(Left) Axial CECT shows no obvious abnormalities. However, there is some subtle infiltration of the subcutaneous tissues in the anterior jaw ➡. *(Right)* Axial fused PET/CT shows a focal area of intense FDG activity ➡ in this patient with jaw pain and a history of a dental abscess being treated with antibiotics.

BENIGN CAUSES OF FDG ACTIVITY

Benign Causes of FDG Uptake in the Neck

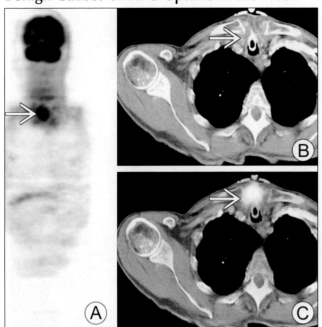

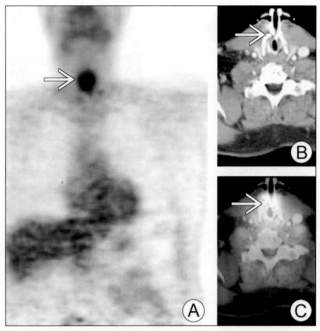

(Left) Approximately 8 weeks after tracheostomy tube placement, coronal PET (A), axial CT (B) and PET/CT (C) demonstrate intense FDG activity surrounding the tube ➡, compatible with inflammation. *(Right)* Coronal PET (A), axial CT (B) and PET/CT (C) demonstrate focal intense FDG activity surrounding this patient's tracheostomy ➡, compatible with inflammation &/or granulation tissue. Almost all tracheostomies will have some degree of increased FDG due to inflammation.

Benign Causes of FDG Uptake in the Neck

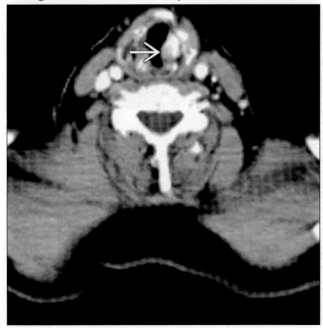

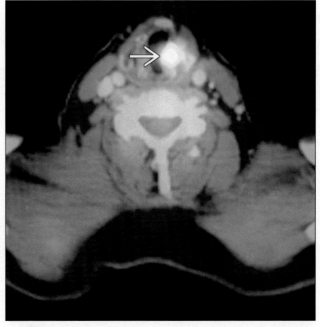

(Left) Axial CECT shows slight asymmetrical fullness in the left false vocal cord ➡. This patient had a history of thyroid carcinoma, status post thyroidectomy, and damage of the left recurrent laryngeal nerve. *(Right)* Axial fused PET/CT shows focal intense FDG activity in the region of left false vocal cord fullness ➡. Additional history revealed a thyroplasty procedure for paralyzed vocal cord. Teflon may cause a chronic granulomatous reaction, creating intense FDG activity indefinitely.

BENIGN CAUSES OF FDG ACTIVITY

Benign Causes of FDG Uptake in the Neck

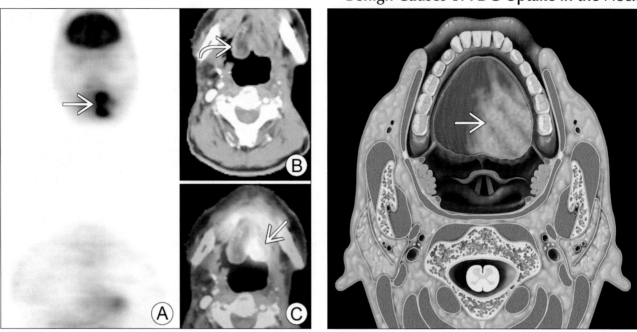

(Left) Coronal PET (A), axial CT (B) and fused PET/CT (C) show intense FDG activity in the left side of the tongue ➥ in this patient with a history of damage to the right XII cranial nerve, now with fatty replacement ➥ and paralysis of the right side. *(Right)* Graphic shows fatty infiltration of the left side of the tongue ➥, seen with cranial nerve VII denervation.

Benign Causes of FDG Uptake in the Chest

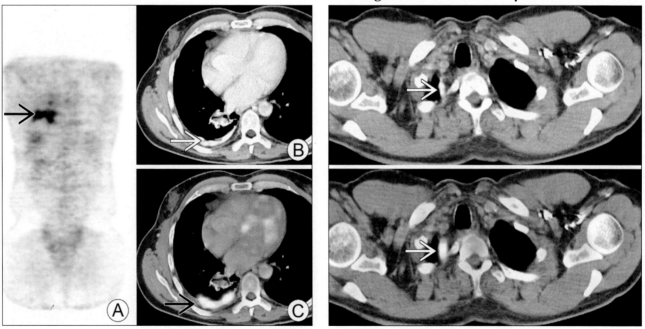

(Left) Coronal PET (A) and PET/CT (C) show linear FDG activity along the pleural surfaces posteriorly on the right ➥ following talc pleurodesis. Inspection of the axial CT (B) shows discontinuous, but linear, areas of high attenuation material, corresponding to talc ➥. *(Right)* Axial CT (top) and PET/CT (bottom) show a focal increased FDG activity, corresponding to a high attenuation focus at the right apex ➥, compatible with talc. Increased metabolic activity may be seen for years following pleurodesis.

BENIGN CAUSES OF FDG ACTIVITY

Benign Causes of FDG Uptake in the Chest

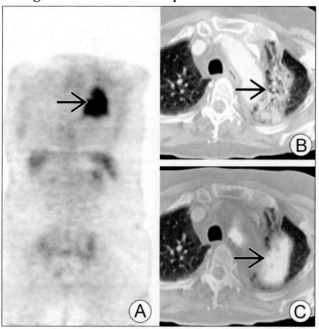
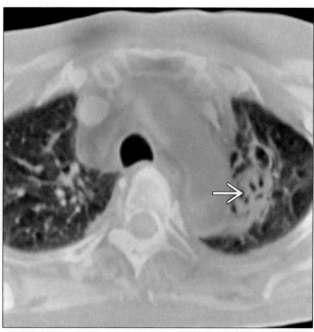

(Left) *Coronal PET (A) and axial fused PET/CT (C) show marked FDG activity* ➨ *within the left upper lobe parenchyma 8 weeks after radiation therapy, compatible with radiation pneumonitis. The axial CECT (B) shows the interstitial changes.* ***(Right)*** *Follow-up 5 months after radiation shows radiation fibrosis* ➨*.*

Benign Causes of FDG Uptake in the Chest

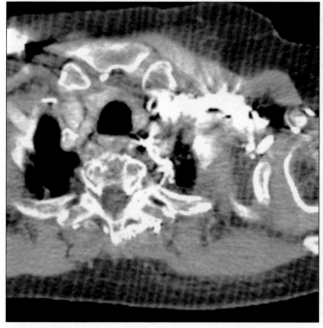
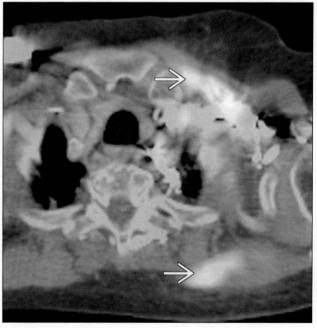

(Left) *Axial CECT shows no definite abnormalities.* ***(Right)*** *Axial fused PET/CT shows linear intense FDG activity in the anterior and posterior upper thoracic musculature* ➨ *in this patient who had recent radiation therapy, compatible with radiation-induced myositis.*

BENIGN CAUSES OF FDG ACTIVITY

Benign Causes of FDG Uptake in the Chest

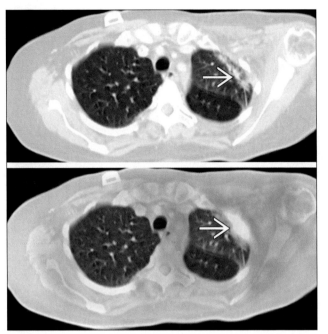

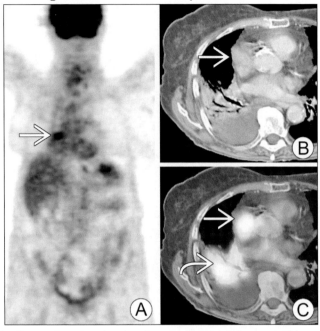

(Left) Axial CT (top) and PET/CT (bottom) in a patient, status post radiation therapy 8 weeks prior, show increased FDG activity, compatible with active radiation pneumonitis ➡. *(Right)* Coronal PET (A), axial CT (B) and PET/CT (C) in a patient who underwent radiation therapy 8 weeks prior demonstrate marked FDG activity in the right lower lobe consolidation ➡ and increased metabolic activity in the region of the right atrial appendage ➡, secondary to inflammation.

Benign Causes of FDG Uptake in the Chest

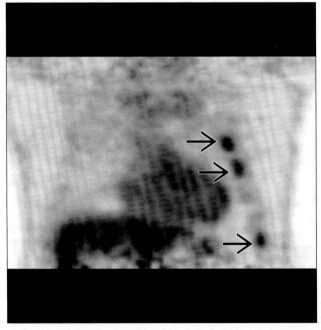

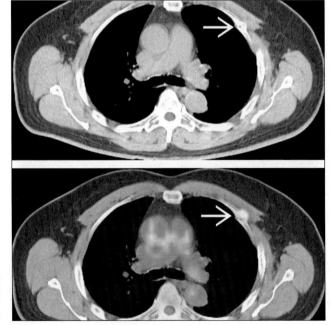

(Left) Coronal PET shows multiple foci of moderate to intense FDG activity ➡ within multiple ribs in this patient with recent trauma and multiple rib fractures. *(Right)* Axial NECT (top) and fused PET/CT (bottom) show focal intense activity within a rib fracture ➡.

BENIGN CAUSES OF FDG ACTIVITY

Benign Causes of FDG Uptake in the Chest

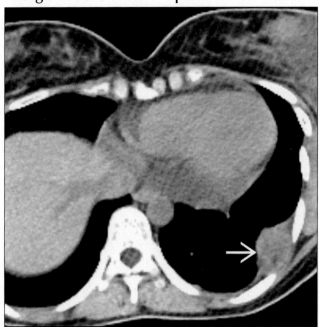
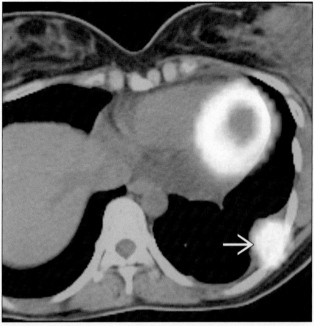

(Left) Axial NECT shows a pleural-based homogeneous soft tissue lesion ➡ with broad-based obtuse borders. This patient has no history of malignancy. *(Right)* Axial fused PET/CT shows markedly increased FDG activity associated with the pleural-based mass ➡, very suggestive of malignancy. However, a subsequent biopsy showed extensive granulomatous reaction without malignant cells.

Benign Causes of FDG Uptake in the Chest

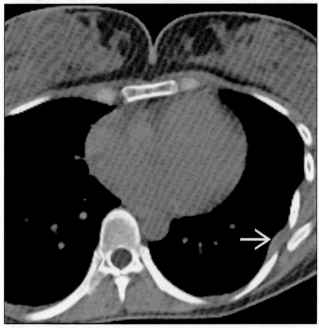
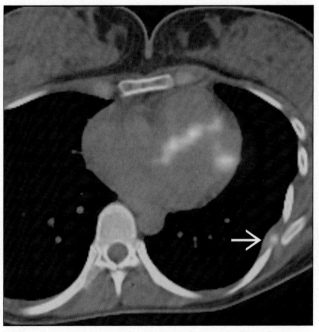

(Left) Axial NECT performed in the same patient as the prior two images demonstrates almost complete resolution of the pleural-based mass ➡ without interval therapy. *(Right)* Axial fused PET/CT shows almost complete resolution of the abnormal metabolic activity as well, with only mild residual metabolic activity remaining ➡.

BENIGN CAUSES OF FDG ACTIVITY

Benign Causes of FDG Uptake in the Chest

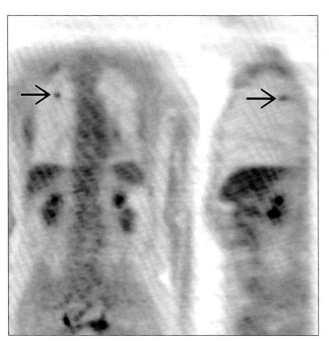

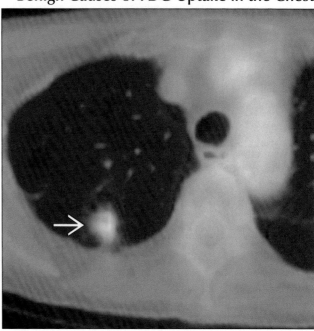

(Left) Coronal (left) and sagittal (right) images show a focal area of intense FDG activity in the right upper lung zone ➡, worrisome for malignancy. *(Right)* Axial fused PET/CT shows intense FDG activity within a slightly spiculated cavitary right lung pulmonary nodule ➡, subsequently proven to be tuberculosis. Unfortunately, infectious/inflammatory processes can mimic malignancy on FDG PET.

Benign Causes of FDG Uptake in the Chest

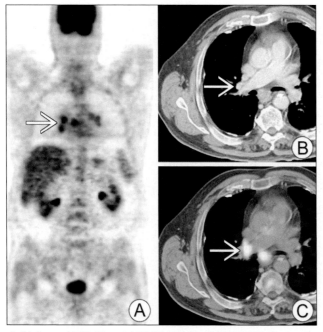

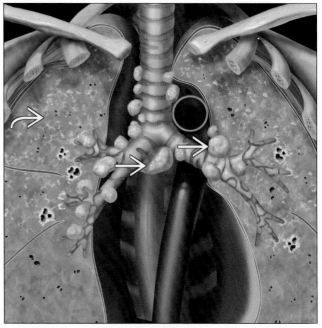

(Left) Coronal PET (A), axial CT (B) and fused PET/CT (C) demonstrate right hilar and subcarinal adenopathy ➡ in a patient with active sarcoidosis. *(Right)* Graphic shows multiple mediastinal enlarged lymph nodes ➡ in this patient with sarcoidosis. Also note predominant upper lobe lung changes along the bronchovascular bundles ➡.

BENIGN CAUSES OF FDG ACTIVITY

Benign Causes of FDG Uptake in the Chest

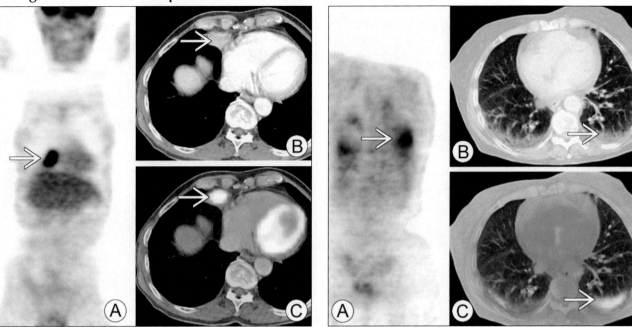

(Left) Coronal PET (A), axial CT (B) and fused PET/CT (C) show intense FDG activity in a new area of consolidation in the right middle lobe ➔, compatible with pneumonia. This resolved on a three-month follow-up. *(Right)* Coronal PET (A), axial CT (B) and fused PET/CT (C) demonstrate increased metabolic activity along the dependent portions of the lower lobes bilaterally ➔, compatible with dependent atelectasis.

Benign Causes of FDG Uptake in the Chest

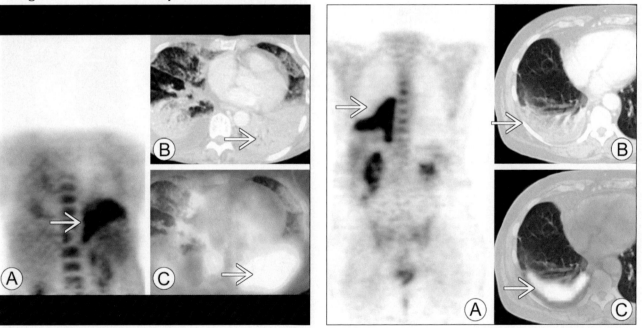

(Left) Coronal PET (A), axial CT (B) and fused PET/CT (C) in a patient with clinical symptoms of diffuse pneumonia show diffusely increased FDG activity bilaterally ➔ in regions of extensive pulmonary consolidation, compatible with pneumonia. *(Right)* Coronal PET (A), axial CT (B) and fused PET/CT (C) of a patient with a clinical history of recent pneumonia demonstrate intense FDG activity within consolidation in the right lower lobe ➔, compatible with pneumonia.

BENIGN CAUSES OF FDG ACTIVITY

Benign Causes of FDG Uptake in the Chest

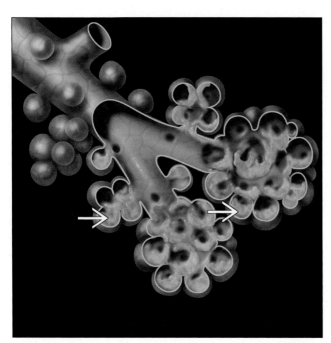

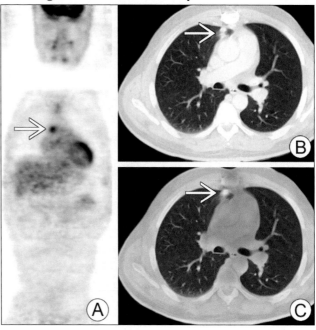

(Left) Graphic shows filling of the alveoli with mucus and pus ➡ in a patient with pneumonia. *(Right)* Coronal PET (A), axial CT (B) and fused PET/CT (C) show a focal area of intense FDG activity correlating with a small focal opacity in the medial aspect of the right upper lobe ➡. Subsequent thorascopic resection showed a focal area of bronchiolitis.

Benign Causes of FDG Uptake in the Chest

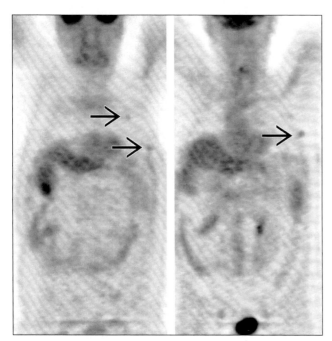

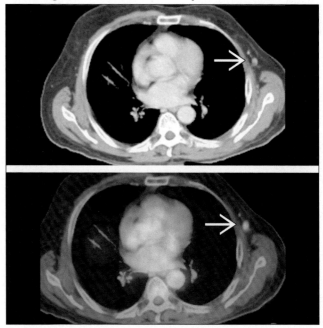

(Left) Coronal PET shows multiple tiny foci of FDG activity in the left anterior chest wall ➡ in this patient with a clinical history of herpes zoster. *(Right)* Axial CT (top) and fused PET/CT (bottom) demonstrate focally increased FDG activity that correlates with tiny left axillary lymph nodes ➡ in this patient with active Herpes zoster.

BENIGN CAUSES OF FDG ACTIVITY

Benign Causes of FDG Uptake in the Chest

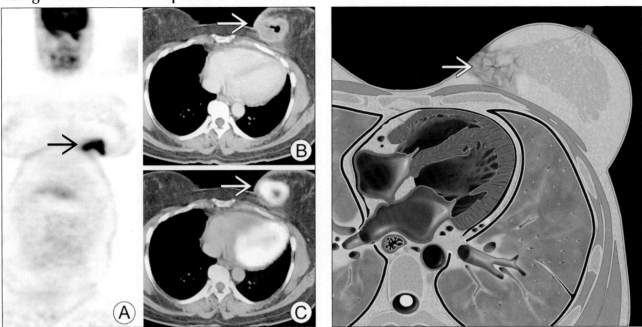

(Left) Coronal PET (A), axial CT (B) and fused PET/CT (C) show intense FDG activity in the medial aspect of the left breast ➡, corresponding to a necrotic mass ➡, compatible with a breast abscess. (Right) Graphic shows inflammation of the medial breast with central abscess ➡.

Benign Causes of FDG Uptake in the Chest

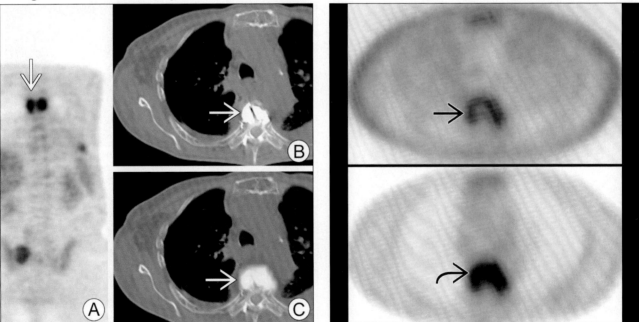

(Left) Coronal PET (A), axial CT (B) and fused PET/CT (C) of a patient who underwent a vertebroplasty approximately 2.5 weeks prior to this examination show intensely increased metabolic activity associated with the high attenuation material ➡. (Right) Axial PET images show increased activity on both the non-attenuation corrected image (top) ➡ as well as the attenuation corrected image (bottom) ➡, proving that the activity was not related to an attenuation correction artifact.

BENIGN CAUSES OF FDG ACTIVITY

Benign Causes of FDG Uptake in the Chest

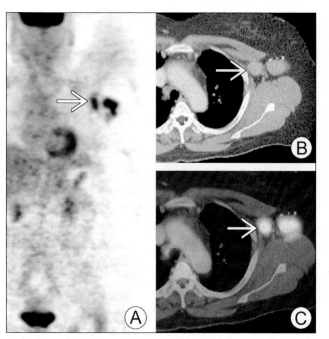
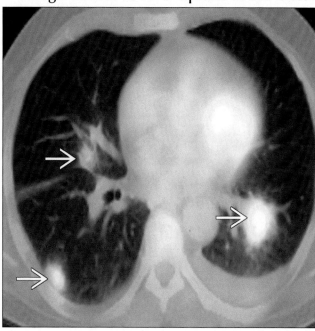

(Left) Coronal PET (A), axial CT (B) and PET/CT (C) in a patient without a known malignancy demonstrate large left hypermetabolic axillary lymph nodes ➡, suspicious for malignancy. However, biopsy revealed benign reactive lymph nodes. A six-month follow-up PET/CT showed complete resolution. *(Right)* Axial fused PET/CT shows multiple FDG-avid lesions in the lungs bilaterally ➡ in this patient without a history of malignancy. Subsequent biopsy and further workup showed Wegener granulomatosis.

Benign Causes of FDG Uptake in the Chest

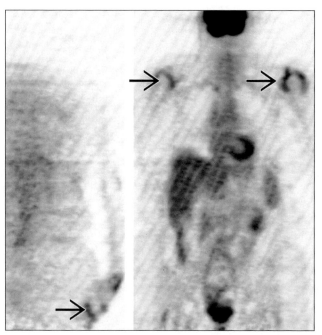
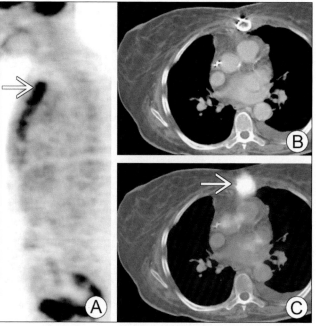

(Left) Coronal PET shows increased metabolic activity in both shoulder joints as well as in the left wrist ➡ in this patient with a known history of rheumatoid arthritis. *(Right)* This patient underwent a CABG approximately 4 weeks prior to this PET/CT exam. Sagittal PET (A), axial CT (B) and fused PET/CT (C) show linear and intense FDG activity along the median sternotomy ➡. This type of activity can be seen for an extended period of time.

BENIGN CAUSES OF FDG ACTIVITY

Benign Causes of FDG Uptake in the Abdomen/Pelvis

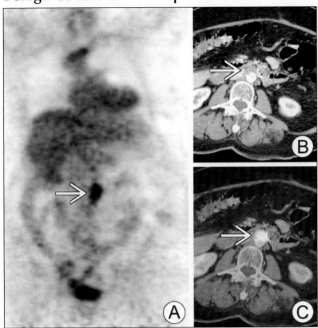

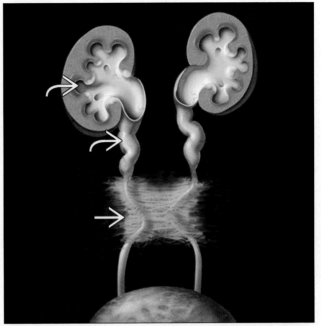

(Left) Coronal PET (A), axial CT (B) and PET/CT (C) demonstrate intense FDG activity surrounding the aorta ➡ in a patient without a history of malignancy. Two biopsies were negative for neoplasm, showing only inflammatory cells; the most likely diagnosis is the active phase of retroperitoneal fibrosis. *(Right)* Graphic shows changes of later stage retroperitoneal fibrosis ➡ with medial displacement of the ureters bilaterally as well as mild hydroureter and hydronephrosis ➡ proximally.

Benign Causes of FDG Uptake in the Abdomen/Pelvis

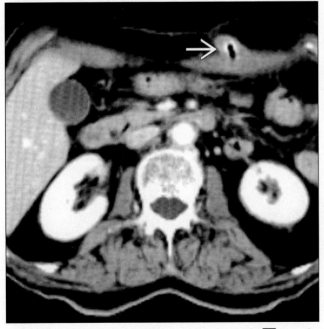

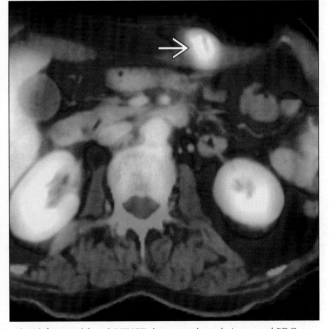

(Left) Axial CECT shows atypical appearance of a G-tube ➡ recently placed. *(Right)* Axial fused PET/CT shows moderately increased FDG activity surrounding the G-tube ➡, compatible with mild inflammation.

BENIGN CAUSES OF FDG ACTIVITY

Benign Causes of FDG Uptake in the Abdomen/Pelvis

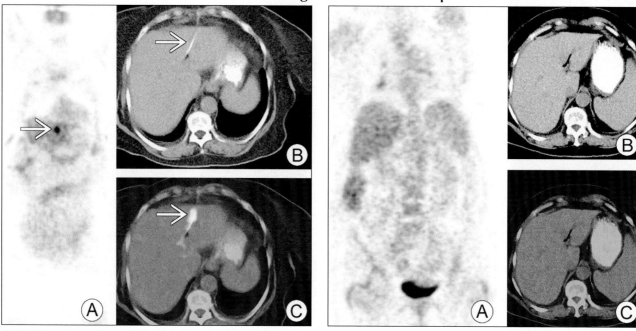

(Left) *This patient underwent a percutaneous insertion of a biliary catheter 2 weeks prior to this exam. Coronal PET (A), axial CT (B) and fused PET/CT (C) show linear increased metabolic activity along the track of the catheter* ➔, *compatible with inflammation.* **(Right)** *Coronal PET (A), axial CT (B) and fused PET/CT (C) from the patient in the previous figure show complete resolution on a six-month follow-up after the biliary drainage catheter was removed.*

Benign Causes of FDG Uptake in the Abdomen/Pelvis

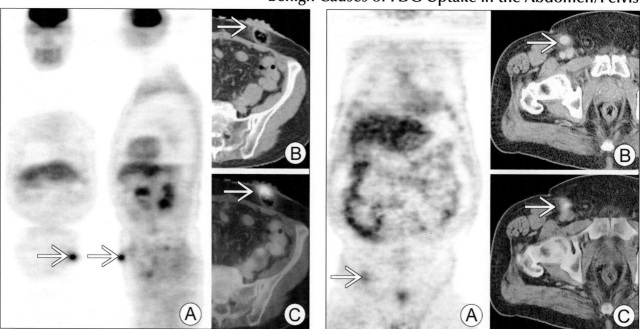

(Left) *Coronal and sagittal PET (A), axial CT (B) and PET/CT (C) show intense activity at the patient's ileostomy* ➔. *Almost all tubes, catheters, and other internal communications with the skin will have increased metabolic activity secondary to inflammation.* **(Right)** *This patient underwent a cardiac catheterization two days prior to this scan. Coronal PET (A), axial CT (B) and PET/CT (C) show increased metabolic activity in the right groin, corresponding to a pseudoaneurysm* ➔.

BENIGN CAUSES OF FDG ACTIVITY

Benign Causes of FDG Uptake in the Abdomen/Pelvis

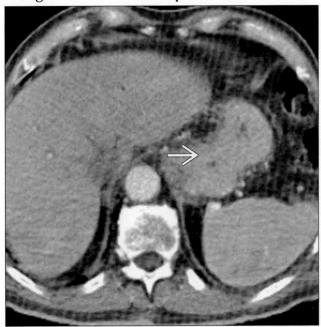
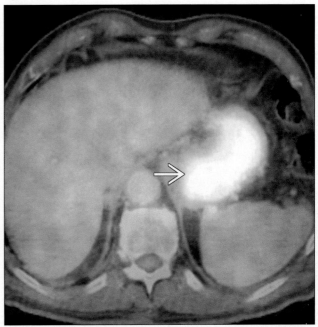

(Left) Axial CECT shows diffusely thickened gastric mucosa ➡ in this patient with a history of severe acute gastritis. However, it is difficult to assess gastric mucosal thickness when the stomach is decompressed. *(Right)* Axial fused PET/CT shows diffuse intense FDG activity throughout the stomach ➡, suggestive but certainly not diagnostic of acute gastritis. Normal physiologic activity within the stomach could have a similar appearance.

Benign Causes of FDG Uptake in the Abdomen/Pelvis

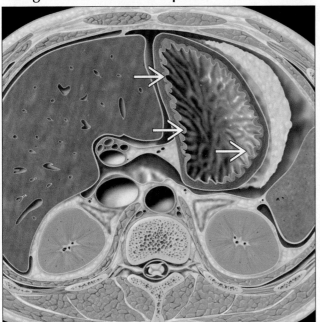
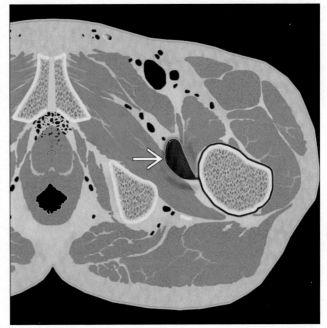

(Left) Graphic shows diffusely thickened gastric mucosal folds ➡, representing changes of acute gastritis. *(Right)* Graphic shows a depiction of a bursal sac/synovial cyst communicating with the left hip joint ➡.

BENIGN CAUSES OF FDG ACTIVITY

Benign Causes of FDG Uptake in the Abdomen/Pelvis

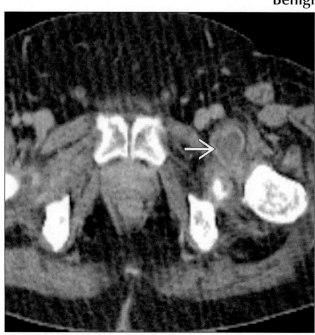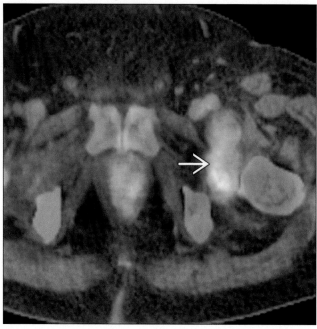

(Left) Axial CECT shows a teardrop-shaped, fluid-filled structure emanating from the left hip joint ➡, representing either an iliopsoas bursa or synovial cyst. *(Right)* Axial fused PET/CT shows moderately increased FDG activity correlating with the bursal sac/synovial cyst ➡, compatible with inflammation.

Benign Causes of FDG Uptake in the Abdomen/Pelvis

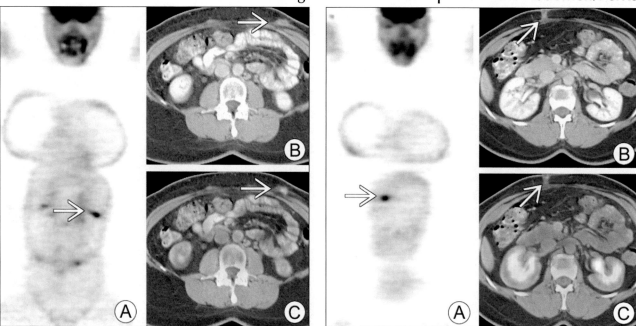

(Left) Coronal PET (A), axial CT (B) and PET/CT (C) demonstrate areas of FDG activity in the anterior subcutaneous fat ➡ in a diabetic patient on subcutaneous injections of insulin, compatible with injection granulomas. *(Right)* Additional images, coronal PET (A), axial CT (B) and fused PET/CT (C), in the same patient show other areas in the subcutaneous fat ➡ that represent injection granulomas.

BENIGN CAUSES OF FDG ACTIVITY

Benign Causes of FDG Uptake in the Abdomen/Pelvis

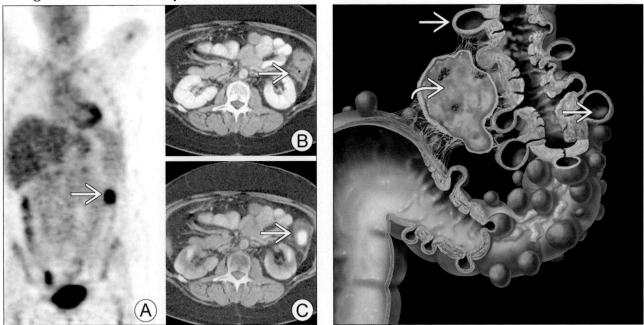

(Left) Coronal PET (A), axial CT (B) and fused PET/CT (C) show focal intense FDG activity in the proximal descending colon ➜ in this patient with active diverticulitis. *(Right)* Graphic shows changes of diverticulosis ➜ and acute diverticulitis with a pericolonic abscess ➜.

Benign Causes of FDG Uptake in the Abdomen/Pelvis

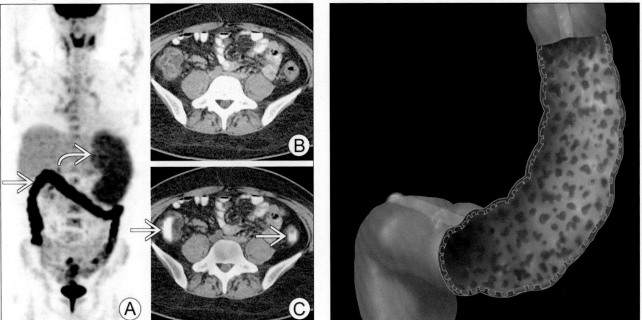

(Left) Coronal PET (A), axial CT (B) and fused PET/CT (C) show intense FDG activity throughout the entire colon ➜ in this patient with ulcerative colitis. Also note diffusely increased metabolic activity in the spleen ➜, secondary to newly diagnosed non-Hodgkin lymphoma. *(Right)* Graphic shows a depiction of the colon in a patient with ulcerative colitis.

BENIGN CAUSES OF FDG ACTIVITY

Benign Causes of FDG Uptake in the Abdomen/Pelvis

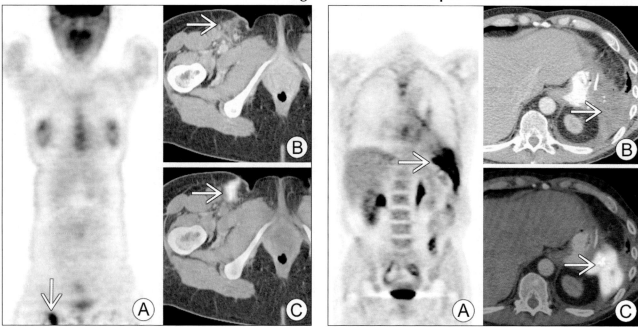

(Left) Coronal PET (A), axial CT (B) and PET/CT (C) in a patient who underwent an excisional biopsy approximately 1 week prior to the scan show intense metabolic activity in the biopsy bed ➡, compatible with inflammation. *(Right)* Coronal PET (A), axial CT (B) and PET/CT (C) demonstrate intensely FDG-avid soft tissue in the splenectomy bed ➡ approximately 8 weeks after splenectomy. Fine-needle aspiration and biopsy showed inflammatory cells and probable infection.

Benign Causes of FDG Uptake in the Abdomen/Pelvis

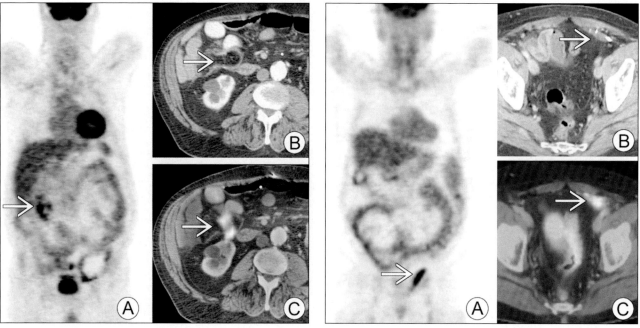

(Left) Coronal PET (A), axial CT (B) and fused PET/CT (C) in a patient 8 weeks after partial colectomy show intense FDG activity associated with a fatty lesion ➡ in the mesentery, compatible with omental infarct. *(Right)* Coronal PET (A), axial CT (B) and fused PET/CT (C) show linear intense FDG activity associated with high attenuation material in the anterior abdominal wall ➡ in a patient with a recent hernia repair and mesh placement, compatible with inflammation.

BENIGN CAUSES OF FDG ACTIVITY

Benign Causes of FDG Uptake in the Abdomen/Pelvis

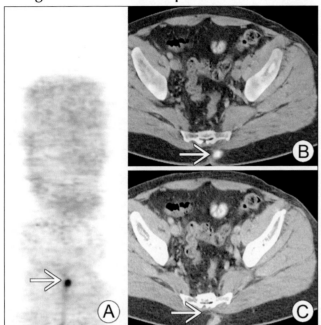 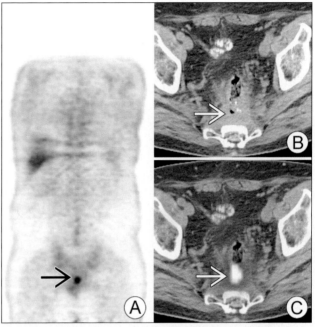

(Left) Coronal PET (A), axial CT (B) and fused PET/CT (C) show intense activity posterior to the sacrum in the subcutaneous tissues ➡ in a patient with a decubitus ulcer. *(Right)* Coronal PET (A), axial CT (B) and fused PET/CT (C) demonstrate focal FDG activity within the presacral area ➡, correlating with presacral inflammatory changes ➡ and a small focus of extraluminal air. The patient had recently had a partial colectomy.

Benign Causes of FDG Uptake in the Abdomen/Pelvis

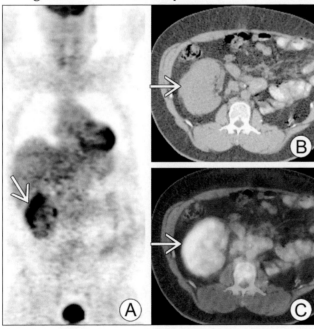 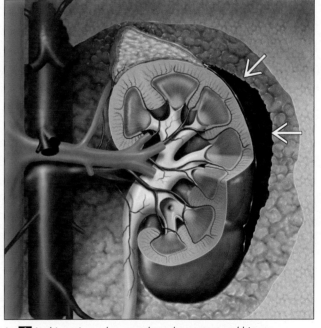

(Left) Coronal PET (A) shows a crescent-shaped area of intense FDG activity ➡ in this patient who recently underwent a renal biopsy. Axial CT (B) shows a very subtle area of slightly increased attenuation localizing to the area of increased metabolic activity on axial PET/CT (C). Narrowing the window width will help visualize subtle areas of blood. *(Right)* Graphic shows typical crescent-shaped appearance of a perinephric hematoma ➡.

INDEX

INDEX

INDEX

INDEX

INDEX

INDEX

INDEX

INDEX

INDEX

INDEX

INDEX

INDEX